Social and Administrative Aspects of Pharmacy in Low- and Middle-Income Countries

Social and Administrative Aspects of Pharmacy in Low- and Middle-Income Countries

Present Challenges and Future Solutions

Edited by

Mohamed Izham Mohamed Ibrahim

Albert I. Wertheimer

Zaheer-Ud-Din Babar

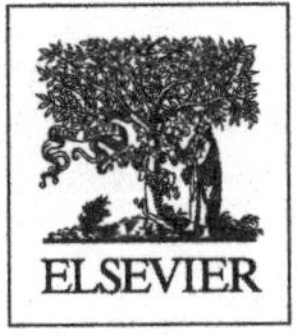

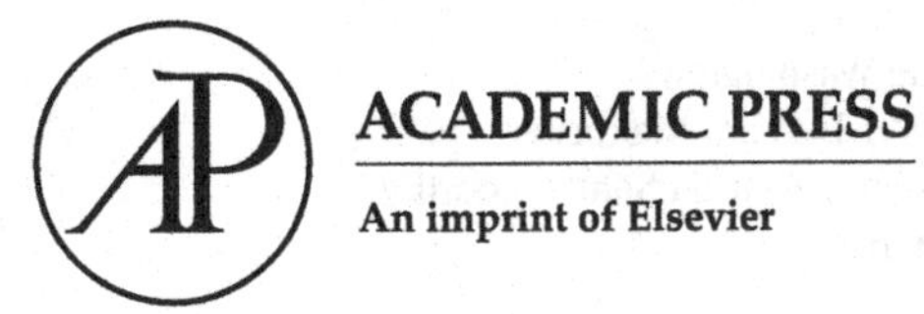

Academic Press is an imprint of Elsevier
125 London Wall, London EC2Y 5AS, United Kingdom
525 B Street, Suite 1800, San Diego, CA 92101-4495, United States
50 Hampshire Street, 5th Floor, Cambridge, MA 02139, United States
The Boulevard, Langford Lane, Kidlington, Oxford OX5 1GB, United Kingdom

Library of Congress Cataloging-in-Publication Data
A catalog record for this book is available from the Library of Congress

British Library Cataloguing-in-Publication Data
A catalogue record for this book is available from the British Library

ISBN: 978-0-12-811228-1

For information on all Academic Press publications visit our website at https://www.elsevier.com/books-and-journals

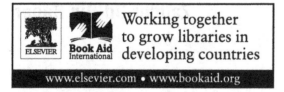

Publisher: Mica Haley
Acquisition Editor: Kattie Washington
Editorial Project Manager: Barbara Makinster
Production Project Manager: Anusha Sambamoorthy
Cover Designer: Greg Harris

Typeset by TNQ Books and Journals

Izham

To my family—Norlela, Syazwan, Fatin, Daniel, Najihah, Imran, Aiman, and my parents—Mohamed Ibrahim and Faridah—for their understanding and support throughout the many hours during which my work keeps me away from those most precious parts of my lives: the persons, the times, and the occasions that I cannot recover after they are missed or gone.

Albert

To Joaquima

Zaheer

To my parents

Contents

SECTION 10 GOOD GOVERNANCE AND PHARMACEUTICAL POLICY IN LOW- AND MIDDLE-INCOME COUNTRIES

List of Contributors

Nada Abdel Rida
Qatar University, Doha, Qatar

Abubakr A. Alfadl
Qassim University, Unaizah, Kingdom of Saudi Arabia

Mukhtar Ansari
University of Hail, Hail, Kingdom of Saudi Arabia

Yara Arafat
Qatar University, Doha, Qatar

Saira Azhar
COMSATS, Abbottabad, Pakistan

Zaheer-Ud-Din Babar
University of Huddersfield, Huddersfield, United Kingdom; University of Auckland, Auckland, New Zealand

Gianluigi Casadei
University of Milan, Milan, Italy

Yu Fang
Xi'an Jiaotong University, Xi'an, China

Ahmed I. Fathelrahman
Qassim University, Buraidah, Kingdom of Saudi Arabia

Omotayo Fatokun
UCSI University, Kuala Lumpur, Malaysia

Mohamed Azmi Hassali
Universiti Sains Malaysia, Minden, Malaysia

Saval Khanal
Griffith University, Nathan, QLD, Australia

Jillian C. Kohler
University of Toronto, Toronto, ON, Canada; Munk School of Global Affairs, Toronto, ON, Canada

Paola Minghetti
University of Milan, Milan, Italy

Mohamed Izham Mohamed Ibrahim
Qatar University, Doha, Qatar

Kathy Moscou
University of Toronto, Toronto, ON, Canada; York University, Toronto, ON, Canada; Brandon University, Brandon, MB, Canada

Chin H. Ng
Universiti Sains Malaysia, Minden, Malaysia

Tuan A. Nguyen
University of South Australia, Adelaide, SA, Australia

Lisa M. Nissen
Queensland University of Technology, Brisbane, QLD, Australia

Benson Njuguna
Moi Teaching and Referral Hospital, Eldoret, Kenya

Guat See Ooi
Asian Institute of Medicine, Science and Technology University, Kedah, Malaysia

Subish Palaian
Gulf Medical University, Ajman, United Arab Emirates

Sonak Pastakia
Purdue University College of Pharmacy, Eldoret, Kenya; Moi Teaching and Referral Hospital, Eldoret, Kenya

Vibhu Paudyal
University of Birmingham, Birmingham, United Kingdom; Robert Gordon University, Aberdeen, United Kingdom

Arjun Poudel
Queensland University of Technology, Brisbane, QLD, Australia

Pathiyil Ravi Shankar
American International Medical University, Gros Islet, Saint Lucia

Elizabeth E. Roughead
University of South Australia, Adelaide, SA, Australia

Shane L. Scahill
Massey University, Auckland, New Zealand

Asrul A. Shafie
Universiti Sains Malaysia, Minden, Malaysia

Dixon Thomas
Gulf Medical University, Ajman, United Arab Emirates

Dan N. Tran
Purdue University College of Pharmacy, Eldoret, Kenya; Moi Teaching and Referral Hospital, Eldoret, Kenya

Dinesh K. Upadhyay
Asian Institute of Medicine, Science and Technology University, Kedah, Malaysia

Albert I. Wertheimer
Nova Southeastern University (NSU), Fort Lauderdale, FL, United States

Zhi Yen Wong
Hospital Teluk Intan, Teluk Intan, Malaysia

Kangkang Yan
Xi'an Jiaotong University, Xi'an, China; Xi'an No. 3 Hospital, Xi'an, China

Kazeem B. Yusuff
King Faisal University, Al-Ahsa, Kingdom of Saudi Arabia

Seeba Zachariah
Gulf Medical University/Thumbay Hospital, Ajman, United Arab Emirates

Acknowledgments

Izham

To academicians who are very important in my career: Prof. Albert I Wertheimer, Prof. Dzulkifli Abdul Razak, the late Prof. Saringat Hj Baie, and the late Prof. Abas Hj Husin.
They motivated and provided encouragement in so many extraordinary ways.

Albert

To Professor Manuel Carvajal for permitting to use my time in the preparation of this book.

Zaheer

I would like to acknowledge researchers, academics and colleagues who have contributed to improve my understanding towards social and administrative aspects of pharmacy.

CHAPTER

INTRODUCTION: DISCOVERING ISSUES AND CHALLENGES IN LOW- AND MIDDLE-INCOME COUNTRIES

1

Mohamed Izham Mohamed Ibrahim[1], **Albert I. Wertheimer**[2]

[1]*Qatar University, Doha, Qatar;* [2]*Nova Southeastern University (NSU), Fort Lauderdale, FL, United States*

What is today greatly depends upon what was yesterday and helps shape the future of what will be tomorrow

Robert V. Evanson et al. (1985)

CHAPTER OUTLINE

INTRODUCTION

Evanson, McEvilla, Hammel, and DeSalvo (1985) reminded us that the major obstacle to the establishment of pharmacy administration is due to the negative attitudes and imbalanced focus and emphasis between professionalism versus business orientation that are inherent in pharmacy practice. The book that was edited by Fathelrahman, Mohamed Ibrahim, and Wertheimer (2016), explored the pharmacy practice in 19 developing countries in Asia, Africa and Latin America and provided an excellent overview of pharmacy practice. The book also provides us with gaps, challenges and possible solutions for various pharmacy stakeholders in the developing countries. There is a great deal of work that needs to be done by the pharmacy stakeholders in order to improve the pharmaceutical health services for fulfilling the needs of the society. It is understood that under the sustainable development goals (SDGs), every country is in need for development (United Nations, 2017). Yet unfortunately, the weak global economy has hindered progress toward the SDGs, especially for countries with lower economic level. Development is everyone's problem and everyone's dream.

Social and Administrative Aspects of Pharmacy in Low- and Middle-Income Countries. http://dx.doi.org/10.1016/B978-0-12-811228-1.00001-7

There is no clear definition of the terms "developed and developing countries" or no consensus on how to categorize these countries. Developing countries include, in decreasing order of economic growth or size of the capital market: newly industrialized countries, emerging markets, frontier markets, and least developed countries. List of developing countries according to the United Nations (2014) can be classified into three categories: developed economies, economies in transition, and developing economies. Geographical regions for developing economies are as follows: Africa, East Asia, South Asia, Western Asia, and Latin America and the Caribbean. According to the O'Sullivan and Sheffrin (2003, p. 471), a developing country is a country with a relatively low standard of living, undeveloped industrial base, and moderate to low Human Development Index. This index is a comparative measure of poverty, literacy, education, life expectancy, and other factors for countries worldwide. For the sake of the discussion, the book will consider the classification of countries based on per capita gross national income (i.e., low- and middle-income countries (LMICs)).

The political, economic, and pharmaceutical sector conditions differ between the countries; some have to do much more and work harder to improve their situations than others. There are significant social and economic differences between developed countries and LMICs. Many of the underlying causes of these differences are rooted in the long history of the development of such nations and include social, cultural, and economic variables; historical, political, and geographical factors; as well as international relations.

Furthermore, it is not the intention of the book to indicate the level of the inferiority of an LMIC or an undeveloped country compared with a developed country or between East and West, but rather to trigger and stimulate the mind of the people in the LMICs about the challenges and problems the societies are facing for decades. No country in this world is free from problems and challenges, but people in the developing world suffer relatively more. The focus of this book is to highlight, discuss, and document policy issues in LMICs and about having best practices in the pharmaceutical sector. So far, to what extent is the contribution of pharmacists to this matter?

Health and public health are essentials for development. Around 50% of the world's population are residing in LMICs and they are still living in poverty with poor health status and inadequate healthcare. In any healthcare system, pharmacy system is one of the core components and pharmacists play a very important role. With the dynamic changes happening in healthcare, disease, information communication technology and regulations, and the roles and responsibilities of pharmacists are becoming more important than before. The expectations on the pharmacists are changing; the societal needs and demands are much greater compared with several decades ago. On the other hand, there are growing problems with medicines, the health system, and human resources, especially in the LMICs. There are countries with high prices of medicines, a wide prevalence of nonquality medicines (i.e., substandard and counterfeit), lack of access to medicines, and absence of a national medicines policy (NMP) even with strong encouragement from World Health Organization (WHO). Poor health and pharmaceutical sectors in a country will increase the vulnerability of the country toward several critical problems at micro- and macrolevels and leaves the society at risk. In the medicines supply system, to ensure access to medicines, the following aspects are critical:

- reliable health and supply systems;
- sustainable financing;
- rational selection; and
- affordable prices of medicines.

The importance of a healthcare system must be looked from three angles: the institutions, organizations, and resources; resources include workforce, financial, and infrastructure. To achieve universal health coverage, the system must function well. The three elements, i.e., institutions, organizations, and resources must be brought together to deliver quality health services to meet the demands of the society. Unfortunately, according to Mills (2014), the goals of universal health coverage in LMICs could not be achieved, child and maternal deaths are still high, financial protection is lacking, and people do not seek care because of lack of financial support.

PUBLIC HEALTH PHARMACY IN LOW- AND MIDDLE-INCOME COUNTRIES: ISSUES AND CHALLENGES

Even though the rational use and quality use of medicines are worldwide issues, but they are particularly pertinent to LMICs. Access to medicines is still crucial, as 400 children suffering from tuberculosis worldwide die daily, largely because of low access to appropriate treatment (WHO, 2016a, 2016b). Ranganathan and Gazarian (2015) reported that there are several key challenges for delivering rational use of medicines (RUM) to children in the developing countries. Among the problems are as follows:

- lack of coordinated NMP to support RUM;
- availability, affordability, and accessibility to medicines' issues;
- inappropriate standards of quality, safe, and efficacy of medicines;
- lack of independent, unbiased, and evidence-based information;
- lack of information, knowledge, and skills among healthcare practitioners who are dealing with medication use process among children;
- lack of proper devices and tools (e.g., calculator and weighing machine) used when deciding on the appropriate dosage for the children; and
- retailers selling prescription medicines extensively over the counter.

Dowse (2016) reported that the likelihood of poor health literacy in developing countries is prevalent. Health literacy is fundamental to the effectiveness of health programs and improvement to the quality of life. The United Nations Educational, Scientific and Cultural Organization Institute for Statistics found that around 7% of countries (13/180) indicate an adult literacy rate below 50%. All these countries are from sub-Saharan Africa, and the lowest adult literacy rate is in Mali with a 26.2% (United Nations, 2009). Another issue is corruption. Corruption (e.g., misinformation, bribery, theft, and bureaucratic corruption) is a global problem and negatively affects the medicines supply chain and the overall healthcare system. The backbone of the health system is formed by well-functioning supply chains that deliver various pharmaceutical products (Yadav, 2015). The Corruption Perception Index 2016 illustrated that none of the LMICs listed top 10 of the transparent (i.e., clean) ranking. On the scale of 0 (highly corrupt) to 100 (very clean), over two-thirds of the 176 countries and territories in this index fall below the midpoint (Transparency International, 2016). People also faced with issues related to substandard medicines, counterfeit drugs, nutrition, tobacco consumption, maternal and child health, and environmental hazards (WHO, 2017). WHO (2014) reported that the environmental hazards such air pollution caused around 7 million premature deaths a year. Most areas affected were densely populated LMICs. The conditions in the developing countries become worse when people suffer from various turmoil conditions such as war, humanitarian conflict, and public health crisis, which further collapse completely the healthcare system. These aspects make working in the healthcare system and the practice of pharmacists more challenging.

In short, the LMICs are facing social, economic, environmental, human capital, political, and infrastructure issues that directly or indirectly affecting the health and pharmaceutical health services. Much needs to be done in LMICs. The following are important elements for functioning global supply systems and availability of safe and effective medical products at prices equitable to all: effective and innovative health and medicines policies, coordinated approaches, international cooperation, and effective oversight. Especially for the pharmacy regulators, policy makers, and practitioners, they must appreciate the complexity of the healthcare system and human life. What is considered fine or rational in one country and society might not be fine or considered irrational among other societies with different cultures, beliefs, and backgrounds. Regulators, policy makers, and practitioners in countries of the developing world should evaluate thoroughly health- and pharmaceutical-related issues in their country and find solutions that are appropriate and relevant according to the environment.

There are several significant initiatives to ensure health for all and RUM in LMICs that were advocated by organizations such as Health Action International Asia Pacific (HAIAP), People Health Movement (PHM), Third World Network (TWN), International Network for Rational Use of Drugs (INRUD) and WHO, just to name a few. Chowdhury (2017) noted that "Since the 1985 Nairobi Conference on the Rational Use of Drugs, for every two steps we have advanced we have gone one step backward. A progressive agenda for people-centred, rational and affordable healthcare continues to be undermined by powerful vested interests." We are getting closer and closer, but are not there yet. The PHM's member developed the People's Charter for Health in 2000. It was established after realizing that vision and goals of Alma-Ata Declaration that was established in 1978 failed to ensure "Health for All by the Year 2000." PHM felt that the health status of the LMICs has not improved as aimed, but instead worsened further. Health crisis happened everywhere, especially in the LMICs. There are significant inequalities between and within countries. New threats to health are continually developing (PHM, n.d.).

According to International Monetary Fund (IMF) (2014), "the world is a healthier place today but major issues continue to confront humanity." The world has improved greatly with eliminating and controlling few of the communicable diseases such as smallpox and polio. Quality and better medicines have been produced to improve the health conditions. People have better sanitation and accessible to clean water. Even with the innovations and cost-effective interventions in healthcare, individuals continue to experience and suffer from health threats such as malaria, dengue, typhoid, chikungunya, severe acute respiratory syndrome, middle east respiratory syndrome–related coronavirus, Ebola virus crisis. In addition, the prevalence of mental disorders and noncommunicable diseases continues to increase. Chronic diseases such as cancer, cardiovascular diseases, and diabetes cause serious ill health and millions of premature death. It is reported that 85% of them are in LMICs. All these threats and disorders negatively affect the public health system and infrastructure, cause disability, and ruin businesses, workforce, and productivity of the affected country (IMF, 2014; WHO, 2011).

Thanks to pharmaceutical industries, which have produced antibiotics to fight against infectious diseases. The practice of medicine has been transformed. But, unfortunately due to the irresponsible and irrational used of antibiotics by healthcare providers and public, it has resulted in an increase in resistance and caused a worldwide decline in antibiotic effectiveness. The primary healthcare sectors failed to play their roles in containing these threats. The primary healthcare providers failed to perform their responsibilities. Pharmacists have a responsibility regarding antibiotic stewardship to help contain or reduce amount of unnecessary antibiotic use especially against viruses and in trivial diseases. We need cost-effective, affordable, and practical interventions. The use of health technology assessment tools becomes helpful at this point.

Where are the pharmacists when the nations are crippled by these threats? Do the pharmaceutical policies fail to curb these problems? The lack of adequate, resilient public health surveillance systems, infrastructure to effectively deploy resources, and a health workforce to provide accessible, quality care where needed leaves us vulnerable to regional and global spread. Despite the progress that has been made in the last two decades, more needs to be done to create enabling regulatory environments. Understanding the social and cultural contexts that may contribute to these problems, plus effective solutions, is also crucial. Health communication often receives less attention and fewer resources than medical, scientific, or policy areas. There is an urgent need for society to value and invest more in evidence-informed public health strategies. The multifactorial nature of broader global health issues poses an enormous challenge to all stakeholders (WHO, 2016b). Effective public health action depends on understanding the scale and nature of threats to health (WHO, 1986). According to the Ottawa patient charter, the public health community has a duty to make the invisible visible. They must measure and assess the burden of diseases, health status, and risk factors including the protection factors. The public health community must make the best use of data to promote health. Public health interventions should be evaluated, using rigorous research methods, and the results disseminated. The public health community must ensure that evidence is used to give voice to those who would otherwise be unheard. Research findings must be disseminated effectively to the different stakeholders in the health sectors, including public, policy makers, practitioners, and (social) media. Findings at times are complex and this information should be delivered in ways that are comprehensible and in a timely manner (Lomazzi, 2016).

Effective public health interventions can save hundreds of millions of lives in LMICs, as well as create broad social and economic benefits. According to Frieden and Henning (2009), it is often assumed that public health interventions applied in developed countries are not appropriate in developing countries. Main public health functions are similar regardless of a country's income level. Many basic public health measures achieved decades ago in developed countries are urgently needed, highly appropriate, extremely cost-effective, and eminently attainable in LMICs today. Further according to Frieden and Henning (2009), a progress of public health in developing countries is possible but will require sufficient funding and human resources; improved physical infrastructure and information systems; effective program implementation and regulatory capacity; and, most importantly, political will at the highest levels of government. Most change is due to money. For instance, robotics, automation, and technicians are widely used to save money. In the hospital setting, unit dose, unit-of-use, etc. are done to save cost. Similarly, medication therapy management is done to save money and that is why most other changes are accepted, provided if they are cost-effective.

Pharmacists are dedicated and in a strategic position to preserve and advance public health. Their efforts enhance the quality of individual's lives by helping people to live as free as possible from disease, pain, and suffering (Jandovitz & Brygider, 2005). With respect to their relationship with the public, pharmacists are often portrayed as an underused resource for health- and medicines-related advice and information. Furthermore, the practice of pharmacy involves both pharmacist and public and can be conceptualized as a social process (Harding & Taylor, 2009, p. 395). Don't we need something about the efforts to locate new pharmacy roles, e.g., in relation to immunizations, patient advisor, educator and advocator for wellness, screening and prevention activities, birth control promotions, and other population health initiatives? Pharmacists have an obligation to educate the public in LMICs, for example, teaching poor rural women about birth control and safe sex especially if their partner has HIV, etc. The other one is to encourage immunizations. In certain places, some cult leader and religious groups discourage their followers not to be immunized and then we end up with local epidemics of preventable conditions such as polio. Hence, understanding the concepts and principles behind social pharmacy disciplines is important and useful. There is a need to apply a socioecological model to public health issues that are impacting the health of the population.

SOCIAL PHARMACY

What is social pharmacy? Social pharmacy is a discipline driven by social needs (Fukushima, 2016) and more focus on the society at large. It is interdisciplinary subject, which helps to understand the interaction between drugs and society. Experts have defined social pharmacy as a discipline concerned with the behavioral sciences relevant to the utilization of medicine by both consumers and healthcare professionals (Wertheimer, 1991). Sørensen, Mount, and Christensen (2003) defined social pharmacy as studying "...the drug/medicine sector... from the social scientific and humanistic perspectives. Topics relevant to Social Pharmacy consist of all the social factors that influence medicine use, such as medicine- and health-related beliefs, attitudes, rules, relationships, and processes."

Almarsdottir and Granas (2016) also agree that social pharmacy is a discipline where there is use of the social sciences in pharmacy to add its usefulness to the society. It is also known as "pharmacy administration" or "social and administrative pharmacy." It has two components: the social sciences and the administrative sciences. The social sciences component includes demography, anthropology, psychology, social psychology, sociology, political sciences, and geography (Mount, 1989), while the administrative sciences component includes areas such as management, marketing, finance, economics, organizational behavior, law, policy, ethics, information technology, and statistics. Social and administrative pharmacy is the integration and application of the social and administrative sciences disciplines in pharmacy, i.e., education and practice. Social pharmacy scientists utilize both sciences to improve clinical practice, enhance the effectiveness of pharmaceutical regulations and policy, advocate political awareness, and promote improvements in pharmaceutical health services and healthcare delivery. Social pharmacy applied a biopsychosocial or socioenvironmental method to understand health and illness conditions (Claire, 2008). Many types of research use either the quantitative or qualitative or a mixed method approach, from simple to complex statistical methods and modeling in pharmacy practice to make changes and improvement in the healthcare system, quality of care, and patient's quality of life. In addition, there are many useful tools from the social and behavioral sciences literature that researchers could use, for example, in helping with patient–pharmacist communication and compliance enhancement efforts.

According to Wertheimer (1989), "there are very few similarities in the education and practice of pharmacy around the world." Many individuals have an ethnocentric, regiocentric, or geocentric approach in which they believe. For example, pharmacy colleges in a country might be reluctant to accept improvement in the curriculum. The pharmacy educators think that they are superior, and the curriculum developed and used, for example, in the last decades was excellent. In some cases, there is an imbalance of focus between the pharmaceutical sciences courses and the pharmacy practice and administration courses. They consider teaching more of the basic pharmaceutical sciences subjects to the undergraduate students or just offering pharmaceutical sciences-related research (i.e., lab-based research) at the MSc and PhD level is adequate to provide the pharmacy graduates knowledge and skill to practice. The regiocentric or geocentric phenomenon in pharmacy practice is quite common and could be observed in the middle east region, for example. Further, political struggle and lack of leadership could hurt the dynamic and mission of the pharmacy profession. According to Morgall and Almarsdóttir (1999), the pharmacy profession could lose its monopoly and become weak due to the internal conflicts. Pharmacists need to advocate locally to upgrade the quality of pharmacy education away from massive amounts of chemistry to applied patient care science and practice and to upgrade the level of standards in each country to work with legislators to ban pharmacies not operated by qualified, licensed personnel.

When Wertheimer and Smith (1989) published the first edition of their book in 1974, social pharmacy or social and administrative pharmacy was a very new discipline and possibly not known in the LMICs. The book includes topics such as the contribution of the social sciences; pharmacy, pharmacist, and the professions; the contribution of psychosocial aspects; the contribution of sociology; and behavioral aspects of drugs and medication use, ethics, pharmacist and public health and the future of pharmacists. In the United Kingdom, according to Harding and Taylor (2015), social pharmacy was introduced in the pharmacy curriculum of UK colleges sometime in the early 2000. The Mills Commission Report in 1975 recognized the importance to develop the behavioral and social sciences aspects in pharmacy (Study Commission on Pharmacy, 1975). But, actually, the social pharmacy components were first experienced in the United States in the 1950s (Wertheimer, 1991). Then later, the UK and European colleges of pharmacy introduced social pharmacy into their curriculum (Claire, 2008).

It is doubtful if pharmacy colleges in the LMICs have successfully introduced this discipline in their pharmacy curriculum. Most of the times, the internal politics and a lack of understanding limit or even counteract the collaboration of clinical and social pharmacy, thus weakening both fields (Almarsdottir & Granas, 2016). However, there are cases, to name a few, which had reported positive experience such as in Malaysia. School of Pharmaceutical Sciences, Universiti Sains Malaysia that was established in 1972, first introduced a course "Drugs in Developing Countries" (Mohamed Izham, Awang, & Abdul Razak, 1998) in the early 1990s. After a long struggle, the discipline was established in 2002 (School of Pharmaceutical Sciences, n.d.). Several important courses (e.g., drug and society, social and public health pharmacy, pharmaceutical management and marketing, and pharmacoeconomics) managed to be included in the pharmacy curriculum. These additions offer a perspective on the pharmacy that balances and complements the behavioral and natural/physical sciences component of the pharmacy curriculum (Hassali et al., 2011) to produce well-rounded graduates. In addition, the department has also produced hundreds pieces of social and administrative pharmacy-related research generated from more than 150 MSc and PhD students from around 15 LMICs. Kostriba, Alwarafi, and Vlcek (2014) identified large differences in approach and scope of teaching social pharmacy courses as a field of study in the undergraduate pharmacy education worldwide. They also identified regional trends connected with the political, economic, and social aspects of particular regions. Basak (2012) expressed concern with the recent changes in the Indian pharmacy education. According to the author, in the introduction of the PharmD program (Pharmacy Council of India, n.d.), social pharmacy is the least developed discipline in the curriculum. It called for cooperation in an attempt to develop social pharmacy components in teaching and research in India. There is a drive to incorporate the social pharmacy topics in the Yemeni pharmacy education even with all the challenges and limitations that the country is experiencing nowadays (Alshakka, Aldubhani, Basaleem, Hassali, & Mohamed Ibrahim, 2015). In Libya, according to Abrika, Hassali, and Abduelkarem (2012), the pharmacy practitioners were supportive with the ideas of inclusion of social pharmacy subjects in the curriculum because it will enhance the pharmacists' professional roles.

In contrast, in the United States, Zorek, Lambert, and Popovich (2013) noted that even though the basic and clinical sciences provide a critical scientific foundation for direct patient care, pharmacists are likely to flounder in the face of social and behavioral challenges without a practical mastery of the relevant principles of modern social and behavioral science. According to the authors, pharmacy education and practice must require greater mastery of social and behavioral science. In the United Kingdom, the incorporation of social and behavioral sciences into the curricula of all schools of pharmacy, reflecting a broad recognition that pharmacy practice does not simply involve supplying medicines and advice to a passive public who take their medicines and follow expert advice without question (Harding & Taylor, 2009, p. 395).

WHY DO WE NEED THIS BOOK?

We know a great deal about pharmacy in the developed world but we know very little about pharmacy practice, education, and science in the lesser developed countries. That is unfortunate because if we in the developed countries understood what the major problems and impediments were in the lesser developed countries, we could be in a better situation to offer advice and aid. Very little has been published in the main stream, international literature about the status of pharmacy in the lesser developed countries. It is possible that some more is published in local journals in local languages that may be of limited help to others outside of that country. There are other problems as well. One is that accurate and timely vital health statistics may not be available for any of many possible reasons, such as budget restrictions, and shame in reporting accurate and precise reports that are not flattering to that country's leaders in the healthcare area.

This book sheds light on various topics that individually and in combination determine the status of pharmacy practice in individual countries. The nature of pharmacy characteristics in a country has a great deal to do with traditions and characteristics from colonial times, the wealth of the country, its political and economic systems, the level of capital available for investment, the extent of technical education among the population, the presence of a middle class and the size of an upper class, if there is one, and the extent of a culture of corruption.

There is one other reason why we need this book. When resources are constrained, sometimes clever persons devise exceptional strategies and schemes that require minimal resources. We are never so good that we cannot learn from our less fortunate colleagues, nor should we be too proud to borrow ideas and systems from nonindustrialized countries.

WHAT DOES IT ADD TO THE PRESENT KNOWLEDGE?

If one of us wanted to learn about some aspects of pharmacy practice, education, or research in Jordan, for example, it would be a time-consuming, complicated task, extracting various parts of our goal from a large array of journals, textbooks, and websites, and often a doomed task since some of the references will be missing, unavailable, obsolete, or in foreign languages. Some citations may only be available through the interlibrary loan organization, requiring several weeks.

One may realize immediately that having all or nearly all of the desired data and information in one, easy-to-use source makes data collection and subsequent analysis far easier, and the work may be performed in a fraction of the time required to search here and there. In addition, relying on a single source for primary data can be dangerous. Governmental statistics offices often spin data-related reports to underreport communicable diseases so as not to discourage tourism or so as not to put a country behind its neighboring nations in its effectiveness in combating health problems, childhood immunizations, etc.

This book incorporates multiple data sources and when outliers are discovered, which may be called to the attention of the reader. This book also provides knowledge and understanding about social and administrative aspects of pharmacy in healthcare in LMICs. It also creates awareness among readers, providing ideas and possible solutions to these obstacles. It is hoped that the pharmacists and other stakeholders will be better equipped to tackle any problems and challenges facing them in practice.

> If I had one hour to save the world, I would spend the first fifty-five minutes defining the problem and the last five minutes solving it.
>
> **Albert Einstein**

REFERENCES

Abrika, O. S. S., Hassali, M. A., & Abduelkarem, A. R. (2012). Importance of social pharmacy education in Libyan pharmacy schools: perspectives from pharmacy practitioners. *Journal of Educational Evaluation for Health Professions*, *9*(6). http://dx.doi.org/10.3352/jeehp.2012.9.6.

Almarsdottir, A., & Granas, A. (2016). Social pharmacy and clinical pharmacy—joining forces. *Pharmacy*, *4*, 1. http://dx.doi.org/10.3390/pharmacy4010001.

Alshakka, M., Aldubhani, A., Basaleem, H., Hassali, M. A., & Mohamed Ibrahim, M. I. (2015). Importance of incorporating social pharmacy education in Yemeni pharmacy school's curriculum. *Journal of Pharmacy Practice and Community Medicine*, *1*(1), 6–11. http://dx.doi.org/10.5530.jppcm.2015.1.3.

Basak, S. C. (2012). *Social pharmacy concept in pharmacy education*. PharmaBiz.com.

Chowdhury, Z. (2017). *HAIAP-PHM ISC meeting*. http://www.haiasiapacific.org.

Claire, A. (Oct–Dec 2008). Social pharmacy- the current scenario. *Indian Journal of Pharmacy Practice*, *1*(1).

Dowse, R. (2016). The limitations of current health literacy measures for use in developing countries. *Journal of Communication in Healthcare*, *9*(1), 4–6. http://dx.doi.org/10.1080/17538068.2016.1147742.

Evanson, R. V., McEvilla, J. D., Hammel, R. W., & DeSalvo, R. J. (1985). *The history of pharmacy*. http://www.pharmacy.umn.edu/sites/pharmacy.umn.edu/files/cop_article_3412601.pdf.

Fathelrahman, A., Mohamed Ibrahim, M. I., & Wertheimer, A. I. (2016). *Pharmacy practice in developing countries: Achievements and challenges* (1st ed.). Cambridge, MA: Academic Press.

Frieden, T. R., & Henning, K. J. (2009). Public health requirements for rapid progress in global health. *Glob Public Health*, *4*(4), 323–337. http://dx.doi.org/10.1080/17441690903089430.

Fukushima, N. (2016). Social pharmacy: Its performance and promise. *Yakugaku Zasshi*, *136*(7), 993–999.

Harding, G., & Taylor, K. (2009). Social dimensions of pharmacy: The social context of pharmacy. *The Pharmaceutical Journal*, *269*, 395.

Harding, G., & Taylor, K. M. G. (June 6, 2015). *Teaching social pharmacy: The UK experience. Pharmacy education, [S.l.]*. Available at: http://pharmacyeducation.fip.org/pharmacyeducation/article/view/104.

Hassali, M. A., Shafie, A. A., Al-Haddad, M. S., Abduelkarem, A. R., Ibrahim, M. I., Palaian, S., & Abrika, O. S. (2011). Social pharmacy as a field of study: The needs and challenges in global pharmacy education. *Research in Social and Administrative Pharmacy*, *7*, 415–420.

International Monetary Fund (IMF). (December 2014). Global health threats of the 21st century finance & development(Vol. 51. , 4. http://www.imf.org/external/pubs/ft/fandd/2014/12/pdf/jonas.pdf.

Jandovitz, L., & Brygider, R. (2005). *Pharmacists: Unsung heroes*. WLIW (Television station: Long Island, N.Y.). WLIW New York ©: American Association of Colleges of Pharmacy.

Kostriba, J., Alwarafi, A., & Vlcek, J. (2014). Social pharmacy as a field of study in undergraduate pharmacy education. *Indian Journal of Pharmaceutical Education and Research*, *48*(1), 0612.

Lomazzi, M. A. (2016). Global charter for the public's health-the public health system: Role, functions, competencies and education requirements. *European Journal of Public Health*, *26*(2), 210–212.

Mills, A. (2014). Health care systems in low- and middle-income countries. *The New England Journal of Medicine*, *370*, 552–557.

Mohamed Izham, M. I., Awang, R., & Abdul Razak, D. (1998). Introducing social pharmacy courses to pharmacy students in Malaysia. *Medical Teacher*, *20*(2), 122–126.

Morgall, J. M., & Almarsdóttir, A. B. (May 1999). No struggle, no strength: How pharmacists lost their monopoly. *Social Science & Medicine*, *48*(9), 1247–1258.

Mount, J. K. (1989). Contributions of the social sciences. In A. I. Wertheimer, & M. C. Smith (Eds.), *Pharmacy practice: Social and behavioral aspects* (3rd ed.). Baltimore MA: Williams & Wilkins.

O'Sullivan, A., & Sheffrin, S. M. (2003). *Economics: Principles in action*. Upper Saddle River, New Jersey 07458: Pearson Prentice Hall.

People Health Movement (PHM). People's charter for health. http://www.phmovement.org/.

Pharmacy Council of India. PharmD Scheme. http://www.pci.nic.in/PDF-Files/Pharm.D.(PB).pdf.

Ranganathan, S. S., & Gazarian, M. (2015). Rational use of medicines (RUM) for children in the developing world: Current status, key challenges and potential solutions. In S. MacLeod, et al. (Ed.), *Optimizing treatment for children in the developing world*. Switzerland: Springer International Publishing. http://dx.doi.org/10.1007/978-3-319-15750-4_20. (Chapter 20).

School of Pharmaceutical Sciences – USM. http://www.pha.usm.my/index.php/en/organization02/academic-staff/discipline-of-social-administrative-pharmacy.

Sørensen, E. W., Mount, J. K., & Christensen, S. T. (2003). The concept of social pharmacy. *Chronic Ill*, *7*, 8–11. Available online http://www.mcppnet.org/publications/issue07-3.pdf.

Study Commission on Pharmacy. (1975). *Pharmacists for the future*. Ann Arbor, MI: Health Administration Press.

Transparency International. (2016). *Corruption perceptions index 2016*. https://www.transparency.org/news/feature/corruption_perceptions_index_2016.

United Nations. (2009). *Human development report*.

United Nations. (2014). *World economic situation and prospects* Country classification. http://www.un.org/en/development/desa/policy/wesp/wesp_current/2014wesp_country_classification.pdf.

United Nations. (2017). *World economic situation and prospects*. https://www.un.org/development/desa/dpad/publication/world-economic-situation-and-prospects-2017/.

Wertheimer, A. I. (1989). International comparisons. In A. I. Wertheimer, M. C. Smith (Eds.), *Pharmacy practice: social and behavioral aspects*. Philadelphia: Williams and Wilkins, Park Press.

Wertheimer, A. I. (1991). Social/behavioural pharmacy: The Minnesota experience. *J Clin Pharm Ther*, *16*, 381–383.

Wertheimer, A. I., & Smith, M. C. (1989). *Pharmacy practice: Social and behavioral aspects*. Philadelphia: Williams and Wilkins, Park Press.

World Health Organization (WHO). (1986). *Ottawa charter for health promotion*. Ottawa. Geneva, Switzerland: WHO.

World Health Organization (WHO). (2011). *World economic forum (wef), 2011, "from burden to 'best buys': Reducing the economic impact of non-communicable diseases in low- and middle-income countries* (Geneva, Switzerland).

World Health Organization (WHO). (2014). *Public health, environmental and social determinants of health.* Geneva: Switzerland.

World Health Organization (WHO). (2016a). *WHO essential medicines and health products. Annual report 2015.* Geneva, Switzerland: WHO/EMP/2016.02. http://www.who.int/medicines/publications/AR2015_links_bookmarks.pdf?ua=1.

World Health Organization (WHO). (2016b). *Global disease outbreaks.* http://reports.weforum.org/global-risks-2016/global-disease-outbreaks/.

World Health Organization (WHO). (2017). *World health report.* Geneva: Switzerland.

Yadav, P. (2015). Health product supply chains in developing countries: Diagnosis of the root causes of underperformance and an agenda for reform. *Health Systems & Reform, 1*(2), 142–154.

Zorek, J. A., Lambert, B. L., & Popovich, N. G. (2013). The 4-year evolution of a social and behavioral pharmacy course. *AJPE, 77*(6) Article 119.

FURTHER READING

The World Bank. World Bank Country and Lending Groups. https://datahelpdesk.worldbank.org/knowledgebase/articles/906519-world-bank-country-and-lending-groups.

SECTION 1

SOCIOBEHAVIORAL ASPECTS OF MEDICINES USE IN LOW- AND MIDDLE-INCOME COUNTRIES

CHAPTER

2

SOCIOBEHAVIORAL ASPECTS OF MEDICINES USE IN DEVELOPING COUNTRIES

Mukhtar Ansari

University of Hail, Hail, Kingdom of Saudi Arabia

CHAPTER OUTLINE

BACKGROUND

Sociobehavioral aspect is an important determinant of effective management of health problems involving pharmacy practice (Rovers, 2011). Various resource materials have been published toward emphasizing the importance of sociobehavioral issues in pharmacy practice (Myers, 1975; Rayes, Hassali, & Abduelkarem, 2015a, 2015b). Some of the important resource materials in the form of books are Social and Behavioral Aspects of Pharmacy Practice by Rickles, Wertheimer, and Schommer (2016) and Social and Behavioral Aspects of Pharmaceutical Care by Rickles, Wertheimer, and Smith (2010). In developed nations, the concept of sociobehavioral science (SBS) is well adopted in pharmacy and other

Social and Administrative Aspects of Pharmacy in Low- and Middle-Income Countries. http://dx.doi.org/10.1016/B978-0-12-811228-1.00002-9

health education curriculum, but developing countries are dawdling in this context (Zorek, Lambert, & Popovich, 2013). Developing nations are enriched with various beliefs, traditions, norms, and values. Thus, they are more in need of adopting and emphasizing considering sociobehavioral aspects of medicine use, however, there are various barriers.

These barriers can be overcome to some extent through applying Engel's "biopsychological model." The model acts as a useful link between the SBS and clinical practice, setting the hierarchy of learning objectives based on priority and teacher training program emphasizing clinical role model (Benbassat, Baumal, Borkan, & Ber, 2003). In 1977, Dr. George Engel highlighted an integrated approach to human behavior and disease (Engel, 1980). His biopsychological model was a call to change the way of understanding the patient and to expand the domain of medical knowledge to address the needs of each patient (Borrell-Carrio, Suchman, & Epstein, 2004).

SBS are theoretically diverse and very important to understand the health education process and the professional context of medicine use. The ways that healthcare professional–patient relationships, health systems, professional obligations, and educational organizations interact and create continuing patterns of influence are revealed by SBS inquiry (Cuff & Vanselow, 2004; Institute of Medicine Committee on & Social Sciences in Medical School, 2004). Although there are various branches of SBS, two branches such as social psychology and medical sociology have widely been discussed.

Social psychology is the understanding of individual behavior in a social context. It is defined as "the scientific field that seeks to understand the nature and causes of individual behavior (e.g., feelings, thoughts) in social situations" (Baron, Byrne, & Suls, 1989). The various markers toward differentiating between groups of people in a given society include education, income and occupation, ethnicity and race, religion, political affiliation, and geographic region. Culture and social well-beings are not similar within a society, and these social inequalities impact the health. For example, in Nepal, reproductive health is an alarming issue and many women die annually due to reproductive health problems. This is mainly among the women of rural Nepal due to early marriage as a culture and low level of education and literacy (Armenakis & Kiefer, 2007).

Medical sociology (i.e., sociology of health and illness) is concerned with the relationship between social factors and health. It also relates with the application of sociological theory and research techniques to the questions related to health and the healthcare system (NLM, 2012). Concisely, medical sociology is the study of relationships between health phenomena (e.g., illness, medical care) and social factors (e.g., social class, gender, stress) (Sigdel, 2012).

The main focus of medial sociology is to investigate about how social inequalities contribute to differences in health and how these relationships over time persist despite ever-changing mechanisms, leading to poorer health among the disadvantaged. The concept of medical sociology tries to solve health problems and improve healthcare such as patient and healthcare provider relationships, social epidemiology of disease, and social factors affecting delivery of health services. More insight on sociobehavioral aspect of medicine use can be achieved through sociobehavioral theories.

SOCIOBEHAVIORAL THEORIES IN PHARMACY

Managing healthcare is a complex phenomenon, and it requires to consider various factors. Sociobehavioral aspects of medicine use are one of the fundamental components of healthcare system. There are various sociobehavioral theories related to healthcare; however, the Health Belief Model (HBM) and Health-Seeking Behavior Model are the two frequently discussed theories.

HEALTH BELIEF MODEL

The health-seeking behavior and compliance with the recommended health action depends on various components of HBM (Fig. 2.1). The HBM is a psychological model used to describe and predict association between beliefs about a particular condition (e.g., disease) and the recommended health action (Becker, 1974). Personal perception about the risk of getting a particular disease and its severity may vary from person to person. Perceived severity provides a force to take action, but it does not define which action is likely to be taken. A person takes action in his own way based on the knowledge, beliefs, norms, and family or social group pressure. If he/she perceives the condition is severe, an immediate action is sought while on contrary, there may be delay or even no action if the condition is perceived as mild or moderate (Becker, 1974; Rosenstock, 1974, 2005).

The next step of the HBM is the comparison between the perceived benefits and barriers of taking action. If the person believes that the benefits of taking health actions are superior to the barriers, he/she will try to adopt it. Actions may not take place due to the barriers, although he may believe that the benefits of taking action are effective. There may be both modifiable barriers (e.g., lack of knowledge about a particular disease, lack of prior exposure or experience, difficulty with starting a new behavior, attitude and family pressure) and nonmodifiable barriers (e.g., availability and accessibility of health services/providers, inconvenience/distance of healthcare facility, out of pocket expenses, location and transportation facilities, culture, education level), which play a negative role about taking the recommended health actions. Only modifiable barriers can be

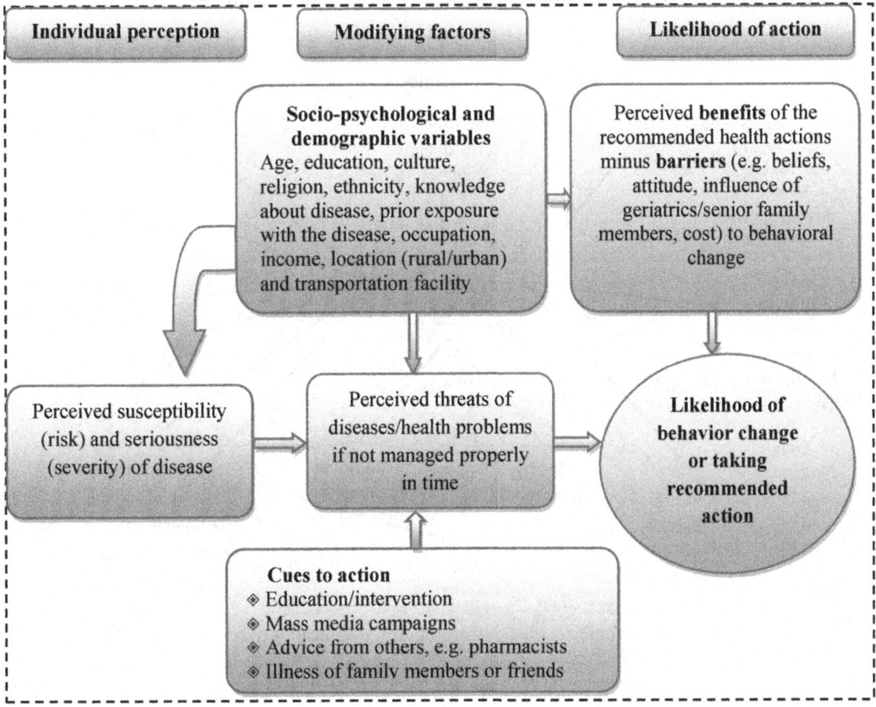

FIGURE 2.1

Adapted conceptual framework of the Health Belief Model.

approached through interventions toward taking advised health actions (Rosenstock, 2005; Rosenstock, Strecher, & Becker, 1988).

The most basic approach to convey health related messages or to improve health-related existing knowledge and practice of the people is through the application of educational intervention or counseling at an individual level. Moreover, there is variability in the level of readiness among them about the acceptance of change in health behavior. When perceptions of susceptibility and severity are high, a very minor stimulus (cue) may initiate the action (Glanz & Rimer, 2005; Rosenstock, 2005; Stretcher & Rosenstock, 1997).

FACTORS CONCERNED WITH SEEKING HEALTHCARE

Decision-making about seeking a particular health action is a complex process involving several components as shown in Fig. 2.2. Although urgency or severity of illnesses acts as a driving force in seeking healthcare, decision for health action may not take place due to poverty, unaffordability, and distance of the healthcare facility (Adegboyega, Onayade, & Salawu, 2005; Luong, Tang, Zhang, & Whitehead, 2007; Mbagaya, Odhiambo, & Oniang'o, 2005). Unavailability or inadequate availability of essential medicines at public healthcare centers is a persistent problem in developing countries. Therefore, patients are compelled to purchase medicines from private outlets that they cannot afford due to excessive price (Babar, Ibrahim, Singh, Bukahri, & Creese, 2007).

Peoples' or caregivers' beliefs pattern that is under the influence of culture, religion, and education has a very strong persuasive role on the nature of seeking healthcare (Shaikh & Hatcher, 2005). Besides,

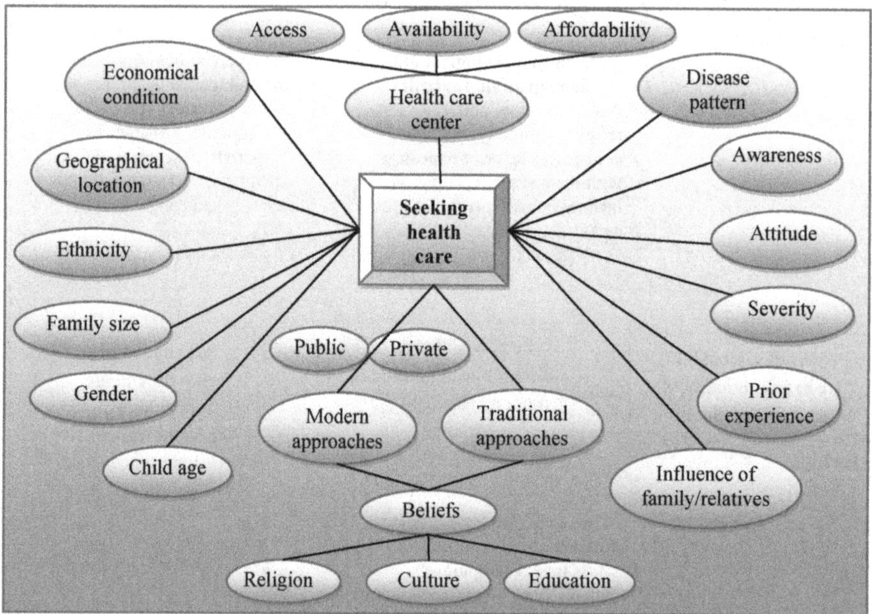

FIGURE 2.2

Adapted conceptual framework of the factors concerned with seeking healthcare.

perceived severity of the illness, financial condition, gender and age, as well as education, also contribute significantly toward seeking healthcare (Amin, Shah, & Becker, 2010; Burton et al., 2011; Ndugwa & Zulu, 2008; Pillai et al., 2003; Taffa & Chepngeno, 2005; Thind, 2004). There is gender inequality in terms of seeking healthcare (Yount, 2003). Interestingly, gender disparity is more pronounced among urban wealthier families compared with the rural one (Larson, Saha, Islam, & Roy, 2006). Financially poor families wish to visit public healthcare centers, whereas wealthier families favor private healthcare institutions as their first choice (Sakisaka, Jimba, & Hanada, 2010). The preference to the private healthcare centers is due to the belief and attitude of getting better treatment with powerful medication (Sudharsanam & Rotti, 2007). Conversely, less inclination toward public healthcare centers is due to poor quality of care, distance, inconvenient service time, and even absence of healthcare providers (Dalal & Dawad, 2009). However, socioeconomically poor people preferably consult unqualified or traditional practitioners due to cost, accessibility, and familiarity (Huq & Tasnim, 2008). Health-seeking behavior also depends on disease pattern, age, and number of children, and even the ethnicity. People of ethnic minority are less likely to seek healthcare (Nuruddin, Hadden, Petersen, & Lim, 2009; Page et al., 2011; Shaikh & Hatcher, 2005; Shawyer, Bin Gani, Punufimana, & Seuseu, 1996; Teerawichitchainan & Phillips, 2008; USAID, 2009).

MEDICINE USE, HEALTH BEHAVIOR, AND BELIEFS

Developing countries are facing various health and behavioral issues, such as high burden of diseases and disease pattern, inadequate health resources, socioeconomic status, illiteracy, cultural beliefs (e.g., a traditional belief that people suffering from diarrhea must not be given water/fluid), psychological distress, history and racism, age, gender biasness, long distance of healthcare facilities, lack of transportation, and problems associated with availability and affordability of essential medicines. These factors lead to discrepancies in health-seeking behavior compelling people toward self-medication, traditional healers, herbal medicines, and so forth (Ahmed, Adams, Chowdhury, & Bhuiya, 2000; Barkley, 2008; Ogunlesi & Olanrewaju, 2010; Shaikh & Hatcher, 2005).

Similarly, other factors that influence medicines use by consumers include perceived need for medicines, ideas about efficacy and safety (e.g., the color and shape of medicines—red medicines are thought to be good for the blood), uncertainty resulting in polytherapy (e.g., consulting a variety of modern and traditional health providers for serious conditions), medicine consumption roles (e.g., mothers in the Philippines decide the medicines for their children; while the contrast is true in Pakistan), the cost of medicines, literacy levels of consumers, and information channels (e.g., radio, television programs, magazines, newspapers, advertisements) (Bledsoe & Goubaud, 1985; Hardon, 1991; Hardon, Hodgkin, & Fresle, 2004; Rasmussen, Rahim, Streefland, & Hardon, 1996).

The following two cases will illustrate issues related to belief and health behavior. **Example 1**: Devi Pariyaar (the name has been changed to protect the privacy of the individual) was a 35-year-old poor illiterate lady living in a hut with a corrugated tin roof, a mud floor, and a single naked light bulb. Her 8-month-old child was having diarrhea and vomiting since the last 8 days. The poor child was skinny, dehydrated, and malnourished. He (the child) was being treated by a witch doctor. The witch doctor had a pinch of ash in his fingers and was saying some "mantras" (holy words believed to have special power and which could eliminate evil spirits). Then he applied the ash on the forehead of the child and blew all over the body of the child to "blow off" the evil spirit from him. In many cases, witch doctors sacrifice a cock or a hen but luckily, it was not done in the present case. Maybe, the family was too poor to afford one (Giri & Shankar, 2006). **Example 2**: There is no role of oral rehydration solution and enough water in diarrhea due to teething. "I applied ash of dried animal dung with finger twice daily at the site of teething for about 1 week and it was cured" (focused group discussion (FGD)-mother 1). **Example 3**: Some mothers' milk is harmful by nature and it should be stopped during diarrhea (FGD-mother 5) (Ansari et al., 2012).

Modifying health behavior at early ages such as during basic health education training or starting of the professional carrier would be fruitful. For example, young-aged people have to face numerous pressures and challenges, including "growing academic expectations, changing social relationships with family and peers and the physical and emotional changes associated with maturation." Young age is vital, as behaviors developed in this transition stage would continue in latter stages of life such as adulthood. Thus, it is emphasized to monitor young people's health behavior and determine effective health improvement interventions (Currie et al., 2012).

Use of mass media campaigns can produce positive change in health behaviors (Wakefield, Loken, & Hornik, 2010). Similarly, academic detailing is another worldwide accepted approach to modify health behaviors of pharmacists and other healthcare professionals. Developing countries are more in need to highlight the issue of academic detailing (Khanal, Palaian, Shankar, Mishra, & Ibrahim, 2009; Shankar et al., 2010).

FAITH HEALING

Faith healing is a ritualistic practice of curing sick people by using the power of prayer and belief. Despite advancements in modern medicine, traditional healing practices are still predominant in rural Nepal and people of rural societies are reluctant to accept changes in their cultural practices (Baniya, 2014). Neurological and psychiatric illnesses are mainly managed by faith healing approaches (Giri & Shankar, 2006). Faith healers are of different types—*dhami-jhakri*, *pandit-lama-gubhaju-pujari*, and *jyotishi* (Shankar, Paudel, & Giri, 2006).

Dhami-jhakri are shamans (witch doctors) and they act as mediators between the spirit world and the material world. During shamanic ceremonies, colorful costumes, drumming, chanting, dancing, and singing and the sacrifice of either a rooster or a black goat depending on the complications are used. Example: An old man came and taught me mantras in my dreams. He asked me to use it to cure patients. I have practiced it to help many people. My maternal grandfather was a *Dhami*. It is said at least one member of family is followed [by the deceased *Dhami*] to become a *Dhami*. Mantra should not be taught to everyone. It can be taught to a disciple or to a family member before my death. You can learn mantras only if the god likes you. First, god makes you sick. Then, if you could identify him you can learn mantras and become a *Dhami*. I use only one mantra. However, methods of applying it are different according to the problems faced by a patient. My Guru taught me the methods. I did as said by my Guru and it cured patients. I have improved it by using for many years with many patients. When I close my eyes and ask my Guru, a kind of shadowed figure appears and I can hear holy voices instructing me the things to be done for a sick person (Tamang & Broom, 2010).

Pandit-lama-gubhaju-pujari are the priests of the different ethnic and religious groups in Nepal. *Gubhaju* are the priest of *Newar*, *Lamas* are the priest of Buddhist, and *Pandit* and *Pujaris* are the Hindu priests. They all diagnose and treat illnesses through prayers and rituals. *Jyotishi* are astrologers and they treat patients by reading their horoscope, palms, and forehead (Gartoulla, 1992; Raut & Khanal, 2011).

In India, studies conducted on mental disorders found that majority (75%–78%) of the patients practices faith healing before seeking medical intervention (Kar, 2008; Rajan, Cherupushpam, Saleem, & Jithu, 2016).

SELF-MEDICATION

Self-medication is an important component of healthcare system and its practice is widespread (Albawani, Hassan, Abd-aziz, & Gnanasan, 2016; Al-Flaiti, Al-Badi, Hakami, & Khan, 2014; James, Handu, Al Khaja, Otoom, & Sequeira, 2006; Jassim, 2010; Selvaraj, Kumar, & Ramalingam, 2014; Sharif, Bugaighis, & Sharif, 2015). However, the major problem with self-medication is the detrimental consequences due to its inappropriate use. Consumers prefer to manage their common health problems using self-medication as it is easier, cost effective, and time efficient (Keshari, Kesarwani, & Mishra, 2014; WHO, 2000).

Use of self-medication is influenced by several factors such as personal, organizational, and environmental factors (de Boer, Versteegen, & van Wijhe, 2007; Sawalha, 2008; Worku & Mariam, 2003). Media, Internet, and extensive advertisement by the pharmaceutical manufacturers also play an important role toward practicing self-medication (Bond & Hannaford, 2003; Klemenc-Ketis, Hladnik, & Kersnik, 2011). Inadequacies in the healthcare delivery systems especially in low income countries such as inaccessibility, unregulated distribution of medicines, inequitable distribution, lack of healthcare professionals, high costs, and patients' attitudes toward healthcare providers are some of the key drivers of self-medication (Esimone, Nworu, & Udeogaranya, 2007; Yousef, Al-Bakri, Bustanji, & Wazaify, 2008).

Although various factors contribute, self-medication is the major reason for the irrational use of medicines (Filho, Lima-Costa, & Uchoa, 2004). This could lead to adverse medicine reactions, development of resistance, medicine dependence, wastage of money, prolonged suffering, and medicine dependence (Clavijo, Baquero, Ulloa, & Morales, 1995; Hughes, McElnay, & Fleming, 2001). In terms of antimicrobial self-medication, the common problems include inadequate dose, short duration of treatment, stopping treatment upon improvement of disease symptoms, sharing of medicines among others, and therapeutic failure (Bennadi, 2013; Skliros et al., 2010). Thus, proper health communication is inevitable to minimize medicine use problems including antimicrobials.

PHARMACY AND HEALTH COMMUNICATION

Communication is the imparting or interchange of thoughts, opinions, or information by speech, writing, or signs. Communication is an important factor in the healthcare system. Medication errors due to lack of proper communication between pharmacists or healthcare providers and patients or their relatives are common problem, and they may even endanger the life through serious adverse medicine reactions (JCR, 2009). Errors "occur because information is unrecorded, misdirected, never received, never retrieved or ignored." Communication will help to heighten collaboration between pharmacists and other healthcare professionals, which in turn enhance teamwork attitude, sharing responsibility for problem-solving, decision–making, and carry out plans for patient care.

Communication does not only mean to speak but also to listen. To have a meaningful communication, pharmacists and other healthcare providers should listen carefully to the primary complaints of the patients to ensure correct diagnosis of the diseases or complications. Once proper diagnosis is made, effective communication between providers as well as between providers and patients would help in rational management of the diseases. Furthermore, patient-centered communication (PCC) will ensure medicine safety, patients' satisfaction, and prevent unwanted emergency situations (Martina, Ummenhoferb, Manserc, & Spiriga, 2010; O'Grady & Jadad, 2010; Wanzer, Booth-Butterfield, & Gruber, 2004). PCC is a vital step in understanding patients' actual health-related problems and to address them accordingly. It involves open-ended questions, active listening to understand patients' feelings, concerns, and expectations, and to respect and support (Hashim, 2017). Example: A young man was prescribed a fentanyl patch to treat pain resulting from a back injury. He was not informed that heat could make the patch unsafe to use. He fell asleep with a heating pad and died. The level of fentanyl in his bloodstream was found to be 100 times the level it should have been and caused life-threatening breathing problem and finally death (FDA, 2007).

COMMUNICATION PROBLEMS IN HEALTHCARE SYSTEM

Most of the communication problems occurring at healthcare centers can broadly be categorized into three types:

1. **Provider-to-provider communication problem**: It includes miscommunication about the patient's condition, poor documentation, workload pressure, personal values and expectations, qualifications and status, hierarchy, failure to read the patient's medical record, and disruptive behavior (Ha & Longnecker, 2010; Leonard, Graham, & Bonacum, 2004).
2. **Provider-to-patient communication problem**: It encompasses unsympathetic response to a patient's complaint, no or wrong information given to patient, differences in schedules and professional routines, incomplete follow-up instructions, language, culture, ethnicity and jargon, and gender (Almutairi, 2015; Bowen, 2001; Saha & Fernandez, 2007).
3. **Miscellaneous communication problem**: This represents differences in accountability, payment, and rewards; concerns regarding clinical responsibility, complexity of care, distraction; differences in requirements, regulations, and norms of professional education; and emphasis on rapid decision-making (O'Daniel & Rosenstein, 2008).

PHARMACY SYSTEMS AND ORGANIZATIONS

In developing countries, most people reside in rural areas where healthcare facilities are scarce (MoHP, 2012). Thus, community pharmacies become the most favored place for those seeking healthcare for general ailments (Gyawali et al., 2014; Miller & Goodman, 2016). Furthermore, consultation is easier and cheaper (Hadi et al., 2016). However, the actual problem is the nonprofessionals, i.e., nonpharmacists who operate the community pharmacies especially in rural areas, and the delivery of healthcare by them can be detrimental in certain instances (Bhuvan, Alrasheedy, & Ibrahim, 2013).

The pharmacy practice is in growing stage with regard to developing countries, and the professional role of pharmacists is not established (Bhuvan et al., 2013; Ibrahim, Palaian, Al-Sulaiti, & El-Shami,

2016b; Rayes et al., 2015a, 2015b). The important factors that hinder the professional role of pharmacists in healthcare system include shortage of qualified pharmacists, lack of separation between dispensing and counseling units, lack of focus on delivering quality services, and lack of standard pharmacy practice guidelines (Hermansyah, Sukorini, Setiawan, & Priyandani, 2012; Hussain, Ibrahim, & Malik, 2013; Malik et al., 2013; Sharma, Kc, Alrasheedy, Kaundinnyayana, & Khanal, 2014).

HUMANISTIC STUDIES OF PHARMACY

Humanistic studies deal with the outcomes measures including health status, patient satisfaction, work outcomes, and patient-based assessments following medicine therapy. The patient-reported outcome about their health status is vital in decision-making about treatment choices and as a monitoring parameter for effectiveness or toxicities of pharmacotherapy (Bungay, 2000; Refolo, Minacori, Mele, Sacchini, & Spagnolo, 2012). There are various clinical and patient-centered indicators toward measuring humanistic outcomes, for example, SF-12 Health Survey, HRQoL, WHO-5 Well-Being Index, Diabetes Empowerment Scale, Problem Areas in Diabetes, Health Care Climate Questionnaire, Patients Assessment of Chronic Illness Care, Barriers to Medications, Patient Support, Diabetes Self-care Activities, and Global Satisfaction for Diabetes Treatment (Fischer et al., 2004; Nicolucci et al., 2014).

In modern healthcare system, pharmacists' role is increasingly getting recognition and thus their contribution is inevitable. Pharmacists especially associated with hospitals, clinics, and community pharmacies can substantially contribute in humanistic outcomes. Pharmacists' interventions have resulted in preventing potential adverse medicine events and to decrease medical expenditure (Hsiao et al., 2012; Touchette et al., 2014).

EDUCATION DISCIPLINES

The understanding of sociobehavioral aspects of patients such as patient's beliefs, health values, and behaviors is critical to a successful clinical encounter. The main purpose of SBS is to integrate mental health and social sciences into healthcare education so as to prepare students to care patients from diverse social and cultural backgrounds (Betancourt, 2003).

In this modern era, the trend of chronic and neuropsychiatric disorders is increasing (Ngui, Khasakhala, Ndetei, & Roberts, 2010). Thus, pharmacy and other allied health sciences curricula need an urgent call for incorporating the concept of SBS such as patient behavior, healthcare provider's role and behavior, pharmacist–patient interactions, social and cultural issues in healthcare, and health policy and economics (Cordingley et al., 2013; Cuff, 2004; Hassali et al., 2011). The concept of SBS has been included in many of the western pharmacy and healthcare schools, but developing nations are still lagging behind in this aspect (Gwee, Samarasekera, & Chay-Hoon; Kallivayalil, 2012; Manickam & Sathyanarayana Rao, 2007; Sreeramareddy et al., 2007; Tsutsumi, 2015). The Institute of Medicine has recommended the following SBS domains to be included in pharmacy and health school's curriculum, which include healthcare professional–patient interaction, patient behavior, health policy and economics, mind–body interactions, healthcare professional role and behavior, and social and cultural issues.

Table 2.1 The Pharmacy Practice Activity Classification

A. Ensuring Appropriate Therapy and Outcomes
- Ensuring appropriate pharmacotherapy
- Ensuring patient's understanding/adherence to his or her treatment plan
- Monitoring and reporting outcomes

B. Dispensing Medications and Devices
- Processing the prescription or medicine order
- Preparing the pharmaceutical product
- Delivering the medication or device

C. Health Promotion and Disease Prevention
- Delivering clinical preventive services
- Surveillance and reporting of public health issues
- Promoting safe medication use in society

D. Health Systems Management
- Managing the practice
- Managing medications throughout the health system
- Managing the use of medications within the health system
- Participating in research activities
- Engaging in interdisciplinary collaboration

BEHAVIORAL RESEARCH IN PHARMACY PRACTICE

There is a paradigm shift in the professional role of pharmacists—from industry-oriented role to patient care. Pharmacists' behavior plays an important role in promoting safe and effective use of medicines. Narrative reviews have demonstrated that pharmacists have a wide range of skills in medication management. However, there are various obstacles toward offering the quality services. Understanding and addressing the barriers would help pharmacists to perform their professional duty with more outcomes (Alhabib, Aldraimly, & Alfarhan, 2016; Rubio-Valera, Chen, & O'Reilly, 2014). Patient counseling is one of the important components of good dispensing practices of pharmacists. However, there are several barriers toward patient counseling such as lack of time, lack of knowledge and confidence, lack of professional fee, poor response from patients, doctors' dispensing and lack of Continuous Professional Development programs (Adepu & Nagavi, 2009; Eades, Ferguson, & O'Carroll, 2011).

In industrialized countries, the professional role of pharmacists is well established compared with the developing countries. In contrast, the services and expertise offered by pharmacists in developing countries are still underutilized (Azhar, Latif, Murtaza, & Khan, 2013). Thus, there is a need of continued pharmacy education and managerial interventions to improve pharmacists' attitude and behavior for better recognition in the healthcare system (Basak & Sathyanarayana, 2010; Ibrahim, Palaian, Al-Sulaiti, & El-Shami, 2016a). Following are the activities that pharmacists can work hard and with honesty to get their professional recognition in the society (Table 2.1) (Wiedenmayer et al., 2006).

ACHIEVEMENTS

The concept of SBSs is getting attention in pharmacy and health education curriculum, as most of the health problems require management from both medical and sociopsychological perspectives. Industrialized countries are leading in this context and the developing nations are also paying interest in this direction. India and China, the two huge countries in Asia region, are also encouraging the implementation of sociobehavioral issues in pharmacy and health curricula. Malaysia is also growing up toward adopting the concept of SBSs in its pharmacy education curriculum. Similarly, various studies in developing countries have drawn a serious attention toward the importance of incorporating the discipline of social pharmacy in pharmacy curricula. Sociobehavioral research interest is proliferating in developing countries. Health communication and humanistic outcomes are also getting attention.

CHALLENGES

Although SBS has been an integral part of pharmacy and health curriculum since 1920s, its integration in clinical practice is still a big challenge and it needs continued reinforcement (Peterson, Rdesinski, Biagioli, Chappelle, & Elliot, 2011; Pickren, 2007; Rameshkumar, 2009). There are several challenges toward teaching SBS in pharmacy and health schools such as lack of perceived relevance of SBS in clinical practice, multiplicity of topics creating confusion about teaching priorities, lack of qualified teachers (i.e., teaching SBS by other professionals who lack experience of both SBS and healthcare), and modern medical pedagogies such as problem-based learning (PBL) (Benbassat et al., 2003; Chur-Hansen et al., 2008; Litva & Peters, 2008). Other challenges represent varieties in traditional beliefs and cultures in developing countries.

RECOMMENDATIONS: THE WAY FORWARD

Sociobehavioral aspects of medicine use are highly neglected issues in developing nations. Furthermore, low-income countries are facing various health and behavioral issues such as high burden of diseases and disease pattern, inadequate health resources, availability and affordability of essential medicines, socioeconomic status, illiteracy, culture and beliefs, psychological distress, history and racism, age, and gender inequality. Modifying health behavior of healthcare professionals at early ages such as during basic health education training or at the starting of the professional carrier is more effective. Thus, incorporating the discipline of SBS in undergraduate pharmacy and other health educational training programs is highly suggestive. Likewise, there is a need of establishing a separate department of SBS in health-related academic and clinical institutions. Pharmacists and other healthcare professionals should consider the social and behavioral factors of patients while treating the patients.

CONCLUSIONS

The emphasis of modern pharmacy and other health education is on modern medical pedagogies (i.e., PBL). Thus, it is hard for the concept of SBS to get its place in health education curriculum. However, the effective management of most of the diseases or disorders in current medical practice requires sociobehavioral and psychological interventions. Developing countries should learn from the industrialized nations and need to strive to adopt SBS in their pharmacy and other health education programs as well as in clinical settings. There is a need of more research in this area and implementation of SBS in modern health education and healthcare.

LESSONS LEARNED

- The concept of social and behavioral issues is quiet familiar within pharmacy and health school's curriculum of Western countries.
- The pharmacy and other health education curricula of developing countries are deficient in realizing the importance of social and behavioral discipline in modern health education and healthcare management.
- SBS is a vast concept and, thus, selection of the contents from SBS to be included in pharmacy and other health education curricula is vital. Furthermore, to have better acceptability and impact, the teaching of SBS should be performed by healthcare professionals experienced in SBS rather than pure sociologists or psychologists.

REFERENCES

Adegboyega, A. A., Onayade, A. A., & Salawu, O. (2005). Care-seeking behaviour of caregivers for common childhood illnesses in Lagos Island local government area, Nigeria. *Nigerian Journal of Medicine: Journal of the National Association of Resident Doctors of Nigeria*, *14*(1), 65–71.

Adepu, R., & Nagavi, B. G. (2009). Attitudes and behaviors of practicing community pharmacists towards patient counselling. *Indian Journal of Pharmaceutical Sciences*, *71*(3), 285–289. http://dx.doi.org/10.4103/0250-474X.56029.

Ahmed, S. M., Adams, A. M., Chowdhury, M., & Bhuiya, A. (2000). Gender, socioeconomic development and health-seeking behaviour in Bangladesh. *Social Science & Medicine*, *51*(3), 361–371.

Albawani, S. M., Hassan, Y. B., Abd-aziz, N., & Gnanasan, S. (2016). Self medication practice among consumers in Sana'a city. *International Journal of Pharmacy and Pharmaceutical Sciences*, *8*(10), 119–124.

Al-Flaiti, M., Al-Badi, K., Hakami, W. O., & Khan, S. A. (2014). Evaluation of self-medication practices in acute diseases among university students in Oman. *Journal of Acute Disease*, *3*(3), 249–252.

Alhabib, S., Aldraimly, M., & Alfarhan, A. (2016). An evolving role of clinical pharmacists in managing diabetes: Evidence from the literature. *Saudi Pharmaceutical Journal*, *24*(4), 441–446. http://doi.org/10.1016/j.jsps.2014.07.008.

Almutairi, K. M. (2015). Culture and language differences as a barrier to provision of quality care by the health workforce in Saudi Arabia. *Saudi Medical Journal*, *36*(4), 425–431. http://dx.doi.org/10.15537/smj.2015.4.10133.

Amin, R., Shah, N. M., & Becker, S. (2010). Socioeconomic factors differentiating maternal and child health-seeking behavior in rural Bangladesh: A cross-sectional analysis. *International Journal for Equity in Health*, *9*, 9. http://dx.doi.org/10.1186/1475-9276-9-9.

Ansari, M., Ibrahim, M. I. M., Hassali, M. A., Shankar, P. R., Koirala, A., & Thapa, N. J. (2012). Mothers' beliefs and barriers about childhood diarrhea and its management in Morang district, Nepal. *BMC Research Notes*, *5*(1), 576. http://dx.doi.org/10.1186/1756-0500-5-576.

Armenakis, A., & Kiefer, C. (2007). *Social & cultural factors related to health part A: Recognizing the impact* Global Health Education Consortium. Retrieved from https://www.cugh.org/sites/default/files/13_Social_And_Cultural_Factors_Related_To_Health_Part_A_Recognizing_The_Impact_-_Copy_0.pdf.

Azhar, S., Latif, U., Murtaza, G., & Khan, S. A. (2013). Mixed methodology approach in pharmacy practice research. *Acta Poloniae Pharmaceutica-Drug Research*, *70*(6), 1123–1130.

Babar, Z. U., Ibrahim, M. I., Singh, H., Bukahri, N. I., & Creese, A. (2007). Evaluating drug prices, availability, affordability, and price components: Implications for access to drugs in Malaysia. *PLoS Medicine*, *4*(3), e82. http://dx.doi.org/10.1371/journal.pmed.0040082.

Baniya, R. (2014). Traditional healing practices in rural Nepal. *Journal of Patan Academy of Health Sciences, 1*(1), 52–53.

Barkley, G. S. (2008). Factors influencing health behaviors in the National Health and Nutritional Examination Survey, III (NHANES III). *Social Work in Health Care, 46*(4), 57–79. http://dx.doi.org/10.1300/J010v46n04_04.

Baron, R. A., Byrne, D. E., & Suls, J. M. (1989). *Exploring social psychology*. Boston (Mass.) [etc.]: Allyn and Bacon.

Basak, S. C., & Sathyanarayana, D. (2010). Evaluating medicines dispensing patterns at private community pharmacies in Tamilnadu, India. *Southern Med Review, 3*(2), 27–31.

Becker, M. H. (1974). *The health belief model and personal health behavior* C. B. Slack.

Benbassat, J., Baumal, R., Borkan, J. M., & Ber, R. (2003). Overcoming barriers to teaching the behavioral and social sciences to medical students. *Academic Medicine, 78*(4), 372–380.

Bennadi, D. (2013). Self-medication: A current challenge. *Journal of Basic and Clinical Pharmacy, 5*(1), 19–23. http://dx.doi.org/10.4103/0976-0105.128253.

Betancourt, J. R. (2003). Cross-cultural medical education: Conceptual approaches and frameworks for evaluation. *Academic Medicine: Journal of the Association of American Medical Colleges, 78*(6), 560–569.

Bhuvan, K. C., Alrasheedy, A. A., & Ibrahim, M. I. M. (2013). Do community pharmacists in Nepal have a role in adverse drug reaction reporting systems? *Australas Med J, 6*(2), 100–103.

Bledsoe, C. H., & Goubaud, M. F. (1985). The reinterpretation of Western pharmaceuticals among the Mende of Sierra Leone. *Social Science & Medicine, 21*(3), 275–282.

de Boer, M. J., Versteegen, G. J., & van Wijhe, M. (2007). Patients' use of the Internet for pain-related medical information. *Patient Education and Counseling, 68*(1), 86–97. http://dx.doi.org/10.1016/j.pec.2007.05.012.

Bond, C., & Hannaford, P. (2003). Issues related to monitoring the safety of over-the-counter (OTC) medicines. *Drug Safety: an International Journal of Medical Toxicology and Drug Experience, 26*(15), 1065–1074.

Borrell-Carrio, F., Suchman, A. L., & Epstein, R. M. (2004). The biopsychosocial model 25 years later: Principles, practice, and scientific inquiry. *Annals of Family Medicine, 2*(6), 576–582. http://dx.doi.org/10.1370/afm.245.

Bowen, S. (2001). *Language barriers in access to health care, health Canada*. Retrieved from http://www.hc-sc.gc.ca/hcs-sss/pubs/acces/2001-lang-acces/index-eng.php.

Bungay, K. M. (2000). Methods to assess the humanistic outcomes of clinical pharmacy services. *Pharmacotherapy: The Journal of Human Pharmacology and Drug Therapy, 20*(10P2), 253S–258S. http://dx.doi.org/10.1592/phco.20.16.253S.35010.

Burton, D. C., Flannery, B., Onyango, B., Larson, C., Alaii, J., Zhang, X., … Feikin, D. R. (2011). Healthcare-seeking behaviour for common infectious disease-related illnesses in rural Kenya: A community-based house-to-house survey. *Journal of Health, Population, and Nutrition, 29*(1), 61–70.

Chur-Hansen, A., Carr, J. E., Bundy, C., Sanchez-Sosa, J. J., Tapanya, S., & Wahass, S. H. (2008). An international perspective on behavioral science education in medical schools. *Journal of Clinical Psychology in Medical Settings, 15*(1), 45–53. http://dx.doi.org/10.1007/s10880-008-9092-0.

Clavijo, H. A., Baquero, J. A., Ulloa, S., & Morales, A. (1995). Self-medication during pregnancy. *World Health Forum, 16*(4), 403–404.

Cordingley, L., Peters, S., Hart, J., Rock, J., Hodges, L., McKendree, J., & Bundy, C. (2013). What psychology do medical students need to know? An evidence based approach to curriculum development. *Health and Social Care Education, 2*(2), 38–47. http://dx.doi.org/10.11120/hsce.2013.00029.

Cuff, P. A. (2004). Enhancing the behavioral and social science content of medical school curricula. *Improving Medical Education.*

Cuff, P. A., & Vanselow, N. A. (2004). *Improving medical education: Enhancing the behavioral and social science content of medical school curricula*. US: National Academies Press.

Currie, C., Zanotti, C., Morgan, A., Currie, D., de-Looze, M., Roberts, C., … Barnekow, V. (2012). *Social determinants of health and well-being among young people: Health Behaviour in School-Aged Children (HBSC) study: International report from the 2009/2010 survey* (Health Policy for Children and Adolescents, No. 6) Copenhagen: WHO Regional Office for Europe. From http://www.euro.who.int/__data/assets/pdf_file/0003/163857/Social-determinants-of-health-and-well-being-among-young-people.pdf.

Dalal, K., & Dawad, S. (2009). Non-utilization of public health care facilities: Examining the reasons through a national study of women in India. *Rural and Remote Health*, *9*(3), 1178.

Eades, C. E., Ferguson, J. S., & O'Carroll, R. E. (2011). Public health in community pharmacy: A systematic review of pharmacist and consumer views. *BMC Public Health*, *11*, 582. http://dx.doi.org/10.1186/1471-2458-11-582.

Engel, G. L. (1980). The clinical application of the biopsychosocial model. *The American Journal of Psychiatry*, *137*(5), 535–544. http://dx.doi.org/10.1176/ajp.137.5.535.

Esimone, C. O., Nworu, C. S., & Udeogaranya, O. P. (2007). Utilization of antimicrobial agents with and without prescription by out-patients in selected pharmacies in South-eastern Nigeria. *Pharm World Sci*, *29*(6), 655–660. http://dx.doi.org/10.1007/s11096-007-9124-0.

FDA. (2007). *Fentanyl transdermal system (patch) (marketed as duragesic and generics)* Full Version. Retrieved from https://www.fda.gov/Drugs/DrugSafety/DrugSafetyPodcasts/ucm078367.htm.

Fischer, J. S., McLaughlin, T., Loza, L., Beauchamp, R., Schwartz, S., & Kipnes, M. (2004). The impact of insulin glargine on clinical and humanistic outcomes in patients uncontrolled on other insulin and oral agents: An office-based naturalistic study*. *Current Medical Research and Opinion*, *20*(11), 1703–1710. http://dx.doi.org/10.1185/030079904X5526.

Gartoulla, R. P. (1992). *Ethnomedicine and other alternativemedication practices, a study in medicalanthropology in Nepal* (Ph D). Darjeeling, India: North Bengal University.

Giri, B. R., & Shankar, P. R. (2006). Faith healing in western Nepal. *Nepal Journal of Neuroscience*, *3*(1), 54–55.

Glanz, K., & Rimer, B. K. (2005). *Theory at a glance: A guide for health promotion practice* (2nd ed.). US Department of Health and Human Services, National Institutes of Health. From. http://www.sbccimplementationkits.org/demandrmnch/wp-content/uploads/2014/02/Theory-at-a-Glance-A-Guide-For-Health-Promotion-Practice.pdf.

Gwee, M.C.E., Samarasekera, D.,, Chay-Hoon, T. Role of basic sciences in 21st century medical education: an Asian perspective. *International Association of Medical Science Educators. 20*(3). http://www.iamse.org/mse-article/role-of-basic-sciences-in-21st-century-medical-education-an-asian-perspective/.

Gyawali, S., Rathore, D. S., Adhikari, K., Shankar, P. R., KC, V. K., & Basnet, S. (2014). Pharmacy practice and injection use in community pharmacies in Pokhara city, Western Nepal. *BMC Health Services Research*, *14*(190).

Ha, J. F., & Longnecker, N. (2010). Doctor-patient communication: A review. *The Ochsner Journal*, *10*(1), 38–43.

Hadi, M. A., Karami, N. A., Al-Muwalid, A. S., Al-Otabi, A., Al-Subahi, E., … Elrggal, M. E. (2016). Community pharmacists' knowledge, attitude, and practices towards dispensing antibiotics without prescription (DAwP): A cross-sectional survey in Makkah Province, Saudi Arabia. *International Journal of Infectious Diseases*, *47*, 95–100. http://dx.doi.org/10.1016/j.ijid.2016.06.003.

Hardon, A. (1991). *Confronting ill health: Medicines, self-care, and the poor in Manila/Anita P. Hardon*. Quezon City: Health Action Information Network.

Hardon, A., Hodgkin, C., & Fresle, D. (2004). *How to investigate the use of medicines by consumers* WHO/EDM/PAR/2004.2. From http://www.who.int/drugresistance/Manual1_HowtoInvestigate.pdf.

Hashim, M. J. (2017). Patient-centered Communication: Basic skills. *American Family Physician*, *95*(1), 29–34.

Hassali, M. A., Shafie, A. A., Al-Haddad, M. S., Abduelkarem, A. R., Ibrahim, M. I., Palaian, S., & Abrika, O. S. (2011). Social pharmacy as a field of study: The needs and challenges in global pharmacy education. *Research in Social and Administrative Pharmacy*, *7*(4), 415–420. http://dx.doi.org/10.1016/j.sapharm.2010.10.003.

Hermansyah, A., Sukorini, A. I., Setiawan, C. D., & Priyandani, Y. (2012). The conflicts between professional and non professional work of community pharmacists in Indonesia. *Pharmacy Practice*, *10*(1), 33–39.

Hsiao, C. L., Lin, Y. M., Chang, Y. T., Chen, C. C., Tsai, C. S., & Liu, H. P. (2012). The financial impacts of pharmacist intervention in in-patient department of a local hospital in Taiwan. Value in health. *The Journal of the International Society for Pharmacoeconomics and Outcomes Research*, A1–A256.

Hughes, C. M., McElnay, J. C., & Fleming, G. F. (2001). Benefits and risks of self medication. *Drug Safety: an International Journal of Medical Toxicology and Drug Experience*, *24*(14), 1027–1037.

Huq, M. N., & Tasnim, T. (2008). Maternal education and child healthcare in Bangladesh. *Maternal and Child Health Journal*, *12*(1), 43–51. http://dx.doi.org/10.1007/s10995-007-0303-3.

Hussain, A., Ibrahim, M. I., & Malik, M. (2013). Assessment of disease management of insomnia at community pharmacies through simulated visits in Pakistan. *Pharmacy Practice*, *11*(4), 179–184.

Ibrahim, M. I., Palaian, S., Al-Sulaiti, F., & El-Shami, S. (2016a). Evaluating community pharmacy practice in Qatar using simulated patient method: Acute gastroenteritis management. *Pharmacy Practice (Granada)*, *14*(4).

Ibrahim, M. I., Palaian, S., Al-Sulaiti, F., & El-Shami, S. (2016b). Evaluating community pharmacy practice in Qatar using simulated patient method:acute gastroenteritis management. *Pharmacy Practice*, *14*(4), 800. http://dx.doi.org/10.18549/PharmPract.2016.04.800.

Institute of Medicine Committee on, B, & Social Sciences in Medical School, C. (2004). The national academies collection: Reports funded by National Institutes of Health. In P. A. Cuff, & N. A. Vanselow (Eds.), *Improving medical education: Enhancing the behavioral and social science content of medical school curricula*. Washington (DC): National Academies Press (US), (National Academy of Sciences).

James, H., Handu, S. S., Al Khaja, K. A., Otoom, S., & Sequeira, R. P. (2006). Evaluation of the knowledge, attitude and practice of self-medication among first-year medical students. *Medical Principles and Practice: International Journal of the Kuwait University, Health Science Centre*, *15*(4), 270–275. http://dx.doi.org/10.1159/000092989.

Jassim, A.-M. (2010). In-home drug storage and self-medication with antimicrobial drugs in Basrah, Iraq. *OMJ*, *25*, 79–87.

JCR. (2009). *The joint commission guide to improving staff communication*. Retrieved from http://www.jcrinc.com/assets/1/14/GISC09_Sample_Pages1.pdf.

Kallivayalil, R. A. (2012). The importance of psychiatry in undergraduate medical education in India. *Indian Journal of Psychiatry*, *54*(3), 208–216. http://dx.doi.org/10.4103/0019-5545.102336.

Kar, N. (2008). Resort to faith-healing practices in the pathway to care for mental illness: A study on psychiatric inpatients in Orissa. *Mental Health, Religion & Culture*, *11*(7), 720–740.

Keshari, S. S., Kesarwani, P., & Mishra, M. (2014). Prevalence and pattern of self-medication practices in rural area of Barabanki. *Indian Journal of Clinical Practice*, *25*(7), 636–639.

Khanal, S., Palaian, S., Shankar, P. R., Mishra, P., & Ibrahim, M. I. M. (2009). Academic detailing as a possible source of drug information in the context of Nepal: A short review. *Journal of Clinical and Diagnostic Research*, *3*(4), 1697–1703.

Klemenc-Ketis, Z., Hladnik, Z., & Kersnik, J. (2011). A cross sectional study of sex differences in self-medication practices among university students in Slovenia. *Collegium Antropologicum*, *35*(2), 329–334.

Larson, C. P., Saha, U. R., Islam, R., & Roy, N. (2006). Childhood diarrhoea management practices in Bangladesh: Private sector dominance and continued inequities in care. *International Journal of Epidemiology*, *35*(6), 1430–1439. http://dx.doi.org/10.1093/ije/dyl167.

Leonard, M., Graham, S., & Bonacum, D. (2004). The human factor: The critical importance of effective teamwork and communication in providing safe care. *Quality and Safety in Health Care*, *13*(Suppl. 1), i85–i90. http://dx.doi.org/10.1136/qshc.2004.010033.

Litva, A., & Peters, S. (2008). Exploring barriers to teaching behavioural and social sciences in medical education. *Medical Education*, *42*(3), 309–314. http://dx.doi.org/10.1111/j.1365-2923.2007.02951.x.

Loyola Filho, A. I., Lima-Costa, M. F., & Uchoa, E. (2004). Bambui project: A qualitative approach to self-medication. *Cadernos de saúde pública*, *20*(6), 1661–1669 doi:/S0102-311x2004000600025.

Luong, D. H., Tang, S., Zhang, T., & Whitehead, M. (2007). Vietnam during economic transition: A tracer study of health service access and affordability. *Int J Health Serv*, *37*(3), 573–588.

Malik, M., Hassali, M. A., Shafie, A. A., Hussain, A., Aljadhey, H., & Saleem, F. (2013). Case management of malaria fever at community pharmacies in Pakistan: A threat to rational drug use. *Pharmacy Practice*, *11*(1), 8–16.

Manickam, L. S. S., & Sathyanarayana Rao, T. S. (2007). Undergraduate medical education: Psychological perspectives from India. *Indian Journal of Psychiatry*, *49*(3), 175–178. http://dx.doi.org/10.4103/0019-5545.37317.

Martina, J. S., Ummenhoferb, W., Manserc, T., & Spiriga, R. (2010). Interprofessional collaboration among nurses and physicians: Making a difference in patient outcome. *Swiss Medical Weekly*.

Mbagaya, G. M., Odhiambo, M. O., & Oniang'o, R. K. (2005). Mother's health seeking behaviour during child illness in a rural western Kenya community. *African Health Sciences*, *5*(4), 322–327. http://dx.doi.org/10.5555/afhs.2005.5.4.322.

Miller, R., & Goodman, C. (2016). Performance of retail pharmacies in low- and middle-income Asian settings: A systematic review. *Health Policy and Planning*. http://dx.doi.org/10.1093/heapol/czw007.

MoHP. (2012). *Nepal demographic and health survey 2011. Kathmandu, Nepal: Ministry of health and population, new era, and ICF international* Calverton, Maryland. http://dhsprogram.com/pubs/pdf/FR257/FR257%5B13April2012%5D.pdf.

Myers, M. J. (1975). Pharmacy practice: Social and behavioral aspects. Edited by A. I. Wertheimer and M. C. Smith. University Park Press, Baltimore, MD 21202, 1974. xv + 556 pp. 16 × 24 cm. Price $15.50. Journal of *Pharmaceutical Sciences, 64*(11), 1898–1898. http://dx.doi.org/10.1002/jps.2600641141.

Ndugwa, R. P., & Zulu, E. M. (2008). Child morbidity and care-seeking in Nairobi slum settlements: The role of environmental and socio-economic factors. *Journal of Child Health Care*, *12*(4), 314–328. http://dx.doi.org/10.1177/1367493508096206.

Ngui, E. M., Khasakhala, L., Ndetei, D., & Roberts, L. W. (2010). Mental disorders, health inequalities and ethics: A global perspective. *International Review of Psychiatry (Abingdon, England)*, *22*(3), 235–244. http://dx.doi.org/10.3109/09540261.2010.485273.

Nicolucci, A., Rossi, M. C., Pellegrini, F., Lucisano, G., Pintaudi, B., Gentile, S., … Vespasiani, G. (2014). Benchmarking network for clinical and humanistic outcomes in diabetes (BENCH-D) study: Protocol, tools, and population. *SpringerPlus*, *3*(1), 83. http://dx.doi.org/10.1186/2193-1801-3-83.

NLM. (2012). *Medical sociology. U.S. National Library of Medicine*. National Institutes of Health. From https://www.nlm.nih.gov/tsd/acquisitions/cdm/subjects59.html.

Nuruddin, R., Hadden, W. C., Petersen, M. R., & Lim, M. K. (2009). Does child gender determine household decision for health care in rural Thatta, Pakistan? *Journal of Public Health*, *31*(3), 389–397. http://dx.doi.org/10.1093/pubmed/fdp038.

O'Daniel, M., Rosenstein, A. H., & Professional Communication and Team Collaboration (2008). In R. G. Hughes (Ed.), *Patient safety and quality: An evidence-based handbook for nurses*. Rockville (MD): Agency for Healthcare Research and Quality (US) (Chapter 33). Available from https://www.ncbi.nlm.nih.gov/books/NBK2637/.

O'Grady, L., & Jadad, A. (2010). Shifting from shared to collaborative decision making: A change in thinking and doing. *Journal of Participatory Medicine*, *2*(e13).

Ogunlesi, T. A., & Olanrewaju, D. M. (2010). Socio-demographic factors and appropriate health care-seeking behavior for childhood illnesses. *Journal of Tropical Pediatrics*, *56*(6), 379–385. http://dx.doi.org/10.1093/tropej/fmq009.

Page, A. L., Hustache, S., Luquero, F. J., Djibo, A., Manzo, M. L., & Grais, R. F. (2011). Health care seeking behavior for diarrhea in children under 5 in rural Niger: Results of a cross-sectional survey. *BMC Public Health*, *11*, 389. http://dx.doi.org/10.1186/1471-2458-11-389.

Peterson, C. D., Rdesinski, R. E., Biagioli, F. E., Chappelle, K. G., & Elliot, D. L. (2011). Medical student perceptions of a behavioural and social science curriculum. *Mental Health in Family Medicine*, *8*(4), 215–226.

Pickren, W. (2007). Psychology and medical education: A historical perspective from the United States. *Indian Journal of Psychiatry*, *49*(3), 179–181. http://dx.doi.org/10.4103/0019-5545.37318.

Pillai, R. K., Williams, S. V., Glick, H. A., Polsky, D., Berlin, J. A., & Lowe, R. A. (2003). Factors affecting decisions to seek treatment for sick children in Kerala, India. *Social Science & Medicine*, *57*(5), 783–790.

Rajan, B., Cherupushpam, S. D., Saleem, T. K., & Jithu, V. P. (2016). Role of cultural beliefs and use of faith healing in management of mental disorders: A descriptive survey. *Kerala Journal of Psychiatry*, *29*(1), 12–18.

Rameshkumar, K. (2009). Ethics in medical curriculum; Ethics by the teachers for students and society. *Indian Journal of Urology : IJU : Journal of the Urological Society of India*, *25*(3), 337–339. http://dx.doi.org/10.4103/0970-1591.56192.

Rasmussen, Z. A., Rahim, M., Streefland, P., & Hardon, A. (1996). *Enhancing appropriate medicine use in the Karakoram Mountains. Community drug use studies*. Amsterdam: Het Spinhuis.

Raut, B., & Khanal, D. P. (2011). Present status of traditional healthcare system in Nepal. *International Journal of Research in Ayurveda and Pharmacy*, *2*(3), 876–882.

Rayes, I. K., Hassali, M. A., & Abduelkarem, A. R. (2015a). Perception of community pharmacists towards the barriers to enhanced pharmacy services in the healthcare system of Dubai: A quantitative approach. *Pharmacy Practice*, *13*(2), 506.

Rayes, I. K., Hassali, M. A., & Abduelkarem, A. R. (2015b). The role of pharmacists in developing countries: The current scenario in the United Arab Emirates. *Saudi Pharmaceutical Journal*, *23*(5), 470–474. http://dx.doi.org/10.1016/j.jsps.2014.02.004.

Refolo, P., Minacori, R., Mele, V., Sacchini, D., & Spagnolo, A. G. (2012). Patient-reported outcomes (PROs): The significance of using humanistic measures in clinical trial and clinical practice. *European Review for Medical and Pharmacological Sciences*, *16*, 1319–1323.

Rickles, N., Wertheimer, A., & Schommer, J. O. N. (2016). *Social and behavioral aspects of pharmacy practice*. Kendall Hunt Publishing Company.

Rickles, N. M., Wertheimer, A. I., & Smith, M. C. (2010). *Social and behavioral aspects of pharmaceutical care*. Jones & Bartlett Publishers.

Rosenstock, I. M. (1974). The health belief model and preventive health behavior. *Health Educ Monogr*, *2*, 354–386.

Rosenstock, I. M. (2005). Why people use health services. *The Milbank Quarterly*, *83*(4). http://dx.doi.org/10.1111/j.1468-0009.2005.00425.x.

Rosenstock, I. M., Strecher, V. J., & Becker, M. H. (1988). Social learning theory and the health belief model. *Health Educ Q*, *15*(2), 175–183.

Rovers, J. (2011). Advancing pharmacy practice through social theory. *Innovations in Pharmacy*, *2*(3) Article 53.

Rubio-Valera, M., Chen, T. F., & O'Reilly, C. L. (2014). New roles for pharmacists in community mental health care: a narrative review. *International Journal of Environmental Research and Public Health*, *11*(10), 10967–10990. http://dx.doi.org/10.3390/ijerph111010967.

Saha, S., & Fernandez, A. (2007). Language barriers in health care. *Journal of General Internal Medicine*, *22*(Suppl. 2), 281–282. http://dx.doi.org/10.1007/s11606-007-0373-3.

Sakisaka, K., Jimba, M., & Hanada, K. (2010). Changing poor mothers' care-seeking behaviors in response to childhood illness: Findings from a cross-sectional study in Granada, Nicaragua. *BMC International Health and Human Rights*, *10*, 10. http://dx.doi.org/10.1186/1472-698x-10-10.

Sawalha, A. F. (2008). A descriptive study of self-medication practices among Palestinian medical and nonmedical university students. *Research in Social & Administrative Pharmacy*, *4*(2), 164–172. http://dx.doi.org/10.1016/j.sapharm.2007.04.004.

Selvaraj, K., Kumar, S. G., & Ramalingam, A. (2014). Prevalence of self-medication practices and its associated factors in Urban Puducherry, India. *Perspectives in Clinical Research*, *5*(1), 32–36. http://dx.doi.org/10.4103/2229-3485.124569.

Shaikh, B. T., & Hatcher, J. (2005). Health seeking behaviour and health service utilization in Pakistan: Challenging the policy makers. *Journal of Public Health*, *27*(1), 49–54. http://dx.doi.org/10.1093/pubmed/fdh207.

Shankar, P. R., Jha, N., Piryani, R. M., Bajracharya, O., Shrestha, R., & Thapa, H. S. (2010). Academic detailing. *Kathmandu University Medical Journal*, *8*(29), 126–134.

Shankar, P. R., Paudel, R., & Giri, B. R. (2006). Healing traditions in Nepal. *Online Journal for the American Association of Integrative Medicine*. http://www.aaimedicine.com/jaaim/sep06/Healing.pdf.

Sharif, S. I., Bugaighis, L. M. T., & Sharif, R. S. (2015). Self-medication practice among pharmacists in UAE. *Pharmacology & Pharmacy*, *6*, 428–435.

Sharma, S., Kc, B., Alrasheedy, A. A., Kaundinnyayana, A., & Khanal, A. (2014). Impact of community pharmacy-based educational intervention on patients with hypertension in Western Nepal. *The Australasian Medical Journal*, *7*(7), 304–313. http://dx.doi.org/10.4066/AMJ.2014.2133.

Shawyer, R. J., Bin Gani, A. S., Punufimana, A. N., & Seuseu, N. K. (1996). The role of clinical vignettes in rapid ethnographic research: A folk taxonomy of diarrhoea in Thailand. *Social Science & Medicine*, *42*(1), 111–123.

Sigdel, R. (2012). Role of medical sociology and anthropology in public health and health system development. *Health Prospect*, *11*, 28–29.

Skliros, E., Merkouris, P., Papazafiropoulou, A., Gikas, A., Matzouranis, G., Papafragos, C., … Sotiropoulos, A. (2010). Self-medication with antibiotics in rural population in Greece: A cross-sectional multicenter study. *BMC Family Practice*, *11*, 58. http://dx.doi.org/10.1186/1471-2296-11-58.

Sreeramareddy, C. T., Shankar, P. R., Binu, V., Mukhopadhyay, C., Ray, B., & Menezes, R. G. (2007). Psychological morbidity, sources of stress and coping strategies among undergraduate medical students of Nepal. *BMC Medical Education*, *7*(1), 26. http://dx.doi.org/10.1186/1472-6920-7-26.

Stretcher, V., & Rosenstock, I. M. (1997). The health belief model. In K. Glanz, F. M. Lewis, & B. K. Rimer (Eds.), *Health behavior and health education: Theory, research and practice*. San Francisco: Jossery-Bass.

Sudharsanam, M., & Rotti, S. (2007). Factors determining health seeking behaviour for sick children in a fishermen community in Pondicherry. *Indian Journal of Community Medicine*, *32*(1), 71–72. http://dx.doi.org/10.4103/0970-0218.53411.

Taffa, N., & Chepngeno, G. (2005). Determinants of health care seeking for childhood illnesses in Nairobi slums. *Tropical Medicine & International Health: TM & IH*, *10*(3), 240–245. http://dx.doi.org/10.1111/j.1365-3156.2004.01381.x.

Tamang, A. L., & Broom, A. (2010). The practice and meanings of spiritual healing in Nepal. *South Asian History and Culture*, *1*(2), 328–340. http://dx.doi.org/10.1080/19472491003593084.

Teerawichitchainan, B., & Phillips, J. F. (2008). Ethnic differentials in parental health seeking for childhood illness in Vietnam. *Social Science & Medicine*, *66*(5), 1118–1130. http://dx.doi.org/10.1016/j.socscimed.2007.10.020.

Thind, A. (2004). Health service use by children in rural Bihar. *Journal of Tropical Pediatrics*, *50*(3), 137–142.

Touchette, D. R., Doloresco, F., Suda, K. J., Perez, A., Turner, S., Jalundhwala, Y., … Hoffman, J. M. (2014). Economic evaluations of clinical pharmacy services: 2006–2010. *Pharmacotherapy*, *34*(8), 771–793.

Tsutsumi, A. (2015). A behavioral science/behavioral medicine core curriculum proposal for Japanese undergraduate medical education. *BioPsychoSocial Medicine*, *9*(1), 24. http://dx.doi.org/10.1186/s13030-015-0051-3.

USAID. (2009). *Health-seeking behavior in rural Uttar Pradesh: Implications for HIV prevention, care, and treatment*. Retrieved from http://www.healthpolicyinitiative.com/Publications/Documents/961_1_UP_Health_Seeking_Behavior_and_HIV_Brief_FINAL_8_31_09_acc.pdf.

Wakefield, M. A., Loken, B., & Hornik, R. C. (2010). Use of mass media campaigns to change health behaviour. *Lancet*, *376*(9748), 1261–1271. http://dx.doi.org/10.1016/S0140-6736(10)60809-4.

Wanzer, M. B., Booth-Butterfield, M., & Gruber, K. (2004). Perceptions of health care providers' communication: Relationships between patient-centered communication and satisfaction. *Health Commun*, *16*(3), 363–383. http://dx.doi.org/10.1207/s15327027hc1603_6.

WHO. (2000). *Guidelines for the regulatory assessment of medicinal products for use in self-medication* (WHO/EDM/QSM/00.1) Geneva: World Health Organization. Retrieved http://apps.who.int/iris/bitstream/10665/66154/1/WHO_EDM_QSM_00.1_eng.pdf.

Wiedenmayer, K., Summers, R. S., Mackie, C. A., Gous, A. G. S., Everard, M., & Tromp, D. (2006). *Developing pharmacy practice-A focus on patient care* Handbook-2006 edition. WHO/PSM/PAR/2006.5.

Worku, S. G., & Mariam, A. (2003). Practice of self-medication in Jimma town. *Ethiopian Journal of Health Development*, *17*(2), 111–116.

Yount, K. M. (2003). Provider bias in the treatment of diarrhea among boys and girls attending public facilities in Minia, Egypt. *Social Science & Medicine*, *56*(4), 753–768.

Yousef, A. M., Al-Bakri, A. G., Bustanji, Y., & Wazaify, M. (2008). Self-medication patterns in Amman, Jordan. *Pharm World Sci*, *30*(1), 24–30. http://dx.doi.org/10.1007/s11096-007-9135-x.

Zorek, J. A., Lambert, B. L., & Popovich, N. G. (2013). The 4-year evolution of a social and behavioral pharmacy course. *American Journal of Pharmaceutical Education*, *77*(6), 119. http://dx.doi.org/10.5688/ajpe776119.

CHAPTER

3

PATIENTS', CONSUMERS', AND HEALTHCARE PROFESSIONALS' PERCEPTIONS, BELIEFS, KNOWLEDGE, ATTITUDES, AND PRACTICES TOWARD THE USE OF MEDICINES

Kazeem B. Yusuff

King Faisal University, Al-Ahsa, Kingdom of Saudi Arabia

CHAPTER OUTLINE

INTRODUCTION

The prime concern of man since the dawn of creation has been consistently focused on the reduction and/or elimination of morbidity and mortality from communicable and noncommunicable diseases. History is replete with detailed accounts of mankind's phenomenal struggle against diseases with only a handful of medicines, which were mostly of plant and animal origin (WHO, 1998). The advent of the age of modern medicines at the end of World War II was the major game changer, as medicines that cure or control diseases in unprecedented ways became widely available (Dukes, 1993). The widespread geographic and economic access to and effective and safe use of modern and highly potent

Social and Administrative Aspects of Pharmacy in Low- and Middle-Income Countries. http://dx.doi.org/10.1016/B978-0-12-811228-1.00003-0

medicines have drastically reduced mortality from infectious and chronic noncommunicable diseases and improved the quality of life of people globally (MSH/WHO/DAP, 1997).

The fundamental principle underlining the use of medicines is the provisos "First, do *no harm.*" This presupposes that the right medication is prescribed, dispensed, and used by the right patient at the right time in the right dose/regimen and dosage form (Jacobson, 2002). This process of ensuring delivery and use of appropriate medications by patients, the medication use process, is complex and involves multiple stages and professionals from different health disciplines. The complex interactions of several factors significantly influence medication use behavior of patients and healthcare professionals (HCPs). Furthermore, the appropriateness, effectiveness, and safety of the medication process are largely determined by several factors attributable to HCPs, patients, and organizational or institutional framework within which the process of medication use exists (Institute of Medicine, 1999). Studies have shown that the medication use process is prone to misadventures such as adverse drug effects (ADEs), adverse drug reactions, and medication errors (ASHP, 1988; Bates et al., 1995). Medication error is the commonest type of medical errors affecting substantial number of people and accounting for staggering healthcare costs (Johnson & Bootman, 1995; Leape, Brennan, & Laird, 1991; Manasse, 1989). This is expected, as drug therapy is the most commonly used medical intervention in patient care.

THE MEDICATION USE PROCESS

This is the process, which determines the necessity and ensures the delivery of appropriate medications to patients for the purpose of achieving definite therapeutic outcomes such as cure of a disease, elimination or reduction of symptoms, arrest or slowing of a disease process and prevention of disease or symptom. It is a complex system involving multiple stages and a network of professionally and functionally interrelated activities during the course of patient care (Institute of Medicine, 1999). The medication use process has been enunciated in literature in various forms, but it essentially consists of six different but functionally interrelated steps (Smith & Knapp, 1992):

- Perception of need for a drug
- Selection of a specific drug product
- Choice of treatment regimen
- Acquisition of the drug product
- Administration/Consumption of the drug product
- Monitoring of the effects of drug therapy

Nadzam (1991) in the process of developing medication use indicators for the accreditation of health institutions in the United States also put medication use processes as consisting of five succeeding steps including prescribing, dispensing, administering, monitoring, systems and management control (Fig. 3.1).

The main objective of an ideal medication use process is to assure a seamless system in which medications are provided efficiently, used effectively and safely, and their movement through the medication use process fully accounted for and adequately documented (Lee & Ray, 2002). In reality, however, the process of medication use is often far from ideal as errors could occur at any of the phases making up the medication use process. Bates et al. (1995) reported that 56% of all preventable ADEs occurred at the prescribing phase followed by administration phase (34%), transcription phase (6%), and dispensing phase (4%). The prescribing phase has been specifically identified as the most critical error-prone focus in the medication use process (Barber, Rawlins, & Dean, 2003; Dean, Schachter, Vincent, & Barber, 2002).

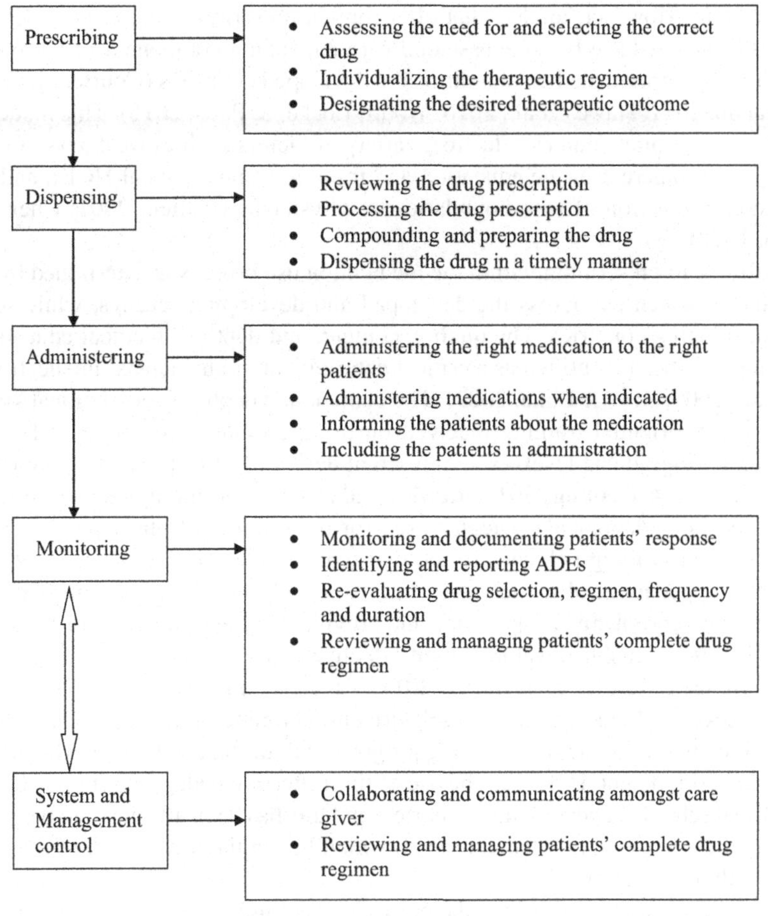

FIGURE 3.1

The medication use process. *ADE*, adverse drug effects.

Adapted from Nadzam Deborah, M. (1991). Development of medication-use indicators by the Joint Commission on Accreditation of Healthcare Organisation. American Journal of Health-System Pharmacy, 48, *1925–1930.*

PHYSICIAN IMPACT ON MEDICATION USE BEHAVIOR

Prescribing is a process, which lies deeply at the very heart of medication use, and this starts with the correct and evidence-based assessment of patient medical condition, determination of an appropriate patient-specific therapeutic goals, and appropriate choice of medicines that will best achieve the set goals. The importance of appropriate prescribing as a major determinant of the effectiveness and safety of the medication use process underscores why it is the most error-prone focus, and where specific interventions can be made to increase the odds of optimal therapeutic outcomes and minimize the risk of potential or actual harms to patients during medication use (Al-Jeraisy, Alanazi, & Abolfotouh, 2011; Bates et al., 1995; Dean, Barber, & Schachter, 2000; Ernawati, Lee, & Hughes, 2014; Leape et al., 1995; Lewis et al., 2009). The responsibility for appropriate prescribing is vested majorly in physicians. However, models that offer limited prescribing role to other HCPs under the supervision of physicians have become essential care-enhancing component of the medication use process especially for chronic medical conditions in developed countries (Courtenay, Carey, Stenner, Lawton, & Petersm, 2011; Hawes et al., 2016; Woolf, Locke, & Potts, 2016). This model is currently a long way off in developing countries due to a variety of factors such as weakness of the healthcare system, inadequacies inherent in the education and training of nonmedical HCPs, and needless in-fighting and fierce protection of task boundaries by physicians (Britten, 2001; Chen et al., 2004; Eaton & Webb, 1979).

Physician attitude to prescribing within the medication use process is determined by a number of key factors some of which cut across the developed and developing settings, while some are very mainly in the developing countries. The quality, content, and depth of medical education and post-graduate training have been identified as a critical determinant of physicians' medication use behavior (Dornan et al., 2009; Ross & Loke, 2009). The content and depth of foundational knowledge and the quality of the experiential training received during the clinical component of training at the undergraduate and postgraduate levels is an important determinant of prescribing behavior (Ajjawi, Thistlethwaite, Aslani, & Cooling, 2010; Lewis et al., 2013). Furthermore, the effectiveness and appropriateness of the pedagogical strategies used for the training of physicians are also key contributory factors to prescribing behavior in the real world of practice (Graber, 2009; Smith et al., 2006). However, the pedagogical models used in most developing countries for medical education and training are often reproductive, superficial, and provide little learning opportunities that are deep, constructive and does not enable development of effective metacognitive skills among medical graduates (Murray, Wenger, Downe, & Terrazas, 2011; Vanderschmidt et al., 1979). Yet, the dynamic nature of the field of medicine demands a self-driven continuous reflective approach to learning, which enables objective assessment of learning progress and the gaps which must be filled within the zone of proximal development. However, the use of this reflective pedagogic approach is few and far between in medical schools in developing countries, and this has been attributed to the overwhelming influence of rote memorization and factual recall, which lies in the lower level of the cognition and is inconsistent with deep learning.

The impact of the hierarchical nature of the prescribing culture on physicians' prescribing behavior especially at the specialist care level are well documented in both developed and developing settings (Lewis et al., 2013; Lewis & Tully, 2009). Physicians at the various levels of the organizational structure within a specialist medical unit are expected to limit their prescribing habit within the limit set by the most senior physician who is usually the consultant in charge of each unit. Such rigid prescribing culture often modulates the prescribing behavior of junior physicians who tend to follow the "prescribing tone" set by the consultant physicians (Duncan et al., 2012; Ross et al., 2013). Deviation of prescribing behavior from this limit is often avoided not to offend senior physicians or damage the working relationship between residents and their consultant physician. Hence, junior physicians limit their prescribing practice within the set boundary (Duncan et al., 2012). The clinical consequences of this rigid prescribing framework on outcomes of medication use become dependent on the appropriateness of the "prescribing tone" set by consultants-in-charge of the medical units. Furthermore, studies have shown that this is a major cause of rule-based mistakes associated with medication error attributable to prescribing by junior physicians (Lewis et al., 2013; Pearson, Rolfe, & Smith, 2002).

Furthermore, personal influence and opinion leadership is also a key factor that influences physicians' attitude to medication use especially in developing setting. This has been attributed to the rigid nature of the prescribing culture within the healthcare system, which places specialist physicians at the top of the prescribing pyramid. Hence, specialist physicians are often regarded as opinion leaders within a define area and may exert significant influence on prescribing behavior of other physicians through the use of personal influence (McGettigan, Golden, Fryer, Chan, & Feely, 2001; Thistlethwaite, Ajjawi, & Aslani, 2010).

The quality, currency, and depth of knowledge of physicians are important determinants of prescribing behavior. Several studies have reported these factors as key factors underlining the frequency of exposure to and severity of medication errors (Ajjawi et al., 2010; Lewis et al., 2013). This is a global phenomenon with a potentially telling impact on outcome of medication use in developing countries. Deficiency in the depth of knowledge of clinical pharmacology has been specifically been identified by several studies, and intervention studies focused on filling this knowledge gap have shown significant improvement in prescribing behavior (Al-Dhawailie, 2011; Graber, 2009; Morey et al., 2002). Furthermore, poor access to facilities that enable regular update of physician knowledge particularly at the primary care level is an important determinant of inappropriate prescribing behavior and medication use (Buchan, Lourey, D'Este, & Sanson-Fisher, 2009). However, institutional interventions focused on improving access to continuous professional development have been made mandatory for registration and annual licensure to practice by the relevant bodies saddled with responsibility of regulating medical education, training, and practice in developing countries. Furthermore, the lack of awareness and/or nonadherence to updated clinical guidelines is an important factor underling medication use behavior by physicians in developing countries. Poor funding of the healthcare system, lack of access to relevant digital medical, medication related resources that enhance evidence-based practice, and the rigid hierarchical nature of prescribing culture are factors that contribute to poor adherence to evidence-based clinical guidelines during medication use in developing countries.

Physicians' attitude to medication use is strongly influenced by system and job-related factors. These include inadequate remuneration, lack of modern clinical facilities, brain drain, heavy work load, and lack of/or nonadherence to essential medicine list or hospital formulary (Ajayi, Olumide, & Oyediran, 2005; Chen et al., 2004; Ndom & Makanjuola, 2004; Talabi, 2003). Several studies have reported the negative impact of these factors on prescribing behavior and frequency of patient exposure to medications errors (Alubo, 1985; Fabrican & Hirschorn, 1987; Salmasi, Khan, Hong, Ming, & Wui Wong, 2016). Furthermore, the weak drug regulatory capacities and the pervasive presence of counterfeiting and adulteration with the medicine distribution network has also impacted significantly on prescribing pattern and medication use in most developing countries (Erhun, Babalola, & Erhun, 2001; Maponga & Odari, 2003, pp. 1–54). Heavy reliance on branded medicine during prescribing due to the perceived quality of the originator products is an important contributory factor. This is due to lack of faith in the quality of generic medicines, psychological association of expensive originator brands with high quality, perceived low quality of relatively cheaper generic medicines and high costs of healthcare (Almuzaini, Choonara, & Sammons, 2013; Ravinetto et al., 2016). The pervasiveness of branded prescribing has contributed to the poor economic access to essential medicines for millions of people, majority of who live below the poverty line in most developing countries.

Finally, the promotional activities of pharmaceutical companies such as engaging in profoundly unethical marketing practices to influence prescribing behavior is also an important contributory factor. In fact, the impact is appeared more in developing countries because of lack of structural mechanisms that are designed to mitigate the effect of this phenomenon on physician prescribing behavior (Erhun & Erhun, 2003; Yusuff & Yusuf, 2009). Such mitigating institutional mechanisms include robust entrenchment of evidence-based practice in the medication use process and a strong system for monitoring and evaluating prescribing practices. This ensures prompt detection and resolution of aberrant prescribing practices, which are inconsistent with the highest level of clinical evidence (Ostini et al., 2009). Sadly, these care-enhancing mechanisms are few and far between in the medication use process in most developing countries.

PHARMACISTS' AND OTHER HEALTHCARE PROFESSIONALS' IMPACT ON MEDICATION USE

The dispensing process is a critical determinant of the effectiveness, safety, and convenience of medication use. The pharmacists play critical care-defining roles in ensuring that medication choice is effective and safe, meet patient-specific therapeutic needs, and will best achieve the set therapeutic goals (Bond & Raehl, 2007; Castelino, Bajorek, & Chen, 2009; Hanlon et al., 1996). The contemporary pharmacists are uniquely qualified, skillful, and competent at delivering effectively on the expanded clinical and direct patient care roles within the medication use process due to the radical changes in the curricular and training paradigm used especially in the developed settings (Jungnickel, Kelley, Hammer, Haines, & Marlowe, 2009). This wave of paradigm change is also slowly wafting through pharmacy education, training, and practice in developing countries and is appeared to become a key determinant of knowledge, attitude, and practice concerning pharmacists' roles within the medication use process. However, the current inadequacies of the training and practice of pharmacy in most developing countries appeared to be a key limiting factor. This has been attributed to the reproductive approach to pedagogy and learning, and lack of strong focus on higher level cognitive processes that the 21st century pharmacists need to function effectively and efficiently in guiding medication use at the individual, institutional, and societal levels (Basak, van Mil, & Sathyanarayana, 2009; Ogaji & Ojabo, 2014; Udeogaranya, Ukwe, & Ekwunife, 2009). This surface approach to learning is inherently inconsistent with the skill set required by contemporary pharmacy graduates. Furthermore, the practice setting in most developing countries are beset with entrenched poorly guided self-medication practices, weakly regulated medicine distribution system, and unfettered access to prescription-only and over-the-counter medicines. The synergy of these aberrant systemic factors continues to make it difficult for pharmacists in developing countries to effectively contribute to improving safe medication use. Hence, the quality, standard, and effectiveness of services provided by pharmacists in developing countries still fall far short (Auta, Strickland-Hodge, & Maz, 2016a; Wibowo, Parsons, Sunderland, & Hughes, 2015).

Job-related factors have been identified as an important determinant of pharmacists' behavior within the medication use process. These include inadequate remuneration, poor work environment, and role overload. These factors have telling impact on job satisfaction, good job experience, and organizational loyalty for pharmacists especially in developing and resource-limited setting (Auta et al., 2016a; Oparah & Eferakeya, 2005). In addition, role conflict, which saddles pharmacists with peripheral tasks that are inconsistent with expanded clinical and direct patient care responsibilities of the contemporary pharmacists is a key factor underlining pharmacists' attitude and practice within the medication use process. Varieties of negative consequences such as poor service delivery, and increased risk of patients' exposure to medication use errors have been reported by several studies. Furthermore, the stifling professional conflict between pharmacists and other HCPs, especially physicians over task boundaries and fierce resistance to pharmacists into the clinical realm appeared to an important factor underlining pharmacists' limited role in the medication use process in developing countries (Auta, Strickland-Hodge, & Maz, 2016b; Eaton & Webb, 1979; Ritchey & Raney, 1981).

The role of nurses within the medication use process is limited to medication administration especially in developing countries. This is notwithstanding the expanded clinical roles and the relevant changes in the training and practice paradigm for nurses in the developed world. However, nurses and other lower level categories of community healthcare workers appear to exert a significant influence on medication use behavior especially at the primary care level in rural communities in most developing countries (Fagbule & Kalu, 1995; Ovbiagele, 2015). This is because the primary care level is closest to the majority of the populace in developing countries, and this is often the first point of contact with formal and orthodox healthcare services. However, poor funding and inequity in the distribution of available healthcare resources appeared to be a key contributory factor to poor geographic access to essential medicines and unguided self-medication practices.

PATIENTS AND CONSUMERS ATTITUDE TO MEDICATION USE

Medication use is an action that involves a change in behavior, and appropriate use of medications by patients involves a desired change in behavior which is consistent with the prescription issued by physicians and/or recommendations by pharmacists. Patient medication use behavior is influenced by several factors, some of which are more prominent in developing countries. Another important determinants of patients' medication use behavior are culture and religious belief, which are often deeply ingrained in personality and significantly influence behavior (Sachs & Tomson, 1992; Van der Geest & Hardon, 2006). Several studies have reported pervasive self-medication with herbal medicines alone or concurrently with orthodox medicines due to entrenched belief in the efficacy and safety of local herbs (Ajayi & Falade, 2006; Yusuff & Omarusehe, 2011). Furthermore, traditional herbal practitioners are often regularly consulted especially in rural areas where the majority of the populace in developing countries resides. These traditional practitioners are perceived as a trusted source of healthcare and thus exert significant influence on medication use behavior sometimes with untoward clinical consequences (Aggarwal & Aides, 2001; Peltzer, Mngqundaniso, & Petros, 2006). However, some public health initiatives have been deployed to mitigate the negative impact of the activities of traditional health practitioners on medication use through capacity building with training interventions (Stokes et al., 2016).

Health literacy, self-efficacy, and the effectiveness of self-management practices have also been reported as key factors that influence patients' medication use behavior in both developed and developing countries (Murphy, Chuma, Mathews, Steyn, & Levitt, 2015; Yusuff, Obe, & Joseph, 2008). High health literacy and self-efficacy significantly increase the odd of effective self-management practices and the achievement of positive therapeutic outcomes especially for patients with chronic medical conditions requiring life-long medication use. Furthermore, a major determinant of health literacy and self-efficacy is the quality and depth of interactions between HCPs and patients, particularly during the prescribing and dispensing phases of the medication use process (Aggarwal et al., 2016). The quality and depth of patient–HCP interactions is enhanced in a democratized practice setting where patients are actively involved in decision-making about the therapeutic goals and choice of appropriate therapeutic management strategies that will best meet patient-specific therapeutic needs. Furthermore, the depth of counseling information provided about the nature and severity of patients' medical conditions, the benefits inherent in good adherence to the appropriately prescribed medicines, and the negative clinical consequences associated with nonadherence or delayed treatment are all significant determinants of patients' medication use behavior and optimal therapeutic outcomes. However, the HCPs–patients interactions in most developing countries often occur in a dictatorial and paternalistic setting, where patients rarely have the opportunities of meaningfully interacting and getting active in clinical decision making about therapeutic management strategies (Aggarwal et al., 2016; Ajayi et al., 2005). This is often linked with aberrant medication use behavior such as intentional nonadherence and unguided self-medication practices. The factors that have been reported as promoting this phenomenon include unfriendly attitude of HCPs especially physicians, poor health infrastructure, heavy patient load, long waiting time, lack of two-way communication during consultation, poor patients' satisfaction with the quality of healthcare service (Ajayi et al., 2005; Ndom & Makanjuola, 2004). Furthermore, patient's deep understanding of the counseling and educational information provided by HCPs and the cognitive association of the therapeutic benefits inherent in using the prescribed medicines and the consequent achievement of specific therapeutic goals are important determinants of patient medication use behavior especially during the management of chronic medical conditions in an ambulatory setting (Lopes Ibanez-Gonzalez, Mendenhall, & Norris, 2014; Mendenhall & Norris, 2015). However, interventions focused on increasing the awareness of HCPs to the strategic importance of this phenomenon in ambulatory medication use is few and far between in developing countries.

Direct-to-consumer advertising (DTCA) of over-the-counter medicines by pharmaceutical manufacturers is a key factor influencing patients' attitude to medication use in developing countries (Consumers International, 2007; Salmasi, Ming, & Khan, 2016). The potential impact of DTCA in fueling inappropriate self-medication in developing countries is particularly telling because of the weak regulatory framework for monitoring the contents of DTCA. Hence, it is difficult to ensure that the content of the direct-to-consumer advertisement is accurate, objective, and balance the information offered to consumers on the benefits and risks of the advertised medicines (Mohiuddin, Rashid, Shuvro, Nahar, Ahmed, 2015; Yusuff & Yusuf, 2009). In addition, the lack of a robust institutional framework focused on empowering patients with objective, accurate, and up-to-date drug information services to guide medication use and mitigate the potential negative impact of biased DTCA is also a strong contributory factor in developing countries.

Finally, the poor financial status and lack of geographic and economic access to essential medicines are important determinants of medication use behavior in developing countries. This is particularly due to the fact that majority of the populace live below the poverty line and often have to make out-of-pocket payments for healthcare service in general and medicines in particular (Buabeng, Matowe, & Plange-Rhule, 2004; Kimani-Muragea, Manderson, Norrise, & Kahn, 2013; Yusuff & Alabi, 2007).

ACHIEVEMENTS

The achievement of an optimal medication use behavior, which is effective, safe, and assures that patient-specific therapeutic needs are met in an efficient manner is still a long way off in most developing countries, and several of the underlining factors have been discussed extensively in the previous sections. However, significant progress has been made in strengthening the various components of the institutional framework that governs medication use at the individual, institutional, and societal levels. This has resulted in the following achievements:

- The synergy achieved with the bilateral and multilateral cooperation between the governments at various levels in developing countries and nongovernmental organizations, donor agencies, and private partners involved in medicine supply management, especially for public health programs that are focused on diseases of priority and public health importance has significantly improved geographic and economic access to essential and life-saving medicines, and strengthen the medication use process to minimize risks and maximize therapeutic benefits. The potential positive public health impact of this public–private interventional synergy in reducing disease burden and improving the prospects of optimal patient outcomes is significantly visible in most developing countries. This concerted effort may also contribute on the long term to reducing aberrant medication use behavior such as unguided self-medication practices, especially among the people with poor financial status who readily turns to irrational health-seeking behavior that are often guided by untrained or poorly trained individuals involved in illicit supply and distribution of medicines in most developing countries.
- Improvement of drug regulatory capacity:
  Effective and robust framework for medicine registration and regulation is critical for guaranteeing safe and effective use of medications at the individual, institutional, and societal levels. This is one of the key national goals of the national medicines policy in developing countries. The ineffectual state of national medicine regulatory authorities and medicine distribution system in most developing countries is well documented. However, significant progress has been made through financial, technical, and infrastructural supports from bilateral and multilateral partner agencies to strengthen regulatory capacity for medicines registration, marketing and sales, and quality assurance in developing countries. This concerted effort made toward safeguarding public health has contributed to improving the effectiveness and safety of the framework that guides medication use by both the patients and HCPs in developing countries. Furthermore, the synergy achieved by donor partners and the relevant organ in the ministries of health in developing countries has strengthen the technical and infrastructural capacities of national medicine regulatory authorities in areas such as medicine registration, marketing authorization, laboratory test for quality, medicine advertising, clinical trial and evaluation, and pharmacovigilance. This cooperation has significantly contributed to reducing the circulation of counterfeit, adulterated, or substandard medicines and their associated negative public health consequences in developing countries. Furthermore, several developing countries have tackled head-on the seemingly intractable problem of chaotic medicine distribution network and unfettered marketing of medicine by untrained hands in places not approved for such. Interventions deployed to energize the various regulatory bodies, saddled with the responsibility of ensuring an orderly network for distribution and sales of medicines in places approved for such, and people legally licensed to handle medicines are positively impacting on the medication use process and behaviors at the individual and societal levels. In addition, intervention programs focused on public enlightenment using both the news and electronic media about the dangers of inappropriate self-medication practices, patronage of untrained individuals for information to guide medicine use, and use of fake and adulterated medicines have become integral part of the overarching national policy for improving medication

use behavior in developing countries. Furthermore, several countries have made concerted effort, sometimes with donor support, to set up pharmacovigilance and poison centers with the aim of ensuring adequate monitoring, detection, assessment, and reporting of adverse drug reactions, which are rare and undetected during premarketing. Most of these centers are affiliated with the WHO center for global monitoring of adverse or beneficial effects of medicines that were previously undetected at the premarketing phase. The potential impact of this pharmacovigilance system, particularly in developing countries, cannot be overstressed.

- The thriving culture of pharmacoepidemiologic research focused on identifying the various gaps in the medication use process at the institutional and societal levels, and determinants of inappropriate medication use behavior by patients and HCPs is becoming deeply entrenched in developing countries. Findings generated from these research efforts have significantly enriched the global body of knowledge in several research areas related to medication use. In addition, these research findings have also served as a compass for governments and partner donor agencies to optimally channel their interventions focused on improving the effectiveness and safety of medication use at the individual, institutional, and societal levels. Furthermore, the increasing fascination with and the bold attempts to incorporate the concept of evidence-based medicines especially in guiding the prescribing process at the institutional level is a significant shift toward improving the effectiveness and safety of medication use in developing countries.
- Finally, curricular changes focused on deepening the knowledge and skills, and sharpening the competencies of HCPs, especially doctors and pharmacists in critical areas such as clinical pharmacology, pharmacoepidemiology, therapeutics, clinical pharmacy, and evidence-based medicines, have received significant attention from medical and pharmacy teachers in developing countries. Strong emphasis is being placed on ensuring that physicians in developing countries imbibe the culture of safe and effective prescribing, rational use of medicines both within the walls of the universities and as critical component of experiential/residency training, continuing professional education, and life-long self-directed learning. Furthermore, significant attention has focused on improving the quality of pedagogical strategies and facilities used for the training of HCPs. This is done with a view to ensure that HCPs are exposed to learning opportunities which enable them master concepts, construct their own learning, and engage in self-directed metacognitive practices that will adequately prepare them for effective delivery of direct patient care services and fulfilling professional career in the world of practice. In addition, the wholesale adoption of the doctor of pharmacy (PharmD) paradigm for the training of pharmacists and the increasing engagement of clinical pharmacists with overseas postgraduate residency training in specialized clinical areas in several developing countries have significantly contributed to the bourgeoning radical change in the training and practice of pharmacy. This is no doubt that a pleasant development can significantly improve the effectiveness and safety of medication use at both individual and societal levels in developing countries.

CHALLENGES

It is incontrovertible that varieties of interventions focused on improving medication use behavior and the framework for delivering medication use have been deployed in several developing countries, and these have resulted in modest gains in this area. However, more significant efforts need to be done as the existing challenges, most of which were extensively discussed in the previous section of this chapter, continue to be an existential threat to ensuring effective and safe use of medications by patients/consumers and HCPS. The followings are the challenges that remain daunting in developing countries:

- Inappropriate health-seeking behavior and unguided self-medication practices continue to underlie irrational medication use habit and potential risks of medication use–related harms to patients/consumers in developing countries. Patients' first response to ill-health often involves consultation of informal and often untrained sources about self-medication to resolve the perceived medical problems, and this habit is associated with potentially harmful clinical consequences. In addition, the lack of an institutionalized system that ensure an excellent audit trail and accurate/complete documentation of patients' use of medications prescribed by physicians and those used during self-medication complicate outcomes of medication use. Hence, prescribing decisions are often made without an access to a detailed and accurate medication history at both the public and private health facilities with the well-documented attendant high risks of patients' exposure to medication errors and other medication use–related harms.
- Despite the significant investment made in expanding the drug regulatory capacity and sanitizing the system for marketing, distribution, and sales of medicines, these factors continue to present a major challenge in several developing countries. The negative clinical consequences of exposure to adulterated and counterfeit medicines are well documented. The attendant increase in morbidity and mortality, and avoidable increase in healthcare cost particularly from priority diseases of public health importance such as malaria, HIV/AIDS, vaccine-preventable diseases, cardiovascular and metabolic disorders are potentially catastrophic. Furthermore, the patients' trust in the effectiveness and safety of the medication use process is threatened due to failure to achieve the therapeutic goals and resolution of medical problems because of the use of counterfeit and adulterated medicines. In addition, their risk of exposure to permanent injury and/or death due to the use of counterfeit medicines is also real. This may yet be a key factor underlining aberrant health-seeking behavior such as unguided self-medication practices. Regular consultation of traditional herbal practitioners and self-medication with herbal medicines that are often regarded as "safe" due to ethos rooted deeply in culture and beliefs are also key features of the attitude and practice to medication use by patients in several developing countries.
- Poor geographic and economic access to essential medicines is an important determinant of medication use behavior in several developing countries. This is linked to poor funding, endemic corruption, and poor management of the healthcare system. The negative impact on medication use habit is especially telling in the rural areas where the majority of the populace who are often poor and live below the poverty line lives. Hence, recourse to unguided self-medication practices, consultation of informal and often untrained sources, and self-medication with herbal medicines or cheap and affordable counterfeit orthodox medicines becomes the only alternative to patients living in these underserved areas.
- Inadequate patients' satisfaction with service delivery by HCPs especially at public health facilities is another major determinant of medication use and health-seeking behavior in developing countries. The poor patients' perception of the quality service delivery threatens patients'

trust in the effectiveness and safety of the medication use process, encourages infrequent clinic attendance especially for chronic medical conditions, and resorts to unguided self-medication practices and/or consultation of unorthodox and untrained sources for health- or medication use–related matters. Several factors that underlie poor patients' satisfaction include poor job-related attitude of HCPs, which is often linked to high patient load, inadequate staffing and infrastructural facilities, poor remuneration, job stress, and job dissatisfaction. In addition, lack of privacy during clinical consultation, long waiting time, paternalistic and domineering attitude especially by HCPs, and inadequate health literacy and commitment to self-management practices by patients have all contributed to poor quality of patients' interactions with HCPs and patients' perception of the quality of healthcare services offered to them at public health facilities in several developing countries. These factors also negatively affect the quality and depth of counseling information and education offered to patients, and patients' understanding of the key counseling information that should enhance appropriate medication use and optimal therapeutic outcomes.

RECOMMENDATIONS: THE WAY FORWARD

- Robust strengthening of the institutional framework for the delivery of medication use based on an effective strategic planning involving all the major stakeholders and focused on achieving a clear vision of ensuring the establishment of a robust medication use system that is safe, is effective, meets patient-specific therapeutic needs, protects patients from harm, and contributes significantly to reducing the morbidity and mortality due to communicable and chronic non-communicable diseases in developing countries. This strategic planning will be predicated on an open and deep discussion of the strengths, weaknesses, opportunities, and threats associated with the current system used for the delivery of medication at the national, local, individual, and institutional levels. This evidence-based systematic approach will ensure a dispassionate analysis of the current state of the medication use process and its impact on medication use behavior; correct assessment of what is needed to close the current existing gaps; determination of activities, responsibilities, and resources needed to put in place an effective and transparent medication use system, which maximizes the therapeutic benefits and minimize the potential risks.
- The critical role of an effective drug regulatory system in promoting rational, effective, and safe use of medicines at the individual, institutional, and societal levels is well documented. Notwithstanding the significant improvement that have been achieved in strengthening the capacities of drug regulatory authorities in developing countries to minimize varieties of unwholesome practices associated with registration, marketing authorization, quality assurance, distribution and sales of medicines, more need to be done in these areas to ensure that the current gains are not jeopardized.
- Massive investments in pharmacoepidemiologic and other clinical research studies to identify aberrant medication use practices, analyze and identify the key determinants, and recommend appropriate and evidence-based interventions to fill the identified gaps, and minimize or mitigate any potential negative clinical consequences will be critical to improving the effectiveness and safety of medication use in developing countries. In addition, governments need to strengthen the curriculum and pedagogical strategies used for the training of HCPs with a

view to ensuring that medical and pharmacy graduates are well rooted in the basic principles of evidence-based medicine in clinical decision making. Furthermore, learning in medical and pharmacy schools must take place in a democratized, participatory, and nonthreatening setting, which encourages deep and active learning; discourages surface, reproductive, and rote learning; and helps imbibe the culture of self-directed metacognitive practices in monitoring progress with learning.

- Effective community engagement and participatory approach in planning, designing, conducting, and monitoring the implementation of public enlightenment campaigns. This initiative must be a key component of the national strategy focused on improving the knowledge, attitude, and practice of the general populace with regard to medication use and must be focused on assessment of medication use practices, analysis and identification of determinants of aberrant medication use behavior, the design and implementation of appropriate interventions, and monitoring and evaluation of the impact on medication use behavior at the individual and societal levels.

CONCLUSION

Despite the incremental gains associated with the varieties of interventions deployed to strengthen the institutional framework used for the delivery of medication use in developing countries, the knowledge, attitude, and practices of patients and HCPs with regard to medication use remain far from ideal and is incomparable with the standards that have been achieved in the developed parts of the world. The framework within which the medication use process is foregrounded in developing countries remains weakened by a variety of systemic factors that compromise the effectiveness and safety of the medication use by the patients and HCPs; negatively influences medication use behavior at the individual, institutional, and societal levels; and exposes patients to potentially harmful clinical consequences.

LESSONS LEARNED

- Significant collaborative interventional strategies have been deployed by governments and bilateral/multilateral donor agencies in developing countries to improve geographic and economic access to essential medicines and strengthen the infrastructural and technical capacities of the medications process to ensure effective and safe medication use behavior by patients and HCPs.
- The plurality of bilateral and multilateral collaborative interventions deployed to strengthen the institutional framework used for the delivery of medication at individual and societal levels have resulted in relatively modest gains in knowledge, attitude, and practices related to medication use by patients and HCPs in developing countries.
- Medication use behavior among patients and HCPs in developing countries is significantly influenced by several systemic factors that increase the risk of exposure to potentially harmful clinical consequences; undermine the effectiveness and safety of the medication use process; and are strong determinants of patients' knowledge, attitude, and practices associated with medication use.

REFERENCES

Aggarwal, A., & Aides, P. A. (2001). Interactions of herbal remedies with prescription cardiovascular medications. *Coronary Artery Disease*, *12*, 581–584.

Aggarwal, N. K., Pieh, M. C., Dixon, L., Guarnaccia, P., Alegría, M., & Lewis-Fernández, R. (2016). Clinician descriptions of communication strategies to improve treatment engagement by racial/ethnic minorities in mental health services: A systematic review. *Patient Education and Counseling*, *99*(2), 198–209.

Ajayi, I. O., & Falade, C. O. (2006). Pre-hospital treatment of febrile illness in children attending the general outpatient clinic, University College Hospital, Ibadan, Nigeria. *African Journal of Medicine and Medical Science*, *35*, 85–91.

Ajayi, I. O., Olumide, E. A., & Oyediran, O. (2005). Patient satisfaction with the services provided at a general outpatient clinic, Ibadan, Oyo state, Nigeria. *African Journal of Medicine and Medical Science*, *34*, 133–140.

Ajjawi, R., Thistlethwaite, J. E., Aslani, P., & Cooling, N. B. (2010). What are the perceived learning needs of Australian general practice registrars for quality prescribing? *BMC Medical Education*, *10*, 92.

Al-Dhawailie, A. (2011). In-patient prescribing errors and pharmacist intervention at a teaching hospital in Saudi Arabia. *Saudi Pharmaceutical Journal*, *19*, 193–196.

Al-Jeraisy, M., Alanazi, M., & Abolfotouh, M. (2011). Medication prescribing errors in a pediatric inpatient tertiary care setting in Saudi Arabia. *BMC Research Notes*, *4*, 294.

Almuzaini, T., Choonara, I., & Sammons, H. (2013). Substandard and counterfeit medicines: A systematic review of the literature. *BMJ Open*, *3*(8), e002923.

Alubo, S. A. (1985). Drugging the people: Pills, profits and underdevelopment in Nigeria. *Studies in Third World Societies*, *24*, 89–113.

American Society of Health-System Pharmacists (ASHP) Reports. (1998). Suggested definitions and relationships among medication misadventures, medication errors, adverse drug events and adverse drug reactions. *American Journal of Health-System Pharmacy*, *55*, 165–166.

Auta, A., Strickland-Hodge, B., & Maz, J. (2016a). Challenges to clinical pharmacy practice in Nigerian hospitals: A qualitative exploration of stakeholders' views. *Journal of Evaluation in Clinical Practice*, *22*, 699–706.

Auta, A., Strickland-Hodge, B., & Maz, J. (2016b). Stakeholders' views on granting prescribing authority to pharmacists in Nigeria: A qualitative study. *International Journal of Clinical Pharmacy*, *38*, 960–967.

Barber, N., Rawlins, M. D., & Dean, F. B. (2003). Reducing prescribing error; competence; control and culture. *Quality and Safety in Health Care*, *12*, 29.

Basak, S. C., van Mil, J. W., & Sathyanarayana, D. (2009). The changing roles of pharmacists in community pharmacies: Perception of reality in India. *Pharmacy World & Science*, *31*(6), 612–618.

Bates, D. W., Cullen, D. J., Laird, N., Petersen, L. A., Small, S. D., Servi, D., … Hallisey, R. (1995). Incidence of adverse drug events and potential adverse drug events in hospitalized adults: Implications for prevention. *Journal of American Medical Association*, *274*, 29–34.

Bond, C., & Raehl, C. L. (2007). Clinical pharmacy services, pharmacy staffing, and hospital mortality rates. *Pharmacotherapy*, *27*(4), 481–493.

Britten, N. (2001). Prescribing and the defence of clinical autonomy. *Sociology of Health & Illness*, *23*(4), 478–496.

Buabeng, O. K., Matowe, L., & Plange-Rhule, J. (2004). Unaffordable drug prices: The major cause of noncompliance with hypertension medication in Ghana. *Journal of Pharmacy & Pharmaceutical Sciences*, *7*(3), 350–352.

Buchan, H., Lourey, E., D'Este, C., & Sanson-Fisher, R. (2009). Effectiveness of strategies to encourage general practitioners to accept an offer of free access to online evidence-based information: A randomised controlled trial. *Implementation Science*, *4*, 68.

Castelino, R. L., Bajorek, B. V., & Chen, T. F. (2009). Targeting suboptimal prescribing in the elderly: A review of the impact of pharmacy services. *Annals of Pharmacotherapy*, *43*(6), 1096–1106.

Chen, L., Evans, T., Anand, S., Boufford, J. I., Brown, H., Chowdhury, M., … Wibulpolprasert, S. (2004). Human resources for health: Overcoming the crisis. *Lancet, 364*, 1984–1990.

Consumers International. (2007). *Drugs, doctors and dinners, how drug companies influence health in the developing world* (London, UK).

Courtenay, M., Carey, N., Stenner, K., Lawton, S., & Petersm, J. (2011). Patients' views of nurse prescribing: Effects on care, concordance and medicine taking. *British Journal of Dermatology, 164*(2), 396–401.

Dean, B., Barber, N., & Schachter, M. (2000). What is a prescribing error? *Quality and Safety in Health Care, 9*, 232–237.

Dean, B., Schachter, M., Vincent, C., & Barber, N. (2002). Prescribing errors in hospital in-patients: Their incidence and clinical significance. *Quality and Safety in Health Care, 11*, 340–344.

Dornan, T., Ashcroft, D. M., Heathfield, H., Lewis, P. J., Miles, J., Taylor, D., … Wass, V. (2009). *An in-depth investigation into causes of prescribing errors by foundation trainees in relation to their medical education – EQUIP study*. FINAL report. United Kingdom: General Medical Council.

Dukes, M. N. G. (1993). Drug utilization studies: Methods and uses. *WHO Regional Publications, European series no. 45* Copenhagen: World Health Organization.

Duncan, E. M., Francis, J. J., Johnston, M., Davey, P., Maxwell, S., McKay, G. A., … Bond, C. (2012). Learning curves, taking instructions, and patient safety: using a theoretical domains framework in an interview study to investigate prescribing errors among trainee doctors. *Implementation Science, 7*, 86.

Eaton, G., & Webb, B. (1979). Boundary encroachment: Pharmacists in the clinical setting. *Sociology of Health and Illness, 1*(1), 69–89.

Erhun, W. O., Babalola, O. O., & Erhun, M. O. (2001). Drug regulation and control in Nigeria: The challenge of counterfeit drugs. *Journal of Health & Population in Developing Countries, 4*(2), 23–34.

Erhun, W. O., & Erhun, M. O. (2003). The Qualitative impact of broadcast media advertisement on the perception of medicines in Nigeria. *Journal of Consumer Behavior, 3*(1), 8–19.

Ernawati, D. K., Lee, Y. P., & Hughes, J. D. (2014). Nature and frequency of medication errors in a geriatric ward: An Indonesian experience. *Therapeutics and Clinical Risk Management, 10*, 413–421.

Fabrican, S. J., & Hirschorn, N. (1987). Deranged distribution, perverse prescription, unprotected use: The irrationality of pharmaceuticals in the developing world. *Health Policy and Planning*, 2, 204–213.

Fagbule, D., & Kalu, A. (1995). Case management by community health workers of children with acute respiratory infections: Implications for national ARI control programme. *Journal of Tropical Medicine and Hygiene, 98*(4), 241–246.

Graber, M. L. (2009). Educational strategies to reduce diagnostic error: Can you teach this stuff? *Advance Health Science Education Theory Practice, 14*(1), 63–69.

Hanlon, J. T., Weinberger, M., Samsa, G. P., Schmader, K. E., Uttech, K. M., Lewis, I. K., … Feussner, J. R. (1996). A randomized, controlled trial of a clinical pharmacist intervention to improve inappropriate prescribing in elderly outpatients with polypharmacy. *American Journal of Medicine, 100*, 428–437.

Hawes, E. M., Misita, C., Burkhart, J., McKnight, L., Deyo, Z. M., Lee, R. A., … Eckel, S. F. (2016). Prescribing pharmacists in the ambulatory care setting: Experience at the university of North Carolina medical center. *American Journal of Health- System Pharmacy, 73*, 1425–1433.

Institute of Medicine. (1999). To err is human: Building a safer health system. In L. T. Kohn, J. M. Corrigan, & M. S. Donaldson (Eds.), *Report of the committee on quality of health care in America*. Washington, DC: National Academy Press.

Jacobson, J. (2002). Ensuring continuity of care and accuracy of patient medication history on hospital admission. *American Journal of Health-System Pharmacy, 59*, 1054–1055.

Johnson, J. A., & Bootman, J. L. (1995). Drug-related morbidity and mortality: A cost of illness model. *Archive of Internal Medicine, 155*, 1949–1956.

Jungnickel, P. W., Kelley, K. W., Hammer, D. P., Haines, S. T., & Marlowe, K. F. (2009). Addressing competencies for the future in the professional curriculum. *American Journal of Pharmaceutical Education, 73*(8), 156.

Kimani-Muragea, E. W., Manderson, L., Norrise, S. A., & Kahn, K. (2013). It's my secret'': Barriers to paediatric HIV treatment in a poor rural South African setting. *AIDS Care, 25*(6), 744–747.

Leape, L. L., Bates, D. W., Cullen, D. J., Cooper, H. J., Demonaco, T., Gallivan, R., ... Laffel, G. (1995). System analysis of adverse drug events. *JAMA, 274*, 35–43.

Leape, L. L., Brennan, T. A., & Laird, N. (1991). The nature of adverse events in hospitalized patients: Results from the Harvard medical practice study 11. *New England Journal of Medicine, 324*, 377–384.

Lee, P., & Ray, M. D. (2002). Qualities of a patient-focused medication-use system. *American Journal of Health-System Pharmacy, 59*, 2103–2105.

Lewis, P. J., Ashcroft, D. M., Dornan, T., Taylor, D., Wass, V., & Tully, M. P. (2013). Exploring the causes of junior doctors' prescribing mistakes: A qualitative study. *British Journal of Clinical Pharmacology, 78*(2), 310–319.

Lewis, P. J., Dornan, T., Taylor, D., Tully, M. P., Wass, V., & Ashcroft, D. M. (2009). Prevalence, incidence and nature of prescribing errors in hospital inpatients. *Drug Safety, 32*, 379–389.

Lewis, P. J., & Tully, M. P. (2009). Uncomfortable prescribing decisions in hospitals: The impact of teamwork. *Journal of the Royal Society of Medicine, 102*, 481–488.

Lopes Ibanez-Gonzalez, D., Mendenhall, E., & Norris, S. A. (2014). A mixed methods exploration of patterns of healthcare utilization of urban women with non-communicable disease in South Africa. *BMC Health Services Research, 14*, 528.

Mannase, H. R., Jr. (1989). Medication in an imperfect world: Drug misdaventuring as an issue of public policy, part 1. *American Journal of Hospital Pharmacy, 46*, 929–944.

Management Sciences for Health/World Health Organization/Action Programme on Essential Drugs (MSH/WHO/DAP). (1997). *Managing drug supply* (2nd ed.). Hartford, C.T.: Kumarian.

Maponga, C., & Odari, C. (2003). The quality of antimalarial: A study in selected African countries. *WHO/EDM/PAR* (Vol. 4). Geneva: World Health Organization.

McGettigan, P., Golden, J., Fryer, J., Chan, R., & Feely, J. (2001). Prescribers prefer people: The sources of information used by doctors for prescribing suggest that the medium is more important than the message. *British Journal of Clinical Pharmacology, 51*, 184–189.

Mendenhall, E., & Norris, S. A. (2015). Diabetes care among urban women in Soweto, South Africa: A qualitative study. *BMC Public Health, 15*, 1300.

Mohiuddin, M., Rashid, S. F., Shuvro, M. I., Nahar, N., & Ahmed, S. M. (2015). Qualitative insights into promotion of pharmaceutical products in Bangladesh: How ethical are the practices? *BMC Medical Ethics, 16*, 80.

Morey, J. C., Simon, R., Jay, G. D., Wears, R. L., Salisbury, M., Dukes, K. A., & Berns, S. D. (2002). Error reduction and performance improvement in the emergency department through formal teamwork training: Evaluation results of the MedTeams project. *Health Service Research, 37*, 1553–1581.

Murphy, K., Chuma, T., Mathews, C., Steyn, K., & Levitt, N. (2015). A qualitative study of the experiences of care and motivation for effective self-management among diabetic and hypertensive patients attending public sector primary health care services in South Africa. *BMC Health Service Research, 15*, 303.

Murray, J. P., Wenger, A. Z., Downe, E. A., & Terrazas, S. B. (2011). *Educating health professionals in low-resource countries: A global approach.* New York: The Carter Centre. Springer Publishing Company.

Nadzam, D. M. (1991). Development of medication-use indicators by the joint commission on accreditation of health organization. *American Journal of Health- System Pharmacy, 48*, 1925–1930.

Ndom, R. J. E., & Makanjuola, A. B. (2004). Perceived stress factors among resident doctors in a Nigerian teaching hospital. *West African Journal of Medicine, 23*(3), 78–81.

Ogaji, J. I., & Ojabo, C. E. (2014). Pharmacy education in Nigeria: The journey so far. *Archives of Pharmacy Practice, 5*(2), 47–60.

Oparah, A. C., & Eferakeya, A. E. (2005). Attitudes of Nigerian pharmacists towards pharmaceutical care. *Pharmacy World & Science*, *27*(3), 208–214.

Ostini, R., Hegney, D., Jackson, C., Williamson, M., Mackson, J. M., Gurman, K., … Tett, E. (2009). Systematic review of interventions to improve prescribing. *Annals of Pharmacotherapy*, *43*, 502–513.

Ovbiagele, B. (2015). Phone-based intervention under nurse guidance after Stroke: Concept for lowering blood pressure after stroke in Sub-Saharan Africa. *Journal of Stroke and Cerebrovascular Diseases*, *24*(1), 1–9.

Pearson, S. A., Rolfe, I., & Smith, T. (2002). Factors influencing prescribing: An intern's perspective. *Medical Education*, *36*, 781–787.

Peltzer, K., Mngqundaniso, N., & Petros, G. (2006). HIV/AIDS/STI/TB knowledge, beliefs and practices of traditional healers in KwaZulu-Natal, South Africa. *AIDS Care*, *18*(6), 608613.

Ravinetto, R., Vandenbergh, D., Macé, C., Pouget, C., Renchon, B., Rigal, J., … Caudron, J. (2016). Fighting poor-quality medicines in low- and middle-income countries: The importance of advocacy and pedagogy. *Journal of Pharmaceutical Policy and Practice*, *9*, 36.

Ritchey, F. J., & Raney, M. R. (1981). Medical role-task boundary maintenance: Physicians' opinions on clinical pharmacy. *Medical Care*, *19*(1), 90–103.

Ross, S., & Loke, Y. K. (2009). Do educational interventions improve prescribing by medical students and junior doctors? A systematic review. *British Journal of Clinical Pharmacology*, *67*, 662–670.

Ross, S., Ryan, C., Duncan, E. M., Francis, J. J., Johnston, M., Ker, J. S., … Bond, C. (2013). Perceived causes of prescribing errors by junior doctors in hospital inpatients: A study from the protect programme. *BMJ Quality & Safety*, *22*, 97–102.

Sachs, L., & Tomson, G. (1992). Medicines and culture–a double perspective on drug utilization in a developing country. *Social Science & Medicine*, *34*(3), 307–315.

Salmasi, S., Khan, T. M., Hong, Y. H., Ming, L. C., & Wui Wong, T. W. (2016). Medication errors in the Southeast Asian countries: A systematic review. *Plos One*, *10*(9), e0136545.

Salmasi, S., Ming, L. C., & Khan, T. M. (2016). Interaction and medical inducement between pharmaceutical representatives and physicians: A meta-synthesis. *Journal of Pharmaceutical Policy and Practice*, *9*, 37.

Smith, M. C., & Knapp, D. A. (1992). *Pharmacy, drugs and medical care* (5th ed.). Maryland: Williams & Wilkins.

Smith, A., Tasioulas, T., Cockayne, N., Misan, G., Walker, G., & Quick, G. (2006). Construction and evaluation of a web-based interactive prescribing curriculum for senior medical students. *British Journal of Clinical Pharmacology*, *62*, 653–659.

Stokes, T., Shaw, E. J., Camosso-Stefinovic, J., Imamura, M., Kanguru, L., & Hussein, J. (2016). Barriers and enablers to guideline implementation strategies to improve obstetric care practice in low- and middle-income countries: A systematic review of qualitative evidence. *Implementation Science*, *11*, 144.

Talabi, O. A. (2003). A questionnaire survey of senior house officers/registrars response to their training at University College Hospital, Ibadan. *West African Journal of Medicine*, *22*(2), 108–111.

Thistlethwaite, J. E., Ajjawi, R., & Aslani, P. (2010). The decision to prescribe: Influences and choice. *InnovAiT*, *3*, 237–243.

Udeogaranya, P. O., Ukwe, C. V., & Ekwunife, O. I. (2009). Assessment of attitudes of University of Nigeria pharmacy students toward pharmaceutical care. *Pharmacy Practice (Internet)*, *7*(3), 145–149.

Van der Geest, S., & Hardon, A. (2006). Social and cultural efficacies of medicines: Complications for antiretroviral therapy. *Journal of Ethnobiology and Ethnomedicine*, *2*, 48.

Vanderschmidt, l., Massey, J. A., Arias, J., Duong, T., Haddad, J., Noche, L. K., … Yepes, F. (1979). Competency-based training of health professions in seven developing countries. *American Journal of Public Health*, *69*, 585–590.

Wibowo, Y., Parsons, R., Sunderland, B., & Hughes, J. (2015). Evaluation of community pharmacy-based services for type-2 diabetes in an Indonesian setting: Pharmacist survey. *International Journal of Clinical Pharmacy*, *37*(5), 873–882.

Woolf, R., Locke, A., & Potts, C. (2016). Pharmacist prescribing within an integrated health system in Washington state. *American Journal of Health-System Pharmacy*, *73*, 1416–1424.

World Health Organization (WHO). (1998). *World health report: Life in the 21st century*. A vision for all. Report of the Director General. Geneva: WHO.

Yusuff, K. B., & Alabi, A. A. (2007). Assessing patient adherence to antihypertensive drug therapy: Can a structured pharmacist-conducted interview separate the wheat from the chaff? *International Journal of Pharmacy Practice*, *15*(2), 295–300.

Yusuff, K. B., Obe, B., & Joseph, Y. B. (2008). Adherence to anti-diabetic drug therapy and self-management practices among type-2 diabetics in a Nigerian tertiary care setting. *Pharmacy World & Science*, *30*, 876–883.

Yusuff, K. B., & Omarusehe, L. (2011). Determinants of self-medication practices among pregnant women in Nigeria. *International Journal of Clinical Pharmacy*, *33*, 868–875.

Yusuff, K. B., & Yusuf, A. (2009). Advertising OTC medicines in a Nigerian urban setting: Content analysis for indications, targets and advertising appeals. *Journal of the American Pharmacists Association*, *49*(1), 86–89.

FURTHER READING

Auta, A., Fredrick, N. C., David, S., Banwat, S. B., & Adeniyi, M. A. (2014). Patients' views on their consultation experience in community pharmacies and the potential prescribing role for pharmacists in Nigeria. *Journal of Pharmaceutical Health Services Research*, *5*, 233–236.

Gilbert, L. (1998). Pharmacy's attempts to extend its roles: A case study in South Africa. *Social Science & Medicine*, *47*(2), 153–164.

Yusuff, K. B. (2013). Perceived challenges associated with prescribed medications and self-initiated coping strategies used by medical outpatients in Nigeria. *International Journal of Clinical Pharmacy*, *35*, 65–71.

CHAPTER

THE USE OF MEASUREMENTS AND HEALTH BEHAVIORAL MODELS TO IMPROVE MEDICATION ADHERENCE

4

Yara Arafat, Mohamed Izham Mohamed Ibrahim
Qatar University, Doha, Qatar

CHAPTER OUTLINE

INTRODUCTION

Medications will not work and disease conditions will not improve if patients do not take their medications as directed; i.e., adherence to treatments is a main determinant of therapy success. Medication nonadherence is a common problem. Issues related to nonadherence in healthcare are increasingly becoming a global concern, especially in developing countries. Nonadherence results when a patient does not initiate or continue care that a provider has recommended. It is a major concern for society; it affects health outcomes and causes wastage in healthcare. Healthcare professionals (HCPs) have relied on the biomedical model to manage patients with chronic illness and to encourage them to adhere to

Social and Administrative Aspects of Pharmacy in Low- and Middle-Income Countries. http://dx.doi.org/10.1016/B978-0-12-811228-1.00004-2

their medications. Patients commonly take fewer medications than prescribed or prematurely discontinue the therapy. The underlying forces have not been thoroughly studied. Slight progress has been made in resolving the problem. It is a difficult and multidimensional healthcare problem.

Adherence improvement is surely needed, but finding the best approach is a challenge. Why do the present clinical approaches fail? What kinds of interventions are needed to overcome this problem? Why do patients not adhere to their providers' orders and advice? Why do they not take their medications as prescribed? Do they not value the treatment that they receive? Is this problem more severe in developing countries than in developed countries? This chapter explores some sociobehavioral models and measurements that are potentially beneficial in addressing nonadherence to medications in patients with chronic illnesses in developing countries.

WHAT IS MEDICATION NONADHERENCE?

The terms "compliance," "concordance," and "adherence" have different meanings (Aronson, 2007). "Compliance" has the meaning of "to fulfill a promise," while "concordance" has the meaning of "agreement." The World Health Organization (WHO) defines "adherence" as "the extent to which a person's behavior – taking medication, following a diet, and/or executing lifestyle changes, corresponds to agreed recommendations from a healthcare provider" (WHO, 2003). According to Aronson (2007), "adherence" is a better and more meaningful term in the context of drug therapy; it means to "cling to, keep close, or remain constant," e.g., to commit to a therapeutic regimen. It is the collaborative involvement of the patient in his/her disease management, particularly the therapeutic regimen, in a mutual relationship between him/her and his/her healthcare provider to achieve a successful health outcome. The behavior of adhering to medications also involves the act of perseverance. Adherence relates to consistency in taking medications. Optimal adherence is recognized as "a patient taking their medication exactly as prescribed, at the exact time, dosage and for the recommended length of time" (Breccia, Efficace, & Alimena, 2011). In this chapter, the term "adherence" will be used throughout the discussion.

On the other hand, "nonadherence" has more than one definition. It could mean that patients are not taking their medications at all, or are taking reduced amounts, or are taking doses at the prescribed frequencies but not matching the medications to food requirements (Altice & Friedland, 1998).

THE PREVALENCE OF NONADHERENCE AND ITS IMPLICATIONS

Nonadherence to appropriately prescribed medications is a global health problem and a major concern in developing countries. It is widespread and associated with factors such as types of diseases and patient characteristics. It is difficult to get reliable statistics on medication nonadherence based on developed versus developing countries. However, due to the economic conditions (e.g., lack of financial resources to supply medicines and make medicines available and affordable) and the environment of the pharmaceutical sector in developing countries (e.g., lack of access to medicines, shortage of medicines), the nonadherence issue is more problematic (i.e., in overall impact and negative consequences) than in developed nations.

The WHO (n.d.) reported that in terms of absolute number of deaths, slightly more than three-fourths of global noncommunicable disease (NCD) deaths occurred in low- and middle-income countries (LMICs). Statistics of more than two decades stated that in developed countries, nonadherence to the medications for chronic diseases ranges between 30% and 50%, and this figure is even greater in developing countries (Lassen, 1989; Morris & Schulz, 1992). Another report noted that approximately 50% of patients with chronic illnesses do not use their medications as prescribed (Lee, Grace, & Taylor, 2006), which in turn leads to an increase in morbidity and death rates (Osterberg & Blaschke, 2005).

Adhering to medications is crucial in order to obtain better patient outcomes among NCD patients. For example, the risk of stroke and ischemic heart disease doubles in patients with hypertension for every 20 mm Hg increase in systolic blood pressure (BP) and every 10 mm Hg increase in diastolic BP (Lewington, Clarke, Qizilbash, Peto, & Collins, 2002). Even though it is well known that adhering to medications will lower the risk of ischemic events (Amarenco & Labreuche, 2009; Baigent et al., 2005), many patients still fail to take their medications consistently (Costa, 1996; Cramer, Benedict, Muszbek, Keskinaslan, & Khan, 2008; Glader, Sjolander, Eriksson, & Lundberg, 2010).

Medication adherence to antiplatelet agents and statins is also poor, and hence, patients develop worse clinical outcomes. Approximately 25%–50% of patients were found to stop taking statins within 6–12 months after having been prescribed them (Deambrosis et al., 2007; Mann, Allegrante, Natarajan, Halm, & Charlson, 2007; Poluzzi et al., 2008), and at the end of 2 years, 75% of the patients were not taking their medications (Chodick et al., 2008; Evans et al., 2009). Moreover, mortality from ischemic heart disease in developing countries is likely to rise by 137% for men and 120% for women between the years 1990 and 2020 (Leeder, Raymond, Greenberg, Liu, & Kathy, 2004), and rates of ischemic heart disease and strokes are expected to almost triple in sub-Saharan Africa, Latin America, and the Middle East. Therefore, these countries currently experience a huge burden of chronic diseases (Frenk, Bobadilla, Sepulveda, & Cervantes, 1989).

The prevalence of nonadherence in patients with type 2 diabetes is high (Cramer, 2004; Fischer et al., 2010), and it appears to be a major cause of increased morbidity and mortality in the diabetic population (Ho et al., 2006). The number of individuals with diabetes is expected to increase to 366 million in 2030, 298 million of whom will live in developing countries (Wild, Roglic, Green, Sicree, & King, 2004). If we factor the estimated proportion of potential nonadherence to medication, the impact will be high. On average, 50% of patients newly prescribed antidiabetic medications during their first year of therapy will fail to take at least 80% of their doses (Grégoire, Sirois, Blanc, Poirier, & Moisan, 2010; Osterberg & Blaschke, 2005), and adherence rates to antidiabetic medications range between 36% and 93% (Cramer, 2004).

It is estimated that the total cost for nonadherence each year in the United States ranges from $100 billion to $300 billion (Berg, Dischler, Wagner, Raia, & Palmer-Shevlin, 1993; Levy, Zamacona, & Jusko, 2000; Senst et al., 2001). Many developed countries have focused on addressing the burden of chronic diseases. However, the increasing burden of chronic diseases on developing countries has received insufficient consideration and is often neglected (Beaglehole & Yach, 2003). Thus, considering the prevalent rates of nonadherence, direct costs, i.e., drug-related expenses, could decrease significantly if adherence is improved.

WHY ARE PATIENTS NOT ADHERING TO MEDICATIONS?

To enhance medication adherence, the multifactorial causes of nonadherence must first be understood, e.g., patient characteristics, patient beliefs, patient–healthcare provider relationships, stigma, therapy schedules, drug regimens, information, side effects, access to medicines, etc. In broad terms, the WHO classifies factors causing nonadherence into three categories: patient-related, physician-related, and health system/team building–related factors (World Health Organization, 2003).

1. Patient-related aspects such as lack of understanding of their disease (Ryan, 1999), lack of participation in the treatment decision-making process (Haynes, McDonald, & Garg, 2002), and suboptimal medical literacy (Raynor, 2008) lead to nonadherence. Other patient-related factors are their previous experiences with pharmacological therapies, their health beliefs regarding the effectiveness of the treatment, and their lack of motivation (Brunner et al., 2009; Joyner-Grantham et al., 2009; Osterberg & Blaschke, 2005). Patients tend to provide reasons for not adhering to their medications, such as "I forgot," "I thought I already took it," "I am tired of it," "I felt fine," "It does not work," "I do not feel like taking it," etc.
2. Physician-related factors can also lead to nonadherence because physicians are often unable to recognize that their patients are not taking their medications consistently and end up prescribing new medications to them without considering the additional costs and the financial burden to the patient (Osterberg & Blaschke, 2005).
3. Health system/team building–related factors influence medication adherence, as some healthcare systems create barriers by restricting the patient's access to care (Bodenheimer, 2008). High-priced medications also lead to medication nonadherence (Pallares et al., 2009). In addition, some healthcare institutions are overcrowded. Physicians have to treat a vast number of patients without spending enough time to properly assess their behavior regarding medication adherence, thus preventing patients from engaging in a discussion on the significance of medication adherence.

MEASURING MEDICATION ADHERENCE

There are several methods to measure medication adherence, i.e., indirectly or directly, and the following are the most common techniques currently used separately or together to measure medication adherence (Lam & Fresco, 2015; Luga & McGuire, 2014). Luga and McGuire (2014) classified the methods as indirect measurements, i.e., medication possession ratio (MPR), proportion of days covered (PDC), self-report, questionnaire, pill counting, dose counting device and electronic prescribing, and direct measurements, i.e., direct observation and drug levels and markers. The measurements could also be categorized (Lam & Fresco, 2015) into the following:

1. Objective measurements, which are obtained by assessing the pharmacy refill records, counting pills, or using electronic medication event monitoring systems;
2. Subjective measurements, which are obtained by questioning the patient, family members, or HCPs about the patient's medication use patterns; and
3. Biochemical measurements, which are obtained by incorporating a nontoxic marker for the medication taken and identifying its presence in blood or urine or measurements of serum drug levels.

The MPR and PDC are widely used in administrative and research settings. The most common indirect method of measuring medication adherence used in clinical settings is patient self-reported measures. They are questionnaires that have a high degree of agreement with electronic medication monitoring devices (Shi et al., 2010), and they are a way to measure medication adherence both simply and effectively (Haynes et al., 1980).

Medication adherence scales are usually validated and compared to an objective measure of medication adherence before they are given to different patient populations with different disease conditions. A good medication adherence scale should be able to identify the beliefs, barriers, or behaviors of the patients regarding taking their medications, and it must be highly accurate and precise (Nguyen, La Caze, & Cottrell, 2014). The problem with questionnaires is that patients could misinterpret the information in them and a distortion of some results could occur through the patients themselves (Osterberg & Blaschke, 2005). Many medication adherence scales are used in clinical settings including the Beliefs about Medication Questionnaire (BMQ) (Horne, Weinman, & Hankins, 1999); the Adherence Self-Report Questionnaire (ASRQ) (Zeller, Schroeder, & Peters, 2008); the Medication Adherence Rating Scale (MARS) (Thompson, Kulkarni, & Sergejew, 2000); and the most commonly used Morisky Medication Adherence Scale (MMAS) (Morisky, Green, & Levine, 1986) that was improved to the eight-item Morisky Medication Adherence Scale (MMAS-8) (Morisky, Ang, Krousel-Wood, & Ward, 2008).

SOCIOBEHAVIORAL MODELS TO ADDRESS NONADHERENCE TO MEDICATIONS

Why do we need sociobehavioral models? Although the treatment of chronic conditions has improved immensely in the past few years, many patients experience a reduced quality of life due to the failure to achieve the desired clinical outcomes. The main reason for the aforementioned problem is that HCPs depend solely on the biomedical model to treat chronic conditions (Engel, 1977). The biomedical model is a conceptual model of illness in which patients are passive recipients of a doctor's instructions. It provides a mechanistic view of any illness, and it requires HCPs to carry out mechanical solutions such as prescribing the correct medicine with the correct dose for the patient. Clinicians who apply this model believe that problems of nonadherence to medications are due to certain characteristics in patients (Blackwell, 1992). According to the WHO, health is defined as "a complete state of physical, social, and mental wellbeing, and not merely the absence of disease of infirmity" (WHO, 1946). Since the biomedical model works only on improving physical well-being, interventions began incorporating sociobehavioral models along with the biomedical model to improve a person's health based on the WHO definition. Furthermore, the biomedical model has significant limitations that fail to associate health behaviors with factors such as patients' opinions of their own illness, psychosocial influences, and socioeconomic conditions (WHO, 2003; Blackwell, 1992). Sociobehavioral models identify what factors influence the behaviors needed for outcome to be achieved and sustained. Such models synthesize complex causes of outcomes, behaviors, and influential factors.

Several sociobehavioral models have been developed to describe the mental and social well-being of patients. Since the inability to adhere to medications is a complex sociobehavioral problem, adding a behavioral intervention might help patients control their disease and achieve better clinical outcomes. Behavioral interventions are targeted to change individual behavior in those aspects related to everyday life. In the case of adherence, they aim to modify patients' behavior toward treatment, i.e., to improve adherence. To improve the health outcome, we need to change the behavior, and to change the behavior, we need to work on the factors that influence the behavior.

Behavioral interventions for enhancing medication adherence have shown conflicting outcomes (Clarkesmith, Pattison, & Lane, 2013; George, Elliott, & Stewart, 2008; Haynes, Ackloo, Sahota,

McDonald, & Yao, 2008). The most effective interventions are those that incorporate multiple components, but unfortunately, they have been proven to be not cost-effective and not easily applicable in clinical practice (Haynes et al., 2008). Hence, the development of effective behavioral interventions, in which behavior counseling is directly offered to patients by HCPs, has become crucial. According to Haynes et al. (2008), strategies to enhance adherence to prescribed medications are more successful for short-term treatments than for long-term chronic diseases. For example, 36 of 83 interventions for adherence to medications for chronic conditions resulted in an increase in medication adherence, and almost all of those interventions were complex and multifactorial.

There are two problems with the current adherence interventions. First, adherence was improved by only approximately 4%–11% in most interventions, so even the most effective interventions did not greatly enhance adherence and patient outcomes (Kripalani, Yao, & Haynes, 2007). Second, the majority of patients take multiple medications for many medical problems, but most interventions focus on a single medication or a particular disease area (Choudhry et al., 2011). Thus, applying the adherence interventions to a real-world setting is likely to be impractical. Hence, multifaceted and tailored adherence interventions are needed to enhance medication adherence and provide global benefits. Although studies and evidence focusing on medication adherence have increased, there are limited recommendations available for enhancing medication adherence. The common ways are simplifying patients' medication regimens if possible and regularly offering reminders to take medications (Zedler, Kakad, Colilla, Murrelle, & Shah, 2011). In general, many of the interventions for long-term medications tend to be exceedingly complicated and expensive. To understand the effects of various interventions on adherence, future research using behavioral models to aim to increase medication adherence, especially in developing countries, is required. The following are the commonly used behavioral models previously used to improve medication adherence, with most studies being conducted in developed countries. According to Newman, Steed, and Mulligan (2008), the health belief model (HBM), the theory of reasoned action (TRA), the theory of planned behavior (TPB), the transtheoretical model (TTM), and the information–motivation–behavioral skills (IMB) model, all of which are potentially amenable to change, have been widely used to develop behavioral interventions.

TRANSTHEORETICAL MODEL

One of the commonly used behavioral models used is the TTM, which is also known as the stages of change (SOC) model. It is commonly used in research and clinical practice. It is an integrative model of intentional change that explains how people acquire a positive behavior or change their unhealthy behavior by focusing on the decision-making process of the individual. The TTM was first used to focus on smoking behavior, but due to its popularity, it has been tested with several other behaviors in areas such as weight loss (Prochaska, Norcross, Fowler, Follick, & Abrams, 1992), cancer screening (Eiser & Cole, 2002), or encouraging stroke victims to exercise (Garner & Page, 2005). It consists of four components: stages of change, processes of change, decisional balance, and self-efficacy.

The progression through the SOC is not linear; people move through these stages in a manner similar to a cyclical pattern. Thus, they may regress to previous stages before moving forward. The SOC of the TTM are precontemplation, contemplation, preparation, action, and maintenance (Prochaska & Norcross, 2010).

To progress through the SOC, individuals apply 10 processes of change, some of which are more relevant to specific SOC than others. The TTM has been used over the years to address medication adherence in different populations with chronic conditions. Some studies have determined that the TTM could enhance medication adherence in patients with hypertension; one study suggested that the TTM could be used as a method to measure SOC for medication adherence in patients receiving antihypertensive drugs (Willey, 1999), and another study found that patients with hypertension who received a TTM intervention were more successful in adhering to their antihypertensive medication regimen compared to patients who received the usual care (Johnson et al., 2006). The TTM was also able to enhance medication adherence in patients taking lipid-lowering medications (Johnson et al., 2006). Moreover, two studies used the TTM on patients with HIV; one reported that using a model such as the TTM, which is tailored to each person, could help HIV patients adhere to their antiretroviral therapy (ART) (Tuldra & Wu, 2002), and the other stated that there was an association between SOC and patients' adherence to ART (Genberg, Lee, Rogers, Willey, & Wilson, 2013). Another study used the TTM framework to describe factors that were thought to have caused patients with multiple sclerosis (MS) to discontinue the use of interferon beta-1a-Biogen. The results suggested that constructs of the TTM were effective in differentiating between MS patients who discontinued the use of the treatment and those who did not (Berger, Hudmon, & Liang, 2004). This suggests that the TTM could effectively be implemented in interventions to enhance adherence to the prescribed treatments for MS.

All the studies provide some degree of evidence to suggest that the TTM can help patients with chronic diseases to change their behaviors in ways that can help them manage their disease. Even though research studies indicate that using the TTM seems promising in enhancing medication adherence, the model has yet to be widely applied in clinical practice. To date, the precise effect of the use of the TTM approach on medication adherence remains only partly examined. Therefore, further research in this area is still required to clarify whether the use of the TTM could assist patients with chronic conditions to enhance medication adherence and improve patient outcomes.

HEALTH BELIEF MODEL

Another commonly used model is the HBM, which suggests that behavior is determined by a number of beliefs about threats to an individual's well-being and the effectiveness of a particular behavior (Becker, 1974; Rosenstock, 1966). The following four perceptions are the main constructs of the model: perceived severity, perceived susceptibility, perceived benefits, and perceived barriers. Two other constructs have been added, and the model has been expanded to include cues to action and self-efficacy. The model suggests that behavior is influenced by a person's perception of a threat resulting from a health problem and the benefits related to reducing the threat. The HBM can be used to predict how patients will behave in relation to their health.

The HBM has been used in studies related to medication adherence. In a study on patients with hypertension, the model suggested that the prevalence of adherence to hypertension management was low in the participants due to inadequate perceived susceptibility, perceived severity, perceived benefit, and poor lifestyle factors, hence suggesting that to improve adherence in patients with hypertension, the value and importance of patient perceptions regarding medications must be clearly acknowledged (Kamran, Sadeghieh Ahari, Biria, Malepour, & Heydari, 2014). The HBM was also reliable in predicting medication adherence in Chinese patients with hypertension. The study suggested that for an intervention to be successfully applied in clinical practice, it should be guided by the association between risk factors and HBM constructs and antihypertensive medication adherence (Yue, Li, Weilin, & Bin, 2015). Another study examined the relationship between health beliefs and the use of prescribed medications among patients who have been diagnosed with hypertension for at least 1 year in a rural South African hospital. The results suggest that nonadherence was associated with the perceived benefits and barriers of antihypertensive medications and some aspects of the quality of the practitioner–patient relationship (Peltzer, 2004).

THEORY OF PLANNED BEHAVIOR

The TPB is also a widely applied behavioral model. It helps us understand how the behavior of people can change. The model assumes that behavior is planned; hence, it predicts deliberate behavior (Ajzen, 1991). The TPB is the descendant of a similar model known as the TRA (Ajzen & Fishbein, 1975). The succession was due to the discovery that behavior is not completely voluntary and cannot always be controlled; therefore, perceived behavioral control was added to the model, and with this addition, the theory was renamed the TPB. According to the TPB, any action a person takes is guided by three types of considerations: behavioral beliefs (beliefs about the probable consequences of the practiced behavior), normative beliefs (beliefs about the normative expectations of other people), and control beliefs (beliefs about the presence of factors that may enable or obstruct the performance of the behavior). Behavioral beliefs normally result in a favorable or unfavorable attitude toward a specific behavior, normative beliefs result in perceived social pressure or subjective norms, and control beliefs trigger perceived behavioral control. Usually, the greater the favorable behavior, subjective norm, and perceived control, the stronger the person's intention to perform the behavior in question.

The TPB was able to explain approximately 25% and 50% of the variance in intention and adherence behavior, respectively. While other constructs that are related to adherence could be added to the TPB to enhance it (Ajzen, 1991), it has been suggested that adding more variables will limit any progress in the development of the model (Sniehotta, Presseau, & Araújo-Soares, 2014). Adherence to prescribed medications is influenced by several factors other than patient-related factors, including social and economic, therapy related, and health system factors (WHO, 2003); thus, for a theory to successfully improve medication adherence, it must be able to accommodate these complex components. The TPB is applicable to many health behaviors, but its ability to predict medication adherence behavior in people with chronic diseases seems to be limited. Therefore, further research must be conducted to test the ability of other theories to predict medication adherence so that they may be incorporated into interventions and applied in clinical practice. The TPB was also able to enhance medication adherence in Mexican American patients with schizophrenia (Kopelowicz et al., 2015). The study demonstrated that the TPB constructs can be used to develop an effective intervention that improves medication adherence in such populations.

INFORMATION–MOTIVATION–BEHAVIORAL SKILLS

The IMB model identifies three components, i.e., information, behavioral skills, and motivation that are required for a specified health behavior (Fisher & Fisher, 1992). Information relates to basic knowledge regarding the medical condition. Motivation, which includes personal and social motivation, results from personal attitudes as well as social support or norms toward engaging in a specific behavior, such as adherence. The third element, behavioral skills, includes factors such as ensuring that patients have the tools, skills, and strategies to perform the behavior as well as a sense of self-efficacy—the belief that they can achieve the behavior. Starace, Massa, Amico, and Fisher (2006) reported that the data and assumptions support the utility of the IMB model as a potential framework for understanding ART adherence. Munro, Lewin, Swart, and Volmink (2007) noted that the advantage and application of the IMB model to ART adherence suggests that it may be a good model for enhancing medication adherence among TB patients.

There are other perspectives, models, and theories that are not part of this discussion: behavioral learning perspectives, the communication perspective, the protection motivation theory, the social cognitive theory, and self-regulation perspectives (Munro et al., 2007; WHO, 2003).

HEALTHCARE PROVIDER'S ROLE IN IMPROVING ADHERENCE

Patients, healthcare providers, and healthcare systems all play an important role in improving medication adherence. Many developing countries have observed an increase in their morbidity and mortality rates due to nonadherence to medications (WHO, 2002), which causes a burden on the society. Therefore, nonadherence has become a growing concern for clinicians and healthcare systems. For example, an improvement of only 20% in medication adherence could lessen total healthcare expenditure by $1074 annually for every patient with diabetes (Sokol, McGuigan, Verbrugge, & Epstein, 2005).

A single technique alone will not be able to improve medication adherence; instead, a combination of various adherence methods should be applied to enhance patients' adherence to their medications. In addition, doctors underestimate the problem of nonadherence in their patients (Roth & Caron, 1978). It is crucial to correctly measure medication adherence in clinical practice. This can be done by pill counting, self-reports, and in some cases determining urine or serum drug levels. Among these, the most practical and extensively used tool is the self-report. In general, if patients are asked honestly and openly, they can be very accurate in telling whether they are adhering to their treatment regimens (Duong et al., 2001).

It is not just the physicians who play an important part in improving medication adherence in chronic populations. All other healthcare providers, such as pharmacists, nurses, and psychologists, perform a major part in helping patients enhance their medication adherence, whether by determining the reasons and causes for nonadherence and how to address these issues, educating patients about the importance and benefits of adhering consistently to medications, or observing whether their medication adherence is enhanced. Even though HCPs understand the significance of adhering to medications, they are unable to help patients adhere to their medication regimen in their clinical practice due to the short time they spend with patients, which does not allow them to implement any interventions or strategies to improve adherence (Ammerman et al., 1993). To educate HCPs on ways to help patients enhance their medication adherence in their short visits, training programs to teach physicians how to educate patients using behavioral models should be developed. Effective communication between healthcare providers and patients depends in part on the providers' confidence in their ability to teach, develop, and improve patient skills as well as the amount of time available to offer preventive services (Wright, 1993).

HCPs should also ensure friendliness and approachability, enhancement of patient centeredness, improvement in teaching and counseling skills and recognition of patients' problems as well as their spiritual and psychological factors that might affect medication adherence.

Furthermore, patients who must visit different providers in multiple settings are usually vulnerable to decreased medication adherence. Institutions that are designed to deliver multiple interventions can help more patients achieve the goals set for them by their providers (Belcher, 1990; DeBusk et al., 1994).

Despite the desire and need to improve care and enhance medication adherence, institutions often lack sufficient knowledge methods to encourage patients to increase their adherence to their prescribed medications. The solution to this problem is to regularly train and educate HCPs about different approaches to improve patient medication adherence, and organizations must be committed to implementing these effective strategies rapidly. Only then will alterations in patient behavior, improvement in medication adherence, and better clinical outcomes be achieved (DeBusk et al., 1994).

Medication technology advancement has managed to assist in developing tools and devices to help patients improve their adherence. Does this really work? If it does, and providers could supply patients with medication adherence devices, are these appropriate and effective for individuals in developing countries, especially LMICs, due to the cost, education level, and health literacy rate?

ACHIEVEMENTS

Although the ability of behavioral models to improve medication adherence has not been widely tested in developing countries, they have been able to enhance medication adherence in developed countries. Thus, there is a true need—now more than ever—to test these models on diverse populations in developing countries. The TTM was able to enhance medication adherence in patients receiving antihypertensive medications, patients taking lipid-lowering drugs, and patients with HIV receiving ART therapy. The HBM, IMB, and TPB also seem promising in enhancing medication adherence, but further research must be conducted to ensure that these behavioral models as well as others (not discussed here) could be used in clinical practice to improve adherence in various populations.

CHALLENGES

The extent and effect of nonadherence to medications in developing countries are assumed to be higher than that in developed countries due to inequities in access to healthcare and limited healthcare resources. Nonadherence to medications is a great challenge for these populations, as long-term adherence to prescribed medications would lead to a significant decrease in morbidity and mortality rates in all populations with chronic diseases. There is a lack of information about the prevalence of nonadherence to medications in developing countries and in important subgroups, such as children and the elderly. With this information, healthcare providers, policy makers, and other relevant parties would be able to develop suitable policies or strategies to enhance medication adherence in diverse populations. In addition, NCDs, HIV, tuberculosis, and mental health disorders combined represented 54% of the burden of all diseases worldwide in 2001 (WHO, 2002). Unexpectedly, NCDs and mental health problems are also common in developing countries, representing 46% of the total burden of diseases for the year 2001 (WHO, 2002), and the prevalence is expected to increase to 56% by 2020 (Murray & Lopez, 1996).

There is a lack of high-quality studies on medication adherence that have been conducted in developing countries. Now more than ever, more studies discussing the reasons for nonadherence and necessary strategies to improve it in these countries are desperately needed to fill the knowledge gap and help design effective interventions for nonadherence.

One study determined the factors associated with self-reported adherence among patients with hypertension in a poor urban community in Nigeria (Osamor & Owumi, 2011). The factors associated with high adherence to medications were attending clinics regularly, using Western prescription medications, and having constant social support from family or friends who care about the patients' medical status and always remind patients to take their medications. The study suggests that the medication adherence in this community is close to ideal. However, more research is required to confirm whether these factors are the same in other developing countries or in other populations with chronic diseases.

Last but not least, developing countries, especially LMICs, need effective and reliable healthcare systems. This will ensure the sustainable financing and a steady supply of medications. These factors could affect availability, affordability, and acceptability as well as accessibility to medicines. A lack of these fundamental aspects of a healthcare system could cause poor medication adherence.

RECOMMENDATIONS: THE WAY FORWARD

Further studies must be conducted to determine the best and most applicable health behavioral models and could be used to enhance medication adherence in various populations that are diverse in terms of ethnic group, culture, lifestyle, and behavior. Researchers and healthcare providers should systematically test the existing health behavior models. Interventions using these theories need to be developed and evaluated appropriately. Studies of interventions to promote adherence to medications for one health issue should be carefully reviewed to explore how these have drawn on health behavior theories and how this could be applied to other health issues.

Once determined, the model must be applied in clinical practice to help patients adhere to their medications and obtain good clinical outcomes and quality of life. Healthcare providers are encouraged to learn and be familiar with these different models.

CONCLUSIONS

The issue of medication adherence should be examined from a wider perspective, i.e., "bio-psycho-socio-environmental" theory. More behavioral interventions are necessary to help chronic populations in developing countries comply with their medication regimens. Studies implementing behavioral models to improve adherence to long-term treatment regimens are needed to create uncomplicated approaches that could be easily implemented in institutions with limited resources. More focus must be given to chronic populations that are underserved and often neglected in developing countries.

Moreover, to improve the clinical outcomes and the health-related quality of life and to decrease morbidity and mortality rates from NCDs, patients and all HCPs must be committed and set optimal medication adherence as their target. There is great pressure to reduce costs and to improve the quality of life and clinical outcomes. Thus, developing and implementing these interventions are extremely important now than ever. The solution to the problem of nonadherence is not as simple as telling patients what they need to do to obtain the desired outcomes. More complex, multilevel interventions that incorporate one of the behavioral models and measurement tools mentioned earlier will be more effective. Moreover, while the economic burden of nonadherence must be addressed, it is also important to address other factors that could influence behavior, such as social, psychological, or cultural factors. Finally, patients, HCPs, and healthcare organizations must collaborate to address the problem of nonadherence, to decrease the economic burden of the problem, and to achieve better patient outcomes.

LESSONS LEARNED

- Poor adherence to medications is still a global problem; developing countries are more vulnerable to a high prevalence of medication nonadherence because of the weaknesses in their healthcare systems.
- The growth of chronic disease has negatively impacted medication adherence, which in turn has caused a burden to healthcare systems due to the increased rate of poor medication adherence.
- More focus and further studies are needed to determine the rates of nonadherence to medications in developing countries.
- Medication-taking behavior is extremely complex, and various multifactorial strategies are required to improve adherence.
- More research must be conducted in developing countries to determine the best behavioral models that could be used to increase medication adherence with low costs in countries with limited resources.

REFERENCES

Ajzen, I. (1991). The theory of planned behavior. *Organizational Behavior and Human Decision Processes*, *50*(2), 179–211. http://dx.doi.org/10.1016/0749-5978(91)90020-T.

Ajzen, I., & Fishbein, M. (1975). *Belief, attitude, intention and behavior: An introduction to theory and research.* Reading, MA: Addison-Wesley.

Altice, F. L., & Friedland, G. H. (1998). The era of adherence to HIV therapy. *Annals of Internal Medicine*, *129*(6), 503–505.

Amarenco, P., & Labreuche, J. (2009). Lipid management in the prevention of stroke: Review and updated meta-analysis of statins for stroke prevention. *Lancet Neurology*, *8*(5), 453–463. http://dx.doi.org/10.1016/s1474-4422(09)70058-4.

Ammerman, A. S., DeVellis, R. F., Carey, T. S., Keyserling, T. C., Strogatz, D. S., Haines, P. S., … Siscovick, D. S. (1993). Physician-based diet counseling for cholesterol reduction: Current practices, determinants, and strategies for improvement. *Preventive Medicine*, *22*(1), 96–109. http://dx.doi.org/10.1006/pmed.1993.1007.

Aronson, J. K. (April 2007). Compliance, concordance, adherence. *British Journal of Clinical Pharmacology*, *63*(4), 383–384. http://dx.doi.org/10.1111/j.1365-2125.2007.02893.x.

Baigent, C., Keech, A., Kearney, P. M., Blackwell, L., Buck, G., Pollicino, C., … Simes, R. (2005). Efficacy and safety of cholesterol-lowering treatment: Prospective meta-analysis of data from 90,056 participants in 14 randomised trials of statins. *Lancet*, *366*(9493), 1267–1278. http://dx.doi.org/10.1016/s0140-6736(05)67394-1.

Beaglehole, R., & Yach, D. (2003). Globalisation and the prevention and control of non-communicable disease: The neglected chronic diseases of adults. *Lancet*, *362*(9387), 903–908. http://dx.doi.org/10.1016/s0140-6736(03)14335-8.

Becker, M. H. (1974). *The health belief model and personal health behavior* (Vol. 2). Thorofare, NJ: Charles B. Slack.

Belcher, D. W. (1990). Implementing preventive services. Success and failure in an outpatient trial. *Archives of Internal Medicine*, *150*(12), 2533–2541.

Berg, J. S., Dischler, J., Wagner, D. J., Raia, J. J., & Palmer-Shevlin, N. (1993). Medication compliance: A healthcare problem. *The Annals of Pharmacotherapy*, *27*(9 Suppl), S1–S24.

Berger, B. A., Hudmon, K. S., & Liang, H. (2004). Predicting treatment discontinuation among patients with multiple sclerosis: Application of the transtheoretical model of change. *Journal of the American Pharmacists Association*, *44*(4), 445–454 (2003).

Blackwell, B. (1992). Compliance. *Psychotherapy and Psychosomatics*, *58*(3–4), 161–169.

Bodenheimer, T. (2008). Coordinating care-a perilous journey through the healthcare system. *The New England Journal of Medicine*, *358*(10), 1064–1071. http://dx.doi.org/10.1056/NEJMhpr0706165.

Breccia, M., Efficace, F., & Alimena, G. (2011). Imatinib treatment in chronic myelogenous leukemia: What have we learned so far? *Cancer Letters*, *300*(2), 115–121.

Brunner, R., Dunbar-Jacob, J., Leboff, M. S., Granek, I., Bowen, D., Snetselaar, L. G., … Wu, L. (2009). Predictors of adherence in the Women's health initiative calcium and vitamin D. *Journal of Behavioral Medicine*, *34*(4), 145–155. http://dx.doi.org/10.3200/bmed.34.4.145-155.

Chodick, G., Shalev, V., Gerber, Y., Heymann, A. D., Silber, H., Simah, V., & Kokia, E. (2008). Long-term persistence with statin treatment in a not-for-profit health maintenance organization: A population-based retrospective cohort study in Israel. *Clinical Therapeutics*, *30*(11), 2167–2179. http://dx.doi.org/10.1016/j.clinthera.2008.11.012.

Choudhry, N. K., Fischer, M. A., Avorn, J., Liberman, J. N., Schneeweiss, S., Pakes, J., … Shrank, W. H. (2011). The implications of therapeutic complexity on adherence to cardiovascular medications. *Archives of Internal Medicine*, *171*(9), 814–822.

Clarkesmith, D. E., Pattison, H. M., & Lane, D. A. (2013). Educational and behavioural interventions for anticoagulant therapy in patients with atrial fibrillation. *The Cochrane Database of Systematic Reviews*, *4*(6), Cd008600. http://dx.doi.org/10.1002/14651858.CD008600.pub2.

Costa, F. V. (1996). Compliance with antihypertensive treatment. *Clinical and Experimental Hypertension: CHE*, *18*(3–4), 463–472.

Cramer, J. A. (2004). A systematic review of adherence with medications for diabetes. *Diabetes Care*, *27*(5), 1218–1224.

Cramer, J. A., Benedict, Á., Muszbek, N., Keskinaslan, A., & Khan, Z. M. (2008). The significance of compliance and persistence in the treatment of diabetes, hypertension and dyslipidaemia: A review. *IInternational Journal of Clinical Practice*, *62*(1), 76–87. http://dx.doi.org/10.1111/j.1742-1241.2007.01630.x.

Deambrosis, P., Saramin, C., Terrazzani, G., Scaldaferri, L., Debetto, P., Giusti, P., & Chinellato, A. (2007). Evaluation of the prescription and utilization patterns of statins in an Italian local health unit during the period 1994-2003. *European Journal of Clinical Pharmacology*, *63*(2), 197–203. http://dx.doi.org/10.1007/s00228-006-0239-3.

DeBusk, R. F., Miller, N. H., Superko, H. R., Dennis, C. A., Thomas, R. J., Lew, H. T., … Taylor, C. B. (1994). A case-management system for coronary risk factor modification after acute myocardial infarction. *Annals of Internal Medicine*, *120*(9), 721–729.

Duong, M., Piroth, L., Grappin, M., Forte, F., Peytavin, G., Buisson, M., … Portier, H. (2001). Evaluation of the patient medication adherence questionnaire as a tool for self-reported adherence assessment in HIV-infected patients on antiretroviral regimens. *HIV Clinical Trials*, *2*(2), 128–135. http://dx.doi.org/10.1310/m3jr-g390-lxcm-f62g.

Eiser, J. R., & Cole, N. (2002). Participation in cervical screening as a function of perceived risk, barriers and need for cognitive closure. *Journal of Health Psychology*, *7*(1), 99–105. http://dx.doi.org/10.1177/135910530200 7001657.

Engel, G. L. (1977). The need for a new medical model: A challenge for biomedicine. *Science*, *196*(4286), 129–136.

Evans, C. D., Eurich, D. T., Lamb, D. A., Taylor, J. G., Jorgenson, D. J., Semchuk, W. M., … Blackburn, D. F. (2009). Retrospective observational assessment of statin adherence among subjects patronizing different types of community pharmacies in Canada. *Journal of Managed Care Pharmacy*, *15*(6), 476–484. http://dx.doi.org/10.18553/jmcp.2009.15.6.476.

Fischer, M. A., Stedman, M. R., Lii, J., Vogeli, C., Shrank, W. H., Brookhart, M. A., & Weissman, J. S. (2010). Primary medication non-adherence: Analysis of 195,930 electronic prescriptions. *Journal of General Internal Medicine*, *25*(4), 284–290. http://dx.doi.org/10.1007/s11606-010-1253-9.

Fisher, J. D., & Fisher, W. A. (1992). Changing AIDS-risk behavior. *Psychological Bulletin*, *111*(3), 455–474. http://dx.doi.org/10.1037/0033-2909.111.3.455.

Frenk, J., Bobadilla, J. L., Sepulveda, J., & Cervantes, L. M. (1989). Health transition in middle-income countries: new challenges for healthcare. *Health Policy Plan*, *4*(1), 29–39.

Garner, C., & Page, S. J. (2005). Applying the transtheoretical model to the exercise behaviors of stroke patients. *Topics in Stroke Rehabilitation*, *12*(1), 69–75. http://dx.doi.org/10.1310/yjw0-fk07-tgn7-avw7.

Genberg, B. L., Lee, Y., Rogers, W. H., Willey, C., & Wilson, I. B. (2013). Stages of change for adherence to antiretroviral medications. *AIDS Patient Care STDS*, *27*(10), 567–572. http://dx.doi.org/10.1089/apc.2013.0126.

George, J., Elliott, R. A., & Stewart, D. C. (2008). A systematic review of interventions to improve medication taking in elderly patients prescribed multiple medications. *Drugs & Aging*, *25*(4), 307–324.

Glader, E. L., Sjolander, M., Eriksson, M., & Lundberg, M. (2010). Persistent use of secondary preventive drugs declines rapidly during the first 2 years after stroke. *Stroke: A Journal of Cerebral Circulation*, *41*(2), 397–401. http://dx.doi.org/10.1161/strokeaha.109.566950.

Grégoire, J.-P., Sirois, C., Blanc, G., Poirier, P., & Moisan, J. (2010). Persistence patterns with oral antidiabetes drug treatment in newly treated patients—a population-based study. *Value in Health: The Journal of the International Society for Pharmacoeconomics and Outcomes Research*, *13*(6), 820–828. http://dx.doi.org/10.1111/j.1524-4733.2010.00761.x.

Haynes, R. B., Ackloo, E., Sahota, N., McDonald, H. P., & Yao, X. (2008). Interventions for enhancing medication adherence. *The Cochrane Database of Systematic Reviews*, *16*(2), Cd000011. http://dx.doi.org/10.1002/14651858.CD000011.pub3.

Haynes, R. B., McDonald, H. P., & Garg, A. X. (2002). Helping patients follow prescribed treatment: Clinical applications. *JAMA*, *288*(22), 2880–2883.

Haynes, R. B., Taylor, D. W., Sackett, D. L., Gibson, E. S., Bernholz, C. D., & Mukherjee, J. (1980). Can simple clinical measurements detect patient noncompliance? *Hypertension*, *2*(6), 757–764.

Horne, R., Weinman, J., & Hankins, M. (1999). The beliefs about medicines questionnaire: The development and evaluation of a new method for assessing the cognitive representation of medication. *Psychology & Health*, *14*(1), 1–24. http://dx.doi.org/10.1080/08870449908407311.

Ho, P. M., Rumsfeld, J. S., Masoudi, F. A., McClure, D. L., Plomondon, M. E., Steiner, J. F., & Magid, D. J. (2006). Effect of medication non-adherence on hospitalization and mortality among patients with diabetes mellitus. *Archives of Internal Medicine*, *166*(17), 1836–1841. http://dx.doi.org/10.1001/archinte.166.17.1836.

Johnson, S. S., Driskell, M. M., Johnson, J. L., Dyment, S. J., Prochaska, J. O., Prochaska, J. M., & Bourne, L. (2006). Transtheoretical model intervention for adherence to lipid-lowering drugs. *Disease Management*, *9*(2), 102–114. http://dx.doi.org/10.1089/dis.2006.9.102.

Johnson, S. S., Driskell, M. M., Johnson, J. L., Prochaska, J. M., Zwick, W., & Prochaska, J. O. (2006). Efficacy of a transtheoretical model-based expert system for antihypertensive adherence. *Disease Management*, *9*(5), 291–301. http://dx.doi.org/10.1089/dis.2006.9.291.

Joyner-Grantham, J., Mount, D. L., McCorkle, O. D., Simmons, D. R., Ferrario, C. M., & Cline, D. M. (2009). Self-reported influences of hopelessness, health literacy, lifestyle action, and patient inertia on blood pressure control in a hypertensive emergency department population. *The American Journal of the Medical Sciences*, *338*(5), 368–372. http://dx.doi.org/10.1097/MAJ.0b013e3181b473dc.

Kamran, A., Sadeghieh Ahari, S., Biria, M., Malepour, A., & Heydari, H. (2014). Determinants of patient's adherence to hypertension medications: Application of health belief model among rural patients. *Annals of Medical and Health Sciences Research*, *4*(6), 922–927. http://dx.doi.org/10.4103/2141-9248.144914.

Kopelowicz, A., Zarate, R., Wallace, C. J., Liberman, R. P., Lopez, S. R., & Mintz, J. (2015). Using the theory of planned behavior to improve treatment adherence in Mexican Americans with schizophrenia. *Journal of Consulting and Clinical Psychology*, *83*(5), 985–993. http://dx.doi.org/10.1037/a0039346.

Kripalani, S., Yao, X., & Haynes, R. B. (2007). Interventions to enhance medication adherence in chronic medical conditions: A systematic review. *Archives of Internal Medicine*, *167*(6), 540–550. http://dx.doi.org/10.1001/archinte.167.6.540.

Lam, W. Y., & Fresco, P. (2015). Medication adherence measures: An overview. *Biomed Research International*, *2015*, 217047. http://dx.doi.org/10.1155/2015/217047.

Lassen, L. C. (1989). Patient compliance in general practice. *Scandinavian Journal of Primary Health Care*, *7*(3), 179–180.

Leeder, S., Raymond, S., Greenberg, H., Liu, H., & Kathy, E. (2004). *A race against time: The challenge of cardiovascular disease in developing economies*. New York: Coumbia University.

Lee, J. K., Grace, K. A., & Taylor, A. J. (2006). Effect of a pharmacy care program on medication adherence and persistence, blood pressure, and low-density lipoprotein cholesterol: A randomized controlled trial. *JAMA*, *296*(21), 2563–2571. http://dx.doi.org/10.1001/jama.296.21.joc60162.

Levy, G., Zamacona, M. K., & Jusko, W. J. (2000). Developing compliance instructions for drug labeling. *Clinical Pharmacology and Therapeutics*, *68*(6), 586–591. http://dx.doi.org/10.1067/mcp.2000.110976.

Lewington, S., Clarke, R., Qizilbash, N., Peto, R., & Collins, R. (2002). Age-specific relevance of usual blood pressure to vascular mortality: A meta-analysis of individual data for one million adults in 61 prospective studies. *Lancet*, *360*(9349), 1903–1913.

Luga, A. O., & McGuire, M. J. (2014). Adherence and healthcare costs. *Risk Management and Healthcare Policy*, *7*, 35–44.

Mann, D. M., Allegrante, J. P., Natarajan, S., Halm, E. A., & Charlson, M. (2007). Predictors of adherence to statins for primary prevention. *Cardiovascular Drugs and Therapy*, *21*(4), 311–316. http://dx.doi.org/10.1007/s10557-007-6040-4.

Morisky, D. E., Ang, A., Krousel-Wood, M., & Ward, H. J. (2008). Predictive validity of a medication adherence measure in an outpatient setting. *The Journal of Clinical Hypertension (Greenwich)*, *10*(5), 348–354.

Morisky, D. E., Green, L. W., & Levine, D. M. (1986). Concurrent and predictive validity of a self-reported measure of medication adherence. *Medical Care*, *24*(1), 67–74.

Morris, L. S., & Schulz, R. M. (1992). Patient compliance-an overview. *Journal of Clinical Pharmacy and Therapeutics*, *17*(5), 283–295.

Munro, S., Lewin, S., Swart, T., & Volmink, J. (2007). A review of health behaviour theories: How useful are these for developing interventions to promote long-term medication adherence for TB and HIV/AIDS? *BMC Public Health*, *7*, 104. http://dx.doi.org/10.1186/1471-2458-7-104.

Murray, C. J. L., & Lopez, A. (1996). *The global burden of disease*. Geneva: World Health Organization.

Newman, S., Steed, E., & Mulligan, K. (2008). *Chronic physical illness: Self-management and behavioral interventions*. Maidenhead, UK: Open University Press.

Nguyen, T. M., La Caze, A., & Cottrell, N. (2014). What are validated self-report adherence scales really measuring?: a systematic review. *British Journal of Clinical Pharmacology*, *77*(3), 427–445. http://dx.doi.org/10.1111/bcp.12194.

Osamor, P. E., & Owumi, B. E. (2011). Factors associated with treatment compliance in hypertension in southwest Nigeria. *Journal of Health, Population, and Nutrition*, *29*(6), 619–628.

Osterberg, L., & Blaschke, T. (2005). Adherence to medication. *The New England Journal of Medicine*, *353*(5), 487–497. http://dx.doi.org/10.1056/NEJMra050100.

Pallares, M. J., Powers, E. R., Zwerner, P. L., Fowler, A., Reeves, R., & Nappi, J. M. (2009). Barriers to clopidogrel adherence following placement of drug-eluting stents. *The Annals of Pharmacotherapy*, *43*(2), 259–267. http://dx.doi.org/10.1345/aph.1L286.

Peltzer, K. (2004). Health beliefs and prescription medication compliance among diagnosed hypertension clinic attenders in a rural South African Hospital. *Curationis*, *27*(3), 15–23.

Poluzzi, E., Strahinja, P., Lanzoni, M., Vargiu, A., Silvani, M. C., Motola, D., … Montanaro, N. (2008). Adherence to statin therapy and patients' cardiovascular risk: A pharmacoepidemiological study in Italy. *European Journal of Clinical Pharmacology*, *64*(4), 425–432. http://dx.doi.org/10.1007/s00228-007-0428-8.

Prochaska, J. O., & Norcross, J. C. (2010). *Systems of psychotherapy: A transtheoretical analysis* (7th ed.). California: Brooks-Cole.

Prochaska, J. O., Norcross, J. C., Fowler, J. L., Follick, M. J., & Abrams, D. B. (1992). Attendance and outcome in a work site weight control program: Processes and stages of change as process and predictor variables. *Addictive Behaviors*, *17*(1), 35–45.

Raynor, D. K. (2008). Medication literacy is a 2-way street. *Mayo Clinic Proceedings*, *83*(5), 520–522. http://dx.doi.org/10.4065/83.5.520.

Rosenstock, I. M. (1966). Why people use health services. *Milbank Mem Fund Q*, *44*(3), 94–127.

Roth, H. P., & Caron, H. S. (1978). Accuracy of doctors' estimates and patients' statements on adherence to a drug regimen. *Clinical Pharmacology and Therapeutics*, *23*(3), 361–370.

Ryan, A. A. (1999). Medication compliance and older people: A review of the literature. *The International Journal of Nursing Studies*, *36*(2), 153–162.

Senst, B. L., Achusim, L. E., Genest, R. P., Cosentino, L. A., Ford, C. C., Little, J. A., … Bates, D. W. (2001). Practical approach to determining costs and frequency of adverse drug events in a healthcare network. *American Journal of Health-system Pharmacy*, *58*(12), 1126–1132.

Shi, L., Liu, J., Fonseca, V., Walker, P., Kalsekar, A., & Pawaskar, M. (2010). Correlation between adherence rates measured by MEMS and self-reported questionnaires: A meta-analysis. *Health Qual Life Outcomes*, *8*, 99. http://dx.doi.org/10.1186/1477-7525-8-99.

Sniehotta, F. F., Presseau, J., & Araújo-Soares, V. (2014). Time to retire the theory of planned behaviour. *Health Psychology Review*, *8*(1), 1–7. http://dx.doi.org/10.1080/17437199.2013.869710.

Sokol, M. C., McGuigan, K. A., Verbrugge, R. R., & Epstein, R. S. (2005). Impact of medication adherence on hospitalization risk and healthcare cost. *Medical Care*, *43*(6), 521–530.

Starace, F., Massa, A., Amico, K. R., & Fisher, J. D. (2006). Adherence to antiretroviral therapy: An empirical test of the information-motivation-behavioral skills model. *Health Psychol.*, *25*(2), 153–162.

Thompson, K., Kulkarni, J., & Sergejew, A. A. (2000). Reliability and validity of a new medication adherence rating scale (MARS) for the psychoses. *Schizophrenia Research*, *42*(3), 241–247.

Tuldra, A., & Wu, A. W. (2002). Interventions to improve adherence to antiretroviral therapy. *Journal of Acquired Immune Deficiency Syndromes*, *31*(Suppl. 3), S154–S157.

WHO. (1946). *Constitution of the World Health Organization*. Geneva: World Health Organization.

WHO. (2002). *The world health report 2002-reducing risks, promoting healthy life*. Geneva: World Health Organization.

WHO. (2003). *Adherence to long-term therapies. Evidence for action* (Geneva).

WHO. (n.d.). The top 10 causes of death. http://www.who.int/mediacentre/factsheets/fs310/en/index1.html.

Wild, S., Roglic, G., Green, A., Sicree, R., & King, H. (2004). Global prevalence of diabetes: Estimates for the year 2000 and projections for 2030. *Diabetes Care*, *27*(5), 1047–1053.

Willey, C. (1999). Behavior-changing methods for improving adherence to medication. *Current Hypertension Reports*, *1*(6), 477–481.

Wright, E. C. (1993). Non-compliance-or how many aunts has Matilda? *Lancet*, *342*(8876), 909–913.

Yue, Z., Li, C., Weilin, Q., & Bin, W. (2015). Application of the health belief model to improve the understanding of antihypertensive medication adherence among Chinese patients. *Patient Education and Counseling*, *98*(5), 669–673. http://dx.doi.org/10.1016/j.pec.2015.02.007.

Zedler, B. K., Kakad, P., Colilla, S., Murrelle, L., & Shah, N. R. (2011). Does packaging with a calendar feature improve adherence to self-administered medication for long-term use? A systematic review. *Clinical Therapeutics*, *33*(1), 62–73. http://dx.doi.org/10.1016/j.clinthera.2011.02.003.

Zeller, A., Schroeder, K., & Peters, T. J. (2008). An adherence self-report questionnaire facilitated the differentiation between non-adherence and nonresponse to antihypertensive treatment. *Journal of Clinical Epidemiology*, *61*(3), 282–288. http://dx.doi.org/10.1016/j.jclinepi.2007.04.007.

SECTION 2

PHARMACEUTICAL PROMOTION IN LOW- AND MIDDLE-INCOME COUNTRIES

CHAPTER

5

ACADEMIC DETAILING IN LOW- AND MIDDLE-INCOME COUNTRIES: PRINCIPLES, USE, IMPACT, AND LESSONS LEARNED

Saval Khanal

Griffith University, Nathan, QLD, Australia

CHAPTER OUTLINE

Social and Administrative Aspects of Pharmacy in Low- and Middle-Income Countries. http://dx.doi.org/10.1016/B978-0-12-811228-1.00005-4

INTRODUCTION

> Academic detailing is not just a 'say no to drugs' programme. It begins with the assumption that prescribing is one of the most useful and challenging things we doctor do, and we crave accessible, unbiased data about the drugs we prescribe.
>
> **Dr Jerry Avorn, inventor of academic detailing and professor of medicine at Harvard Medical School**

Evidence-based practice is an integral part of the rational use of medicine. In many circumstances, clinical practice guidelines are implemented to promote the evidence-based practice (Sackett, 1997). These guidelines are made and promulgated at any level, from institutional level to national and international levels, with an aim to promote the rational use of medicines (Abula & Kedir, 2017; Falzon et al., 2017; Freeland et al., 2015; Royal Australian and New Zealand College of Psychiatrists, 2017). However, translation of such guidelines into real practice is often challenging, especially in low- and middle-income countries (LMICs) (Oliver, Innvar, Lorenc, Woodman, & Thomas, 2014). Failure to adopt such recommended clinical guidelines may lead to different negative consequences, such as, but not limited to, reduction in the quality of life of patients; or may increase the economic burden of diseases (or its treatment) to the payers; or in much worse scenario they may lead to disabilities or deaths (Haegerich, Paulozzi, Manns, & Jones, 2014; van Boven et al., 2014). Evidence suggests that there is a huge gap between evidence-based guidelines and their implementation (Ersek et al., 2016; Williams, Petrov, Kennedy, Halpenny, & Doherty, 2017). In recent years, much attention had been given to find the way to improve the implementation of such clinical guidelines. Numerous types of interventions had been studied to improve the adherence of healthcare professionals toward such guidelines. Educational reminders to the healthcare professionals, academic detailing sessions, and feedback to prescribers about the prescribing are some researched educational interventions to improve the practice of the healthcare professionals (Grimshaw et al., 2002).

In this chapter, we aim to discuss different aspects of academic detailing, including its similarities and differences with pharmaceutical detailing, its principle, current status in developed and LMICs, and achievements and challenges to implement academic detailing in LMICs.

WHAT IS AN ACADEMIC DETAILING?

Academic detailing is a structured educational outreach program in which a trained health professional visits practicing healthcare professionals in their practice settings to deliver tailored evidence-based information (Soumerai & Avorn, 1990). It is also known as educational outreach, educational detailing, or educational visiting. Academic detailing programs are usually funded by the university or not-for-profit organizations. Traditionally, it involved face-to-face education of healthcare professionals by trained academic detailers, but recently alternative modes, such as video conferencing or web-based platform are being explored. Academic detailers are usually healthcare professionals, such as pharmacists, healthcare professionals, nurses, or any trained people on the subject matter. The main aim of academic detailing program is to increase the knowledge of the healthcare professionals on particular topic, change prescribing of targeted drugs to be consistent with medical evidence, provide medical care in a cost-effective way, or minimize the patients' risks due to wrong practice The traditional (face-to-face) form of academic detailing is very similar to that of pharmaceutical/medical representative visiting a healthcare professional. The information provided during academic detailing should be free from economic interest, unlike pharmaceutical detailing, which is narrowly targeted to promote the sales of particular medical product/s. There have been reports that in many circumstances, information provided by pharmaceutical representatives may not cover negative aspects of their product/s (Spurling et al., 2010), which puts healthcare professionals potentially at higher risk to receive biased information. However, information provided by academic detailers is based on extensive literature survey and its critical appraisal. A person affiliated with academic detailing centers, such as academic detailers, administrative staff, and program developers should not ideally have any financial relationships with pharmaceutical companies (Kondro, 2007; Soumerai & Avorn, 1990). Usually, academic detailing program is conducted on a one-to-one basis; however, in some cases, it can even be conducted to the small group of healthcare professionals with a similar type of clinical background. Table 5.1 summarizes basic similarities and difference between academic detailing and pharmaceutical detailing.

Table 5.1 Similarities and Differences Between Academic Detailing and Pharmaceutical Detailing

	Academic Detailing	Pharmaceutical Detailing
Modality of detailing	A trained academic detailer visits healthcare professionals in his/her clinical setting to provide information. The approach is very similar to pharmaceutical detailing.	Academic detailing was originated from the concept of pharmaceutical detailing. Therefore, both approaches are similar in this aspect.
Objective of detailing	Usually, academic detailing sessions are conducted to promote the evidence-based practice, such as optimizing prescribing behavior of healthcare professionals, providing information on new medicine/guidelines to the practitioners, as a reinforcement to different interventions aiming to improve the outcomes, etc.	Mostly targeted to provide information about the particular pharmaceutical company's products; may have agenda to promote sales volume of the products manufactured by that company.
Source of funding	Mostly funded by the government, university, charity, or other not-for-profit organizations.	Usually funded by pharmaceutical companies.
Types of information provided	Systematic, unbiased, balanced information to assist clinical decision-making	Information targeted to influence the sales of products. There are reports that pharmaceutical companies do not highlight negative aspects of their pharmaceutical products during detailing visits.
Mode of providing information	Follows traditional methods of pharmaceutical detailing—mostly face-to-face. However, there have been recent research studies on the use of web-based platform to provide academic detailing.	Face-to-face is highly recommended than the other modes.

Continued

Table 5.1 Similarities and Differences Between Academic Detailing and Pharmaceutical Detailing—cont'd

	Academic Detailing	Pharmaceutical Detailing
Detailers and remuneration	Detailers are usually effective communicator and trained in academic and clinical aspects of the topic. Academic detailers are generally healthcare professionals or medical educators. They should possess a high level of pharmacotherapy knowledge because they are meant to provide unbiased evidence-based information.	Detailers are supposed to have good knowledge of the topic and should have persuasive ability to promote the sales of the project. However, in practice, the former quality is often sacrificed.
Potential conflicts of interest	They should not have any potential conflicts of interest, which might influence themselves from not providing unbiased information. The materials they provide to healthcare professionals should not have any relevant potential conflict of interest. Usually, they, including their near family members, are not associated with any pharmaceutical companies.	Detailers usually have the interest to promote the sales of products of a pharmaceutical company. The materials supporting detailing may not be unbiased in many circumstances.

PRINCIPLES OF ACADEMIC DETAILING

After coining the term "academic detailing" in the early 1980s (Avorn & Soumerai, 1983), same people, Jerry Avorn and Stephen B. Soumerai, published an article including principles of academic detailing to improve clinical decision-making (Soumerai & Avorn, 1990). They believed academic detailing should follow a similar approach to that of pharmaceutical detailing, which has been influential in changing the behavior of healthcare professionals. They suggested that academic detailing model should be based largely on successful approaches developed and practiced by pharmaceutical company marketing departments. Detailers, who are commonly clinical pharmacists, nurses, or physicians, are trained to employ a variety of the same social marketing strategies as their industry counterparts. Ideally, an academic detailer should be a good communicator with an art to persuade healthcare professionals to change their behavior. He or she should also possess a strong knowledge on the pharmacotherapy of the topic for which detailing will be delivered. He or she along with his or her near family members should not have any associated potential conflict of interest. Academic detailers are the most important tool of academic detailing intervention; therefore they must be trained properly. They also summarized some essential techniques for an effective implementation of academic detailing program (Table 5.2).

USE OF ACADEMIC DETAILING

Academic detailing was first practiced by Jerry Avorn and Stephen B. Soumerai, as an intervention to optimize prescribing behavior as a randomized controlled trial (RCT) in four states of the United States (Avorn & Soumerai, 1983), the academic detailing has since then been applied to

Table 5.2 Techniques Used in Academic Detailing to Improve Clinical Decision-Making (Soumerai & Avorn, 1990)

Techniques Used in Academic Detailing
Conduct interviews with the target audience to investigate baseline knowledge and motivations for current prescribing and practice patterns.
Focus programs on specific groups of prescribers and opinion leaders.
Define clear educational and behavioral objectives.
Establish credibility through a respected organizational identity, referencing authoritative and unbiased sources of information, and presenting both sides of controversial issues.
Stimulate active physician participation in educational interactions.
Use concise graphic educational materials.
Highlight and repeat the essential messages.
Provide positive reinforcement of improved practices in follow-up.

other areas, such as, but not limited to, increasing the knowledge, attitude, and practice of healthcare professionals, screening of diseases, smoking cessation, reducing hospital readmissions, disseminating new clinical information, and to changing health practitioners' behavior. The concept of academic detailing started gaining momentum in Europe and other countries in the 1990s and early 2000s. Till date, there are many reports about the use of academic detailing in many countries, which are explained later in this chapter. Some of the major uses of academic detailing programs are explained below briefly.

TO PROVIDE HEALTH AND MEDICINE INFORMATION TO HEALTHCARE PROFESSIONALS

In this era, one can find multiple sources for health and medicine information, either electronically, verbally, or in a hard paper written forms. These sources may range from huge international databases, journals, bulletins, a pharmaceutical representative, direct-to-consumer advertisements, and so on (Hesse et al., 2005). Most of this information, in most cases, is commercially driven by pharmaceutical companies with a lot of expenditure in pharmaceutical promotion (Spurling et al., 2010). This information is many times aimed at increasing the sales of the product; in some cases, healthcare professionals are not provided negative aspects (adverse drug reactions, side effects, etc.) of the products. Coupled with this, there are reports that healthcare professionals in many LMICs do not have access to an unbiased source of information. This makes healthcare professionals, especially those in LMICs, in vulnerable situations on obtaining some unbiased information. Academic detailing can be used as a tool to provide information in such countries. Academic detailing can also be used for tailoring information according to the healthcare professional knowledge and needs. Therefore, academic detailing can be used effectively to provide healthcare professionals in LMICs with unbiased, reliable, and tailored health and medicine information.

TO IMPROVE KNOWLEDGE, ATTITUDE, AND PRACTICE OF HEALTHCARE PROFESSIONALS AND PATIENTS

Academic detailing has known to improve the knowledge, attitude, and practice of healthcare professionals Khanal (2010) (Markey & Schattner, 2001; Ross-Degnan et al., 1996). RCTs conducted in Kenya and Indonesia evaluated the short-term impact of academic detailing on the knowledge and practice of pharmacists on the management of childhood diarrhea. Findings from those trials suggested marked improvement in knowledge and performance of pharmacists regarding the topic. The study had considered a pharmacy as a unit of analysis for RCTs in both countries (n = 107 pharmacies in Kenya; n = 87 in Indonesia) (Ross-Degnan et al., 1996). Another report from Australia suggested the significant improvement in knowledge and self-perceived understanding of evidence-based medicine among the randomly stratified 132 physicians; however, the intervention had limited influence on attitudes toward it (Markey & Schattner, 2001). Another RCT conducted in a district of Nepal assessed the impact of academic detailing on the knowledge, attitude, and practice of healthcare professionals. The findings from this trial also demonstrated the marked improvement in knowledge, attitude, and practice of government health workers and private practitioners toward the use of oral rehydration solution and zinc tablets for childhood diarrhea (Khanal, 2010). The same study also measured the prescribing behavior of healthcare professionals and reported an improvement—particularly increased the prescription of ORS and zinc tablets and minimized the use of antimicrobials in childhood diarrhea, which did not require antimicrobials (Khanal, Ibrahim, Shankar, Palaian, & Mishra, 2013). Hence, comprehensive discussion between academic detailers and healthcare professionals on a particular topic during academic detailing sessions can substantially improve the knowledge, attitude, and practice of healthcare providers. However, in some cases, it may be difficult to attain desired change in their behavior, so some reinforcement program parallel to academic detailing is recommended.

TO IMPROVE PRESCRIBING BEHAVIOR

One of the main objectives of inventing academic detailing program was to influence the prescribing behavior of healthcare professionals. In one of the early published on academic detailing, Avorn and colleagues demonstrated that academic detailing was able to decrease the prescribing of certain not needed medicines—cephalexin, propoxyphene, and papaverine (Avorn & Soumerai, 1983; Soumerai & Avorn, 1990). Subsequently, many studies on the impact of academic detailing on the prescribing behaviors were conducted elsewhere as well. Most of them documented the marked improvement in prescribing behavior of healthcare professionals following one or more academic detailing sessions. Such improvements in prescribing behavior improved the rational use of medicines, such as use of psychoactive drugs, cardiovascular medicines, medicines for respiratory tract infection, rational antimicrobial use, and so on (Awad, Eltayeb, & Baraka, 2006; Davey et al., 2013; Pittenger, Williams, Mecklenburg, & Blackmore, 2015). O'Brien et al. (2008) had conducted meta-analysis about the impact of academic detailing program in the prescribing behavior. From included 69 studies, they concluded that academic detailing can significantly improve the prescribing behavior of healthcare professionals. Most of the available evidence suggests academic detailing is one of the powerful tools to influence the prescribing behavior of the healthcare professionals. So, it can be used to improve the prescribing behavior of the healthcare professionals.

TO INTRODUCE OR PROMOTE CLINICAL GUIDELINES

In many LMICs, evidence has been limited to research or trials. This evidence has not been implemented due to various reasons. Translating such evidence into practice requires implementation of such guidelines. This step has always been a challenge, especially in LMICs. Academic detailing program has been used to help to implement and to promote treatment guidelines in many high-income countries (Davies & Taylor-Vaisey, 1997; Katz et al., 2013; Mold et al., 2014; Silva et al., 2013). Subsequently, academic detailing program has been used in some LMICs to promote clinical guidelines as well. For example, academic detailing program was trialed in a district of Nepal to improve the adherence of healthcare professionals toward the childhood diarrhea management guidelines (Khanal, 2010; Khanal et al., 2013). The aim of the guidelines was to increase the use of oral rehydration salts and zinc tablet in childhood diarrhea and decrease the unnecessary use of antimicrobials. Academic detailing was successful in improving all prescribing indicators, thus helping to promote clinical guidelines among the healthcare providers. Hence, academic detailing can be used as informational or educational intervention to facilitate the implementation of clinical guidelines.

ACCEPTANCE OF ACADEMIC DETAILING PROGRAMS AMONG HEALTHCARE PROVIDERS

One-on-one educational sessions such as academic detailing are recognized to be more effective than orthodox educational interventions to get behavior changes in healthcare professionals (Davies, 1998; Davies & Taylor-Vaisey, 1997; Davies, Thomson, Oxman, & Haynes, 1995). These programs cannot be implemented properly until it is accepted by the participants. Healthcare providers are the participants of academic detailing program. Therefore, the way how academic detailing programs are perceived by healthcare professionals will have a direct impact on their willingness to change the behavior. There are some studies that were conducted on evaluating perception and/or acceptability of academic detailing programs by healthcare professionals. Evidence suggests healthcare professionals had a positive attitude toward academic detailing programs; they told academic detailing programs, which comprise informational sessions with evidence supported information, are more effective than other traditional educational forms (Davies & Taylor-Vaisey, 1997). Some surveys done on the participants of academic detailing program suggested that the healthcare professionals appreciated academic detailing as a good means to obtain new information and update their knowledge on recent advancement in their field (Habraken et al., 2003; Janssens et al., 2005; Shankar, Jha, Shrestha, Bajracharya, & Thapa, 2009). A Belgian study about the perception of healthcare professionals on academic detailing program suggested that the participants rated academic detailing very highly and most of them also mentioned they are willing to participate in such types of programs again in the future (Habraken et al., 2003). A report from a teaching hospital of Nepal suggested that the initial feedback of healthcare professionals toward the academic detailing was positive and encouraging (Shankar et al., 2009). Although many participants regarded academic detailing programs highly, one study reported that healthcare professionals found academic detailing program time-consuming despite providing valuable information (Allen, Ferrier, O'Connor, & Fleming, 2007). From the available evidence, we can assume that academic detailing is highly regarded and widely accepted by participants; however, academic detailing sessions should be tailored in such a way that it is concise but comprehensive.

TRAINING OF PHARMACISTS AS ACADEMIC DETAILERS

Academic detailers should possess good communication skills and good knowledge in health and therapeutics (Soumerai & Avorn, 1990). Pharmacists ideally can be good academic detailers with their training and expertise in pharmacology and health and medicine information (Jin et al., 2012). However, pharmacists should be trained properly on communication skills. Ideally, they should be trained how to influence behavior in healthcare professionals. Usually, this behavioral change training is very similar to that of pharmaceutical detailing, which includes the art of effective oral communication and art of convincing (Jin et al., 2012; Soumerai & Avorn, 1990). They should also know about the latest development in forms or mode of academic detailing. The mode of detailing has been evolved from its basic (face-to-face intervention) into more modern complex form (e-academic detailing). The success of academic detailing program is based on its planning before implementation. There has been evidence suggesting academic detailing has a greater chance of success if combined with other educational and/or managerial interventions (Axon et al., 2014; Newton-Syms et al., 1992; Pittenger et al., 2015; Yourman, Concato, & Agostini, 2008). Hence, they should be trained in using different multimedia and development of educational tools as well. Their participation in the development of educational tools will help them understand the topic much better.

ACADEMIC DETAILING PROGRAMS IN HIGH-INCOME COUNTRIES

Academic detailing programs since the inception in the early 1980s have been implemented in many high-income countries. Information on academic detailing programs of few high-income countries is mentioned below.

UNITED STATES

Academic detailing centers exist in many states of the United States. They are commonly university based. More recently in 2010, National Resource Centre for Academic Detailing (NaRCAD) was established with the funding from Agency for Health Research and Quality (AHRQ)—a government organization. NaRCAD helps the organizations in the United States with limited resources to develop and improve the academic detailing programs (Avorn, 2017; Fischer, 2016). It also aims to create a network of academic detailing program.

CANADA

Canadian Academic Detailing Collaboration (CADC) was formed in 2003 by the networking of academic detailing centers in six provinces of Canada (Jin et al., 2012). This was funded by

Canadian Agency for Drug and Technologies in Health (CADTH). CADC and CADTH had collaborated to develop and disseminate useful evidence reviews to the healthcare professionals to improve their prescribing behavior. Two among six members of CADC were discontinued due to financial constraints.

AUSTRALIA

Australian Government provided a fund to Drug and Therapeutic Information Services (DATIS) to investigate the usefulness of academic detailing programs to support the better outcomes from the use of diagnostic technologies (Broadhurst et al., 2007). DATIS has also focused on various therapeutic issues in addition to diagnostic technologies, such as the rational use of nonsteroidal antiinflammatory drugs, antihyperlipidemic drugs, and antidepressants (Rowett, 2002; Weller et al., 2003).

UNITED KINGDOM

Academic detailing programs in the United Kingdom is well documented (Duerden et al., 2004; Paton, Adebowale, & Okocha, 2008; Walley, Mrazek, & Mossialos, 2005). National Health Services (NHS) has funded a university and center to develop academic detailing aids. These academic detailing aids aim to support the discussion with healthcare professionals one or more key priorities for implementing various National Institute of Health and Care Excellence (NICE) guidelines.

OTHER COUNTRIES

Many other high-income countries have good academic detailing programs. European countries, such as Norway, the Netherlands, and Belgium, has well-established academic detailing programs to support their healthcare professionals (Dyrkorn, Gjelstad, Espnes, & Lindbæk, 2016; Gjelstad et al., 2006, 2013; Habraken et al., 2003). Japan has also started academic detailing program in 2014 (Yamamoto, 2013). Initially, through a school of pharmacy in Tokyo University of Science, the government aims to develop academic detailing database. The database is supposed to be used to provide information about most appropriate medicine for patients.

ACADEMIC DETAILING PROGRAMS IN LOW- AND MIDDLE-INCOME COUNTRIES

Although academic detailing was introduced more than three and half decades ago, it is not still common in LMICs. In many LMICs, it is still conducted as a research or as a pilot study. They do not have government- or state-funded national programs and they also do not have a network of different academic detailing centers within their country. However, in Brazil, there has been a huge discussion to promote academic detailing programs to implement and disseminate clinical protocols and guidelines (Costa et al., 2015, 2016). There is also a local Brazilian academic detailing guideline, which comprises

Stage 1: Prospection and identification of problems
Stage 2: Definition of the AD purpose
Stage 3: Budget estimate, elaboration of schedule, and technical team designation
Stage 4: Elaboration and purchase of the support material
Stage 5: Identification of prescribers and organization of visitation goals
Stage 6: Recruitment of facilitators and workshop training
Stage 7: Prescribers' visiting for AD
Stage 8: Release of the support material
Stage 9: Evaluation of results
Stage 10: Release of the results

FIGURE 5.1

Recommended process to develop and implement academic detailing in Brazil (SUS Collaborating Centre for Technology Assessement and Excellence in Health, 2015). *AD*, academic detailing.

following recommended processes (Fig. 5.1) (SUS Collaborating Centre for Technology Assessement and Excellence in Health, 2015).

Besides the encouraging story from Brazil, there are not many national level programs from LMICs. However, there are some research studies, few of them are mentioned in Table 5.3:

SUSTAINABILITY OF ACADEMIC DETAILING CENTERS

Academic detailing centers should not be funded by pharmaceutical industries or any potential donors, which may have a conflict of interest to promote the sales of particular medicine or group of medicines manufactured by particular companies. So, sustainability of academic detailing centers is a challenge, especially in LMICs, where there are inadequate resources to fund the healthcare system. Since the introduction of academic detailing program in 1983 in the United States, many high-income countries such as the United States, Canada, Sweden, and Australia adopted the program and they currently have good academic detailing centers and programs in their settings as mentioned in previous section of this chapter. There are several economic analyses of academic detailing programs, and many studies have reported that benefits of academic detailing program overcome the operating cost of the academic detailing program (Gandjour & Lauterbach, 2005; Naughton, Feely, & Bennett, 2009; Shaw et al., 2003;

Table 5.3 Some Examples of Academic Detailing Programs in Low- and Middle-Income Countries

Country (References)	Description of Academic Detailing Programs
Sudan (Awad et al., 2006)	Twenty health centers in Sudan were classified into four different groups: (1) no intervention, (2) audit and feedback, (3) audit and feedback + academic detailing, and (4) audit and feedback + seminars. The impact of these interventions was studied in the prescribing practices of antimicrobials. Academic detailing when combined with audit and feedback improved antimicrobials prescribing behavior of healthcare professionals.
Argentina and Uruguay (Althabe et al., 2008)	A multifaceted intervention (including academic detailing) was conducted in 19 maternity hospitals of Argentina and Uruguay. The main objective of intervention was to improve obstetrical care. Academic detailing significantly increased the prophylactic use of oxytocin and decreased the use of episiotomy, thus improving obstetrical care.
Brazil (Silva et al., 2013)	A randomized controlled trial was conducted in a medical cooperative in Brazil. This study examined the effectiveness of academic detailing of obstetricians compared with clinical practice guidelines mailshot and no intervention, on the screening of pregnant women for Group B *Streptococcus*. Academic detailing increased the prevalence of Group B *Streptococcus* screening in pregnant women.
India (Bhargava, Greg, & Shields, 2010)	Academic detailing program coupled with provision of generic medication voucher was provided as the intervention. The main objective of the trial was to determine whether supplementing existing academic detailing initiatives with a generic voucher program would increase the generic dispensing ratio compared with academic detailing alone. Result suggested academic detailing coupled with generic medication voucher program was more effective when compared with academic detailing alone.
Nepal (Khanal, 2010)	Academic detailing was conducted to the primary healthcare providers in a district of Nepal on the management of childhood diarrhea. Academic detailing was successful in improving knowledge, attitude, and practice of healthcare providers about the management of childhood diarrhea. There was also a marked improvement in their prescribing behavior and decrease in the out-of-pocket payment for the patients.

Simon et al., 2007; Soumerai & Avorn, 1986); however in some cases it may not be most cost-effective means, and thus we need to consider other outcomes as well. Hence, many academic detailing programs are generally funded by the governments, not-for-profit organizations, or other charity organizations to make the program sustainable. However, one article reported that one of the academic detailing centers in Canada was closed and some were on the verge of closing because expected outcomes were not profitable when compared with the investment (Kondro, 2007). This is one of the challenges for sustainability of centers. Although there is documentation regarding the long history and good practice of academic detailing in high-income countries, there is a lack of such studies from LMICs. Therefore, the economic feasibility and sustainability of academic detailing in LMICs are still a matter of research.

ACHIEVEMENTS

Academic detailing in high-income countries has been evolved from its infancy state to more developed models within the last four decades. They are now one of the means to promote rational prescribing, provide unbiased healthcare information, and promote evidence-based practice in such countries. However, in LMICs, the concept of academic detailing is slowly emerging. Although there are not many evidence on the establishment of large-scale academic detailing programs in LMICs, there is evidence about the academic detailing as a pilot project or a research in some LMICs. Recent advances in academic detailing from LMICs, such as Brazil, Argentina, Uruguay, Sudan, India, Nepal and others, have suggested there is the scope of academic detailing programs in LMICs as well (Althabe et al., 2008; Bhargava et al., 2010; Costa et al., 2015, 2016; Khanal, 2010; Khanal et al., 2013; Shankar et al., 2009). Academic detailing conducted in such LMICs had contributed to providing health- and medicine-related information, improving knowledge, attitude, and practice of healthcare professionals and improving the prescribing behavior of healthcare professionals.

CHALLENGES

Some barriers on academic detailing have been documented from high-income countries. For example, healthcare professionals in the Netherlands identified that the information in academic detailing was not new and could have been obtained by other means. They also felt that the information provided to them was politically colored and was designed to cut the government healthcare expenditure. They perceived that the educational visits were time-consuming (Allen et al., 2007; Habraken et al., 2003). This type of opinion brings the question mark on the acceptability of academic detailing programs among the healthcare providers. These types of limitations can also be expected in LMICs; however, this type of barrier may not be applicable to many LMICs. In many countries, patients pay for the treatment out of their pocket. In addition to aforementioned challenges, some other potential challenges in LMICs can be as follows.

POOR HEALTH INFORMATION SYSTEM IN LOW- AND MIDDLE-INCOME COUNTRIES

The information provided in the academic detailing is usually tailored according to the need of the place. The information can be evidence based if there are local data about the epidemiology of the diseases, use of medicines, evidence of medicines efficiency/adverse drug reactions on the local population, and so on. Many LMICs have poor health information system (Jones, Rudin, Perry, & Shekelle, 2014; Ledikwe et al., 2014; Mills, 2014; Sheikh, 2014). This may lead to difficulty in selecting the potential topic for academic detailing and also limits evidence that should be provided to the healthcare professionals.

LACK OF TRAINED HUMAN RESOURCES

Due to globalization, many LMICs are facing emigration of capable human resources to high-income countries in search of high income and better quality of life or other reasons (Docquier, Lohest, & Marfouk, 2007; Girma et al., 2016; Kuehn, 2007). They face many challenges to retain capable human resources. Academic detailing requires highly educated and trained personnel. Therefore, brain drain can be one of the major challenges of implementing academic detailing programs in LMICs.

UNAWARENESS ABOUT EVIDENCE-BASED PRACTICE AND POORLY REGULATED HEALTHCARE PROFESSIONALS PRACTICE

There have been reports of lack of evidence-based practice in many LMICs (Behague, Tawiah, Rosato, Some, & Morrison, 2009). This can be attributed either to unawareness of healthcare professionals about evidence-based practice or poorly regulated health professional practice in LMICs (Hogerzeil, 1995; Mills & Colclough, 1997; Reardon, 2014). In many instances, we find their prescribing methods are either motivated by commercial interest or by their personal judgment and/or experience for clinical decision-making. In such case, it is necessary to make aware healthcare professionals about the importance of evidence-based practice and regulate the practice properly prior to planning academic detailing programs (Chow et al., 2013; Mills & Colclough, 1997).

COMMERCIAL INTEREST OF PHARMACEUTICAL COMPANIES

Pharmaceutical companies spend a lot of amount in the promotion of their product (Ahmed & Saeed, 2014; Kohler, Mackey, & Ovtcharenko, 2014; Street, 2015). They may influence prescribing behavior of healthcare professionals by giving any incentives or by influencing them through other means, for example, by providing detailing through their representatives. The aim of both pharmaceutical companies and academic detailers is to bring changes in the prescribing behavior of healthcare professionals, but it may not be in different directions. Academic detailing may find it difficult to compete with the financial strength of pharmaceutical companies, especially in LMICs where pharmaceutical promotions and marketing are less regulated.

LACK OF FINANCIAL RESOURCES

Academic detailing constitutes of different expenses, such as salaries to staffs, travel allowances to academic detailers, bursaries to participants, printing of different educational tools, and a good source of health and medicine information. Academic detailing centers cannot be funded by pharmaceutical companies or other bodies, which may have a potential conflict of interest. They should ideally fund by government, not-for-profit organizations, or universities. Government, nongovernment organizations, and universities in LMICs do not usually have adequate financial resources. Therefore, economic problems may limit academic detailing programs.

RECOMMENDATIONS: THE WAY FORWARD

Many types of research on academic detailing programs from LMICs are required to prove that academic detailing in LMICs can be as effective as high-income countries. As any intervention, academic detailing should be planned, implemented, and evaluated properly to make it successful. Combination of models suggested by Khanal, Palaian, Shankar, Mishra, and Ibrahim (2009) and Brazilian Group (SUS Collaborating Centre for Technology Assessement and Excellence in Health, 2015) can be helpful on proposing a simple implementation and evaluation model to investigate the feasibility of academic detailing centers in the countries (Fig. 5.2).

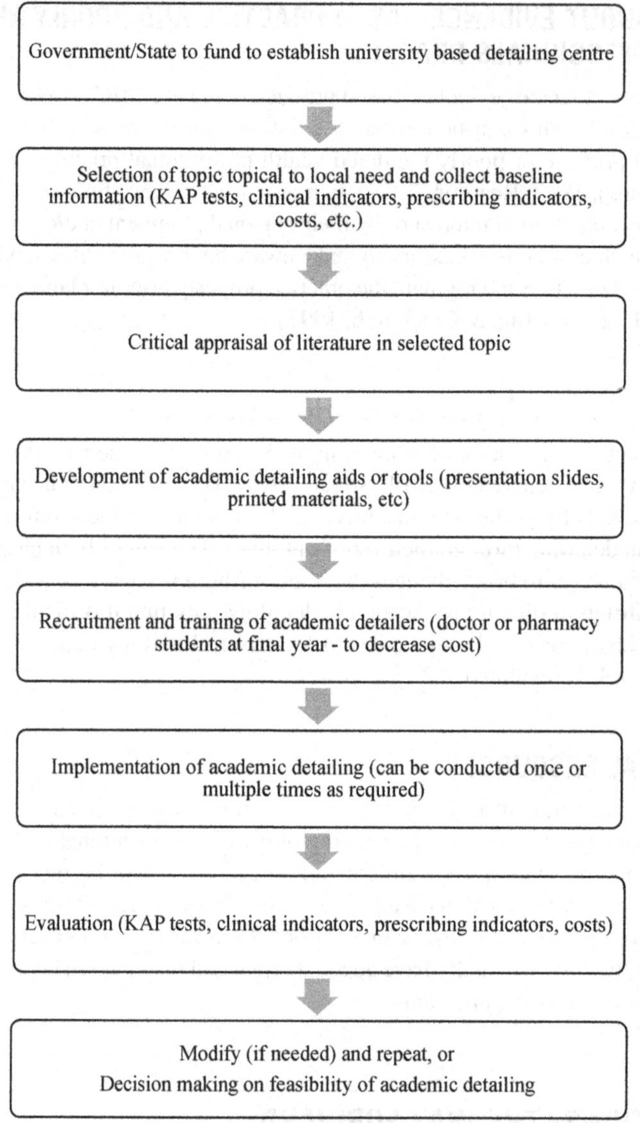

FIGURE 5.2

Proposed model to evaluate the feasibility of academic detailing in low- and middle-income countries. *KAP*, knowledge, attitude, and practice.

If implementation and evaluation of academic detailing as a pilot/trial shows promising results, attention should be given to scale it and make it sustainable. Some seed money from government or not-for-profit organizations or charitable organizations should be sought as the capital investment to fund the program. More sources should be sought to manage operational costs. One of the potential ways to make academic detailing programs sustainable is spending money on such academic detailing programs, which could result in cost saving, for example, using academic detailing to promote generic prescribing, thus directly saving money and discouraging healthcare professionals from prescribing less safe and obsolete medicine (Bhargava et al., 2010; Kersnik & Peklar, 2006). Another topic where academic detailing can be implemented to save cost is discouraging the healthcare professionals prescribing antimicrobials when not needed. It helps global fight against antimicrobial resistance and also directly saves the cost (Smith & Coast, 2013; World Health Organization, 2014). Cost saved from these improvements in prescribing behavior can be potentially used for sustaining academic detailing centers in LMICs.

CONCLUSION

Academic detailing is a tailored educational outreach program in which a trained health professional visits healthcare professionals in their practice settings. It is similar as pharmaceutical representatives visiting the healthcare professionals but to deliver the unbiased evidence-based information. Since its discovery in the early 1980s in the United States, it has been practicing in many high-income countries. Academic detailing programs are used for various purposes including providing information to healthcare professionals; improving their knowledge attitude and practice; influencing their prescribing; and promoting evidence-based practice. These programs are well developed in high-income countries, but they are at a very fundamental stage in the LMICs. They are only conducted as the pilot level or as a research. There are no recognized academic detailing bodies in almost all LMICs. But early evidence from LMICs suggests that the academic detailing if implemented can be as effective as those of high-income countries. Recent evidence from LMICs suggests that research studies in academic detailing will likely grow, and in this process we can assume that few countries are likely to develop academic detailing programs in their settings. There are some challenges to implementing academic detailing programs in LMICs, which include lack of funding, lack of human resources, lack of health information, and probable strong influence of pharmaceutical detailing.

LESSONS LEARNED

Following lessons were learned from this chapter:

- Academic detailing is one of the proven strategies to provide information to healthcare professionals, influence their prescribing, and promote evidence-based practice.
- Academic detailing though has been practiced in high-income countries since a long time, and many high-income countries already have to exit academic detailing structure; however, the concept is still at a premature level in the LMICs.
- Academic detailing should be promoted in LMICs to provide unbiased information to healthcare professionals, thus promoting the rational use of medicine.
- Academic detailing in LMICs can be a challenge, mostly due to economic reasons; governments and other relevant stakeholders should investigate whether academic detailing centers are economically feasible in their countries.

REFERENCES

Abula, T., & Kedir, M. (2017). The pattern of antibiotic usage in surgical in-patients of a teaching hospital, northwest Ethiopia. *The Ethiopian Journal of Health Development (EJHD)*, *18*(1).

Ahmed, R. R., & Saeed, A. (2014). Pharmaceutical drug promotion practices in Pakistan: Issues in ethical and non-ethical pharmaceutical practices. *Middle-east Journal of Scientific Research*, *20*(11), 1630–1640.

Allen, M., Ferrier, S., O'Connor, N., & Fleming, I. (2007). Family physicians' perceptions of academic detailing: A quantitative and qualitative study. *BMC Medical Education*, *7*(1), 36. http://dx.doi.org/10.1186/1472-6920-7-36.

Althabe, F., Buekens, P., Bergel, E., Belizan, J., Campbell, M., Moss, N., … Guidelines Trial, G. (2008). A behavioral intervention to improve obstetrical care. *New England Journal of Medicine*, *358*(18), 1929–1940. http://dx.doi.org/10.1056/NEJMsa071456.

Avorn, J. (2017). Academic detailing: "marketing" the best evidence to clinicians. *Journal of American Medical Association*, *317*(4), 361–362. http://dx.doi.org/10.1001/jama.2016.16036.

Avorn, J., & Soumerai, S. B. (1983). Improving drug-therapy decisions through educational outreach: A randomized controlled trial of academically based detailing. *New England Journal of Medicine*, *308*(24), 1457–1463.

Awad, A., Eltayeb, I., & Baraka, O. (2006). *European Journal of Clinical Pharmacology*, *62*(2), 135–142. http://dx.doi.org/10.1007/s00228-005-0089-4.

Axon, R. N., Penney, F. T., Kyle, T. R., Zapka, J., Marsden, J., Zhao, Y., … Moran, W. P. (2014). A hospital discharge summary quality improvement program featuring individual and team-based feedback and academic detailing. *American Journal of Medical Sciences*, *347*(6), 472–477. http://dx.doi.org/10.1097/MAJ.0000000000000171.

Behague, D., Tawiah, C., Rosato, M., Some, T., & Morrison, J. (2009). Evidence-based policy-making: The implications of globally-applicable research for context-specific problem-solving in developing countries. *Social Science & Medicine*, *69*(10), 1539–1546. http://dx.doi.org/10.1016/j.socscimed.2009.08.006.

Bhargava, V., Greg, M. E., & Shields, M. C. (2010). Addition of generic medication vouchers to a pharmacist academic detailing program: Effects on the generic dispensing ratio in a physician-hospital organization. *Journal of Managed Care Pharmacy*, *16*(6), 384–392. http://dx.doi.org/10.18553/jmcp.2010.16.6.384.

van Boven, J. F., Chavannes, N. H., van der Molen, T., Rutten-van Molken, M. P., Postma, M. J., & Vegter, S. (2014). Clinical and economic impact of non-adherence in COPD: A systematic review. *Respiratory Medicine*, *108*(1), 103–113. http://dx.doi.org/10.1016/j.rmed.2013.08.044.

Broadhurst, N. A., Barton, C. A., Rowett, D., Yelland, L., Martin, D. K., Gialamas, A., & Beilby, J. J. (2007). A before and after study of the impact of academic detailing on the use of diagnostic imaging for shoulder complaints in general practice. *BMC Family Practice*, *8*(1), 12.

Chow, C. K., Teo, K. K., Rangarajan, S., Islam, S., Gupta, R., Avezum, A., … Investigators, P. S. (2013). Prevalence, awareness, treatment, and control of hypertension in rural and urban communities in high-, middle-, and low-income countries. *Journal of American Medical Association*, *310*(9), 959–968. http://dx.doi.org/10.1001/jama.2013.184182.

Costa, J. D. O., Almeida-Brasil, C. C., Godman, B., Fischer, M. A., Dartnell, J., Heaney, A., … Guerra, A. A. (2016). Implementation of clinical guidelines in Brazil: Should academic detailing be used? *Journal of Pharmaceutical Health Services Research*, *7*(2), 105–115.

Costa, J., Almeida-Brasil, C., Lemos, L., Gomes, R., Acurcio, F., Alvares, J., & Guerra Junior, A. (2015). Brazilian guideline for academic detailing: A need to improve health care. *Value in Health*, *18*(7), A854. http://dx.doi.org/10.1016/j.jval.2015.09.451.

Davey, P., Brown, E., Charani, E., Fenelon, L., Gould, I. M., Holmes, A., … Wilcox, M. (2013). Interventions to improve antibiotic prescribing practices for hospital inpatients. *Cochrane Database Syst Rev*, *30*(4), CD003543. http://dx.doi.org/10.1002/14651858.CD003543.pub3.

Davies, D. A. (1998). Does CME work? An analysis of the effect of educational activities on physician performance or health care outcomes. *The International Journal of Psychiatry in Medicine*, *28*(1), 21–39.

Davies, D., & Taylor-Vaisey, A. (1997). Translating guidelines into practice: A systematic review of theoretic concepts, practical experience and research evidence in the adoption of clinical practice guidelines. *Canadian Medical Association Journal*, *157*(4), 408–416.

Davies, D. A., Thomson, M. A., Oxman, A., & Haynes, R. B. (1995). Changing physician performance. A systematic review of the effect of continuing medical education strategies. *Journal of American Medical Association*, *274*(9), 700–705.

Docquier, F., Lohest, O., & Marfouk, A. (2007). Brain drain in developing countries. *The World Bank Economic Review*, *21*(2), 193–218.

Duerden, M., Gogna, N., Godman, B., Eden, K., Mallinson, M., & Sullivan, N. (2004). Current national initiatives and policies to control drug costs in Europe: UK perspective. *The Journal of Ambulatory Care Management*, *27*(2), 132–138.

Dyrkorn, R., Gjelstad, S., Espnes, K. A., & Lindbæk, M. (2016). Peer academic detailing on use of antibiotics in acute respiratory tract infections. A controlled study in an urban Norwegian out-of-hours service. *Scandinavian Journal of Primary Health Care*, *34*(2), 180–185.

Ersek, M., Neradilek, M. B., Herr, K., Jablonski, A., Polissar, N., & Du Pen, A. (2016). Pain management algorithms for implementing best practices in nursing Homes: Results of a randomized controlled trial. *Journal of the American Medical Directors Association*, *17*(4), 348–356. http://dx.doi.org/10.1016/j.jamda.2016.01.001.

Falzon, D., Schunemann, H., Harausz, E., Gonzalez-Angulo, L., Lienhardt, C., Jaramillo, E., & Weyer, K. (2017). World Health Organization treatment guidelines for drug-resistant tuberculosis, 2016 update. *European Respiratory Journal*, *49*(3), 1602308. http://dx.doi.org/10.1183/13993003.02308-2016.

Fischer, M. A. (2016). Academic detailing in Diabetes: Using outreach education to improve the quality of care. *Current Diabetes Reports*, *16*(10), 98.

Freeland, K. N., Cogdill, B. R., Ross, C. A., Sullivan, C. O., Drayton, S. J., VandenBerg, A., … Garrsion, K. L. (2015). Adherence to evidence-based treatment guidelines for bipolar depression in an inpatient setting. *American Journal of Health System Pharmacists*, *72*(23 Suppl. 3), S156–S161. http://dx.doi.org/10.2146/sp150023.

Gandjour, A., & Lauterbach, K. W. (2005). How much does it cost to change the behavior of health professionals? A mathematical model and an application to academic detailing. *Medical Decision Making*, *25*(3), 341–347.

Girma, S., Kitaw, Y., Ye-Ebiy, Y., Seyoum, A., Desta, H., & Teklehaimanot, A. (2016). Human resource development for health in Ethiopia: challenges of achieving the millennium development goals. *The Ethiopian Journal of Health Development (EJHD)*, *21*(3).

Gjelstad, S., Fetveit, A., Straand, J., Dalen, I., Rognstad, S., & Lindbaek, M. (2006). Can antibiotic prescriptions in respiratory tract infections be improved? A cluster-randomized educational intervention in general practice–the Prescription Peer Academic Detailing (Rx-PAD) Study [NCT00272155]. *BMC Health Services Research*, *6*(1), 75.

Gjelstad, S., Hoye, S., Straand, J., Brekke, M., Dalen, I., & Lindbaek, M. (2013). Improving antibiotic prescribing in acute respiratory tract infections: Cluster randomised trial from Norwegian general practice (prescription peer academic detailing (Rx-PAD) study). *British Medical Journal*, *347*, f4403. http://dx.doi.org/10.1136/bmj.f4403.

Grimshaw, J., Shirran, L., Thomas, R., Mowatt, G., Fraser, C., Bero, L., … O'Brien, M. A. (2002). *Changing provider behaviour: An overview of systematic reviews of interventions to promote implementation of research findings by healthcare professionals. Getting research findings into practice* (2nd ed.). .

Habraken, H., Janssens, I., Soenen, K., Van Driel, M., Lannoy, J., & Bogaert, M. (2003). Pilot study on the feasibility and acceptability of academic detailing in general practice. *European Journal of Clinical Pharmacology*, *59*(3), 253–260. http://dx.doi.org/10.1007/s00228-003-0602-6.

Haegerich, T. M., Paulozzi, L. J., Manns, B. J., & Jones, C. M. (2014). What we know, and don't know, about the impact of state policy and systems-level interventions on prescription drug overdose. *Drug and Alcohol Dependence, 145*, 34–47.

Hesse, B., Nelson, D., Kreps, G., Croyle, R., Arora, N., Rimer, B., & Viswanath, K. (2005). Trust and sources of health information: The impact of the Internet and its implications for health care providers: Findings from the first health information national trends survey. *Archives of Internal Medicine, 165*(22), 2618–2624. http://dx.doi.org/10.1001/archinte.165.22.2618.

Hogerzeil, H. V. (1995). Promoting rational prescribing: An international perspective. *British Journal of Clinical Pharmacology, 39*(1), 1–6.

Janssens, I., De Meyere, M., Habraken, H., Soenen, K., Van Driel, M., Christiaens, T., & Bogaert, M. (2005). Barriers to academic detailers: A qualitative study in general practice. *European Journal of General Practice, 11*(2), 59–63.

Jin, M., Naumann, T., Regier, L., Bugden, S., Allen, M., Salach, L., ... Dolovich, L. (2012). A brief overview of academic detailing in Canada: Another role for pharmacists. *Canadian Pharmacists Journal/Revue des Pharmaciens du Canada, 145*(3), 142–146. e142.

Jones, S. S., Rudin, R. S., Perry, T., & Shekelle, P. G. (2014). Health information technology: An updated systematic review with a focus on meaningful use. *Annals of Internal Medicine, 160*(1), 48–54.

Katz, D. A., Holman, J., Johnson, S., Hillis, S. L., Ono, S., Stewart, K., ... Vander Weg, M. (2013). Implementing smoking cessation guidelines for hospitalized veterans: Effects on nurse attitudes and performance. *Jornal of General Internal Medicine, 28*(11), 1420–1429. http://dx.doi.org/10.1007/s11606-013-2464-7.

Kersnik, J., & Peklar, J. (2006). Attitudes of Slovene general practitioners towards generic drug prescribing and comparison with international studies. *Journal of Clinical Pharmacy and Therapeutics, 31*(6), 577–583.

Khanal, S. (2010). A study assessing the impact of academic detailing program on childhood diarrhoea management among the primary healthcare providers. In *Banke region*. Nepal: Universiti Sains Malaysia.

Khanal, S., Ibrahim, M. I. M., Shankar, P. R., Palaian, S., & Mishra, P. (2013). Evaluation of academic detailing programme on childhood diarrhoea management by primary healthcare providers in Banke district of Nepal. *Journal of Health, Population and Nutrition, 31*(2), 231–242.

Khanal, S., Palaian, S., Shankar, P. R., Mishra, P., & Ibrahim, M. I. M. (2009). Academic detailing as a possible source of drug information in the context of Nepal: A short review. *Journal of Clinical and Diagnostic Research, 3*(4), 1697–1703.

Kohler, J. C., Mackey, T. K., & Ovtcharenko, N. (2014). Why the MDGs need good governance in pharmaceutical systems to promote global health. *BMC Public Health, 14*(1), 63. http://dx.doi.org/10.1186/1471-2458-14-63.

Kondro, W. (2007). *Academic drug detailing: An evidence-based alternative*. Can Med Assoc.

Kuehn, B. M. (2007). Global shortage of health workers, brain drain stress developing countries. *Journal of American Medical Association, 298*(16), 1853–1855. http://dx.doi.org/10.1001/jama.298.16.1853.

Ledikwe, J. H., Grignon, J., Lebelonyane, R., Ludick, S., Matshediso, E., Sento, B. W., ... Semo, B.-W. (2014). Improving the quality of health information: A qualitative assessment of data management and reporting systems in Botswana. *Health Research Policy and Systems, 12*(1), 7. http://dx.doi.org/10.1186/1478-4505-12-7.

Markey, P., & Schattner, P. (2001). Promoting evidence-based medicine in general practice-the impact of academic detailing. *Family Practice, 18*(4), 364–366.

Mills, A. (2014). Health care systems in low- and middle-income countries. *New England Journal of Medicine, 370*(6), 552–557. http://dx.doi.org/10.1056/NEJMra1110897.

Mills, A., & Colclough, C. (1997). Improving the efficiency of public sector health services in developing countries: Bureaucratic versus market approaches. *Marketizing Education and Health in Developing Countries: Miracle or Mirage*, 245–274.

Mold, J. W., Fox, C., Wisniewski, A., Lipman, P. D., Krauss, M. R., Harris, D. R., ... Frame, P. (2014). Implementing asthma guidelines using practice facilitation and local learning collaboratives: A randomized controlled trial. *The Annals of Family Medicine, 12*(3), 233–240.

Naughton, C., Feely, J., & Bennett, K. (2009). A RCT evaluating the effectiveness and cost-effectiveness of academic detailing versus postal prescribing feedback in changing GP antibiotic prescribing. *Journal of Evaluation in Clinical Practice*, *15*(5), 807–812. http://dx.doi.org/10.1111/j.1365-2753.2008.01099.x.

Newton-Syms, F. A., Dawson, P. H., Cooke, J., Feely, M., Booth, T. G., Jerwood, D., & Calvert, R. T. (1992). The influence of an academic representative on prescribing by general practitioners. *British Journal of Clinical Pharmacology*, *33*(1), 69–73.

O'brien, M., Rogers, S., Jamtvedt, G., Oxman, A., Odgaard-Jensen, J., Kristoffersen, D., … Davis, D. (2008). Educational outreach visits: Effects on professional practice and health care outcomes (review). *The Cochrane Library*, *3*, 1–64.

Oliver, K., Innvar, S., Lorenc, T., Woodman, J., & Thomas, J. (2014). A systematic review of barriers to and facilitators of the use of evidence by policymakers. *BMC Health Services Research*, *14*(1), 2.

Paton, C., Adebowale, O., & Okocha, C. I. (2008). The use of academic detailing to improve evidence based prescribing of risperidone long acting injection. *International Journal of Psychiatry in Clinical Practice*, *12*(3), 210–214.

Pittenger, K., Williams, B. L., Mecklenburg, R. S., & Blackmore, C. C. (2015). Improving acute respiratory infection care through nurse phone care and academic detailing of physicians. *The Journal of the American Board of Family Medicine*, *28*(2), 195–204.

Reardon, S. (2014). Antibiotic resistance sweeping developing world: Bacteria are increasingly dodging extermination as drug availability outpaces regulation. *Nature*, *509*(7499), 141–143.

Ross-Degnan, D., Soumerai, S. B., Goel, P. K., Bates, J., Makhulo, J., Dondi, N., … Hogan, R. (1996). The impact of face-to-face educational outreach on diarrhoea treatment in pharmacies. *Health Policy and Planning*, *11*(3), 308–318.

Rowett, D. (2002). Formation of an SHPA academic detailing/educational outreach COSP. *Journal of Pharmacy Practice and Research*, *32*(2), 87–89.

Royal Australian and New Zealand College of Psychiatrists. (2017). Royal Australian and New Zealand College of Psychiatrists clinical practice guidelines for the treatment of schizophrenia and related disorders. *Australian & New Zealand Journal of Psychiatry*.

Sackett, D. L. (1997). *Evidence-based medicine* Paper presented at the seminars in perinatology.

Shankar, P., Jha, N., Shrestha, R., Bajracharya, O., & Thapa, H. (2009). Academic detailing at KIST Medical College, Lalitpur, Nepal: Initial experiences. *Hong Kong Medical Journal*, *15*, 403–404.

Shaw, J., Harris, P., Keogh, G., Graudins, L., Perks, E., & Thomas, P. (2003). Error reduction: Academic detailing as a method to reduce incorrect prescriptions. *European Journal of Clinical Pharmacology*, *59*(8–9), 697–699.

Sheikh, M. (2014). Digital health information system in Africa's resource poor countries: Current challenges and opportunities. *Journal of Health Informatics in Developing Countries*, *8*(1).

Silva, J. M., Stein, A. T., Schunemann, H. J., Bordin, R., Kuchenbecker, R., & de Lourdes Drachler, M. (2013). Academic detailing and adherence to guidelines for group B streptococci prenatal screening: A randomized controlled trial. *BMC Pregnancy and Childbirth*, *13*(1), 68. http://dx.doi.org/10.1186/1471-2393-13-68.

Simon, S. R., Rodriguez, H. P., Majumdar, S. R., Kleinman, K., Warner, C., Salem-Schatz, S., … Prosser, L. A. (2007). Economic analysis of a randomized trial of academic detailing interventions to improve use of antihypertensive medications. *The Journal of Clinical Hypertension*, *9*(1), 15–20.

Smith, R., & Coast, J. (2013). The true cost of antimicrobial resistance. *British Medical Journal*, *346*, f1493.

Soumerai, S. B., & Avorn, J. (1986). Economic and policy analysis of university-based drug" detailing. *Medical Care*, 313–331.

Soumerai, S. B., & Avorn, J. (1990). Principles of educational outreach ('academic detailing') to improve clinical decision making. *Journal of American Medical Association*, *263*(4), 549–556.

Spurling, G. K., Mansfield, P. R., Montgomery, B. D., Lexchin, J., Doust, J., Othman, N., & Vitry, A. I. (2010). Information from pharmaceutical companies and the quality, quantity, and cost of physicians' prescribing: A systematic review. *PLoS Medicine*, *7*(10), e1000352. http://dx.doi.org/10.1371/journal.pmed.1000352.

Street, A. (2015). Food as pharma: Marketing nutraceuticals to India's rural poor. *Critical Public Health*, *25*(3), 361–372.

SUS Collaborating Centre for Technology Assessement and Excellence in Health. (2015). *Gudeline: Academic detailing*. Retrieved from Minas Gerais, Brazil http://www.ccates.org.br/content/_pdf/en_PUB_1437678333.pdf.

Walley, T., Mrazek, M., & Mossialos, E. (2005). Regulating pharmaceutical markets: Improving efficiency and controlling costs in the UK. *International Journal of Health Planning and Management*, *20*(4), 375–398.

Weller, D., May, F., Rowett, D., Esterman, A., Pinnock, C., Nicholson, S., … Silagy, C. (2003). Promoting better use of the PSA test in general practice: Randomized controlled trial of educational strategies based on outreach visits and mailout. *Family Practice*, *20*(6), 655–661.

Williams, J., Petrov, G., Kennedy, U., Halpenny, J., & Doherty, C. P. (2017). Moving evidence based guidelines for seizures into practice in the emergency department: What's stopping us? *Epilepsy & Behavior*, *72*, 72–77.

World Health Organization. (2014). *Antimicrobial resistance: Global report on surveillance*. World Health Organization.

Yamamoto, M. (2013). Academic detailing for best practice and pharmacists' role. *Yakugaku Zasshi: Journal of the Pharmaceutical Society of Japan*, *134*(3), 355–362.

Yourman, L., Concato, J., & Agostini, J. V. (2008). Use of computer decision support interventions to improve medication prescribing in older adults: A systematic review. *The American Journal of Geriatric Pharmacotherapy*, *6*(2), 119–129.

SECTION 3

ECONOMIC EVALUATION AND MEDICINES EXPENDITURE IN LOW- AND MIDDLE-INCOME COUNTRIES

CHAPTER

ECONOMIC EVALUATION AND MEDICINES EXPENDITURE IN DEVELOPING COUNTRIES

6

Gianluigi Casadei, Paola Minghetti
University of Milan, Milan, Italy

CHAPTER OUTLINE

INTRODUCTION

People's healthcare is a major commitment for all national governments. Setting and implementing policies on access to medicines is therefore a priority in progressing toward equitable access to drugs and their appropriate use, monitoring affordability, and preserving the medium- to long-term sustainability of the insurance service. The pillars of any effective policy aimed to provide a comprehensive framework for the development of a national pharmaceutical sector should be: (1) medicine selection, use, and quality; (2) sustainable financing, affordable prices, and comparable availability in public and private sectors, (3) governance; (4) monitoring on appropriate use; and (5) deployment of trained personnel for health. Identification of innovations that effectively improve availability, social

Social and Administrative Aspects of Pharmacy in Low- and Middle-Income Countries. http://dx.doi.org/10.1016/B978-0-12-811228-1.00006-6

acceptability, and financial accessibility of underserved communities to essential medicines is the most important area to focus on to progress on medicine access equity (Bigdeli, Javadi, Hoebert, Laing, & Ranson, 2013).

This task is complex especially for low- and middle-income countries (LMICs) where poor availability of essential medicines[1] is a major problem. The publication of WHO guidelines in 1988 (WHO, 1988) and 2001 (WHO, 2001) has enabled many nations to develop and implement their national medicine policies (Hoebert, van Dijk, Mantel-Teeuwisse, Leufkens, & Laing, 2013). A positive correlation has been shown between the number of implemented policies in 2002–08 and quality improvement in the use of essential medicines. This correlation was the strongest in the countries with the lowest per capita national wealth levels (Holloway & Henry, 2014). Four in five LMICs, which responded to a survey carried out by the WHO in 2015, reported a formal or at least informal health technology assessment (HTA) process supporting their decision-making path. This proportion was fully comparable with that reported by upper middle–income and high-income countries (62 out of 73). All 15 low-income and 85% of the 23 middle-income countries said they used HTA for planning and budgeting. These results seem quite reassuring, although it should be considered that 42 out of 80 LMICs did not participate in the survey, and that lack of anonymity of respondents may have encouraged favorable responses. In fact, only 13 (34%) LMICs reported having a national HTA organization or committee that produced HTA reports for the ministry of health. This percentage is probably more representative of the actual implementation of HTA in LMICs (WHO, 2015).

AFRICA

Availability and affordability of essential medicines are a problem in developing countries; it is a pressing issue particularly for inhabitants of sub-Saharan Africa (WHO, 2016; Zainol, Amin, Jusoff, Zahid, & Akpoviri, 2011). Although a low-income country such as Ethiopia has achieved remarkable progress in reducing maternal and child mortality (Desalegn, Solberg, & Kim, 2015), the access to essential medicines free of charge from public sector for the treatment of commonly prevalent diseases is a difficult challenge. Drugs are sold in both public and private sector even at higher prices compared with international references and are unaffordable for the lowest paid government unskilled workers (Abiye, Tesfaye, & Hawaze, 2013; Sado & Sufa, 2016).

Among low-income countries, Tanzania has made substantial advancement in access to quality essential medicines, which are supplied from public health facilities free of charge to the poorest, children below the age of 5 years, pregnant women, and elderly. A copayment (usually 50%) is requested to patients covered by the national insurance. This represents a considerable financial burden for the moderately poor.

Tanzania established its first list of essential medicine in the 1970s and introduced its Standard Treatment Guidelines and National Essential Medicine List in 1991. This guideline is periodically updated by committees of experts from referral hospitals and the Ministry of Health and Social

[1]Essential medicines are those that satisfy the priority healthcare needs of the population. They are selected with due regard to disease prevalence and public health relevance, evidence of clinical efficacy and safety, and comparative costs and cost-effectiveness. Essential medicines are intended to be available within the context of functioning health systems always in adequate amounts, in the appropriate dosage forms, with assured quality, and at a price the individual and the community can afford.

Welfare. The most frequently used criteria for assessment are efficacy, safety, availability, and affordability. International guidelines and drug promotion may be influential. Decision-making process is primarily based on observational experience on efficacy and safety rather than evidence, thus increasing the risk of adopting inefficient interventions. Only products available in Tanzania are selected and generics are favored to allow availability and affordability even when not available at public healthcare facilities. The total cost of treatment, rather than the unit price of single drugs, is considered especially for chronic diseases (Mori, Kaale, Ngalesoni, Norheim, & Robberstad, 2014). Few pharmacoeconomic studies have been conducted in Tanzania and their impact on the listing of drugs in the national list is minimal. Consistent adoption of HTA may represent a further step for improving the efficiency of the selection process and, overall, the availability and affordability of essential drugs (Mori & Robberstad, 2012).

The need for improving resource allocation and utilization is evident considering that in many African countries, funds are largely focused on major infectious diseases, leaving important gaps in treatment of noncommunicable diseases, which are rapidly spreading.

Pharmacoeconomic guidelines are implemented in two middle-income countries, South Africa and Egypt. Introduced after the demise of apartheid, the National Drug Policy for South Africa was focused on equity and access limited by high prices, unsustainable by most of the black population (Hoebert et al., 2013; Zuma, 1997). The policy document was first committed to arrange a transparent pricing structure, and the vast political support led to its implementation despite it was challenged in court by the pharmaceutical industry.

In 2013 the Ministry of Health and Population established a pharmacoeconomic unit entrusted to support pricing and reimbursement process to optimize resource allocation. Economic evaluation guidelines have been adopted shortly after Elsisi et al. (2013).

A comparative analysis of the guidelines in force in South Africa and Egypt is reported in Table 6.1 (EDA, 2016; Department of Health, 2012; ISPOR).

The two guidelines share the main parameters: perspective of the third-party payer; evaluation of approved indications; standard of care as main comparator; and pharmacoeconomic assessment techniques, which include cost-efficacy analysis, cost-minimization analysis, and cost-utility analysis (CUA) (thus targeting quality of life among primary outcomes). Direct medical costs are preferred and modeling is allowed if simple and applicable to real life. Egyptian guidelines seem less well defined, and this is probably explained by their recent introduction and the need to gain experience. The main problems encountered in Egypt are the lack of resources and funding and a fragmented healthcare system characterized by multiple sources of financing (Elmahdawy, 2016). Suboptimal capacity and fragmentation make guideline implementation difficult also in South Africa, where efforts are being made to standardize HTA process and to integrate it into the health system (McGee, 2016).

ASIAN REGION

The largest proportion of the world's population, about 4.2 billion people, resides in the Asia Pacific region. Due to the variety of administrations and economic contexts, health services are quite diversified, ranging from public-governed to private-dominated systems, and have achieved different results. South Korea, Malaysia, Taiwan, and Thailand have already accomplished almost full health coverage for more than 15 years, while other countries, such as China, Indonesia, and Vietnam, propose to reach

Table 6.1 Comparative Analysis of Pharmacoeconomic National Guidelines in South Africa and Egypt

	South Africa (2013) (Department of Health, 2012)	Egypt (2013) (EDA, 2016)
Technology	NCEs, label expansion.	–
Perspective	Third-party payer. Option to use a broader perspective where justified per specific considerations.	Relevant to research question and adapted to benefits for the healthcare service.
Indication	Approved indications only.	Primarily in approved indications.
Comparator	Standard of care for local practice.	Reimbursed healthcare technology for a given patient group.
Time horizon	Based on the natural course of the disease. Short-term analysis may be required based on the primary efficacy end point.	A period sufficient to observe the chosen outcome and resource consumption of the treatment alternatives.
Preferred analytical techniques	CMA, CEA, CUA, and CBA (choice should be justified). Sensitivity analyses required.	CMA, CEA, and CUA. Deterministic sensitivity analysis recommended.
Costs	Direct (indirect generally excluded).	Direct medical. Direct nonmedical and indirect assessed only in the sensitivity analysis.
Source of costs	No preferred source.	Preferably primary data collection; secondary data sources can be used.
Modeling	Allowed, but complex models are discouraged.	Allowed, if corresponds to real practice.
Financial impact analysis	Not specified.	Recommended.
PE assessment submission	Voluntary, may be required.	Recommended (expected to be mandatory in few years).

CBA, *cost-benefit analysis;* CEA, *cost-efficacy analysis;* CMA, *cost-minimization analysis;* CUA, *cost-utility analysis;* NCE, *new chemical entity;* PE, *pharmacoeconomic.*
Modified from ISPOR. (2016). Pharmacoeconomic guidelines around the world. Comparative table. *Available from https://www.ispor.org/PEguidelines/COMP1.asp.*

this goal at the beginning of the next decade. Full coverage is associated with significant results on public health. Reported life expectancy at birth and infant mortality rate, proxies of public health, are 81 years and 3/1000 live births, respectively, in South Korea compared with 71 years and 25/1000 in Indonesia. The resource demand is a critical issue for this gap considering coverage of 50 and 280 million people, respectively. The difficulty in finding additional resources to expand health services also affects the most advanced countries, such as China and Thailand, which already spend 12.5% and 14.2%, respectively, of government funding for health (Chootipongchaivat, Tritasavit, Luz, Teerawattanon, & Tantivess, 2015).

Therefore, the demand for HTA to support cost-effective allocation of resources, scarce by definition, is increasing, nourished by the health service reforms that have been implemented over the last two decades in the Asian region (Pharmacoeconomic and Outcomes Research are steadily moving forward in Asia, 2016).

MALAYSIA

The first HTA agency was established in Malaysia in 1995. The Malaysian Health Technology Assessment Section (MaHTAS) has the mandate to assess safety, cost-effectiveness, and overall efficiency of a wide range of health technologies, mainly programs, procedures, and medical devices. Recommendations are supporting the development of clinical guidelines and purchasing decisions within the public healthcare service, which covers all residents. A national drug formulary has been adopted recently, under the supervision of the Formulary and Pharmacoeconomic Unit in the Pharmaceutical Services Division (PSD). A pharmacoeconomic guideline has been introduced in 2012 (Pharmaceutical Services Division. Pharmacoeconomic guideline for Malaysia, 2012). Economic evaluations, mainly focused on societal costs, are now mandatory to support marketing authorization process (Table 6.2A), although pricing recommendations are not provided. The critical issues reported to

Table 6.2A Key Features of Pharmacoeconomic National Guidelines in Malaysia and South Korea

	Malaysia (2012) (Pharmaceutical Services Division. Pharmacoeconomic guideline for Malaysia, 2012)	**South Korea (2009–13) (Bae and Lee, 2009, 2013)**
Technology	Health technologies.	NCEs.
Perspective	Provider or funder. Patient and societal are encouraged.	Limited societal perspective.
Indication	Approved indications.	Approved indications.
Comparator	Most relevant alternative, including nondrug therapy. Placebo should not be used.	Most prevalent drug. Indirect comparison acceptable if it is not possible to acquire head-to-head data.
Time horizon	Long enough to capture all changes in cost and outcome of the intervention.	Sufficiently long to reflect all important differences in costs and outcomes. However, short-term analysis should be presented.
Preferred analytical techniques	CEA and CUA. Choice should be justified. Sensitivity analyses of all key parameters required (best and worst scenario).	CUA, CEA, and CMA. Sensitivity analysis required (multivariate recommended for critical parameters).
Costs	All (local) costs relevant to the chosen perspective. Societal cost preferred in any analysis.	All costs appropriate from a societal perspective. Cost of lost productivity should be presented separately.
Source of costs	Must be identified.	Low bias sources are preferred. Expert opinion should be avoided.
Modeling	Allowed, if clearly detailed and transparent.	Allowed, if simple and transparent.
Financial impact analysis	Required.	Budget impact required.
PE assessment submission	Mandatory.	Mandatory.

CEA, *cost-efficacy analysis;* CMA, *cost-minimization analysis;* CUA, *cost-utility analysis;* NCE, *new chemical entity;* PE, *pharmacoeconomic.*
Modified from ISPOR. Pharmacoeconomic guidelines around the world 2016. *Available from https://www.ispor.org/peguidelines/index.asp.*

slow down the full implementation of the guideline are quite common to several other developing countries: lack of funding, need to gain technical expertise, necessity of building up updated databases and setting continuous exchange of information, process transparency, and, overall, a defined role of HTA in decision-making (Aljunid, 2014).

SOUTH KOREA

In 2007, the Korean government began to implement a positive list system (PLS) to rationalize drug expenditure. Only new medicines offering good value for money are listed and selectively reimbursed at a negotiated price by the Korean National Health Insurance (NIH). The introduction of the PLS has been accompanied by the publication of the first version of Korean Pharmacoeconomic Evaluation guidelines; so, South Korea became the first Asian country to adopt economic assessment as part of the reimbursement decision-making process (Bae & Lee, 2009). A revised version has been released in 2013 (Table 6.2A). The preferred perspective is societal; consequently, CUA is the reference method, although local health utility data are almost missing; cost-effectiveness can be used when the quality-adjusted life year (QALY) is not an appropriate outcome measure (Bae, Lee, Bae, & Jang, 2013). Pricing recommendations are made on a case-by-case basis. For transparency, each assessment is made publicly available.

THAILAND

In Thailand, the Health Intervention and Technology Assessment Program (HITAP) has been introduced in 2007, as part of the National Drug Policy set in 1971 to ensure availability and affordability of all medicines. The first edition of Thai HTA guidelines was released in 2008 (Teerawattananon & Chaikledkaew, 2008) and then revised in 2012 (Chaikledkaew & Kittrongsiri, 2014). The current guidelines share the main characteristics of those adopted in other Asian countries: social perspective, CUA, and inclusion of direct and indirect costs (Table 6.2B). Nowadays, HITAP is reported to be part of the decision-making process in the development of the national list of essential medicines and the health coverage package (Chootipongchaivat et al., 2015). In 2007–11, several economic assessments have been made available on drugs for primary prevention of cardiovascular diseases, treatment of hepatitis B and C, osteoporosis, Alzheimer disease, chronic myeloid leukemia and colorectal cancer, and rare diseases. In selected cases, the negotiation of reimbursement price has referred to the cost per QALY threshold (Tantivess, 2013).

TAIWAN

The experience gained since 2007 in Taiwan sets a model for other countries that want to implement the HTA to support pricing and reimbursement decisions. The National Institute of Health Technology Assessment (NIHTA) is a nonprofit organization that assesses new drugs, medical devices, and medical services independently from governmental bodies and manufacturers. The NIHTA evaluates comparative cost-effectiveness and budget impact of the new technologies. HTA guidelines, summarized in Table 6.2B, are aligned with international methodologic standards (CDE, 2006). From 2007 to 2013, 250 HTA reports have supported the National Health Administration for reimbursement decisions (Chiu, Pwu, & Gau, 2015).

Table 6.2B Key Features of Pharmacoeconomic National Guidelines in China, Taiwan, and Thailand

	China (2011) (ISPOR, 2011)	Taiwan (2006) (CDE, 2006)	Thailand (2008–12) (Chaikledkaew & Kittrongsiri, 2014; Teerawattananon & Chaikledkaew, 2008)
Technology	NCEs.	NCEs.	NCEs, label expansion.
Perspective	Primarily societal.	Mainly societal (payer and others).	Depending on user, including patient.
Indication	Primarily approved indications.	Approved indications.	Approved indications.
Comparator	Primarily standard of care or conventional treatment.	Most effective and most frequently used (first choice).	The most effective alternative.
Time horizon	Long enough to capture main outcomes and major costs of the intervention.	Long enough to all significant outcomes and costs directly related to the new technology.	Long enough to capture full cost of the intervention.
Preferred analytical techniques	Primarily CUA. Sensitivity analyses for all assumptions.	CEA and CUA, depending on expected outcomes. Sensitivity analyses for all assumptions.	CUA recommended. One-way and probabilistic sensitivity analyses for each parameter (and all other sources of uncertainty).
Costs	Primarily direct medical costs; direct nonmedical cost and indirect cost if data available.	All costs relevant to the chosen perspective. Human capital approach for estimating indirect costs.	All costs relevant to the chosen perspective. Direct and indirect costs, if societal perspective is adopted.
Source of costs	–	Direct cost from the Bureau of National Health Insurance (BNHI); sources should be clearly identified and reflect local situation.	Reference unit cost and setting specific cost.
Modeling	Accepted: both decision tree and econometric framework.	Accepted; detailed description requested.	Accepted.
Financial impact analysis	Required. BIA recommended.	Required.	Required.
PE assessment submission	Initially voluntary, then recommended.	Voluntary.	Mandatory.

BIA, *budget impact analysis;* CEA, *cost-efficacy analysis;* CUA, *cost-utility analysis;* NCE, *new chemical entity;* PE, *pharmacoeconomic.*
Modified from ISPOR. Pharmacoeconomic guidelines around the world 2016. *Available from https://www.ispor.org/peguidelines/index.asp.*

CHINA (MAINLAND)

In 2009 the Chinese government launched a new, comprehensive healthcare reform nationwide with a systematic plan to reach universal health coverage in 2020. The reform is mainly focused on establishing a National Essential Medicine Policy (NEMP) to face poor accessibility and affordability of drugs, which have affected the Chinese people for decades, although China issued its first essential medicine list in 1982. The NEMP included specific policies on reimbursement, procurement, pricing, financing, quality, and rational use of medicines (Barber et al., 2013). Chinese healthcare facilities are classified as public and private, further divided into three levels: primary, secondary, and tertiary, depending on the specialization of the health services provided. Patients can buy drugs from either public or private facilities. Since the early 1980s, drug revenue has become an essential financial resource especially for primary healthcare centers. The 2009 reform is mainly focused on primary healthcare: urban and rural institutions receive government subsidies to sell essential medicines to patients for procurement prices plus a fixed distribution fee (zero-profit drug policy). The Essential Drug List included 307 generic medicines for common treatable diseases. Several surveys have been carried out to assess whether from 2009 to 2011 the reform has ameliorated their accessibility in primary healthcare and reduced patients' economic burden for purchasing.

The mean availability at primary care facilities of lowest-priced generics was 100% in Jiangsu Province, in eastern China, and their prices resulted almost comparable with International references. Treatments of common diseases, including diabetes, hypertension, hypercholesterolemia, asthma, respiratory infections, and depression, were affordable at costs ranging from 0.1 to 0.7 days' wages (Xi et al., 2015). In underdeveloped western China, two cross-sectional surveys showed that inflation-adjusted medicine prices have lowered, but the availability of the lowest-priced generics has decreased over time (Fang et al., 2013). Drug prices were reduced significantly in 2010, but a modest decrease was recorded in 2011, suggesting that more expensive branded medicines were preferred in the postreform period (Song, Bian, Petzold, Li, & Yin, 2014a). The rational use of medicine improved; however, the overprescription of antibiotics and injectable drugs was still common practice (Song, Bian, Petzold, Li, & Yin, 2014b; Yang, Liu, Ferrier, Zhou, & Zhang, 2013).

These results show that the "zero-profit" policy is favoring access and affordability of essential drugs. However, this concept is not yet widely accepted and there is room for improvement through the implementation of treatment guidelines, intense supervision, and continuing training for professionals and consumers (Hogerzeil & Jing, 2013; Song et al., 2014b). Extending this policy to secondary and tertiary levels can give a new impetus to progress on equitable access to health services (Xi et al., 2015).

As part of the healthcare reform, the Chinese government increased healthcare funding to ~US$63 billion in 2012—12-fold the expenditure in 2004—making cost-effective management of this impressive budget as a top priority for the success of the reform (Koh, Glaetzer, Chuen Li, & Zhang, 2016). China has four academic HTA institutes and the Center for Health Policy Evaluation and Technology Assessment (CHPETA) under the National Health and Family Planning Commission, the former MoH. The CHPETA has carried out several HTAs (Chootipongchaivat et al., 2015; Chen, Banta, & Tang, 2009). HTA guidelines have been released in 2011 (Table 6.2B) (ISPOR, 2011) and are not mandatory. A panel of experts has anticipated that economic evaluations will exploit when the Chinese market will open to noncommunicable diseases (Koh et al., 2016).

INDIA

Inequitable access to medicines characterizes the Indian healthcare service (Kotwani, 2013). More than a half of Indian population has no access to essential medicines in public hospitals. The private sector accounts for more than 80% of total healthcare spending and is mostly paid out of pocket by citizens, mainly to buy medicines. Although it is common notion that drug prices in India are low, they are reported to be overpriced and relatively unaffordable by most patients (Ahmad, Khan, & Patel, 2015). It is estimated that each year 20 million people in India fall below poverty threshold because of the purchase of medicines (Oberoi & Oberoi, 2014). Drug Price Control Order (DPCO) has been introduced in 1979 to control prices of 347 essential medicines. Since then the number of products under control decreased progressively (they were only 34 in 2002), until 2013, when the National Pharmaceutical Pricing Authority (NPPA) cut the prices of all the drugs originally included in the 1979 national list of essential medicines (NPPA, 2013). In 2014, a following attempt by NPPA to extend price control to additional 108 lifesaving medicines, including cancer drugs, cardiovascular treatments, and hypoglycemic agents, has been blocked by the Indian Government (Ahmad et al., 2015). The Draft Pharmaceutical Policy 2017, released by the Department of Pharmaceuticals in August 2017, may be a step forward in fostering the discussion on the need for a new health policy that makes essential drugs accessible at affordable prices to the common masses in an economic framework that promotes the development of the Indian pharmaceutical sector.

There is a lack of awareness about the concepts and the methodology of HTA in India (Nair, 2015). This situation is likely due to the dominance of the private health sector.

The HTA would have a *raison d'etre* only if the Indian government entrusted to extend the public health coverage. In that scenario, the HTA could play a role in setting drug pricing, prioritizing health interventions, and supporting development of clinical guidelines (Oberoi & Oberoi, 2014). This contribution would be key to provide equitable access to essential medicines to the expected most populous country in the world in 2030.

LATIN AMERICA

Latin American healthcare services are fragmented. In several countries, social security is the largest healthcare financier and provider, complemented by public and private systems. Health services consist mainly of compulsory benefits packages and formularies of essential medicines for public subsidy (Augustovski, Melendez, Lemgruber, & Drummond, 2011).

A comparative analysis of six Latin American countries confirms an overall fragmented scenario (Table 6.3), where: (1) reimbursement policies cover essential medicines, ranging from lack of reimbursement to compulsory benefit packages; (2) pricing is fifty–fifty administered or uncontrolled; and (3) financial control policies are based on different parameters, local cost indicators, or international pricing references.

Pharmacoeconomic guidelines have been introduced in Latin American countries where prices are administered. In fact, cost-effectiveness evaluation and financial impact analysis are increasingly recommended or made mandatory for supporting the reimbursement of new drugs, devices, or medical procedures (Table 6.4).

Table 6.3 Comparative Analysis of Pricing, Reimbursement, and Financial Control Policies in a Group of Latin American Countries

Country	Pricing Policy	Reimbursement Policy	Financial Control Policy
Argentina (Augustovski et al., 2011)	No formal price regulation. Direct agreements between insurance companies and manufacturers.	Essential medicines available in all primary care centers and subsidized in a variable proportion. Social security covers most high-cost technologies.	National reference pricing.
Colombia (Augustovski et al., 2011)	Administered maximum prices. Private arrangements between providers and manufacturers.	All services included in the compulsory benefit package (*Plan Obligatorio de Salud*) are reimbursed.	Per capita unit payment updated yearly. Budget impact analysis.
Guatemala (Augustovski et al., 2011)	Multilateral agreements for open contracting and a bidding process for essential drugs.	No reimbursement for the public sector.	–
Uruguay (Augustovski et al., 2011)	No price regulation.	Drugs listed in the compulsory formulary are paid by providers. Copayments requested in private sector.	Cost indicators.
Mexico (ISPOR, 2010; Moise and Docteur, 2007)	Administered prices (reference and maximum retail) for patented medicines. Price-oriented public tenders.	Social insurances provide health services at no cost.	International reference pricing.
Brazil (PMLiV, 2012)	Administered prices of drugs listed in the National List of Essential Drugs (RENAME).	Essential drugs, including selected antihypertensives and hypoglycemic supplied free through a nationwide network of public (*Farmácia Popular*) and partly private pharmacies.	International reference pricing.

BIA, *budget impact analysis.*

BRAZIL

The Brazilian experience represents a case study of HTA implementation in the framework of a national access project to essential medicines. In 1988, Brazil established the *Sistema Único de Saúde* (SUS) aimed to guarantee healthcare services for everybody. Drug prices have been regulated since the end of 2000. In 2004 the Brazilian government launched the program *Farmácia Popular* (popular pharmacies) to make available at 90% discounted prices a list of essential medicines to treat common disorders. The size of the program— it is noteworthy that about 51 million potential patients may benefit from the addition of selected antihypertensives and antidiabetics in 2011— accounts for the difficulties encountered during implementation. A survey conducted in 2008–09 showed that a main problem was limited availability of generic drugs at public facilities (Bertoldi, Helfer, Camargo, Tavares, & Kanavos, 2012). The development of the Brazilian HTA guidelines began in 2006 under the auspices of the

Table 6.4 Comparative Analysis of Pharmacoeconomic National Guidelines in Brazil, Colombia, and Mexico

	Brazil (2014) (MoH, 2014)	Colombia (2014)	México (2015)
Technology	Health technologies.	Health technologies.	Drugs to be listed into the national formulary.
Perspective	Public payer. Societal is also possible.	Healthcare service.	Public stakeholders.
Indication	Approved indications.	Approved indications.	Approved indications.
Comparator	Most used alternative in the public service.	Alternatives used in common practice.	Alternatives already listed in the national formulary.
Time horizon	Based on the natural course of the disease.	Sufficiently long to reflect all important differences in costs and outcomes.	Based on the natural course of the disease.
Preferred analytical techniques	CMA, CEA, CUA, and CBA. Sensitivity analyses required for all uncertain parameters.	CUA. Probabilistic or deterministic sensitivity analysis.	CEA, CUA, CBA, and CMA. Probabilistic or deterministic sensitivity analysis for key parameters.
Costs	Direct costs, indirect optional.	Direct medical costs. Indirect and nonmedical direct costs should be excluded.	Direct only.
Source of costs	Government or public databases.	Official databases.	Published cost lists.
Modeling	Allowed, but complex models are discouraged.	Accepted. All assumptions should be clearly described.	Only if available data are not sufficient to assess cost-effectiveness. Data should be based on trials and metaanalyses.
Financial impact analysis	Required.	Not required for the base case assessment. BIA requested for listing in the *Plan Obligatorio de Salud.*	Required. Mandatory for orphan drugs.
PE assessment submission	Recommended.	Recommended.	Mandatory.

BIA, *budget impact analysis;* CBA, *cost-benefit analysis;* CEA, *cost-efficacy analysis;* CMA, *cost-minimization analysis;* CUA, *cost-utility analysis;* PE, *pharmacoeconomic.*
Modified from ISPOR. (2016). Pharmacoeconomic guidelines around the world. Comparative table. *Available from https://www.ispor.org/PEguidelines/COMP1.asp.*

Ministry of health, which were officially launched in 2009, after an extensive review process, including a public consultation. A revised version has been released in 2014 (MoH, 2014). In December 2011, an institutional framework for HTA has been established by law and the National Committee for Incorporation of Technologies (CONITEC, *Comissão Nacional de Incorporação de Tecnologias*) was created. The CONITEC is accountable for assessing all requests for coverage of health technologies. The CONITEC approved 43 of 82 applications of drugs and vaccines evaluated in 2012 and 2013. Most of them have been listed in the National List of Essential Drugs (RENAME). Refusals have been based mainly on lack of sufficient data on the risk–benefit ratio and the availability of less expensive alternatives (Bellanger, Picon, & Stuwe, 2015).

COLOMBIA

In Colombia, provision of healthcare services and essential medicines is progressing apace: out-of-pocket expenses dropped from 50% in 1995 to 16% in 2015, below the Latin America average of 37%. This advance is partly correlated to the institutionalization of HTA, approved in the healthcare reform of 2011 and launched a year later. The Institute of Health Technology Assessment (IETS) has carried out 148 evaluations, mainly related to drugs. The 2014–18 national development plan provides for linking HTA to pricing and reimbursement policies (Vanegas, 2016).

ACHIEVEMENTS

In recent decades, the contribution of HTA to the implementation of healthcare policies in developing countries is increasingly being acknowledged. Currently, 11 pharmacoeconomic guidelines are published (Brazil, Colombia, Cuba, Egypt, Malaysia, Mexico, South Africa, South Korea, and Taiwan) or publicly available (Thailand) (ISPOR, 2016). There are several successful cases where economic evaluations play a defined role in the decision-making process on pricing and reimbursement of essential medicines. In other countries, there is a positive trend toward their enforcement. The growing support by the international community on pharmacoeconomic and outcomes research in developing countries may accelerate the ongoing processes by reducing the learning curve.

CHALLENGES

Providing equitable access to essential medicines is a complex task especially for LMICs, where it is very difficult to reconcile the size of health needs with the available resources. This statement finds confirmation even in those countries where government investment in health services is high in absolute and relative terms. However, it is evident that a strong political and financial commitment to people's healthcare is the precondition. Instead, the predominance of the private health sector seems to represent a factor hindering the launch of HTA.

In countries where health priorities have already been established, the institutionalization of HTA in the framework of the pricing and reimbursement policies is a necessary step to streamline the allocation of resources.

RECOMMENDATIONS: THE WAY FORWARD

First, setting up of HTA body requires adequate investment in terms of resources and timing. Enrollment of trained personnel is strongly recommended. Although the basic methodology is quite simple, the choice of the most appropriate technique in accordance with the chosen perspective and with the availability and reliability of (local) data sources requires a solid experience.

The startup phase takes time because HTA guidelines must be shared with all stakeholders involved in the pricing and reimbursement process. Consequently, governmental authority should accept that the return on investment in the HTA is at best in the medium term.

Strengthening relationship with the national academia and medical societies, and with international institutions, is important to improve technical expertise. However, the development of institutional HTA should be focused on concrete and verifiable objectives, based on priorities endorsed by governmental authorities.

The independence of HTA is a pillar concept. In practice, a careful monitoring to avoid any significant conflict of interest as well as public disclosure of assessments are mandatory as well as assuring the full transparency of evaluations.

CONCLUSIONS

HTA is a valuable tool to support the equitable and sustainable access to healthcare services in LMICs. Although the overall framework is fragmented and the available information is not fully consolidated, there are several examples of countries where economic evaluations have become an integral part of national health policies to allocate government funding cost-effectively. The positive cases and the continuous exchange of expertise promoted by international HTA organizations can accelerate the progress of economic evaluation in developing countries.

LESSONS LEARNED

- There are successful cases where economic evaluations have become an integral part of healthcare policies, giving a valuable contribution to their implementation.
- Political endorsement, sufficient medium-term investments, and sharing with all stakeholders are key success factors for setting HTA.
- HTA agencies should be institutionalized and independent. Minimization of any significant conflict of interest and transparency of economic evaluations are mandatory.

ACKNOWLEDGMENTS

This chapter would not have been written without referring to the information published by the World Health Organization and the International Society for Pharmacoeconomics and Outcomes.

REFERENCES

Abiye, Z., Tesfaye, A., & Hawaze, S. (2013). Barriers to access: Availability and affordability of essential drugs in a retail outlet of a public health center in south western Ethiopia. *Journal of Applied Pharmaceutical Science, 3*(10), 11.

Ahmad, A., Khan, M., & Patel, I. (2015). Drug pricing policies in one of the largest drug manufacturing nations in the world: Are affordability and access a cause for concern. *Journal of Research in Pharmacy Practice, 4*(1), 1–3.

Aljunid, S. M. (2014). Pharmacoeconomics guidelines in Malaysia: Development, content and applications. In *ISPOR 6th Asia-Pacific Conference*. Beijing, China: International Society for PharmacoEconomics and Outcomes.

Augustovski, F., Melendez, G., Lemgruber, A., & Drummond, M. (2011). Implementing pharmacoeconomic guidelines in Latin America: Lessons learned. *Value in Health, 14*(Suppl. 5), S3–S7.

Bae, E. Y., & Lee, E. K. (2009). Pharmacoeconomic guidelines and their implementation in the positive list system in South Korea. *Value in Health, 12*(Suppl. 3), S36–S41.

Bae, S., Lee, S., Bae, E. Y., & Jang, S. (2013). Korean guidelines for pharmacoeconomic evaluation (second and updated version): Consensus and compromise. *Pharmacoeconomics, 31*(4), 257–267.

Barber, S., Huang, B., Santoso, B., Laing, R., Paris, V., & Wu, C. (2013). The reform of the essential medicines system in China: A comprehensive approach to universal coverage. *Journal of Global Health, 3*(1), 010303.

Bellanger, M., Picon, P., & Stuwe, L. (2015). A perspective on health technology assessment activities in Brazil. In *News across Latin America [Internet] USA: ISPOR Latin America development editorial office* Available from https://www.ispor.org/consortiums/LatinAmerica/articles/Health-Policy-Series.pdf.

Bertoldi, A., Helfer, A., Camargo, A., Tavares, N., & Kanavos, P. (2012). Is the Brazilian pharmaceutical policy ensuring population access to essential medicines. *Global Health, 8*, 6.

Bigdeli, M., Javadi, D., Hoebert, J., Laing, R., & Ranson, K. (2013). Alliance fHPaSRNoRoAtM. Health policy and systems research in access to medicines: A prioritized agenda for low- and middle-income countries. *Health Research Policy and Systems, 11*, 37.

CDE. (2006). *Guidelines of methodological standards for pharmacoeconomic evaluations in Taiwan*. Center for Drug Evaluation. Available from https://www.ispor.org/PEguidelines/source/2006_PEG_EN_2009.pdf.

Chaikledkaew, U., & Kittrongsiri, K. (2014). Guidelines for health technology assessment in Thailand (second edition) - the development process. *Journal of the Medical Association of Thailand, 97*(Suppl. 5), S4–S9.

Chen, Y., Banta, D., & Tang, Z. (2009). Health technology assessment development in China. *International Journal of Technology Assessment in Health Care, 25*(Suppl. 1), 202–209.

Chiu, W. T., Pwu, R. F., & Gau, C. S. (2015). Affordable health technology assessment in Taiwan: A model for middle-income countries. *Journal of the Formosan Medical Association, 114*(6), 481–483.

Chootipongchaivat, S., Tritasavit, N., Luz, A., Teerawattanon, Y., & Tantivess, S. (2015). Factors conducive to the development of health technology assessment in Asia. *Policy Brief, 4*(2), 1–57.

Department of Health. (December 2012). *Guidelines for pharmacoeconomic submissions*. Government Gazette, 1–72. 2013.

Department of Pharmaceuticals. (August 2017). *Draft Pharmaceutical Policy* – 2017.

Desalegn, H., Solberg, E., & Kim, J. (2015). The global financing facility: Country investments for every woman, adolescent, and child. *Lancet, 386*(9989), 105–106.

EDA. (2016). *Guidelines for reporting pharmacoeconomic evaluations*. Egyptian Drug Authority. Available from http://www.eda.mohp.gov.eg/Files/402_Egyptian_Pharmacoeconomic_guidelines.pdf.

Elmahdawy, M. M. (2016). *The current capacity for HTA in Africa: Its role in local policies and decision making. Local landscape* [updated May 23]. Available from http://www.ispor.org/AfricaNetwork/documents/HTA-Egypt_Elmahdawy.pdf.

Elsisi, G. H., Kaló, Z., Eldessouki, R., Elmahdawy, M. D., Saad, A., Ragab, S., ... Abaza, S. (2013). Recommendations for reporting pharmacoeconomic evaluations in Egypt. *Value in Health Regional Issues, 2*, 319–327.

Fang, Y., Wagner, A., Yang, S., Jiang, M., Zhang, F., & Ross-Degnan, D. (2013). Access to affordable medicines after health reform: evidence from two cross-sectional surveys in Shaanxi Province, western China. *Lancet Glob Health, 1*(4), e227–e237.

Hoebert, J., van Dijk, L., Mantel-Teeuwisse, A., Leufkens, H., & Laing, R. (2013). National medicines policies - a review of the evolution and development processes. *Journal of Pharmaceutical Policy and Practice, 6*, 5.

Hogerzeil, H., & Jing, S. (2013). Health-sector reform in China and access to essential medicines. *The Lancet Global Health*, e174–e175.

Holloway, K., & Henry, D. (2014). WHO essential medicines policies and use in developing and transitional countries: An analysis of reported policy implementation and medicines use surveys. *PLoS Medicine*, *11*(9), e1001724.

ISPOR. (2010). *Medical device pricing and coverage in Mexico*. International Society for Pharmacoeconomics and Outcome Research. Available from https://www.ispor.org/HTARoadMaps/MexicoMD.asp-4.

ISPOR. (2011). *China guidelines for pharmacoeconomic evaluations: Ministry of Human Resources and Social Security (MHRSS), Ministry of Health, and National Development and Reform Commission (NDRC)*. Available from https://www.ispor.org/PEguidelines/countrydet.asp?c=28&t=4.

ISPOR. (2016). *Pharmacoeconomic guidelines around the world* Comparative table. Available from https://www.ispor.org/PEguidelines/COMP1.asp.

ISPOR. Pharmacoeconomic guidelines around the world 2016 Available from https://www.ispor.org/peguidelines/index.asp.

Koh, L., Glaetzer, C., Chuen Li, S., & Zhang, M. (2016). Health technology assessment, international reference pricing, and budget control tools from China's perspective: What are the current developments and future considerations? *Value in Health Regional Issues*, *9*, 15–21.

Kotwani, A. (2013). Where are we now: Assessing the price, availability and affordability of essential medicines in Delhi as India plans free medicine for all. *BMC Health Services Research*, *13*, 285.

McGee, S. (2016). *HTA is included in South Africa's health reforms – how are we preparing for it?*. Available from http://www.ispor.org/AfricaNetwork/documents/HTA-in-Africa_Shelley_McGee_2016DC.pdf.

MoH. (2014). *Methodological guideline: Economic evaluation of health technologies*. Brasilia: Ministry of Health.

Moise, P., & Docteur, E. (2007). *Pharmaceutical pricing and reimbursement policies in Mexico*. OECD.

Mori, A., Kaale, E., Ngalesoni, F., Norheim, O., & Robberstad, B. (2014). The role of evidence in the decision-making process of selecting essential medicines in developing countries: The case of Tanzania. *PLoS One*, *9*(1), e84824.

Mori, A., & Robberstad, B. (2012). Pharmacoeconomics and its implication on priority-setting for essential medicines in Tanzania: A systematic review. *BMC Medical Informatics and Decision Making*, *12*, 110.

Nair, S. R. (2015). Relevance of health economics to the indian healthcare system: A perspective. *Perspectives in Clinical Research.*, *6*(4), 225–226.

NPPA, & Notified Prices Under DPCO. (2013). *New Delhi (India): National Pharmaceutical Pricing Authority* 2014. Available from http://nppaindia.nic.in/.

Oberoi, S. S., & Oberoi, A. (2014). Pharmacoeconomics guidelines: The need of hour for India. *Int J Pharm Investig*, *4*(3), 109–111.

Pharmaceutical Services Division. (2012). *Pharmacoeconomic guideline for Malaysia*. Available from http://www.pharmacy.gov.my/v2/sites/default/files/document-upload/pharmacoeconomic-guideline-malaysia.pdf.

PMLiVE. (2012). *Country report: The healthcare market in Brazil*. Available from http://www.pmlive.com/pharma_intelligence/country_report_the_healthcare_market_in_brazil_409950.

Pharmacoeconomic and Outcomes Research are steadily moving forward in Asia. *Value in Health Regional Issues*, *9*, (2016), 112.

Sado, E., & Sufa, A. (2016). Availability and affordability of essential medicines for children in the western part of Ethiopia: Implication for access. *BMC Pediatrics*, *16*, 40.

Song, Y., Bian, Y., Petzold, M., Li, L., & Yin, A. (2014a). Effects of the national essential medicine system in reducing drug prices: An empirical study in four Chinese provinces. *Journal of Pharmaceutical Policy and Practice*, *7*(1), 12.

Song, Y., Bian, Y., Petzold, M., Li, L., & Yin, A. (2014b). The impact of China's national essential medicine system on improving rational drug use in primary health care facilities: An empirical study in four provinces. *BMC Health Services Research*, *14*, 507.

Tantivess, S. (2013). Health technology assessment and policymaking in Thailand. In *1st World Health Summit, regional meeting – Asia*. Singapore: World Health Summit.

Teerawattananon, Y., & Chaikledkaew, U. (2008). Thai health technology assessment guideline development. *Journal of the Medical Association of Thailand, 91*(Suppl. 2), S11–S15.

Vanegas, G. (2016). *The institutionalization of health technology assessment in Colombia: Advancements and future challenges. News across Latin America: ISPOR Latin America consortium.* Available from http://press.ispor.org/LatinAmerica/2016/05/the-institutionalization-of-health-technology-assessment-in-colombia-advancements-and-future-challenges-2/.

WHO. (1988). *Guidelines for developing national drug policies.* Available from http://apps.who.int/medicinedocs/documents/s19151en/s19151en.pdf.

WHO. (2001). *How to develop and implement a national drug policy* (2nd ed.). Available from. http://apps.who.int/medicinedocs/pdf/s2283e/s2283e.pdf.

WHO. (2015). *Global survey on health technology assessment by national authorities* Main findings. Available from http://www.who.int/health-technology-assessment/MD_HTA_oct2015_final_web2.pdf?ua=1.

WHO. (2016). *Essential medicines and health products* Annual report 2015. Available from http://www.who.int/medicines/publications/AR2015_links_bookmarks.pdf?ua=1.

Xi, X., Li, W., Li, J., Zhu, X., Fu, C., Wei, X., & Chu, S. (2015). A survey of the availability, prices and affordability of essential medicines in Jiangsu Province, China. *BMC Health Services Research, 15*, 345.

Yang, L., Liu, C., Ferrier, J., Zhou, W., & Zhang, X. (2013). The impact of the National Essential Medicines Policy on prescribing behaviours in primary care facilities in Hubei province of China. *Health Policy Plan, 28*(7), 750–760.

Zainol, Z. A., Amin, L., Jusoff, K., Zahid, A., & Akpoviri, F. (2011). Pharmaceutical patents and access to essential medicines in sub-Saharan Africa. *African Journal of Biotechnology, 10*(58), 12376–12388.

Zuma, N. (1997). South Africa's new national drug policy. Interview by Daphne Fresle. *Journal of Public Health Policy*, 98–105.

CHAPTER 7

MEDICINES PRICING POLICY AND STRATEGIES IN DEVELOPING COUNTRIES: A REVIEW

Nada Abdel Rida, Mohamed Izham Mohamed Ibrahim

Qatar University, Doha, Qatar

CHAPTER OUTLINE

BACKGROUND

Effective pharmaceutical pricing policies in developing countries are important to ensure accessibility and affordability of essential medicines for most people within a society. These policies should be part of the country's National Medicines Policy.

Why do we need National Medicines Policy? The pharmaceutical sector is a platform where various parties participate and coordinate to deliver medicines to needed patients. The overall process of procuring, distributing, prescribing, and dispensing is as important as the health outcome of medicines in a society. In regulating this sector, efforts to remedy any individual stage of this process is pointless if not accompanied with a well-planned strategy to cover all parties and regulate their activities. Since 1970, efforts have been undertaken to tackle various problems observed worldwide. In 1986, the 39th World Health Assembly resulted in a call for governments to implement national drug policies. This later referred to as National Medicine Policies (NDP or NMP) (Laing, Waning, Gray, Ford, & t Hoen, 2003; World Health Organization, 2012b) and thereafter, a World Health Organization (WHO) guideline on the previously named National Drug Policy (NDP) was disseminated in 1988 (Hoebert, van

Social and Administrative Aspects of Pharmacy in Low- and Middle-Income Countries. http://dx.doi.org/10.1016/B978-0-12-811228-1.00007-8

Dijk, Mantel-Teeuwisse, Leufkens, & Laing, 2013). Some of the earliest adopters of NDP were low- and middle-income countries (LMICs) in the mid-1980s, whereas high-income countries (HICs) started implementing such policies in the mid-1990s and frequently updated their NDP (Hoebert et al., 2013). LMICs implemented NMP due to their urgent need to improve access to medicines, especially the essentials within their limited resources (Laing et al., 2003). Although NMP has not been adopted by all HICs, various components of such policies do exist and are well regulated (Hoebert et al., 2013).

NMP should take the form of a government policy enforced by regulation covering both the private and public sector. NMP is a governance process under which governments ensure that all stakeholders in the pharmaceutical sector are collaborating to ensure that quality medicines (especially the essential) are available, affordable, rationally prescribed, and used.

Although NMPs are implemented in many countries, the components of such policies change based on national characteristics and needs (Hoebert et al., 2013; World Health Organization, 2012b). Developing a comprehensive NMP requires a level of financial resources and human capital (World Health Organization, 2012b).

What is the significance of essential medicines list? A fundamental component of any NMP is the establishment of an essential medicines list. In 1975, the World Health Assembly passed resolution WHA28.66 calling the WHO to assist in a program that supports member states in developing a list of essential medicines (Laing et al., 2003).

During the 1970s, countries were facing difficulties controlling pharmaceutical budgets especially in countries with limited resources. By 1977, the first Essential Drug List (EDL) of 205 items (186 medicines) was issued by the WHO (Laing et al., 2003). The included drugs were selected based on their efficacy and cost (Eom, Grootendorst, & Duffin, 2016; Hogerzeil, 2004; World Health Organization, 2016b). In 2002, the name of the list changed from EDL to Essential Medicines List (EML) to reflect that not all included remedies are pharmaceutical (Eom et al., 2016). One of the main aims behind its conception was to improve availability and equitable access to medication in LMIC (Seuba, 2006). However, countries of all income levels, which have implemented EML, especially in the public procurement of medicines, have benefited from improved availability, quality of use, rational selection of medicines, large cost savings, and affordable pharmaceutical treatment (Bazargani, Ewen, de Boer, Leufkens, & Mantel-Teeuwisse, 2014; Eom et al., 2016; Hogerzeil, 2004). As per Bazargani et al.(2014), the availability of essential medicines compared to nonessential medicines in public facilities is inversely proportional to level of income as poorer countries tend to adhere to the procurement of medicines on the EML, while richer countries sometimes have tailored formularies (Bazargani et al., 2014; Hogerzeil, 2004). Nevertheless, equitable access to essential medicines is still suboptimal and questionable (Bazargani et al., 2014).

Prior to 2000, EML medicines were selected based on the recommendation of the World Health Assembly and national committees; however, the current selection process is mostly reliant on evidence-based research (Hogerzeil, 2004; Holloway & Henry, 2014; Laing et al., 2003). The shape, content, and size of the EML changed since its conception and have been subject to revisions and updates every 2 years (Hogerzeil, 2004; Laing et al., 2003). The latest WHO Model List of 2015 includes 30 categories and more than 500 drugs. The WHO releases a Model List that is subject to addition and deletion as per the country/regional priorities. With the improvement of the EML inclusion criteria, it is of note that the list not only includes the most essential cheapest medicines for LMIC (e.g., core medicines) (Hogerzeil, 2004; Laing et al., 2003) but also complimentary medicines whose administration requires specialization and are often expensive (Laing et al., 2003).

Essential medicines are deemed substantial for well-functioning healthcare systems. They encompass the most prevalent diseases such as HIV, malaria, and chronic diseases (e.g., diabetes and cardiovascular diseases) (World Health Organization, 2010). These medicines are selected for their efficacy, safety, quality, and cost-effectiveness. Due to their relevance in treating fundamental illnesses they inherit the value of being essential, and consequently their availability and affordability for communities and individuals are fundamental (World Health Organization, 2016a, 2016b).

Nevertheless, the development and establishment of essential medicines lists face some criticism especially from the pharmaceutical industry, prescribing doctors, and NGOs as being restrictive (Laing et al., 2003).

MEDICINE VALUE

While medicines and drugs are being used interchangeably, some people may argue that they differ in meaning and action. By definition, the two terms are interchangeable, and in this document, they are mostly referred to as a medicine based on the medicinal class or category described in this chapter.

Any medicine whether traditional or modern has value to different stakeholders. It is qualified as a product to manufacturers, a pharmaceutical product for prescribers, and finally a therapeutic mean for consumers or patients. This last connotation confers an emotional and psychological value to pharmaceuticals in treating and alleviating pain or combating morbidity and mortality. Of the various values that patients look for in medicines, safety and efficacy are at the top of the list (Callen, 2012; Wertheimer, Radican, & Jacobs, 2010). The healing value conferred to medicines is consistent with the literature, where in most cases medicines have been proven to exert better efficacy than other non-pharmaceutical treatment or to no treatment at all (Coyle & Drummond, 1993; Grootendorst, Pierard, & Shim, 2009).

MEDICINES ACCESS

Access can be defined by the ability of citizens to reach and use pharmaceuticals that are of good quality and affordable, when needed (World Health Organization, 2012c). Access to quality medicine is a basic human right, simply the right to health. Achieving and fulfilling this right enhances the quality of an individual's life and sustains an adequate standard of health. About one-third of the world's population lacks sustainable access to essentially needed medication. Poor access is not always related to technical issues. Others factors influencing access include social beliefs or values, economic interests, and political process (Frost & Reich, 2009). WHO identifies hindrances to access as being one or all the following: medicine price, quality, availability, and affordability (World Health Organization/Health Action International, 2008). This is most pronounced in poor countries where people face difficulties due to medicine price and availability whether in the public or private sector. While the right to be treated should be a basic right for people around the world, this is not the case in LMICs. In these countries, people are purchasing medicine out-of-pocket because of the lack of a comprehensive health insurance system and inadequate publicly subsidized pharmaceutical services (Cameron, Hill, & Whyte 2015; Institute for Healthcare Informatics, 2014; Peters et al., 2008). Therefore, strategies to ameliorate access should take into account improving affordability (Frost & Reich, 2009). In 1990, several public and nongovernmental organizations, such as WHO, Health Action International (HAI), Médecins Sans Frontières (MSF) (Ho et al., 2008), collaborated their efforts to provide afflicted population with reliable access to medication and to combat health inequity which was a common issue in both developed and developing countries.

MEDICINES PRICES: POLICY AND STRATEGIES

A medicine like any other commercial product is available in a market and is subject to supply and demand forces. This theory is dominated and directed by two main forces: producers and consumers, and their market behavior. The price for most goods is generally shaped by demand; however, this should not be the case for pharmaceuticals. Although patients have willingness-to-pay for an indispensable treatment, allowing market dynamics to set pharmaceutical prices could prove unethical and unhealthy. Given the maxim that "health is priceless," controversy arises between manufacturers that aim at making the most benefit of their research and development (Hassall et al., 2015) and the highest return-on-investment (Enzmann & Broich, 2013) and the patients who, whenever capable, would not spare any resource to access medicines that improve health, well-being, and could be life-saving in cases such as chronic diseases treatment.

In the pharmaceutical sector, these forces should not neglect the unique properties of this essential product (medicine) that set it apart from other traded products (Almarsdottir & Traulsen, 2005; de Joncheere, 2003). In this context, physicians or prescribers usually interfere to decide what would be the most rational medicine to use.

A common misconception is the belief that pharmaceutical prices are reflective of the manufacturing cost. The retail price at which a consumer buys the medicine is the result of cumulative add-on costs along the distribution chain (Babar, Ibrahim, Singh, & Creese, 2007; World Health Organization, 2012a; World Health Organization/Health Action International, 2008):

1. Stage 1: The manufacturer selling price (MSP)—the price covers the production cost and manufacturer profit,
2. Stage 2: Landed price,
3. Stage 3: Wholesale selling price,
4. Stage 4: Retail selling price, and
5. Stage 5: Dispensing selling price.

Controlling the various mark-up components at these different stages is essential for any price reduction. Price variation within and between countries exists and could be attributed to poorly regulated pharmaceutical sectors and lack of comprehensive pharmaceutical policy (Babar et al., 2007; World Health Organization, 2012a). Different procurement processes for different pharmaceutical and health sectors in a country can also influence it. Moreover, the literature deduces that differences in the price of medicines exist between countries, even those of the same income level (Kaló et al., 2015; Morel, McGuire, & Mossialos, 2011; Vogler & Habimana, 2014; Vogler, Kilpatrick, & Babar, 2015).

International price variations are therefore due to (World Health Organization, 2012a):

1. different MSP of the same product,
2. various pricing policies and mark-up schemes applied to distinct stages of pharmaceutical supply chain, and
3. differential pricing, also referred to as equity pricing, to increase affordability in the least developed and poor countries.

Given the different players involved in these stages, a rigid national medicine policy encompassing the whole process in addition to a nation-specific pharmaceutical pricing policy are key determinants of the final retail prices, access, and health equity. A common conclusion is always reached: the inexistence of a "magic bullet" or a one-size-fits-all solution as different countries have diverse needs, challenges, and policy environment.

It is reported that LMICs spend between 20 and 60% of the total healthcare expenditure on medicines in comparison to less than 18% in HICs (Cameron et al., 2015). To tackle this disparity, an assortment of joint experts' efforts must be exploited on various levels worldwide, nationally, and locally.

Having all these tools to assist in shaping better pharmaceutical pricing policies does not exclude the key role played by national governments to enforce and regulate the pharmaceutical sector. Evidence-based national policies and programs must be developed.

The government intervention in determining the price of medicine is undebatable, given the value of medicine from different perspectives. Countries adopt varying strategies to manage the pharmaceutical market. Some countries such as Malaysia (Babar et al., 2007; Babar, Ibrahim, & Bukhari, 2005) prefer minimal intervention, allowing for an equilibrium based on health sectors, suppliers, and patient. Other countries get fully engaged and intervene by either subsidizing medicines or offering them for free to their population. The latter case is what is encountered in industrialized countries that are members of the Organization of Economic and Co-operation and Development (Docteur, Paris, & Moise, 2008).

A REVIEW ON MEDICINES PRICING POLICY AND STRATEGIES

To identify the pharmaceutical pricing policies adopted in the developing countries, a systematic review of the literature was conducted. The first aim was to identify governmental pricing policies or strategies implemented to control the prices of pharmaceuticals and to explore their effects on the pharmaceutical sector in the adopting nations. Then, it was followed by mapping pricing policies to WHO guidelines. The social and economic impacts of such policies were then assessed in studies of eligible designs.

A literature review was conducted to evaluate whether the inefficiency of the pharmaceutical sector is a result of absence of policies or lack of implementation and enforcement of policies in developing countries. The review covered English and Arabic scientific journals (including both experimental and observational studies), and government publications published between January 2000 and March 2016 covering pharmaceutical pricing policies and their effect. The search was conducted across several databases, including PubMed, PQ Central, EconLit, ProQuest, CINAHL, Scopus, ScienceDirect, Cochrane, WHOLIS, WHOCC, and Web of Knowledge. The search terms used were "drug," "medicine," "pharmaceutical," "price, pricing," "price containment," "price control," "pricing strategy," "pricing policy," and "developing countries" or "LMICs" where applicable. Gray literature search was also conducted through government publications, WHO/HAI reports, and Open Grey database in addition to using the search engine Google Scholar. This search yielded 1250 studies. To be eligible, studies needed to include a policy and an evaluation of its effects on at least one relevant outcome. For the qualitative synthesis in the systematic review, only studies that quantify the impact of policies were included; e.g., pre/post, longitudinal, and interrupted time series studies.

Only 21 articles fulfilled our objectives and were included in the explorative synthesis, of which 6 studies were qualitatively synthesized (Table 7.1). The studies were done in several countries. Sixteen studies covered Asian countries, three covered African countries, and three from Latin and South America. China had the highest coverage with eight studies addressing its policies. All studies were published between 2004 and 2015. By mapping the identified pricing policies to WHO guidelines, it was noted that some countries opt to more than one strategy to contain pharmaceutical prices. Mark-up regulation was the most commonly used pricing policy accounting for 30%, followed by external reference pricing (ERP) and cost-plus at 26% and 22%, respectively, and generic promotion at 13%. Tax exemption was the least used, accounting for only 9%. After accounting for multiple studies from the same country, two of the countries were classified as HICs, five were upper-middle income countries (UMICs), two were LMICs, and two were LICs. The targeted medicines under the policies or initiatives included essential medicines (Ahmed & Islam, 2012; Bertoldi, Helfer, Camargo, Tavares, & Kanavos, 2012; Fang et al., 2013; Hu, 2013; Maiga & Williams-Jones, 2010; Nobrega Ode et al., 2007; Yang, Dib, Zhu, Qi, & Zhang, 2010; Zhou et al., 2015), antiretroviral drugs (Ford, Wilson, Costa Chaves, Lotrowska, & Kijtiwatchakul, 2007), or covering all classes of medicines (Abbott et al., 2012; Ball, Tisocki, & Al-Saffar, 2009; Han, Liang, Su, Xue, & Shi, 2013; Meng et al., 2005; Moïse & Docteur, 2007; Russo & McPake, 2010).

Of the 21, only 6 studies exhibited the eligible study designs to measure the impact of pricing strategies. The majority were pre-/poststudies measuring impacts of newly implemented pricing policies, while one was a longitudinal study. While the studies aimed at measuring the impact of new cost and price containment strategies, the outcomes measured varied. This made it difficult to have a quantitative comparison. Policies in China were effective in reducing prices (Fang et al., 2013; Han et al., 2013; Meng et al., 2005; Zhou et al., 2015), however, drug expenditure remained high due to irrational drug utilization (Han et al., 2013; Meng et al., 2005). In Indonesia, the prices were reduced for both drug types but did not reach the targeted maximum prices (Anggriani, Ibrahim, Suryawati, & Shafie, 2013). Mali achieved its policy aims, although it took several years for the effects to be measureable (Maiga & Williams-Jones, 2010).

ACHIEVEMENTS

Within the context of the retrieved articles, developing countries are using pharmaceutical pricing policies as internationally recommended, often combining two or more policies. Strategies are adopted in similar ratios, i.e., high usage of ERP and mark-up regulation policies, to those implemented in developed countries.

Most of the industrialized countries are endeavoring to apply aggressive strategies to control pharmaceutical expenditures (Vogler et al., 2016). ERP is widely implemented for in-patent medicines (Leopold et al., 2012; Vogler & Habimana, 2014). As of 2011, 24 out of the 27 European Union countries (EU) covered in the RAND report used ERP with the exception of Sweden, the UK, and

Table 7.1 Pharmaceutical Pricing Policies Adopted in Developing Countries, Target Medicines, Year of Adoption, and Key Findings

Author and Country	Policy	Target Medicines	Year of Adoption	Key Findings
7 ME countries: Egypt, Kuwait, Jordan, Lebanon, Qatar, Saudi Arabia, United Arab Emirates [31]	• Use of external reference pricing	Mainly branded patented medicines	NA	• More stringent external reference pricing in countries adopting the lowest price among ≥25 countries • Referencing higher-income countries negatively affected the prices in Egypt and Lebanon • 27.5% of price variability (reduction) explained by larger population size, a basket of >5 countries, and mandate of lowest price
Bangladesh [38]	• Promotion of use of generic medicines	Essential medicines	1982	• Poor availability of essential drugs • Higher number of dispensed drugs in rural clinics • 50% of the facilities presenting the EML • Frequent incorrect ATB prescription • Prices of branded > 500% higher
Brazil [40]	• Regulation of mark-ups in the pharmaceutical supply and distribution chain • Application of cost-plus pricing formulae for pharmaceutical price setting	Essential medicines	NA	• Variable availability of essential medicines in the public sector leading to out-of-pocket expenditure • All medicine types MPR ≥ 8 • The launch of CMED started downward trend of prices
Brazil [84]	• Regulation of mark-ups in the pharmaceutical supply and distribution chain • Tax exemptions/reductions for pharmaceutical products	Essential medicines	2000	• Prices were 1.9 and 13.1 times more expensive than those in Sweden and international suppliers, respectively
Brazil and Thailand [44]	• Promotion of use of generic medicines	Antiretrovirals	2006–07 Thailand; 2003 Brazil	• Decrease in spending on some old ART but not on new ART, which is problematic in case of drug resistance • Negotiations with drug companies insufficient to control prices • Compulsory licensing was more effective in reducing prices
China [36]	• Regulation of mark-ups in the pharmaceutical supply and distribution chain	Essential medicines	2010	• Although inflation-adjusted prices were lower, availability of LPG was decreased to lower than the poor availability in 2010 • Decrease in prices of branded medicines was greater than that of LPG

Continued

Table 7.1 Pharmaceutical Pricing Policies Adopted in Developing Countries, Target Medicines, Year of Adoption, and Key Findings

Author and Country	Policy	Target Medicines	Year of Adoption	Key Findings
China [45]	• Regulation of mark-ups in the pharmaceutical supply and distribution chain	60% of all medicines of which systemic antibacterial	1996	• 2005 expenditure 205.7% higher than 1996, even though prices are almost halved • Prescriber behavior and limited government funding of hospitals are key determinants of drug expenditure
China [39]	• Regulation of mark-ups in the pharmaceutical supply and distribution chain	Essential medicines	2009–11	• 25% reduction in the average price of medicines and reduction in the average cost per visit/hospitalization • Expansion of EML by up to 455 medicines based on the characteristics of clinical use and medical requirement, indicating the EML loss of authority
China [41]	• Regulation of mark-ups in the pharmaceutical supply and distribution chain • Application of cost-plus pricing formulae for pharmaceutical price setting	Essential medicines	2009	• Overall reduction of relative expenses by 11% for both outpatients and inpatients
China [48]	• Regulation of mark-ups in the pharmaceutical supply and distribution chain	All medicines	2000	• No positive impact on containment of hospital drug expenditure in the two hospitals • Drug expenditure affected by utilization more than price
China [42]	• Regulation of mark-ups in the pharmaceutical supply and distribution chain	Essential medicines	2009	• Low availability of LPG in public and private sectors (38.9 and 44.4%, respectively) • MPR of procurement prices for IB and LPG in public sector were 9.78 and 0.74 the IRP. Median MPR of LPG in retail public outlets was higher than that in the private (0.68) • Prices for general population are affordable, however, not so for low-income segment
China [85]	• Regulation of mark-ups in the pharmaceutical supply and distribution chain • Application of cost-plus pricing formulae for pharmaceutical price setting	All medicines	2000; 2001; 2005	• Poor access to essential drugs due to irrational supply and distribution systems • Ineffective pricing regulation • Lack of promotion of generics

China and Taiwan [65]	• Application of cost-plus pricing formulae for pharmaceutical price setting	Brand names medicines	2009	• 54/70 medicines of same generic name and dose have a higher price in Mainland China • 47/54 also have the same manufacturing source besides names and dose have higher prices in Mainland China
Indonesia [51]	• Application of cost-plus pricing formulae for pharmaceutical price setting • Use of external reference pricing • Promotion of use of generic medicines	Generic medicines	2010	• Price reduction of LPG by >2000% for some and to a less extent for branded (5–35 times of IRP) due to the absence of policy regulating the price of IB • Unbranded prices are higher than the maximum retail price • The implementation of the pricing policy is not optimal • Local manufacturer of unbranded generic stopped their production
Jordan [49]	• Regulation of mark-ups in the pharmaceutical supply and distribution chain • Use of external reference pricing	All medicines	2000–01	• Increase of overall annual drug expenditure and the price of originator brands • Decline of the weighted average price of generics • Increased medications cost due to delayed generic entry
Kuwait [86]	• Regulation of mark-ups in the pharmaceutical supply and distribution chain	All medicines	NA	• Public sector procurement is efficient • Medicine prices in the private sector two times more expensive with reference to MSH prices • Some medicines are unaffordable in the private sector, with limited penetration of generics whose prices are not efficiently regulated
Mali [37]	• Application of cost-plus pricing formulae for pharmaceutical price setting	Essential medicines	2006	• Availability was unaffected by enforcement, however, prices decreased significantly by 25.6%
Mexico [47]	• Application of cost-plus pricing formulae for pharmaceutical price setting • Use of external reference pricing	All medicines	2004	• Drug price levels are higher compared to Latin American countries and others of the same economic level • Similar availability of medicines to that in developed countries

Continued

Table 7.1 Pharmaceutical Pricing Policies Adopted in Developing Countries, Target Medicines, Year of Adoption, and Key Findings

Author and Country	Policy	Target Medicines	Year of Adoption	Key Findings
Mozambique [46]	• Regulation of mark-ups in the pharmaceutical supply and distribution chain • Tax exemptions/reductions for pharmaceutical products	All medicines	1990, 1998–2003	• Market dominated by generics with availability varying significantly between the capital city and other areas • Controlled generic prices in the public sector • IB prices reach ≥ 23 times the IRP • Ineffective policy due to lack of enforcement and corruption
Oman [87]	• Regulation of mark-ups in the pharmaceutical supply and distribution chain • Use of external reference pricing	All medicines	1990	• Regulation of drug prices especially in the private sector • Prices of less than 50% of medicines are comparable to international prices, the remaining is 2–28 times higher • 100% availability across sectors • Affordable treatment in the private sector to lowest paid employees (especially for children)
Turkey [88]	• Use of external reference pricing	All medicines	Revised in 2011	• Decrease in pharmaceutical expenditure as percentage of total healthcare expenditure from 36% in 2004 to 27% in 2011

MPR, *medicine price ratio;* ART, *antiretroviral treatment;* MSH, *Management Sciences for Health;* IB, *innovator brand;* IRP, *international reference price;* ATB, *antibiotics;* LPG, *lowest price generics;* NA, *not available.*

Modified with permission from Rida, N. M. A., & Ibrahim, M. I. M. (2017). Pricing strategies for pharmaceuticals in developing countries: What options do we have? Generics and Biosimilars Initiative Journal (GaBI Journal), *6(1), 4–6. http://dx.doi.org/10.5639/gabij.2017.0601.002.*

Denmark (Ruggeri & Ellen, 2013). As previously mentioned, ERP is a dynamic process to price in-patent and prescription only medicines including reimbursable medicines (Ruggeri & Ellen, 2013; Vogler & Habimana, 2014). Moreover, the trend is toward including countries of similar income levels as the country applying the policy (Leopold et al., 2012). The supply chain remuneration (mark-ups) is also relatively regulated in these countries through either a fixed fee (a fixed percentage) or fee-for-service (Vogler & Habimana, 2014; Vogler, Vitry, & Babar, 2016; Vogler, Zimmermann, & Habl, 2013). The margins added vary between linear or regressive mark-up schemes, with regressive scheme being applied more often in recent times (Vogler, Lepuschütz, & Schneider, 2015). To curb the total drug expenditure for patients and third parties, regulators are focusing on the transparency and enforcement of the fixed profit margins for the different players in the distribution chain (Leopold et al., 2012).

Likewise, generic medicines promotion policy that curbs pharmaceutical expenditure as in Canada and most OECD countries (Acosta et al., 2014; Docteur et al., 2008; Dylst, Vulto, & Simoens, 2013, 2014; Vogler et al., 2013) is among the pricing policies less likely adopted and surveyed in developing countries.

Tax exemption strategies adopted in Mozambique (Russo & McPake, 2010) and Brazil (Nobrega Ode et al., 2007) are comparable to taxation schemes adopted in developed countries where taxes are imposed on medicinal products at varying levels depending on medicine category and country (Docteur et al., 2008; Vogler & Habimana, 2014).

Countries endeavor to frequently update their policies based on continuous monitoring as was evident in the articles relating to China. Most of the pricing strategies encountered were targeted at all categories of medicines, while some were limited to essential medicines. A remarkable improvement in reducing either the pharmaceutical prices or expenditure was achieved in some developing countries after implementation of adequate pharmaceutical pricing policies such as in Kuwait, Mexico, Mozambique (Ball et al., 2009), and Oman. Higher availability of drugs was detected in some countries, especially in the public sector; however, this cannot be exclusively attributed to the pricing policy. No significant relationship between income level and types of policies implemented was identified, although statistical confirmation was not possible due to the limited sample size.

CHALLENGES

Although developing countries are implementing policies as recommended by WHO guidelines, such policies have not always been successful, as reported in China (Meng et al., 2005) and Indonesia (Anggriani et al., 2013). ERP which uses benchmarking against a basket of countries is one of the most widely used policies (De Lima, Pastrana, Radbruch, & Wenk, 2014). However, it comes with some limitations, which were evident in Mexico (Moïse & Docteur, 2007), Egypt, and Lebanon (Kaló et al., 2015). Optimal ERP should be benchmarked against countries with similar economic status. In many cases, countries with lower income such as Lebanon and Egypt in this study are benchmarked against developed and HICs, resulting in higher medicine prices for local consumers (Kaló et al., 2015).

The efficiency of a pharmaceutical supply chain and commitment of different stakeholders involved is always questionable as demonstrated by this review. Weak MSP negotiation (Ford et al., 2007), irregular supply (Ahmed & Islam, 2012; Anggriani et al., 2013; Meng et al., 2005), and adherence to pricing policies were reflective of such incidences (Russo & McPake, 2010; Weng, Han, Pu, Pan, & Shi, 2014).

A recurrent theme when investigating initiatives adopted to reduce prices and pharmaceutical expenditures is the resistance to generic medicines use. This resistance could be attributed to various factors, some of which are patient and prescriber attitudes and beliefs, financial incentive in selling higher priced innovators, and most importantly the lack of regulatory initiatives to promote the use of generics (Hassali et al., 2014; Kaplan, Ritz, Vitello, & Wirtz, 2012). Evidence supports that incorporating a pro-generic medicine policy in developing countries can immensely reduce the pharmaceutical expenditure and lessen the economic burden on consumers (Cameron, Mantel-Teeuwisse, Leufkens, & Laing, 2012; King & Kanavos, 2002).

Differential pricing, or "tiered pricing," adjusts the pharmaceutical prices to the purchasing power of the population and can result in an increase of market share and sales for the pharmaceutical industries (Henry & Lexchin, 2002). Despite its theoretical potential for reducing prices, tiered pricing is not commonly applied (Kaló, Annemans, & Garrison, 2013) as it requires confidential rebates, controlling of parallel trade and external referencing (Danzon & Towse, 2003). Differential pricing has most commonly been used by NGOs such as UNICEF and Global Alliance for Vaccines and Immunization (GAVI) for vaccines, oral contraceptives, and antiretrovirals in LMICs, particularly in Africa (Babar & Atif, 2014).

While health technology assessment has been implemented and is gaining ground in several industrialized countries (Chalkidou, 2012; Claxton et al., 2012; Lee, Bloor, Hewitt, & Maynard, 2012; Vogler & Habimana, 2014), its use in developing countries is limited. This is mainly due to high level of skill required in design and implementation, as well as transparency in results assessment and decision-making (Acharya, 2014; Chaikledkaew, Lertpitakpong, Teerawattananon, Thavorncharoensap, & Tangcharoensathien, 2009; Hammad, 2016).

Prescribers' commitment and adherence to treatment guidelines is essential to reduce pharmaceutical expenditure. The irrational use of drugs is affecting both budgets and therapeutic outcomes (Han et al., 2013; Meng et al., 2005). Additionally, the low availability of essential medicines especially in the public sector is influencing the affordability and access to treatment for the poor (Bertoldi et al., 2012; Yang et al., 2010).

The abovementioned challenges observed in the retrieved studies emphasize the vital role that an NMP can play in regulating the pharmaceutical sector. The effect of several issues such as prescribing patterns, rational use of drugs, availability of affordable essential medicines, and continuous supply of medicines can be minimized if not eradicated with a sound NMP and governance.

Most countries for which the pharmaceutical pricing policies were reviewed are classified as either HICs or UMICs, whereas few studies were conducted in LMICs. Moreover, the data confirmed a scarcity of pharmaceutical pricing evaluative studies in developing countries as compared to developed countries (Acosta et al., 2014; Cameron et al., 2015; Nguyen, Knight, Roughead, Brooks, & Mant, 2015).

RECOMMENDATIONS: THE WAY FORWARD

After reviewing the impact of policies and the reality of the pharmaceutical sector status in developing countries to the extent permitted by the reviewed studies, more robust research targeting the analysis of pharmaceutical and pricing policies in the developing countries should be conducted, taking into consideration policy reform and adoption. Conducting regular studies is essential for decision-makers to evaluate and take appropriate action.

The implementation of well-established pricing policies can be undermined by the behavior of other stakeholders as the case of prescribers in China (Meng et al., 2005) and lack of enforcement (Anggriani et al., 2013). As such, an effective pharmaceutical pricing policy should be tailored to the social and economic dynamics of a nation, supported by strong governance and legal and administrative frameworks to control the pharmaceutical supply chain at all levels, while ensuring availability of technical knowhow.

The ultimate solution in developing countries may be the implementation of universal health coverage (UHC) under which most medicines are included (World Health Organization, 2012d) as in the case in many OECD countries.

CONCLUSIONS

In this present chapter, we reviewed the pharmaceutical pricing policies and initiatives adopted in the developing countries to contain the price of pharmaceuticals. Governments in developing countries are implementing several strategies to control medicine prices. The scope of policies used varies from disease-specific to essential, and some countries extend it to all medicine classes. With the exception of a few success cases, policies have not been effective due to poor enforcement of regulations, inadequate monitoring, corruption, and noncompliance by stakeholders. Pricing policies adopted are of international recognition; however, they are not optimally implemented and enforced.

LESSONS LEARNED

- Ensuring availability and affordability of quality essential medicines in various sectors is elemental for equitable access to healthcare services.
- No silver bullet pricing policy that can be applied universally.
- In order to tackle the multiple complex issues influencing access to innovators and generic brands, a mix of policies is required with mandatory pre-/postlaunch activities and monitoring.
- Tiered pricing is a suitable choice in poor countries in addition to competition and negotiations.
- Optimal solution is the implementation of UHC with high coverage of essential medicines.

REFERENCES

Abbott, R., Bader, R., Bajjali, L., Abu ElSamen, T., Obeidat, T., Sboul, H., … Alabbadi, I. (2012). The price of medicines in Jordan: The cost of trade-based intellectual property. *Journal of Generic Medicines*, *9*(2), 75–85 (Retrieved from).

Acharya, M. (2014). Pharmacoeconomic studies in Nepal: The need of the hour. *Frontiers in Pharmacology*, *5*, 272. http://dx.doi.org/10.3389/fphar.2014.00272.

Acosta, A., Ciapponi, A., Aaserud, M., Vietto, V., Austvoll-Dahlgren, A., Kosters, J. P., … Oxman, A. D. (2014). Pharmaceutical policies: Effects of reference pricing, other pricing, and purchasing policies. *The Cochrane Database of Systematic Reviews*, *10*, Cd005979. http://dx.doi.org/10.1002/14651858.CD005979.pub2.

Ahmed, S. M., & Islam, Q. S. (2012). Availability and rational use of drugs in primary healthcare facilities following the national drug policy of 1982: Is Bangladesh on right track? *Journal of Health, Population, and Nutrition*, *30*(1), 99–108.

Almarsdottir, A. B., & Traulsen, J. M. (2005). Cost-containment as part of pharmaceutical policy. *Pharmacy World & Science*, *27*(3), 144–148. http://dx.doi.org/10.1007/s11096-005-6953-6.

Anggriani, Y., Ibrahim, M., Suryawati, S., & Shafie, A. (2013). The impact of Indonesian generic medicine pricing policy on medicine prices. *Journal of Generic Medicines*, *10*(3–4), 219–229 (Retrieved from).

Babar, Z., & Atif, M. (2014). Differential pricing of pharmaceuticals: A bibliometric review of the literature. *Journal of Pharmaceutical Health Services Research*, *5*(3), 149–156. http://dx.doi.org/10.1111/jphs.12061.

Babar, Z., Ibrahim, M. I., & Bukhari, N. I. (2005). Medicine utilisation and pricing in Malaysia: The findings of a household survey. *Journal of Generic Medicines*, *3*(1), 47–61 (Retrieved from).

Babar, Z., Ibrahim, M., Singh, N., & Creese, A. (2007). Evaluating drug prices, availability, affordability, and price components: Implications for access to drugs in Malaysia. *PLoS Medicine*, *4*(3). http://dx.doi.org/10.1371/journal.pmed.0040082.

Ball, D., Tisocki, K., & Al-Saffar, N. (2009). *Medicine prices, availability, affordability and price components, Kuwait*. Retrieved from http://haiweb.org/wp-content/uploads/2015/07/Kuwait-Summary-Report-Pricing-Surveys.pdf.

Bazargani, Y. T., Ewen, M., de Boer, A., Leufkens, H. G., & Mantel-Teeuwisse, A. K. (2014). Essential medicines are more available than other medicines around the globe. *Plos One*, *9*(2), e87576. http://dx.doi.org/10.1371/journal.pone.0087576.

Bertoldi, A. D., Helfer, A. P., Camargo, A. L., Tavares, N. U., & Kanavos, P. (2012). Is the Brazilian pharmaceutical policy ensuring population access to essential medicines? *Global Health*, *8*, 6. http://dx.doi.org/10.1186/1744-8603-8-6.

Callen, T. (2012). *Purchasing power parity: Weights matter*. Retrieved from http://www.imf.org/external/pubs/ft/fandd/basics/ppp.htm.

Cameron, A.Hill, S., & Whyte, P. (2015). *WHO guideline on country pharmaceutical pricing policies. Geneva, Switzerland: World Health Organization*. Retrieved from http://apps.who.int/medicinedocs/documents/s21016en/s21016en.pdf.

Cameron, A., Mantel-Teeuwisse, A. K., Leufkens, H. G., & Laing, R. O. (2012). Switching from originator brand medicines to generic equivalents in selected developing countries: How much could be saved? *Value in Health*, *15*(5), 664–673. http://dx.doi.org/10.1016/j.jval.2012.04.004.

Chaikledkaew, U., Lertpitakpong, C., Teerawattananon, Y., Thavorncharoensap, M., & Tangcharoensathien, V. (2009). The current capacity and future development of economic evaluation for policy decision-making: A survey among researchers and decision-makers in Thailand. *Value in Health*, *12*, S31–S35. http://dx.doi.org/10.1111/j.1524-4733.2009.00624.x.

Chalkidou, K. (2012). Evidence and values: Paying for end-of-life drugs in the British NHS. *Health Econ Policy Law*, *7*(4), 393–409. http://dx.doi.org/10.1017/s1744133112000205.

Claxton, K., Palmer, S., Longworth, L., Bojke, L., Griffin, S., McKenna, C., … Youn, J. (2012). Informing a decision framework for when NICE should recommend the use of health technologies only in the context of an appropriately designed programme of evidence development. *Health Technology Assessment*, *16*(46), 1–323. http://dx.doi.org/10.3310/hta16460.

Coyle, D., & Drummond, M. (1993). Does expenditure on pharmaceuticals give good value for money?: current evidence and policy implications. *Health Policy*, *26*(1), 55–75. http://dx.doi.org/10.1016/0168-8510(93)90078-4.

Danzon, P. M., & Towse, A. (2003). Differential pricing for pharmaceuticals: Reconciling access, R&D and patents. *International Journal of Health Economics and Management*, *3*(3), 183–205.

de Joncheere, C. (2003). *Prices, affordability and cost containment* (7th ed.). Amsterdam, The Netherlands: IOP Press.

De Lima, L., Pastrana, T., Radbruch, L., & Wenk, R. (2014). Cross-sectional pilot study to monitor the availability, dispensed prices, and affordability of opioids around the globe. *Journal of Pain and Symptom Management*, *48*(4), 649–659. e641 http://dx.doi.org/10.1016/j.jpainsymman.2013.12.237.

Docteur, E., Paris, V., & Moise, P. (2008). *Pharmaceutical pricing policies in a global market*. OECD Health policy studies. Retrieved from http://www.keepeek.com/Digital-Asset-Management/oecd/social-issues-migration-health/pharmaceutical-pricing-policies-in-a-global-market_9789264044159-en.

Dylst, P., Vulto, A., & Simoens, S. (2013). Demand-side policies to encourage the use of generic medicines: An overview. *Expert Review of Pharmacoeconomics & Outcomes Research*, *13*(1), 59–72. http://dx.doi.org/10.1586/erp.12.83.

Dylst, P., Vulto, A., & Simoens, S. (2014). Analysis of French generic medicines retail market: Why the use of generic medicines is limited. *Expert Review of Pharmacoeconomics & Outcomes Research*, *14*(6), 795–803. http://dx.doi.org/10.1586/14737167.2014.946011.

Enzmann, H., & Broich, K. (2013). Cancer: Is it really so different? Particularities of oncologic drugs from the perspective of the pharmaceutical regulatory agency. *Zeitschrift für Evidenz, Fortbildung und Qualität im Gesundheitswesen*, *107*(2), 120–128. http://dx.doi.org/10.1016/j.zefq.2013.02.003.

Eom, G., Grootendorst, P., & Duffin, J. (2016). The case for an essential medicines list for Canada. *CMAJ*, *188*(17–18), E499–e503. http://dx.doi.org/10.1503/cmaj.160134.

Fang, Y., Wagner, A. K., Yang, S., Jiang, M., Zhang, F., & Ross-Degnan, D. (2013). Access to affordable medicines after health reform: Evidence from two cross-sectional surveys in Shaanxi Province, western China. *The Lancet Global Health*, *1*(4), e227–237. http://dx.doi.org/10.1016/s2214-109x(13)70072-x.

Ford, N., Wilson, D., Costa Chaves, G., Lotrowska, M., & Kijtiwatchakul, K. (2007). Sustaining access to antiretroviral therapy in the less-developed world: Lessons from Brazil and Thailand. *AIDS*, *21*(Suppl. 4), S21–S29. http://dx.doi.org/10.1097/01.aids.0000279703.78685.a6.

Frost, L. J., & Reich, M. R. (2009). Creating access to health technologies in poor countries. *Health Affairs*, *28*(4), 962–973. Retrieved from http://0-search.proquest.com.mylibrary.qu.edu.qa/docview/204619147?accountid=13370.

Grootendorst, P., Pierard, E., & Shim, M. (2009). Life-expectancy gains from pharmaceutical drugs: A critical appraisal of the literature. *Expert Review of Pharmacoeconomics & Outcomes Research*, *9*(4), 353–364. http://dx.doi.org/10.1586/erp.09.35.

Hammad, E. A. (2016). The use of economic evidence to inform drug pricing decisions in Jordan. *Value in Health*, *19*(2), 233–238. http://dx.doi.org/10.1016/j.jval.2015.11.007.

Han, S., Liang, H., Su, W., Xue, Y., & Shi, L. (2013). Can price controls reduce pharmaceutical expenses? A case study of antibacterial expenditures in 12 Chinese hospitals from 1996 to 2005. *International Journal of Health Services*, *43*(1), 91–103.

Hassali, M. A., Alrasheedy, A. A., McLachlan, A., Nguyen, T. A., Al-Tamimi, S. K., Ibrahim, M. I., & Aljadhey, H. (2014). The experiences of implementing generic medicine policy in eight countries: A review and recommendations for a successful promotion of generic medicine use. *Saudi Pharm J*, *22*(6), 491–503. http://dx.doi.org/10.1016/j.jsps.2013.12.017.

Hassall, E., Dib, H., Shepherd, R., Koletzko, S., Radke, M., Henderson, C., & Lundborg, P. (2015). Long-term maintenance treatment with omeprazole in children with healed erosive oesophagitis: A prospective study. *Alimentary Pharmacology & Therapeutics*, *35*(3), 368–379. http://dx.doi.org/10.1111/j.1365-2036.2011.04950.x.

Henry, D., & Lexchin, J. (2002). The pharmaceutical industry as a medicines provider. *Lancet*, *360*(9345), 1590–1595. http://dx.doi.org/10.1016/s0140-6736(02)11527-3.

Hoebert, J. M., van Dijk, L., Mantel-Teeuwisse, A. K., Leufkens, H. G., & Laing, R. O. (2013). National medicines policies - a review of the evolution and development processes. *J Pharm Policy Pract*, *6*, 5. http://dx.doi.org/10.1186/2052-3211-6-5.

Hogerzeil, H. V. (2004). The concept of essential medicines: Lessons for rich countries. *British Medical Journal*, *329*(7475), 1169–1172. http://dx.doi.org/10.1136/bmj.329.7475.1169.

Holloway, K. A., & Henry, D. (2014). WHO essential medicines policies and use in developing and transitional countries: An analysis of reported policy implementation and medicines use surveys. *PLos Medicine*, *11*(9), e1001724. http://dx.doi.org/10.1371/journal.pmed.1001724.

Ho, P. M., Magid, D. J., Shetterly, S. M., Olson, K. L., Maddox, T. M., Peterson, P. N., … Rumsfeld, J. S. (2008). Medication nonadherence is associated with a broad range of adverse outcomes in patients with coronary artery disease. *American Heart Journal*, *155*(4), 772–779. http://dx.doi.org/10.1016/j.ahj.2007.12.011.

Hu, S. (2013). Essential medicine policy in China: Pros and cons. *Journal of Medical Economics*, *16*(2), 289–294. http://dx.doi.org/10.3111/13696998.2012.751176.

Institute for Healthcare Informatics. (2014). *Understanding the pharmaceutical value chain*. Retrieved from https://www.imshealth.com/files/web/IMSH%20Institute/Healthcare%20Briefs/Understanding_Pharmaceutical_Value_Chain.pdf.

Kaló, Z., Alabbadi, I., Al Ahdab, O. G., Alowayesh, M., Elmahdawy, M., Al-Saggabi, A. H., … Kanavos, P. (2015). Implications of external price referencing of pharmaceuticals in Middle East countries. *Expert Review of Pharmacoeconomics & Outcomes Research*, *15*(6), 993–998. http://dx.doi.org/10.1586/14737167.2015.1048227.

Kaló, Z., Annemans, L., & Garrison, L. P. (2013). Differential pricing of new pharmaceuticals in lower income European countries. *Expert Review of Pharmacoeconomics & Outcomes Research*, *13*(6), 735–741. http://dx.doi.org/10.1586/14737167.2013.847367.

Kaplan, W. A., Ritz, L. S., Vitello, M., & Wirtz, V. J. (2012). Policies to promote use of generic medicines in low and middle income countries: A review of published literature, 2000-2010. *Health Policy*, *106*(3), 211–224. http://dx.doi.org/10.1016/j.healthpol.2012.04.015.

King, D. R., & Kanavos, P. (2002). Encouraging the use of generic medicines: Implications for transition economies. *Croatian Medical Journal*, *43*(4), 462–469.

Laing, R., Waning, B., Gray, A., Ford, N., & t Hoen, E. (2003). 25 years of the WHO essential medicines lists: Progress and challenges. *Lancet*, *361*(9370), 1723–1729. http://dx.doi.org/10.1016/s0140-6736(03)13375-2.

Lee, I. H., Bloor, K., Hewitt, C., & Maynard, A. (2012). The effects of new pricing and copayment schemes for pharmaceuticals in South Korea. *Health Policy*, *104*(1), 40–49. http://dx.doi.org/10.1016/j.healthpol.2011.09.003.

Leopold, C., Vogler, S., Mantel-Teeuwisse, A. K., de Joncheere, K., Leufkens, H. G., & Laing, R. (2012). Differences in external price referencing in Europe: A descriptive overview. *Health Policy*, *104*(1), 50–60. http://dx.doi.org/10.1016/j.healthpol.2011.09.008.

Maiga, D., & Williams-Jones, B. (2010). Assessment of the impact of market regulation in Mali on the price of essential medicines provided through the private sector. *Health Policy*, *97*(2–3), 130–135. http://dx.doi.org/10.1016/j.healthpol.2010.04.001.

Meng, Q., Cheng, G., Silver, L., Sun, X., Rehnberg, C., & Tomson, G. (2005). The impact of China's retail drug price control policy on hospital expenditures: A case study in two Shandong hospitals. *Health Policy Plan*, *20*(3), 185–196. http://dx.doi.org/10.1093/heapol/czi018.

Moïse, P., & Docteur, E. (2007). *Pharmaceutical pricing and reimbursement policies in Mexico*. OECD Health Working Papers 25. Retrieved from https://www.oecd.org/mexico/38097348.pdf.

Morel, C. M., McGuire, A., & Mossialos, E. (2011). The level of income appears to have no consistent bearing on pharmaceutical prices across countries. *Health Affairs*, *30*(8), 1545–1552. Retrieved from http://0-search.proquest.com.mylibrary.qu.edu.qa/publichealth/docview/887281241/5FBF549C54704A76PQ/1?accountid=13370.

Nguyen, T. A., Knight, R., Roughead, E. E., Brooks, G., & Mant, A. (2015). Policy options for pharmaceutical pricing and purchasing: Issues for low- and middle-income countries. *Health Policy Plan*, *30*(2), 267–280. http://dx.doi.org/10.1093/heapol/czt105.

Nobrega Ode, T., Marques, A. R., de Araujo, A. C., Karnikowski, M. G., Naves Jde, O., & Silver, L. D. (2007). Retail prices of essential drugs in Brazil: An international comparison. *Revista Panamericana de Salud Pública*, *22*(2), 118–123.

Peters, D. H., Garg, A., Bloom, G., Walker, D. G., Brieger, W. R., & Hafizur Rahman, M. (2008). Poverty and access to health care in developing countries. *Annals of the New York Academy of Sciences*, *1136*(1), 161–171. http://dx.doi.org/10.1196/annals.1425.011.

Ruggeri, K., & Ellen, N. (2013). *Pharmaceutical pricing – the use of external reference pricing* RAND Corporation research report.. Retrieved from http://www.rand.org.

Russo, G., & McPake, B. (2010). Medicine prices in urban Mozambique: A public health and economic study of pharmaceutical markets and price determinants in low-income settings. *Health Policy Plan*, *25*(1), 70–84. http://dx.doi.org/10.1093/heapol/czp042.

Seuba, X. (2006). A human rights approach to the WHO Model list of essential medicines. *Bulletin of the World Health Organization*, *84*(5), 405–407. http://dx.doi.org/10.1590/S0042-96862006000500022. discussion 408-411.

Vogler, S., & Habimana, K. (2014). *Pharmaceutical pricing policies in European countries*. Retrieved from http://whocc.goeg.at/Literaturliste/Dokumente/BooksReports/GOe_FP_Pharmaceutical_Pricing_Europe_CtW_final_forPublication.pdf.

Vogler, S., Kilpatrick, K., & Babar, Z. U. (2015). Analysis of medicine prices in New Zealand and 16 European countries. *Value in Health*, *18*(4), 484–492. http://dx.doi.org/10.1016/j.jval.2015.01.003.

Vogler, S., Lepuschütz, L., & Schneider, P. (2015). Pharmaceutical distribution remuneration in Europe. *Journal of Pharmaceutical Policy and Practice*, *8*(Suppl. 1), P23. http://dx.doi.org/10.1186/2052-3211-8-S1-P23.

Vogler, S., Vitry, A., & Babar, Z. (2016). Cancer drugs in 16 European countries, Australia, and New Zealand: A cross-country price comparison study. *The Lancet Oncology*, *17*(1), 39–47. http://dx.doi.org/10.1016/S1470-2045(15)00449-0.

Vogler, S., Zimmermann, N., Ferrario, A., Wirtz, V. J., de Joncheere, K., Pedersen, H. B., … Babar, Z. (2016). Pharmaceutical policies in a crisis? Challenges and solutions identified at the PPRI Conference. *Journal of Pharmaceutical Policy and Practice*, *9*, 9. http://dx.doi.org/10.1186/s40545-016-0056-8.

Vogler, S., Zimmermann, N., & Habl, C. (2013). Understanding the components of pharmaceutical expenditure—overview of pharmaceutical policies influencing expenditure across European countries. *Generics and Biosimilars Initiative Journal (GaBI Journal)*, *2*(4), 178–187. http://dx.doi.org/10.5639/gabij.2013.0204.051.

Weng, G., Han, S., Pu, R., Pan, W. H., & Shi, L. (2014). Exploration of approaches to adjusting brand-name drug prices in Mainland of China: Based on comparison and analysis of some brand-name drug prices of Mainland and Taiwan, China. *Chinese Medical Journal (England)*, *127*(12), 2222–2228.

Wertheimer, A., Radican, L., & Jacobs, M. R. (2010). Assessing different perspectives on the value of a pharmaceutical innovation. *Southern Medical Journal*, *3*(1), 24–28.

World Health Organization. (2010). *A successful joint Lebanon WHO good governance in medicines programme. Increasing transparency and good governance in the pharmaceutical sector: Lebanon a country case study*. Retrieved from http://www.who.int/alliance-hpsr/projects/alliancehpsr_governance_lebanon.pdf.

World Health Organization. (2012a). *Financing and sustainability* Chapter 9: Pharmaceutical pricing policy. Retrieved from http://apps.who.int/medicinedocs/documents/s19585en/s19585en.pdf.

World Health Organization. (2012b). *Policy and economic issues – Chapter 4-National medicine policy*. Retrieved from http://apps.who.int/medicinedocs/documents/s19581en/s19581en.pdf.

World Health Organization. (2012c). *Target 8e: Access to affordable essential medicines* Delivering on the global partnership for achieving the MDGs. Retrieved fromhttp://www.who.int/medicines/mdg/MDG08ChapterEMedsEn.pdf.

World Health Organization. (2012d). *World Health Statistics*. Retrieved from http://apps.who.int/iris/bitstream/10665/44844/1/9789241564441_eng.pdf.

World Health Organization. (2016a). *Essential medicines and health products – essential medicines*. Retrieved fromhttp://www.who.int/medicines/services/essmedicines_def/en/.

World Health Organization. (2016b). *Fact file – 10 facts on essential medicines*. Retrieved from http://www.who.int/features/factfiles/essential_medicines/essential_medicines_facts/en/.

World Health Organization. *Essential medicines - Health topics*. Retrieved from http://www.who.int/topics/essential_medicines/en/.

World Health Organization/Health Action International. (2008). *Measuring medicine prices, availability, affordability and price components* (2nd ed.). Retrieved fromhttp://www.who.int/medicines/areas/access/OMS_Medicine_prices.pdf.

Yang, H., Dib, H., Zhu, M., Qi, G., & Zhang, X. (2010). Prices, availability and affordability of essential medicines in rural areas of Hubei Province, China. *Health Policy Plan*, *25*(3), 219–229. http://dx.doi.org/10.1093/heapol/czp056.

Zhou, Z., Syu, Y., Campbell, B., Zhou, Z., Gao, J., Yu, Q., … Pan, Y. (2015). The financial impact of the 'zero-markup policy for essential drugs' on patients in county hospitals in western rural China. *PLos One*, *10*(3), e0121630. http://dx.doi.org/10.1371/journal.pone.0121630.

CHAPTER

ECONOMIC EVALUATION OF PREDOMINANT DISEASE IN DEVELOPING COUNTRIES: DIABETES MELLITUS

8

Asrul A. Shafie, Chin H. Ng

Universiti Sains Malaysia, Minden, Malaysia

CHAPTER OUTLINE

INTRODUCTION

The global disease burden has drastically changed between the years 1990 and 2010, whereby the mortality from communicable diseases decreased by 17%, whereas the mortality from noncommunicable diseases increased by 30% (Lozano et al., 2012). The trend is reflective of the underlying changes in the global pattern of diseases over the last four decades, particularly the significant reduction of communicable diseases affecting children and the rapid increase of circulatory causes among adults over the age of 50 years.

Two of the most important factors affecting this change include population growth (contributing 31.8% of the change) and aging, which, on its own, attributes to the decrease of communicable diseases by 11.2% and the increase of noncommunicable diseases by 39.2%.

Hence, the change is more prominent in developing countries, which accounts for 97% of the global population growth (United Nations Population Division, 2011). Their rapid growth, driven by high birth rates and young demographics, is expected to reach a population of 8 billion by 2050, making it three-fourths of the global population.

Therefore, the impact of changes in the affliction of diseases can be more devastating to developing countries because they are more limited in resources and possess an underdeveloped healthcare system, which had already taken a heavy beating from multiple economic recessions over the years. The crisis

Social and Administrative Aspects of Pharmacy in Low- and Middle-Income Countries. http://dx.doi.org/10.1016/B978-0-12-811228-1.00008-X

in the economies of developing countries had manifested because of mounting deficits in trade and payment balances, dwindling currency reserves, currency devaluations, increasing rates of inflation, higher indebtedness, and soaring public budget deficits (Gurtner, 2010). Their average income per capita had dropped one-fifth because of this crisis. Hence, economic evaluation should be increasingly applied to improve efficiency in the health system. This tool allows the maximization of resources at the lowest cost. However, its use in developing countries is challenged by the technical capacity of users (e.g., Health Technology Assessment (HTA) agency, the ministry, or researchers). This limits its uptake in decision-making processes.

In this chapter, the quality and outcome of economic evaluation studies concerning the use of the insulin analogue among diabetic patients in developing countries were reviewed. This will provide an understanding of how the results can be employed, as well as the existing capacity of developing countries to conduct such research.

Diabetes is a major contributor to the global health burden from diseases. There is a 76.5% increase of deaths from diabetes, urogenital disorders, blood, and endocrine disorders over the past four decades. The prevalence of diabetes among all age groups was estimated to be 2.8% in 2000 and 4.4% in 2030, which affects 366 million of the population (Wild, Roglic, Green, Sicree, & King, 2004). Ninety-five percent of cases are type 2 diabetes mellitus (T2DM) and the majority of this increase is likely to occur in developing countries due to population growth, aging, unhealthy diet, obesity, and a sedentary lifestyle.

In symptomatic hyperglycemic patients with metabolic decompensation, or those that fail to achieve targeted HbA1c level with a maximum dose of OADs, human insulin is conventionally initiated in combination with oral antidiabetic drugs (OADs) (UK Diabetes, 2016). It is made by extractions from *Escherichia coli*. The genetic modification of the protein in the DNA of *E. coli* allows production of insulin that mimics the body's natural insulin (Bolli, Di Marchi, Park, Pramming, & Koivisto, 1999), commonly referred to as insulin analogues. It has better postprandial glycemia level control and pharmacokinetic characteristics, and it is as effective as human insulin. Compared with human insulin, the short-acting insulin analogue has a more rapid subcutaneous absorption, postpeak decrease, and earlier and greater insulin peak (Rolla, 2008). The long-acting insulin analogue, on the other hand, is peakless compared with the intermediate-acting human insulin; hence, it is associated with lower risks of nocturnal hypoglycemia. Insulin analogue is recommended for type 1 diabetic patients in the United Kingdom by the National Institute for Health and Care Excellence (NICE), whereas Canada recommends the long-acting insulin analogue as the primary choice for basal insulin regimen, initiated with OADs, instead of the intermediate-acting human insulin.

There are now more varieties of insulin analogues suited for various treatment strategies; however, their uptake remains slow and contentious in developing countries because the price for insulin analogues are at least three to four times more expensive compared with the conventional insulin.

REVIEWING METHODS

Economic evaluation studies published in English until September 30, 2015, were identified by searching electronic databases and reference lists in selected HTA agencies' databases (Canadian Agency for Drugs and Technologies in Health (CADTH), the Centre for Reviews and Dissemination at the University of York, and the Malaysian HTA Section), technical reports, and electronic databases (EMBASE, PubMed, the NHS Economic Evaluation Database, EconLit, and the CEA Registry by Tufts University). The search terms include "insulin," "cost," "benefit," "effective," "utility," and "minimization." The full search terms and strategies were described by Shafie, Ng, Tan, and Chaiyakunapruk (2016). Only full economic evaluations (cost-effectiveness analysis, cost-benefit analysis, and cost-utility analysis) with complete methodological descriptions that evaluated insulin analogues in humans were included.

Selected studies were abstracted and appraised using the CHEERS checklist (Cooper, Coyle, Abrams, Mugford, & Sutton, 2005; Husereau et al., 2013). The costs cited in the original studies were converted to the USD 2015 value using the gross domestic product deflator index and purchasing power parities.

Fifty articles were identified from the full text review to fulfill the inclusion criteria (Fig. 8.1). Only six of them were studies based on developing countries.

PROFILE OF REVIEWED ECONOMIC EVALUATION

Table 8.1 summarized the key elements of the included studies. All studies focused on the population of T2DM and used insulin analogues as an add-on therapy with oral or other injectable antidiabetic agents. There is no research that evaluated short-acting insulin analogues. There are an equal number

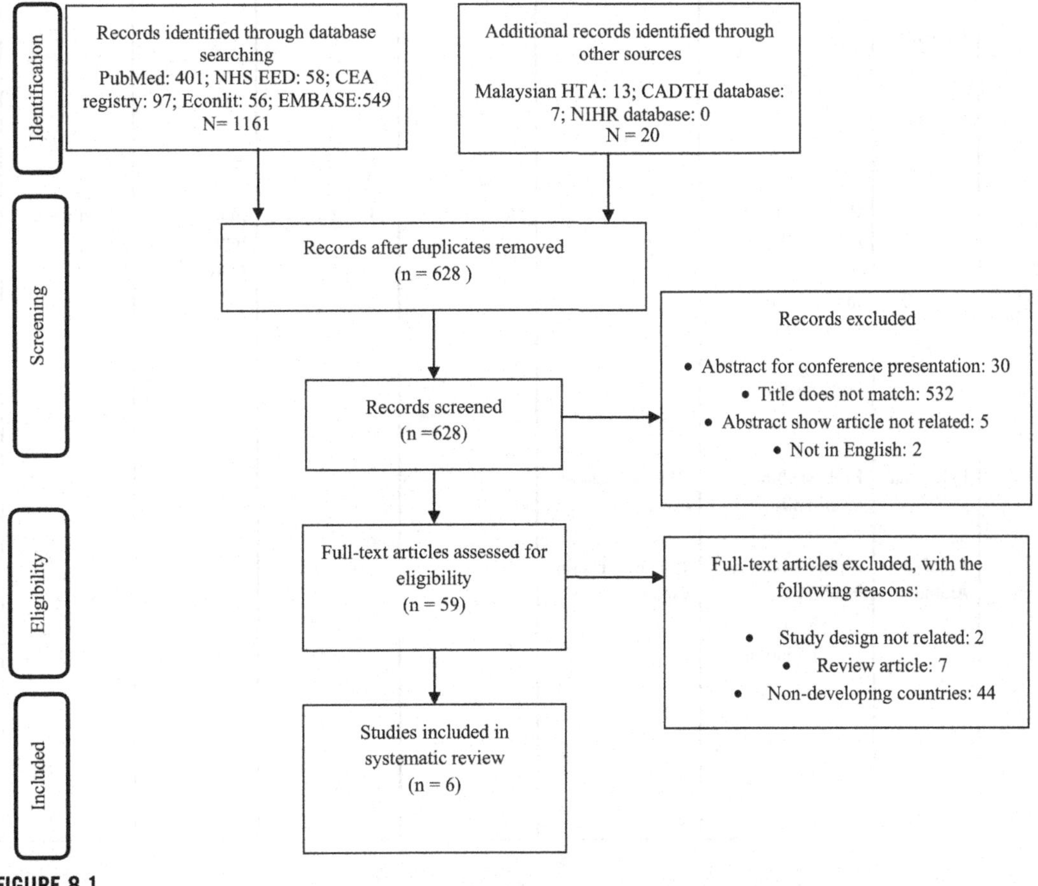

FIGURE 8.1

PRISMA flow diagram describing the study selection process.

Table 8.1 Cost-Effectiveness Analysis in Developing Countries for Insulin

References	Country	Comparator	Intervention	Perspective	Type of Economic Evaluation	Choice of Model	Cost Type	Time Horizon
Palmer et al. (2008)	China	Biphasic human insulin 30	Biphasic insulin aspart 30	Third-party payer	CEA, CUA	State transition model	Healthcare cost	30 years
Palmer, Beaudet, White, Plun-Favreau, and Smith-Palmer (2010)	China	Insulin glargine	Biphasic insulin aspart once daily Biphasic insulin aspart twice daily	Not mentioned	CEA, CUA	State transition model	Healthcare cost	30 years
Shafie et al. (2016)	Saudi Arabia India Indonesia Algeria	OAD	Biphasic insulin aspart	Not mentioned	CEA, CUA	State transition model	Healthcare cost	30 years
Gupta, Baabbad, Hammerby, Nikolajsen, and Shafie (2015)	India	Biphasic human insulin 30 Insulin glargine NPH insulin	Biphasic insulin aspart 30	Not mentioned	CEA, CUA	State transition model	Healthcare costs	35 years
	Indonesia	Biphasic human insulin 30	Biphasic insulin aspart 30					
	Saudi Arabia	Biphasic human insulin 30 Insulin glargine NPH insulin	Biphasic insulin aspart 30					

Discount Rate (Costs and Benefit Both)	Total Costs per Patient		Incremental Effects		Incremental Cost-Effectiveness Ratio	
	Intervention	Comparator	Life Year Gain (LY)	Quality-Adjusted Life Year (QALY)	Incremental Cost per LY	Incremental Cost per QALY
3%	USD 63,281	USD 62,736	0.38	0.91	USD 1450	USD 600
3%	USD 66,466	USD 83,727	0.04	–0.03	Dominant	Cost saving
	USD 87,636	USD 118,670	0.08	–0.01	Dominant	Cost saving
3%	30 years: USD 51,094	30 years: USD 53,060	30 years: 1.9	30 years: 2.77	30 years: Dominant	
	Not mentioned					1 year: USD 1753
	30 years: USD 7674	30 years: USD 5925	30 years: 1.3	30 years: 4.57	30 years: USD 1346	30 years: USD 384
	Not mentioned					1 year: USD 635
	30-years: USD 30,158	30 years: USD 25,177	30 years: 1.8	30 years: 2.73	30 years: USD 2767	30 years: USD 1693
	Not mentioned					1 year: USD 4,206
	30 years: USD 17,457	30 years: USD 12,322	30 years: 1.5	30 years: 2.65	30 years: USD 3423	30 years: USD 2028
	Not mentioned					1 year: USD 3,210
Not mentioned	30 years: USD 7229	30 years: USD 6321		30 years: 2.52		30 years: USD 363
	1-year incremental cost: USD 129			1 year: 0.21		1 year: USD 602
	30 years: USD 7852	30 years: USD 10,490		30 years: 2.82		Dominant
	1-year incremental cost: Cost saving			1 year: 0.24		Dominant
	30 years: USD 6954	30 years: USD 6404		30 years: 2.74		30 years: USD 201
	1-year incremental cost: USD 99			1 year: 0.23		1 year: USD 194
	30 years: USD 31,816	30 years: USD 27,864		30 years: 0.83		30 years: USD 4774
	1-year incremental cost: USD 458			1 year: 0.04		1 year: USD 11,190
	30 years: USD 55,567	30 years: USD 55,103		30 years: 2		30 years: USD 224
	1-year incremental cost: USD 512			1 year: 0.14		1 year: USD 3454
	30 years: USD 54,814	30 years: USD 63,858		30 years: 2.08		Dominant
	1-year incremental cost: USD 355			1 year: 0.24		Dominant
	30 years: USD 49,644	30 years: USD 52,065		30 years: 1.74		Dominant
	1-year incremental cost: USD 30 USD 31			1 year: 0.12		1 year: USD 2661

(Continued)

Table 8.1 Cost-Effectiveness Analysis in Developing Countries for Insulin—cont'd

References	Country	Comparator	Intervention	Perspective	Type of Economic Evaluation	Choice of Model	Cost Type	Time Horizon
Yang, Christensen, Sun, and Chang (2012)	China	Insulin glargine	Insulin detemir	Societal	CEA, CUA	State transition model	Healthcare costs	35 years
Home, Baik, Galvez, Malek, and Nikolajsen (2015)	Mexico South Korea Indonesia India Algeria	OAD	Insulin detemir	Third party payer	CEA, CUA	State transition model	Healthcare costs	30 years

All costs are converted to USD 2015 value.

CEA, *cost-effectiveness analysis;* CUA, *cost-utility analysis;* NPH, *neutral protamine Hagedorn;* OAD, *oral antidiabetic drug.*

Adapted From Shafie, A.A., Ng, C.H., Tan, Y.P., Chaiyakunapruk, N. (2016). Systematic review of the cost effectiveness of insulin analogues in type 1 and type 2 diabetes mellitus. Pharmacoeconomics, *1–22. http://dx.doi.org/10.1007/s40273-016-0456-2.*

Discount Rate (Costs and Benefit Both)	Total Costs per Patient		Incremental Effects		Incremental Cost-Effectiveness Ratio	
	Intervention	**Comparator**	**Life Year Gain (LY)**	**Quality-Adjusted Life Year (QALY)**	**Incremental Cost per LY**	**Incremental Cost per QALY**
3%	USD 48,310	USD 48,768	0.061	0.484	Dominant	
3%	30 years: USD 80,740	30 years: USD 81,295	30 years: 1.19	30 years: 2.57	30 years: Dominant	
	1-year incremental cost: USD 707			1 year: 0.15		1 year: USD 5172
	30 years: USD 42,736	30 years: USD 42,719	30 years: 0.60	30 years: 1.07	30 years: USD 28	30 years: USD 15
	1-year incremental cost: USD 259			1 year: 0.06		1 year: USD 4210
	30 years: USD 25,708	30 years: USD 24,177	30 years: 0.61	30 years: 1.83	30 years: USD 2,510	30 years: USD 444
	1-year incremental cost: USD 272			1 year: 0.11		1 year: USD 2547
	30 years: USD 10,308	30 years: USD 6553	30 years: 0.90	30 years: 4.97	30 years: USD 4172	30 years: USD 756
	1-year incremental cost: USD 362			1 year: 0.322		1 year: USD 1128
	30 years: USD 16,883	30 years: USD 11,300	30 years: 0.50	30 years: 1.18	30 years: USD 11,166	30 years: USD 4948
	1-year incremental cost: USD 507			1 year: 0.064		1 year: USD 8299

of publications that evaluated biphasic (biphasic insulin aspart) and long-acting (detemir, glargine) insulin analogues that covered seven developing countries, which includes Algeria, China, India, Indonesia, Mexico, Saudi Arabia, and South Korea. All studies were sponsored by pharmaceutical companies, specifically Novo Nordisk.

Only two studies had clearly stated their perspectives. One study (Yang et al., 2012) took a societal perspective, whereas another study used the third-party payer perspective. However, the former did not provide clear information regarding the cost accounted for the undertaken societal perspective. Comparators were clearly identified in all studies, although not many had fully justified their choices. Insulin analogues were compared with

- other insulin analogues of a different onset type (biphasic insulin analogue vs. long-acting insulin analogue),
- other insulin analogues of the same onset type (glargine vs. detemir),
- human insulin of the same onset type (e.g., biphasic insulin aspart 30 vs. biphasic human insulin 30),
- human insulin of a different onset type (e.g., biphasic insulin aspart 30 vs. neutral protamine Hagedorn (NPH) insulin), and
- OADs.

The comparison was conducted to evaluate either a switching strategy (three studies), whereby the insulin analogue was assessed on insulin-experienced patient population, or an initiation strategy (three studies), whereby the insulin analogue was assessed on insulin-naïve patient population.

The time horizon was typically stated and justified based on the country's published guideline suggestion or the duration required for capturing all costs and consequences of diabetes-related complications. Most studies had evaluated the intervention for 30 years, except for one study that had selected 35 years in the time horizon. The discount rate for the cost and benefit was selected at 3% for all studies, except for one that did not specify any discount rate despite their 35-year time horizon.

All studies had evaluated their intervention using the proprietary Markov-based IMS CORE Diabetes Model. The model consists of 17 interdependent submodels that simulate the progression of diabetes and its complications, including angina, myocardial infarction, congestive heart failure, and stroke. The model is well validated and continuously updated with new modules and underlying equations. However, none of the published works had described the version of the CORE Diabetes Model used.

These models can bring together data from a variety of sources including randomized controlled trials, observational studies, case registries, public health statistics, and quality-of-life surveys, simulating disease progression and related costs through time in a population. A model may require several sources for its economic, epidemiological, or clinical parameter input. The sources employed to input the study model were appraised using Cooper's checklist (Cooper et al., 2005), where a lower score indicates a higher quality of the evidence. Fig. 8.2 presented the input quality results. The majority of studies (n=5) derived their clinical effects from the same cohort study, whereas their baseline clinical data and resource utilization were mostly estimated from analyzing data from the same study jurisdiction.

The disutility value for hypoglycemia was derived from numerous sources. However, the source for disutility value for mild (−0.0035), moderate (−0.0118), and severe hypoglycemia was less varied with the utility for the two former states taken from Palmer et al. (2004), whereas the last state was taken from Currie et al. (2006). Some studies, however, replaced the default CORE value with the cohort study value.

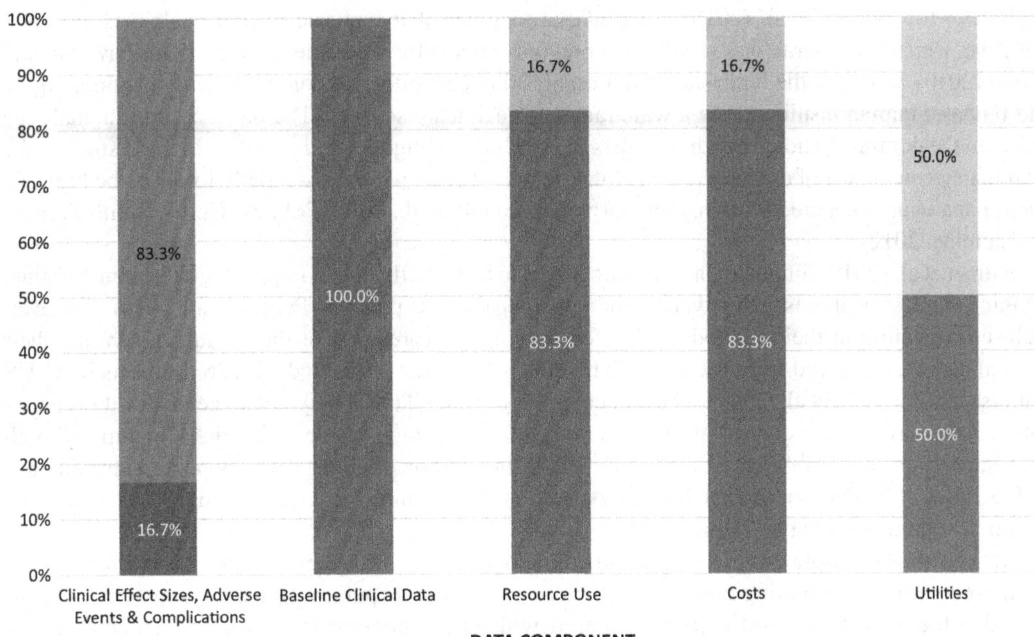

FIGURE 8.2

Stacked bar chart showing the ranks of the evidence used in the decision model. * Not related: It means the study did not required the input from the particular data component.

All articles described handling uncertainty by conducting a sensitivity analysis. The most common parameter variances were the time horizon, annual discount rate, HbA1c effect of the insulin analogue, incidence of hypoglycemia episodes, dose of insulin, and utility value.

All studies reported additional gain of life years (0.04–1.9 LY) of biphasic insulin analogue over comparators. There were mixed results on the changes in quality-adjusted life years (QALY) where some reported to have gained up to 4.57 QALY, whereas one study reported a decrease of QALY between −0.01 and −0.03. Among the insulin-experienced population, switching from insulin glargine to biphasic insulin analogue is consistently a dominant strategy. Switching from NPH insulin provided a variety of incremental cost-effectiveness ratio (ICER) ranging from dominant to USD201/QALY gained over a 30-year time horizon. Switching from biphasic human insulin to a biphasic human analogue, however, has a higher ICER, ranging from USD 224 to USD 4774/QALY gained. Among insulin-naïve patients, initiating biphasic insulin analogue is more cost-effective than OADs with ICER between dominant and USD 3423/QALY gained.

The changes in the clinical benefits (hypoglycemia incidence) for biphasic insulin analogue had the highest impact on the ICER value. The ICER value increased 729% higher than the base-case result when the biphasic insulin aspart was assumed to have no improvement in the hypoglycemia rate (Palmer et al., 2008). Other parameters, such as complications, management costs, time horizon, and number of patient visits, did not have a substantial influence on the ICER values or were not explored in the studies.

Except for Palmer et al. (2010), all studies concluded that biphasic insulin analogues are cost-effective, which, in general, was similar to a previous review by Valentine, Pollock, Plun-Favreau, and White (2010), whereby the biphasic insulin aspart 30 is cost-effective compared with insulin glargine and biphasic human insulin across a wide range of healthcare settings. The biphasic insulin analogue was also the dominant choice in other studies in the United Kingdom and Sweden. In these studies, the total management cost of diabetes and the total treatment costs were substantially lower in the biphasic insulin analogue compared with insulin glargine (Goodall et al., 2008; Pollock, Curtis, Smith-Palmer, & Valentine, 2012).

Palmer et al. (2010) found biphasic insulin aspart to be less effective compared with insulin glargine, bringing to question its cost-effectiveness for managing diabetic patients (Palmer et al., 2010). However, a closer inspection of their methods called for cautious interpretation of their results given that their clinical data were derived from the INITIATE study, which was conducted with 263 subjects in 23 US centers (Yki-Jarvinen et al., 2007). The clinical findings in INITIATE may not be generalized to Asians who usually have poorer control of diabetes and exhibit less improvements in HbA1c compared with whites, Africans, or Caribbeans (James et al., 2012). In addition, the East Asian population usually has earlier onset of T2DM and earlier β-cell dysfunction that require earlier insulin treatment compared with other ethnicities (Ma & Chan, 2013).

Among the available long-acting insulin analogues, insulin detemir is the dominant option compared with the remaining on insulin glargine for insulin-experienced patients. Insulin detemir was also found to be cost-effective compared with OADs among insulin-naïve patients (ICER dominant–USD 11,166/QALY). The cost-effectiveness of long-acting insulin analogue was sensitive to the changes in the HbA1c effect and hypoglycemic event rate. Home et al. (2015) had demonstrated that the application of the first quartile distribution of the HbA1c treatment effects in the model caused the ICER to increase by more than 230-fold (USD 15–USD 3453 per QALY gained) in contrast to the base-case result (Home et al., 2015). Assuming similar hypoglycemia event rates between insulin detemir and glargine increased the ICER by 216%. In terms of cost, inclusion of self-monitoring blood glucose strips increased the ICER by sixfold in Indonesia (Home et al., 2015).

ACHIEVEMENTS

Insulin is the mainstay treatment for type 1 and advanced-stage type 2 diabetes mellitus. Results from the Diabetes Control Trial and United Kingdom Prospective Study confirmed the value of glycemic control conferred by insulin in preventing diabetes complications. However, the pharmacokinetic and pharmacodynamics profile of conventional insulin pose safety risks that limit its use in the population. The newer insulin analogue's ability to more closely match the basal and mealtime components of endogenous insulin secretion than the conventional insulin had resulted in more flexible treatment regiments with a lower risk of hypoglycemia events. Access to safer and more effective innovative treatment is the cornerstone of modern healthcare and is key to managing chronic disease epidemics such as diabetes. However, the higher price of insulin analogues necessitates a careful evaluation of its economic evidence, in addition to efficacy and safety evidences.

Hence, the availability of six published studies that cover seven developing countries provided essential evidences for their decision-makers to determine the cost-effectiveness of insulin analogues for treating diabetic patients in their respective countries. The countries may be able to relate more from studies of neighboring countries with similar macroeconomic levels. In addition, the fairly moderate quality evidences provide further confidence in the decision-making process. Investigation of three types of insulin analogues provided strategic options for decision-makers and clinicians in designing optimum insulin treatments for patients.

CHALLENGES

Although the body of evidence that support safety and efficacy are abundant, the same cannot be said for economic evidence. There are far fewer economic evaluation studies for insulin analogues in developing countries compared with the 44 published studies in developed countries. One of the factors that hinder its availability could be the limited resources accessible to conduct such research in developing countries. Much of the public research funding target hard science research that focus on producing commercially viable products. Most of the funding in HTA agencies or the Ministry of Health in countries are also usually meant for operational or internal purposes. Hence, it is not surprising to find that all studies found in this review were sponsored by manufacturers.

Only three types of insulin analogues and limited treatment strategies were evaluated in developing countries. There are no studies that examined rapid-acting insulin analogues or assessed the type 1 population. This will severely limit the evidence-based choices for developing countries. To meet the domestic demand of clinicians and HTA practitioners, they may need to resort to applying studies of developed countries into their own countries. However, transferability of economic evaluation results from developed countries to developing countries is vulnerable to system bias. The healthcare system in developing countries is different in which the out-of-pocket payment is the principal means to finance healthcare compared with the third-party payer system that is prevalent in developed countries such as the United Kingdom or the United States. In addition, utility values that form the bulk of cost-utility analysis in developed countries might be substantially different to developing countries' population preferences.

There are also significant variations in scope, approach, and quality of information reported between all six studies in developing countries. The majority of economic evaluation studies did not report all information required by the CHEERS statement, particularly in regard to the study perspective, the source of utility, and cost. Consequently, it prevents direct comparisons of the existing cost-effectiveness study results and challenges the study's internal validity. This could severely jeopardize the study's credibility for essential decision-making.

RECOMMENDATIONS: THE WAY FORWARD

The lack of quality studies in developing countries could be a reflection on the gap of the local capacity to conduct and use economic evaluation studies in such countries. International societies (e.g., International Societies for Pharmacoeconomic and Outcomes Research) and developed countries (e.g., NICE International) could assist developing countries to improve this capacity through training and partnership. Because many of the decision-making topics are common among developing countries, they could jointly collaborate in regional network initiatives (e.g., HTAsiaLink) to conduct research and share information.

It is important for developing countries to allocate sufficient resources to fund local economic evaluation studies and proactively detect new technologies through horizon scanning activities. This would limit commercially motivated studies and ensure research integrity.

CONCLUSIONS

At present, there is no evidence on the cost-effectiveness of short-acting insulin analogues for T2DM in developing countries. There is moderate evidence of the cost-effectiveness of long-acting insulin analogues, particularly insulin detemir in T2DM when switched from insulin glargine. However, given the small incremental benefit gained with the insulin analogue, it is critical for future studies to investigate the impact of varying the effectiveness on their results.

Biphasic insulin analogue is a cost-effective option compared with all comparators (all types of conventional insulin and OADs) for T2DM patients, particularly patients who do not have compliance issues. Nevertheless, additional real-world evidence is necessary to consider the implication of patient compliance as a result of the twice daily injection dosage required to achieve the maximum benefits on its cost-effectiveness.

LESSONS LEARNED

- There are six economic evaluation studies on the use of insulin analogues conducted in seven developing countries.
- Only three types of insulin analogues were evaluated.
- There are no studies that had evaluated short-acting insulin analogues for those in type 1 diabetes population.
- Biphasic insulin analogue is a cost-effective option compared with all comparators (all types of conventional insulin and OADs) for T2DM patients.
- There are gaps in quantity and quality of economic evaluation studies in developing countries that could be remedied by increasing public funding and human capital to conduct such researches.

ACKNOWLEDGMENTS

The author appreciates the help of Tan Yui Ping and Nathorn Chaiyakunapruk for their earlier assistance in the review.

REFERENCES

Bolli, G. B., Di Marchi, R. D., Park, G. D., Pramming, S., & Koivisto, V. A. (1999). Insulin analogues and their potential in the management of diabetes mellitus. *Diabetologia, 42*(10), 1151–1167. http://dx.doi.org/10.1007/s001250051286.

Cooper, N., Coyle, D., Abrams, K., Mugford, M., & Sutton, A. (2005). Use of evidence in decision models: An appraisal of health technology assessments in the UK since 1997. *Journal of Health Services Research & Policy, 10*(4), 245–250.

Currie, C. J., Morgan, C. L., Poole, C. D., Sharplin, P., Lammert, M., & McEwan, P. (2006). Multivariate models of health-related utility and the fear of hypoglycaemia in people with diabetes. *Current Medical Research and Opinion*, 22. http://dx.doi.org/10.1185/030079906x115757.

Goodall, G., Jendle, J. H., Valentine, W. J., Munro, V., Brandt, A. B., Ray, J. A., … Palmer, A. J. (2008). Biphasic insulin aspart 70/30 vs. insulin glargine in insulin naive type 2 diabetes patients: Modelling the long-term health economic implications in a Swedish setting. *International Journal of Clinical Practice*, *62*(6), 869–876. http://dx.doi.org/10.1111/j.1742-1241.2008.01766.x.

Gupta, V., Baabbad, R., Hammerby, E., Nikolajsen, A., & Shafie, A. A. (2015). An analysis of the cost-effectiveness of switching from biphasic human insulin 30, insulin glargine, or neutral protamine Hagedorn to biphasic insulin aspart 30 in people with type 2 diabetes. *Journal of Medical Economics*, *18*(4), 1–10. http://dx.doi.org/10.3111/13696998.2014.991791.

Gurtner, B. (2010). *The financial and economic crisis and developing countries*. https://poldev.revues.org/144.

Home, P., Baik, S. H., Galvez, G. G., Malek, R., & Nikolajsen, A. (2015). An analysis of the cost-effectiveness of starting insulin detemir in insulin-naive people with type 2 diabetes. *Journal of Medical Economics*, *18*(3), 230–240. http://dx.doi.org/10.3111/13696998.2014.985788.

Husereau, D., Drummond, M., Petrou, S., Carswell, C., Moher, D., Greenberg, D., … CHEERS Task Force (2013). Consolidated health economic evaluation reporting standards (CHEERS) statement. *BMC Medicine*, *11*(1), 80.

James, G. D., Baker, P., Badrick, E., Mathur, R., Hull, S., & Robson, J. (2012). Type 2 diabetes: A cohort study of treatment, ethnic and social group influences on glycated haemoglobin. *BMJ Open*, *2*(5). http://dx.doi.org/10.1136/bmjopen-2012-001477.

Lozano, R., Naghavi, M., Foreman, K., Lim, S., Shibuya, K., Aboyans, V., … Murray, C. J. L. (2012). Global and regional mortality from 235 causes of death for 20 age groups in 1990 and 2010: A systematic analysis for the global burden of disease study 2010. *The Lancet*, *380*(9859), 2095–2128.

Ma, R. C., & Chan, J. C. (2013). Type 2 diabetes in East Asians: Similarities and differences with populations in Europe and the United States. *Annals of the New York Academy of Sciences*, *1281*, 64–91. http://dx.doi.org/10.1111/nyas.12098.

Palmer, J. L., Beaudet, A., White, J., Plun-Favreau, J., & Smith-Palmer, J. (2010). Cost-effectiveness of biphasic insulin aspart versus insulin glargine in patients with type 2 diabetes in China. *Advances in Therapy*, *27*(11), 814–827. http://dx.doi.org/10.1007/s12325-010-0078-6.

Palmer, J. L., Gibbs, M., Scheijbeler, H. W., Kotchie, R. W., Nielsen, S., White, J., & Valentine, W. J. (2008). Cost-effectiveness of switching to biphasic insulin aspart in poorly-controlled type 2 diabetes patients in China. *Advances in Therapy*, *25*(8), 752–774. http://dx.doi.org/10.1007/s12325-008-0080-4.

Palmer, A. J., Roze, S., Valentine, W. J., Minshall, M. E., Foos, V., Lurati, F. M., … Spinas, G. A. (2004). The CORE diabetes model: Projecting long-term clinical outcomes, costs and cost-effectiveness of interventions in diabetes mellitus (types 1 and 2) to support clinical and reimbursement decision-making. *Current Medical Research and Opinion*, *20*(Suppl. 1), S5–S26. http://dx.doi.org/10.1185/030079904X1980.

Pollock, R. F., Curtis, B. H., Smith-Palmer, J., & Valentine, W. J. (2012). A UK analysis of the cost-effectiveness of Humalog Mix75/25 and Mix50/50 versus long-acting basal insulin. *Advances in Therapy*, *29*(12), 1051–1066. http://dx.doi.org/10.1007/s12325-012-0065-1.

Rolla, A. (2008). Pharmacokinetic and pharmacodynamic advantages of insulin analogues and premixed insulin analogues over human insulins: Impact on efficacy and safety. *The American Journal of Medicine*, *121*(6 Suppl.), S9–s19. http://dx.doi.org/10.1016/j.amjmed.2008.03.022.

Shafie, A. A., Ng, C. H., Tan, Y. P., & Chaiyakunapruk, N. (2016). Systematic review of the cost effectiveness of insulin analogues in type 1 and type 2 diabetes mellitus. *Pharmacoeconomics*, 1–22. http://dx.doi.org/10.1007/s40273-016-0456-2.

UK Diabetes. (2016). *Analogue insulin*. http://www.diabetes.co.uk/insulin/analogue-insulin.html.

United Nations Population Division. (2011). *World population prospects: The 2010 revision*. http://www.prb.org/publications/Datasheets/2012/world-population-data-sheet/fact-sheet-world-population.aspx.

Valentine, W. J., Pollock, R. F., Plun-Favreau, J., & White, J. (2010). Systematic review of the cost-effectiveness of biphasic insulin aspart 30 in type 2 diabetes. *Current Medical Research and Opinion*, *26*(6), 1399–1412. http://dx.doi.org/10.1185/03007991003689381.

Wild, S., Roglic, G., Green, A., Sicree, R., & King, H. (2004). Global prevalence of diabetes: Estimates for the year 2000 and projections for 2030. *Diabetes Care, 27*, 1047–1053.

Yang, L., Christensen, T., Sun, F., & Chang, J. (2012). Cost-effectiveness of switching patients with type 2 diabetes from insulin glargine to insulin detemir in Chinese setting: A health economic model based on the PREDICTIVE study. *Value in Health, 15*(1 Suppl.), S56–S59. http://dx.doi.org/10.1016/j.jval.2011.11.018.

Yki-Jarvinen, H., Juurinen, L., Alvarsson, M., Bystedt, T., Caldwell, I., Davies, M., … Vähätalo, M. (2007). Initiate insulin by Aggressive Titration and Education (INITIATE): A randomized study to compare initiation of insulin combination therapy in type 2 diabetic patients individually and in groups. *Diabetes Care, 30*(6), 1364–1369. http://dx.doi.org/10.2337/dc06-1357.

SECTION 4

PHARMACOVIGILANCE AND PATIENT SAFETY IN LOW- AND MIDDLE-INCOME COUNTRIES

CHAPTER

9

PHARMACOVIGILANCE PRACTICES AND ACTIVITIES: ISSUES, CHALLENGES, AND FUTURE DIRECTION

Subish Palaian

Gulf Medical University, Ajman, United Arab Emirates

CHAPTER OUTLINE

Social and Administrative Aspects of Pharmacy in Low- and Middle-Income Countries. http://dx.doi.org/10.1016/B978-0-12-811228-1.00009-1

IMPORTANCE OF PHARMACOVIGILANCE IN DEVELOPING COUNTRIES

Recently, there has been a rise in awareness among various stakeholders regarding the safe use of medicines. It is not unusual that medications considered safe endanger patient safety and get discontinued from use in society. The past two decades have seen a rise in awareness among developing countries on improving safety mechanisms to ensure patient safety. The World Health Organization (WHO) emphasizes on improving drug safety mechanisms worldwide. Developing countries often rely on the drug safety information available from the developed world that is often documented in standard drug information resources, which do not necessarily incorporate observations from the developing world.

Of late (more than three decades after the thalidomide tragedy), developing countries have sought to have their own national pharmacovigilance systems (NPSs) to handle several practice- and system-related issues. The need for an indigenous adverse drug reaction (ADR) reporting program arises because of the prevalence of unique diseases; use of alternative medicines; dosage forms; poor drug information; variation in the excipients used; unique package inserts; lack of drug information; use of fixed-dose drug combinations (FDCs); poor patient compliance; lack of hospital drug and therapeutics committees (DTCs); poor digitalization of medical data; self-medication practices; nondoctor prescribing; absence of computerization; physician-centered healthcare systems; medication errors; genetic makeup differences; poor data on drug-use pattern; and poor quality, counterfeit, spurious, and adulterated medications; among others. The ethnicity of patients is known to often influence drug allergies (McDowell, Coleman, & Ferner, 2006); hence, a local database on drug safety is substantiated.

At times, developing countries have had to depend on data from the developed world while making decisions on approving and banning harmful drugs. These data thus differ in terms of geography, drug utilization pattern, prescription cultures, and multiple factors, making it difficult to extrapolate findings. Hence, it is necessary to have a local pharmacovigilance program in every country, and countries with a large population should even have a decentralized program. The drug-use problems in developing countries are very unique and special and should therefore be viewed in a different manner from those of developed countries. There are also issues related to substandard medicines and lack of quality control laboratories that may make the safety requirement in developing countries more special and unique. A standard view on pharmacovigilance, keeping in mind these conditions of developing countries, may thus not yield fruitful outcomes and accordingly requires special consideration from the developing world's perspectives.

ADVERSE DRUG REACTION REPORTING SYSTEM IN DEVELOPING COUNTRIES

As mentioned earlier, the importance of an indigenous pharmacovigilance system has been widely recognized, and many countries have started their own pharmacovigilance programs. As of 2014, there were more than 140 countries in the WHO Programme for International Drug Monitoring (national pharmacovigilance guidelines). A broader look at the developing country perspective reveals varying success of the programs.

LATIN AMERICA (BRAZIL)

The NPS of Brazil was established in 2001 (Moscou, Kohler, & MaGahan, 2016) because of two major incidents: the thalidomide tragedy that affected 300 children in Brazil and the meglumine tragedy that caused nearly 300 serious ADRs and even associated deaths (Uppsala Reports, 2002). Brazil's NPS runs under the National Health Surveillance Agency (ANVISA), which was successful in incorporating several standards in ADR reporting. It is now mandatory to report ADRs within a stipulated timeline, and all suspected deaths must be reported (De Carvalho, Varallo, & Dagli-Hernandez, 2016). Brazil's achievements in a short span of nearly 16 years are commendable.

AFRICAN COUNTRIES

Morocco and South Africa became the first African members of the WHO Programme for International Drug Monitoring in 1992 (Isah, Pal, Olsson, Dodoo, & Bencheikh, 2012). In the recent past, there has been substantial development in African countries to promote pharmacovigilance. In 2010, the WHO designated the University of Ghana Medical School as a WHO Collaborating Centre for improving pharmacovigilance in the continent. This center is expected to provide technical support and other requirements in conducting an efficient pharmacovigilance program among African nations (Uppsala Monitoring Centre, n.d.-a, n.d-b). To foster PV culture and strengthen drug safety issues, the Africa Pharmacovigilance Meeting 2012 was conducted, with 110 participants from 32 countries (Africa Pharmacovigilance Meeting, 2012).

As of September 2015, there were 35 member countries from Africa in the WHO Programme (Ampadu et al., 2016). A broader look reveals that these countries face major challenges related to underreporting, poor understanding of the system, lack of coordination, etc.

ASIA—WEST

Iran

Iran became a member of the WHO Programme for International Drug Monitoring in July 1998. It has a comprehensive pharmacovigilance program, and a good number of ADR reports are being collected. Furthermore, manufacturers are required to report ADRs (Shalviri, n.d). The pharmacovigilance activities in Iran are being controlled by the Adverse Drug Reaction Monitoring Center (ADRMC), which received 17,967 ADR reports in the first 10 years of its inception, and the country's pharmacovigilance program was instrumental in sending 86 drug safety alerts to various health professionals, 23 product recalls, 30 product labeling changes, 8 medicine distribution suspensions, and 4 product removals (terfenadine, phenylpropanolamine, iron dextran, and cisapride suspension) from the national list of essential medicines (Shalviri, Valadkhani, & Dinarvand, 2009).

ASIA—SOUTH

India

In India, there have been many attempts to initiate a successful pharmacovigilance program, starting from 1986 (Gupta, n. d.). India became a member of the WHO Programme for International Drug Monitoring in 1997. Most recently, the Central Drugs Standard Control Organization (CDSCO) has started a program emphasizing on safeguarding the general public. It originally had 22 ADR monitoring centers, and a year later, the center shifted to the Indian Pharmacopoeia Commission for effective management (Pharmacovigilance Program of India, n.d.). The pharmacovigilance program has been successful in identifying serious ADRs; nevertheless, underreporting is a major challenge (Lihite & Lahkar, 2015).

Bangladesh

The history of pharmacovigilance in Bangladesh can be traced back to 1996, when a pharmacovigilance cell was established by the Directorate of Drug Administration (Rahman & Haque, n.d.). There are reports of the deaths of 28 children linked to use of improper solvents in paracetamol syrup, as propylene glycol was replaced by diethylene glycol (DEG). In the early 1990s, 339 people in Bangladesh died because of paracetamol syrup contaminated with DEG from propylene glycol (Al-Mustansir, Saha, Paul, Rahim, & Hosen, 2013). In 2014, Bangladesh became a member of the WHO Programme for International Drug Monitoring (Uppsala Reports, 2015).

China

An ADR center was established by the China Food and Drug Administration (CFDA) under the Ministry of Health in 1989, and China became a member of the WHO Programme for International Drug Monitoring in 1998. By 2002, there were 31 provincial ADR monitoring centers (Yan-Min, n.d.). As of 2013, there were 34 provincial centers and more than 400 municipal centers, along with a four-level pharmacovigilance network covering the national, provincial, municipal, and county levels. By 2013, the number of ADR reports exceeded 600,000 (Zhang, Wong, He, & Wong, 2014). Because the country relies on voluntary reporting, there are still challenges associated with underreporting, and because the denominator value is not present (Yan-Min, n.d.), the actual incidence of ADRs is difficult to calculate.

Sri Lanka

The Department of Pharmacology, Faculty of Medicine, Colombo University, is Sri Lanka's national collaborating center. In terms of ADR monitoring, reporting, and prevention, Sri Lanka is way behind like most other developing countries. Prescribers and pharmacists should initiate and sustain remedial actions. Sri Lanka has been a member of the WHO Programme for International Drug Monitoring since 2001 (Uppsala Reports, 2001). Coordination of the National Centre was recently taken over by the National Regulatory Authority, but resources are still quite limited and pharmacovigilance is not a priority.

Nepal

The initiative of starting pharmacovigilance in Nepal was taken in 2002, and the system was functional by 2004; in the same year, Nepal became a member of the WHO Programme for International Drug Monitoring. There is a national center and six regional centers under the Ministry of Health's Department of Drug Administration (Santosh, Tragulpiankit, Gorsanan, Edwards, & Alam, 2013). The initial years of establishment have demonstrated an increasing tendency of ADR reporting, and underreporting of ADRs is a major challenge.

ASIA—EAST

Thailand

Thailand established a pharmacovigilance system and a national pharmacovigilance center in 1983 and became a member of the WHO Programme for International Drug Monitoring in 1984. By 2014, over 600,000 reports were reported to the Thai pharmacovigilance program. Among developing countries, Thailand has one of the most developed pharmacovigilance systems (Suwankesawong, 2015).

Malaysia

The pharmacovigilance activities in Malaysia are managed by the Malaysian Adverse Drug Reactions Advisory Committee (MADRAC), which functions under the drug control authority and monitors registered products in the country. Malaysia became a member of the WHO Programme for International Drug Monitoring in 1990 (National Pharmaceutical Regulatory Agency, Malaysia, n.d.). The center has also developed guidelines for vaccine safety (Guidelines for the Pharmacovigilance on Safety of Vaccines in Malaysia, n.d.).

Philippines

An ADR monitoring system was established in the Philippines in 1994, and the Bureau of Food and Drugs (BFAD) was authorized as the focal point for pharmacovigilance activities in 1997. The Philippines became a member of the WHO Programme for International Drug Monitoring in July 1998 (Hartigan-Go, 2002). By 2002, the center received 1600 ADR reports. Since its establishment, the country has achieved significant progress in safety monitoring issues (Cruz, n.d.).

GUIDELINES FOR SETTING UP A PHARMACOVIGILANCE PROGRAM IN A DEVELOPING COUNTRY

The WHO has established the minimum requirements for setting up a pharmacovigilance center from a developing country perspective. This guideline can be taken as a model for any developing country while setting up or strengthening its national pharmacovigilance program. The WHO guidelines provide information on basic requirements related to technical manpower, infrastructure, resources, and policy guidance (Minimum Requirements for a Functional Pharmacovigilance System, n.d.; Safety Monitoring of Medicinal Products, 2002). The inclusion of various health professionals is important in the program. Often, the programs center on pharmacists, physicians, or pharmacologists. A successful initiation would need to address the following issues, and the program depends on the following:

1. Inclusion of every stakeholder
2. Awareness program so that everyone understands the process goals and objectives
3. Feedback provided to the reporter in the report
4. Results published to a larger group
5. Action taken on the basis of the ADR reports
6. Constant encouragement and appreciation of the reporters

ADVERSE DRUG REACTION REPORTING FORMS: CONSIDERATIONS FOR A DEVELOPING COUNTRY

Because ADR reporting largely varies among countries, the organization and content of ADR reporting forms are crucial. To maximize the reporting rate, the ADR reporting form should be simple. In general, there has been considerable confusion regarding the nature of the forms and is perceived to have simple ADR reporting forms. The information obtained from the forms is often inadequate, and the causality and severity assessment cannot be completed with the available information. As per the WHO, the minimum requirements for an ADR reporting form involve the following information: patient-related information, medicine-related information (suspected drug[s] as well as concomitant drugs), information on the suspected ADR(s), and information related to the reporter (Safety Monitoring of Medicinal Products, 2002). Different countries have their own unique way of presenting their ADR forms. Some of the widely used ADR forms from developed countries are the one from U.S. Food and Drug Administration (U.S. FDA), the Australian blue card system, and the UK yellow cards. In the recent past, many developing countries, such as India, China, Iran, Nepal, and Malaysia, have also created national ADR forms.

Because the underreporting of ADRs is a common problem in developing countries, extensive consideration is needed to ensure that the design of a proper ADR report form accounts for the nature of the healthcare system targeted as well as that of the reporter. However, ADR reporting forms often lack critical information, which makes it difficult to make any decision and take actions based on the reports. Thus, it is a huge challenge to obtain as much data as possible but still keep the reporting form easy and quick to fill in. Hence, it would be advisable to have a simple form in the places where patient tracking/file tracing is available, and a relatively more elaborate form is warranted in places without such an option. Ideally, there should be a mechanism incorporated into the patient records system that enables the doctor to quickly send an ADR report electronically without having to fill in all patient data manually.

A suitable and well-developed ADR reporting form could be developed by taking the following aspects into consideration:

1. Target audience (physicians, pharmacists, nurses, other paramedics, students, and consumers)
2. Nature of the institute (hospitals, clinics)
3. Availability of electronic form
4. Work nature and busy nature of the reporters
5. Legal obligations

6. If consumers are being targeted, local language is a must
7. Simple and quick to fill in

IMPLEMENTATION OF THE WHO PROGRAMME FOR INTERNATIONAL DRUG MONITORING IN DEVELOPING COUNTRIES

Although many developing countries have started pharmacovigilance programs, they often fail in implementing the programs successfully. This is clearly revealed by the low number of ADR reports received by the Uppsala Monitoring Centre (UMC). Failure in implementation of pharmacovigilance occurs in various stages, as discussed below:

1. *Individual level:* Pharmacovigilance activities are often initiated through the enthusiasm of one dedicated person or a few people. The success and failure of the program depends on this/these individual(s).
2. *Institutional level:* ADR monitoring programs often do not get institutionalized and remain an individual interest. People at the higher levels in an institute may also not support the programs. The reasons for resistance range from fear of litigation to poor awareness. In many hospitals, the hospital DTCs play an important role in promoting the programs. Successful implementation depends on the availability of resources, leadership, and inclusive policy of the members associated with the program.
3. *National level:* Incorporation of the pharmacovigilance programs at national levels is crucial. It depends on the commitment from the drug regulatory authority, provisions in national medicine policies, and vision of the people associated with the health ministries.

ADVERSE DRUG REACTION REPORTING STATISTICS IN DEVELOPING COUNTRIES

A previous review of VigiBase, the WHO global database of Individual Case Safety Reports (ICSRs), revealed that there are very few ADR reports from developing countries received by the UMC. For example, in Africa, the number of member countries of the WHO Programme for International Drug Monitoring increased from 2 in 1995 to 35 in 2015, but the number of ADR reports increased by less than 1% (Ampadu et al., 2016).

However, recent data from UMC shows that the LMIC share of ICSRs in VigiBase has grown substantially in the last few years, from 6.7% in 2011 to 12.5% in mid-2017, which is very encouraging. Looking at LMICs alone, the number of ICSRs has increased by over 300% (from 465,000 to almost 2 million ICSRs) between 2011 and mid 2017.

AUTOMATED ADVERSE DRUG REACTION REPORTING SYSTEM AND ITS POTENTIAL ROLE IN A DEVELOPING COUNTRY

Because information technology developments have considerably surpassed advancements in healthcare systems, it is worth utilizing automated online ADR reporting programs. Mobile phones could be customized to report ADRs, and there is a huge potential for using social media in ADR reporting.

Using automated reporting can be beneficial in terms of time management, and a quick reporting time could help in overcoming underreporting. Typical online reporting for a developing country should be as follows:

1. Easy and simple
2. Preferably in local language
3. Linked to the hospital database
4. Able to provide alert messages on similar ADRs to the reporters

However, while using electronic reporting, even social media, one should be careful regarding the validity of the data obtained (Banerjee & Ingate, 2012). Moreover, there should be clear guidelines and specifications that are needed to improve the ADR reporting procedures through social media. All these measures would minimize the possibility of underreporting of ADRs.

HINDRANCE TO ADVERSE DRUG REACTION REPORTING

USE OF LOCAL LANGUAGE IN ADVERSE DRUG REACTION REPORTING

If the target audience also includes consumers, then it would be wiser to prepare the reporting in local languages. The terminologies and procedures for ADR reporting are often in English, which may be understood only by a few. Hence, it is of immense importance to have them in a local language. In India, the ADR dictionary of WHO, WHO Adverse Reactions Terminology (WHOART), has been translated into the local language, Hindi (Mohan, Sharma, Tandon, Semwal, & Agrawal, 2011).

COMPLICATED TERMINOLOGIES CAN BE A HINDRANCE TO ADVERSE DRUG REACTION REPORTING

The process of ADR reporting is often complicated because of the advanced medical terminologies that make it difficult for health professionals, especially paramedical and consumers, to participate in ADR reporting. These terminologies may be essential in carrying out the causality assessment of ADRs as well as categorizing the ADR reports. This poses a real challenge in ADR reporting as whole. Hence, one should use simple and reporter-friendly terminologies.

MYTHS ASSOCIATED WITH GLOBAL REPORTING

At times, healthcare providers do not seem to worry about reporting ADRs and feel that doing so might affect the growth of pharmaceutical companies in the particular country. A product that caused an ADR could be taken as an inferior or "risky" product. In addition, it is felt that the ADR reports might provide benefits only to the developed world and hence do not justify reporting to the WHO global database of ICSRs. Much awareness is needed to address these issues.

EXTENDED ROLE OF PHARMACOVIGILANCE CENTERS

In developing countries, the role of pharmacovigilance should go beyond ADR reporting of commonly used medications.

PHARMACOVIGILANCE OF HERBAL MEDICATION

The use of herbal medicines often complicates ADRs. The general public normally feels that herbal medicines are free from ADRs. However, the literature suggests that a significant number of ADRs are associated with herbal medications.

Hence, in the preview of developing countries:

1. Herbal medicines need a database.
2. They should have clearly defined herbal terminologies.
3. They possess classification of active ingredients.
4. They should be validated for the variation in active ingredients owing to seasonal changes.
5. They should develop experts on training in the area of herbal pharmacovigilance.
6. They must have more reliance on consumer reporting.

There have been serious challenges associated with herbal pharmacovigilance, making it more difficult. Some of them include lack of provision of ADR reporting, many of which are nonprescription drugs; they are often used in the community and as over-the-counter (OTC) products and hence escape from monitoring by health professionals in the hospital (Shetti, Kumar, Sriwastava, & Sharma, 2011).

It is also difficult for the causality assessment. Herbal anatomic–therapeutic–chemical (HATC) classification by the WHO may be useful to obtain a better understanding of herbal terminologies. The general public also believes that there is no expiry date for traditional medicines (Wal, Singh, Mehra, Rizvi, & Vajpayee, 2014). Hence, it is clear that there is a lack of knowledge and awareness on ADRs associated with traditional medicines. There also seems to be less technical expertise and standardization of traditional medicines and establishment of a good pharmacovigilance system in relation to herbal medications.

PHARMACOVIGILANCE OF FIXED-DOSE DRUG COMBINATIONS

The wide availability of FDCs is a common problem that is often discussed in countries like India. Many challenges associated with FDCs exist, although the rationality of many of them has been questioned. An 2016 estimate suggests the presence of more than 6000 FDCs in India (Gupta & Ramachandran, 2016). Similarly, there are even more FDCs in countries such as Nepal (Poudel, Subish, Mishra, Mohamed Izham, & Jayasekera, 2010).

Because there are many FDCs, it is necessary to incorporate pharmacovigilance for FDCs. The challenges associated with pharmacovigilance of FDCs are as follows:

1. Difficulty in identifying the impending drug
2. Difficulty in conducting causality assessment
3. Challenging and dechallenging, an important step to confirm the possible drug causing the ADRs is often difficult
4. Difficulty in predicting the possibility of drug interactions

Thus, these challenges pose a serious problem, and it is difficult to conduct pharmacovigilance studies for FDCs. However, there is a need for pharmacovigilance of FDCs in developing countries.

PHARMACOVIGILANCE OF FOOD SUPPLEMENTS

The regulatory requirements of food supplements in developing countries are often much simpler compared to those of medicinal products. Hence, there is an increasing number of products sold under the banner of "food supplements," including protein powders, amino acids, and antioxidants.

In addition to the abovementioned food supplements, there has recently been an increase in the use of energy drinks. Although they are believed to be safe and people often consume them as food supplements (Stoev, Kalaidjiev, Lebanova, & Getov, 2015), the safety of these products is not clear. In countries where drunk driving is banned, people have the habit of using energy drinks while driving. The safety profile of these energy drinks needs to be closely evaluated.

There is also an increased use of microbial products (probiotics) along with antibiotics, keeping in mind the possible reduction in ADRs. However, the ADRs of these products need to be evaluated.

Moreover, the pharmacovigilance of food supplements should not only focus on their safety but also on their rationality, cost effectiveness, and therapeutic potency and efficacy.

PHARMACOVIGILANCE OF NEGLECTED AND TROPICAL DISEASES

Neglected and tropical diseases affect poor and remote populations that are often neglected by the major healthcare system. Examples of these diseases include trypanosomiasis, dengue, chikungunya, echinococcosis, leprosy, leishmaniasis, schistosomiasis, and leptospirosis. There are frequent outbreaks of these diseases and the focus is more on tackling, curing, and preventing the spread of the disease. Mass administration of drugs in a quicker manner also occurs without considering individual variations. In this course, the safety of the medicines gets neglected. Moreover, in these types of diseases, drug donations are possible, which makes the scrutiny of drug safety much more essential (Isah et al., 2012).

PHARMACOVIGILANCE OF MEDICAL DEVICES

The scope of medical devices has increased in the recent past and ranges from a simple tissue cutter to a complicated life-saving device such as heart valves and coronary stents. A review by Gupta et al. reported the vigilance systems in India, the United States, the United Kingdom, and Australia for medical devices. It is evident that developed countries have a good safety evaluation mechanism in place, and in India, the medical devices are classified under "drugs" (Gupta, Janodia, Jagadish, & Udupa, 2010).

Pharmaceutical companies often monitor the safety of the devices that they manufacture and market (Medical Device Vigilance, n.d.). The U.S. FDA has mandatory reporting (MDR) for medical devices (Medical Device Reporting, n.d.).

Considering the limitations associated with ADR reporting with respect to medications, it can be assumed that there is a possibility of poor vigilance mechanisms for medical devices. With the advancement of technology, there is a possibility for a wider scope of the use of medical devices; hence, device utilization requires special attention and care in terms of the safety of such devices.

PHARMACOVIGILANCE TRAINING OPTIONS FOR DEVELOPING COUNTRIES

Strong technical knowledge can be an asset in the successful running of a pharmacovigilance program. In developing countries, the curriculum of medical, pharmacy, nursing, and other paramedical students do not emphasize the technical aspects of pharmacovigilance. Pharmacovigilance encompasses knowledge on pharmacology, pharmacotherapy, drug information, etc. Causality assessment is another important aspect of pharmacovigilance, which again needs knowledge on drug information and pharmacology.

Since 1993, the UMC has annually conducted an international pharmacovigilance training course in Uppsala, Sweden, and also in Mysore, India, in recent years. These courses cover operational aspects of all the necessary skills and competency needed for pharmacovigilance center staff. Many lectures on the Uppsala course have been filmed, and the recordings are freely available on the UMC YouTube channel. The Asia Pacific Pharmacovigilance Training course is conducted in collaboration with JSS University, Mysore, India, and is tailored to the needs of the region, which may be more relevant to developing countries. This could be a potential program for aspirants hoping to run a pharmacovigilance program.

The UMC newsletter "Uppsala Reports" provides a list of conferences and trainings related to pharmacovigilance. However, only a few may be of significance to developing countries.

An outline of a general pharmacovigilance training program has been created by Olsson (2008) and could be considered as a model for developing countries. The Indian Institute of Health Management Research (IIHMR) from Jaipur, India, also conducts training programs on pharmacovigilance and drug safety.

Furthermore, the national pharmacovigilance program of India occasionally conducts pharmacovigilance trainings.

In addition, international organizations such as International Society of Pharmacovigilance (ISoP) and International Society of Pharmacoepidemiology (ISPE) periodically conduct training programs. The ISoP courses mainly reach out to pharmacovigilance professionals working in the pharmaceutical industry. However, sometimes ISoP and UMC conduct joint courses.

UMC offers a wide range of web lectures freely available on YouTube. In addition, UMC is developing a distance learning course on signal detection and causality assessment. These online training resources are valuable to all who are unable to travel and/or attend live courses. Furthermore, there are other pharmacovigilance courses, such as the training courses provided by the WHO-CCs of Ghana and Morocco, that could be useful. The annual technical briefing seminar conducted by the WHO headquarters could also be useful for attaining comprehensive knowledge on patient safety and appropriate use of medicines.

The current training opportunities in pharmacovigilance, however, do not meet the extensive needs. Moreover, the costs involved may be bothersome for people from developing countries that may be a major barrier in attaining pharmacovigilance training among members of these countries. Therefore, there is a need for more distance training.

PHARMACOVIGILANCE-RELATED POLICY IN DEVELOPING COUNTRIES

Sustainability and functioning of pharmacovigilance programs largely depends on the government's involvement in and commitment toward a pharmacovigilance policy. The government's role is of paramount importance in terms of drug registration, drug bans, labeling changes, usage restrictions, and, more importantly, funding and logistic support for the program.

The WHO stresses on multidisciplinary collaboration among ministries of health, universities, NGOs, pharmaceutical industries, and other stakeholders to establish better ADR monitoring activities. The WHO also lists the key elements of pharmacovigilance in national medicines policy, including national and, if needed, regional pharmacovigilance centers; legislation for medicine monitoring; continuing education programs on safe and effective use of medications; policy development on costing, budgeting, and financing; drug information on ADRs to professionals and consumers; and methods to monitor the outcomes of pharmacovigilance activities (Pharmacovigilance: Ensuring the Safe Use of Medicines, 2004). In recent decades, many countries have brought their pharmacovigilance policies under the national medical policy. The list of pharmacovigilance guidelines for LMIC is listed on the UMC website (National Pharmacovigilance Guidelines, n.d.). These guidelines from developing countries would serve as a model for other countries that may be developing their guidelines in the near future.

ADVERSE DRUG REACTION REPORTING BY PHARMACEUTICAL INDUSTRIES: DEVELOPING COUNTRIES PERSPECTIVE

Developed countries have well-established pharmacovigilance centers (Talbot & Nilsson, 1998), and it is often mandatory for pharmaceutical companies to report ADRs on the products marketed by them. If companies report ADRs, it would be beneficial in a number of ways. Many developing countries do not conduct postmarketing surveillance (PMS) studies on their citizens. They depend on data obtained from developed countries that are provided by the pharmaceutical companies. Such companies have their marketing personnel throughout and maintain good coordination with physicians; therefore, they are in a better place to collect the ADRs and report to the ADR monitoring center. Moreover, they have a technical team and more information of the particular product, its excipients, and pharmacokinetic profile, which make them more unique in monitoring their own drug products.

Because multinational companies already have a well-established pharmacovigilance system in developed countries, it is better for them to come up with technical support in developing the pharmacovigilance in resource-limited countries.

PMS studies in developing countries: There is often a voluntary reporting program in developing countries (Meirik, 1998), and no safety data are generally available to the general public. PMS studies provide information on the real-world scenario and are therefore an important aspect of drug evaluation (A Report of the Safety and Surveillance Working Group, n.d.). There are many ethical issues associated with clinical trials in developing countries.

Legislations on manufacturer reporting: It is often debated that these medicines are already tested and approved by the original innovator and why they need to be monitored again. Thus, it is important to have strict legislation to make manufacturers report ADRs. In India, there are mandatory requirements for pharmaceutical companies to report ADRs (Arora, 2008), and it is recommended to involve medical representatives in ADR reporting (Reporting of Adverse Event Reports, n.d.).

CONSUMER PHARMACOVIGILANCE AND ITS STATUS IN DEVELOPING COUNTRIES

In general, a small percentage of people get admitted to hospitals. ADRs often occur while the patient is away from contact with healthcare professionals. Hence, it becomes important to monitor the medicine use process that takes place outside of contact with healthcare professionals. Thus, involvement of consumers in direct ADR reporting becomes mandatory and could serve as a rich source of information on medicine use scenarios. Consumer reporting captures the ADRs caused by OTC medications, herbal medications, and medicines prescribed by unqualified professionals (commonly seen in developing countries). The concept of consumer pharmacovigilance is new in developing countries and is not well established. The various challenges associated with consumer reporting in three developing countries—Malaysia, Nepal, and Yemen—are listed by Alshakka et al. (Ahmed, Izham, & Subish, 2010; Alshakka et al., 2014). It would be also beneficial to involve community pharmacists in consumer reporting (Jha et al., 2014) to enhance the reporting of ADRs occurring in the community. In developed countries, this concept is well developed, and in Australia, consumer reporting started as early as 1964 (van Hunsel, Härmark, Pal, Olsson, & van Grootheest, 2012).

ADDITIONAL BENEFITS OF HAVING A PHARMACOVIGILANCE CENTER

From a developing country perspective, a well-structured pharmacovigilance program could offer many advantages for the healthcare system. Patient safety is an integral part of every healthcare system, and pharmacovigilance programs could offer a strong linkage between all the stages of the system in an integrated manner. This also provides a platform for resource sharing and maximization of benefits among various services related to medicine use process. Some of the additional benefits could be as follows:

1. *Local database:* It provides a local database on disease prevalence, drug utilization, and safety profile of available drugs.
2. *Drug information services:* There is a huge scope for integrating drug information services along with pharmacovigilance centers. More than half of the ADRs could be prevented with appropriate drug information.
3. *Antimicrobial surveillance programs:* Pharmacovigilance of antimicrobials could provide a strong link between ADRs and improper antimicrobials in terms of dosage, duration, dosage adjustment in renal and hepatic impaired patients, etc.
4. *Tackling unethical drug promotion:* Unethical drug promotion and irrational prescription are common causes of ADRs, and a stringent pharmacovigilance program could offer potential benefits in tackling the same.

5. *Medication error monitoring:* Many ADRs are frequently linked with medication errors. Hence, having a strong pharmacovigilance center would also help in running and strengthening a good medication error reporting and monitoring program.

ACHIEVEMENTS

Despite all the limitations and challenges, the pharmacovigilance programs in developing countries have achieved a lot. Somc of the achievements are as follows:

1. *Raising awareness:* Considerable awareness has been created in developing countries in relation to pharmacovigilance and safe use of medicines. Many countries have their own policies in place so as to ensure the safe use of medicines.
2. *Involvement of all health professionals:* It has also been well understood that patient safety and pharmacovigilance is a team effort and requires participation of all healthcare members and other stakeholders.
3. *Pharmacovigilance in student curriculum:* There have been attempts to teach pharmacovigilance in developing countries, which is a positive sign. Pharmacovigilance is also perceived as a separate discipline of science.
4. *National medicines policies:* The national medicine policies of many developing countries have incorporated pharmacovigilance as one of their major objectives.
5. *Knowledge, attitude, and practice (KAP) studies on ADR reporting and pharmacovigilance*: There has been an increase in the number of KAP studies in the field of ADR reporting and pharmacovigilance.
6. *Student research:* Students are conducting research in pharmacy, nursing, and medical institutes in developing countries, which shows that the field is receiving attention and growing.

CHALLENGES

Like any other health-related activity, pharmacovigilance is not free of challenges. The challenges associated with pharmacovigilance in developing countries are well documented in the literature (Ahmed et al., 2010; Alshakka et al., 2014; Alshammari & Alshakka, 2004). The major challenges are related to technical manpower, underreporting, funding, sustainability, and commitment from the regulatory authority.

RECOMMENDATIONS: THE WAY FORWARD

Given the above findings, the following recommendations are being made:

1. *Government support:* Commitment from the government is strongly needed to have stringent pharmacovigilance activities. Such support may be in the form of policy changes, funding, and on relevant issues that may enhance better pharmacovigilance.
2. *Promoting consumer reporting:* The establishment and strengthening of consumer reporting of ADRs could provide a significant amount of useful information on medicine use process.

3. *Teaching pharmacovigilance to future health professional:* Training future health professionals can be an easy and simple strategy to improve knowledge and awareness on pharmacovigilance.
4. *ADR reporting by manufacturers:* If necessary, the government can make it mandatory for manufacturers to report ADRs associated with their products.
5. *Reporting by retail and community pharmacists:* In many developing countries, the number of retail and community pharmacists outnumber other health professionals and are distributed throughout the community. Hence, involving them could provide a better coverage for ADR monitoring programs.
6. *Reporting by consumer organizations:* Consumer organizations could be encouraged to report suspected ADRs.
7. *Collaborative approach:* All key professionals, such as doctors, nurses, pharmacists, and other paramedical staff, should be involved in making pharmacovigilance a combined responsibility and collaborative approach. For example, laboratory personnel are in a better position to report the hepatotoxicity of drugs by observing the abnormalities in liver enzymes.
8. *Clinical pharmacy:* The concept of pharmacy practice may be beneficial in ADR reporting. Because clinical pharmacists attend ward rounds with clinicians, they are in a better position to report ADRs. In the recent past, many developing countries have come up with Doctor of Pharmacy (PharmD) education, which results in more clinical pharmacists.

CONCLUSIONS

A broader look at the existing literature reveals an increase in the number of developing countries becoming members of the WHO Programme for International Drug Monitoring. Although many developing countries have established pharmacovigilance programs, providing meaningful benefits in improving patient safety requires more reforms. The focus on pharmacovigilance in these countries is often limited to policy levels, and the implementation needs more commitment from governments. Technical expertise, reporting procedures, and options for feedback to reporters need improvement to sustain and strengthen the existing programs. Considerable advancements are required for meaningful pharmacovigilance activities, ensuring patient safety in developing countries.

LESSONS LEARNED

- Awareness regarding pharmacovigilance and safe use of medicines is increasing in developing countries, and many countries have incorporated drug safety in their national medicine policies.
- Although the number of countries with pharmacovigilance programs has increased, a systematic and scientific approach on ADR reporting leading to patient safety is still lacking.
- A collaborative approach involving all stakeholders is needed to improve ADR reporting and strengthen the existing pharmacovigilance programs.
- The sustainability of pharmacovigilance is a crucial area that needs much emphasis.

ACKNOWLEDGMENTS

The author acknowledges Anna Hegerius, MSc Pharm, Senior Specialist, Education and Training, Uppsala Monitoring Centre (UMC), Sweden, for reviewing the initial and subsequent versions of the chapter and suggesting modifications.

REFERENCES

Africa Pharmacovigilance Meeting. (October 2012). *Meeting proceedings*. Retrieved from http://apps.who.int/medicinedocs/documents/s21029en/s21029en.pdf.

Ahmed, A. M., Izham, I. M., & Subish, P. (2010). Importance of consumer pharmacovigilance system in developing countries: A case of Malaysia. *Journal of Clinical and Diagnostic Research*, *4*, 2929–2935.

Al-Mustansir, M. D., Saha, D., Paul, S., Rahim, Z. B., & Hosen, S. M. Z. (2013). Studies on pharmacovigilance in Bangladesh: Safety issues. *International Journal of Pharmacy Teaching & Practices*, *4*, 613–621.

Alshakka, M., Jha, N., Algefril, S., Ibrahim, M. I. M., Hassali, M. A., Abdorabbo, A., & Shankar, P. R. (2014). Problems and challenges faced in consumer reporting of adverse drug reactions in developing countries-a case study of Yemen, Nepal and Malaysia. *Indian Journal of Pharmaceutical and Biological Research*, *2*, 37–43.

Alshammari, T. M., & Alshakka, M. A. (2004). Unhelpful information about adverse drug reactions. *BMJ: British Medical Journal*, *349*, g5019.

Ampadu, H. H., Hoekman, J., de Bruin, M. L., Pal, S. N., Olsson, S., Sartori, D., … Dodoo, A. N. (2016). Adverse drug reaction reporting in Africa and a comparison of individual case safety report characteristics between Africa and the rest of the world: Analyses of spontaneous reports in VigiBase®. *Drug Safety*, *39*, 335–345.

Arora, D. (2008). Pharmacovigilance obligations of the pharmaceutical companies in India. *Indian J Pharmacol*, *40*, S13–S16.

Banerjee, A. K., & Ingate, S. (2012). Web-based patient-reported outcomes in drug safety and risk management. Challenges and opportunities? *Drug Safety*, *35*, 437.

Cruz, N. (n.d.). *Pharmacovigilance (PV) in the Philippine setting*. Retrieved from http://pappi.ph/sites/default/files/Pharmacovigilance%20in%20the%20Philippine%20Setting%20-%20NOEL%20CRUZ.pdf.

De Carvalho, P. M., Varallo, F. R., & Dagli-Hernandez, C. (2016). Brazilian regulation in pharmacovigilance: A review. *Pharmaceut Reg Affairs*, *5*, 164.

Guidelines for the Pharmacovigilance on Safety of Vaccines in Malaysia (n.d.). Retrieved from http://apps.who.int/medicinedocs/documents/s18592en/s18592en.pdf.

Gupta, Y.K. (n.d). *Pharmacovigilance programme for India*. Retrieved from http://www.ipc.gov.in/PvPI/20.%20Pharmacovigilance%20programme%20for%20India.pdf.

Gupta, P., Janodia, M. D., Jagadish, P. C., & Udupa, N. (2010). Medical device vigilance systems: India, US, UK, and Australia. *Medical devices (Auckland)*, *3*, 67–79.

Gupta, Y. G., & Ramachandran, S. S. (2016). Fixed dose drug combinations: Issues and challenges in India. *Indian Journal of Pharmacology*, *48*, 347–349.

Hartigan-Go, K. (2002). Developing a pharmacovigilance system in the Philippines, a country of diverse culture and strong traditional medicine background. *Toxicology*, *2002*, 103–107.

van Hunsel, F., Härmark, L., Pal, S., Olsson, S., & van Grootheest, K. (2012). Experiences with adverse drug reaction reporting by patients. An 11-country survey. *Drug Safety*, *35*, 45–60.

Isah, A. O., Pal, S. N., Olsson, S., Dodoo, A., & Bencheikh, R. S. (2012). Specific features of medicines safety and pharmacovigilance in Africa. *Therapeutic Advances in Drug Safety*, *2012*, 25–34.

Jha, N., Rathore, D. S., Shankar, P. R., Thapa, B. B., Bhuju, G., & Alshakka, M. (2014). Need for involving consumers in Nepal's pharmacovigilance system. *Australasian Medical Journal*, *7*, 191–195.

Lihite, R. L., & Lahkar, M. (2015). An update on the pharmacovigilance programme of India. *Frontiers in Pharmacology*, *6*, 194.

McDowell, S. E., Coleman, J. J., & Ferner, R. E. (2006). Systematic review and meta-analysis of ethnic differences in risks of adverse reactions to drugs used in cardiovascular medicine. *BMJ: British Medical Journal*, *332*, 1177–1181.

Medical Device Reporting. (n.d). *US FDA*. Retrieved from http://www.fda.gov/MedicalDevices/Safety/ReportaProblem/ucm2005291.htm.

Medical Device Vigilance (n.d.). *Panacea*. Retrieved from http://www.panaceapharmaprojects.com/medical-device-vigilance/.

Meirik, O. (1998). Postmarketing surveillance in developing countries. *Network Research Triangle Park*, *9*, 6.

Minimum Requirements for a Functional Pharmacovigilance System (n.d.). Retrieved from https://www.who-umc.org/media/1483/pv_minimum_requirements_2010_2.pdf.

Mohan, G., Sharma, S., Tandon, S., Semwal, B. C., & Agrawal, N. (2011). Pharmacovigilance: A new era for herbal safety. *Journal of Pharmacovigilance Drug Safety*, *8*, 1–08.

Moscou, K., Kohler, J. C., & MaGahan, A. (2016). Governance and pharmacovigilance in Brazil: A scoping review. *Journal of Pharmaceutical Policy and Practice*, *9*, 3.

National Pharmaceutical Regulatory Agency, Malaysia (n.d.). Retrieved from http://npra.moh.gov.my/index.php/about-npcb/malaysian-adverse-drug-reactions-advisory-committee-madrac/introduction.

National Pharmacovigilance Guidelines (n.d.). Uppsala Monitoring Centre. Retrieved from http://www.who-umc.org/DynPage.aspx?id=127878&mn1=7347&mn2=7252&mn3=7253&mn4=7745.

Olsson, S. (2008). Pharmacovigilance training with focus on India. *Indian Journal of Pharmacology*, *40*, s28–s30.

Pharmacovigilance Program of India (n.d.). *National Coordination Centre, Indian Pharmacopoeia Commission, Ghaziabad, India*. Retrieved from http://www.ipc.gov.in/PvPI/pv_home.html.

Pharmacovigilance: Ensuring the Safe Use of Medicines. (2004). *WHO policy perspectives on medicines*.

Poudel, A., Subish, P., Mishra, P., Mohamed Izham, M. I., & Jayasekera, J. (2010). Prevalence of fixed-dose drug combinations in Nepal: A preliminary study. *Journal of Clinical and Diagnostic Research*, *4*, 2246–2252 [Serial online].

Rahman, S, Haque, M. (n.d.). *International conference and CME cum workshop on pharmacovigilance systems and rational use of medicines: An integrated approach*. Retrieved from https://www.researchgate.net/publication/209390286_Pharmacovigilance_Bangladesh_Situation.

A Report of the Safety and Surveillance Working Group. (n.d.) Bill and Melinda Gates Foundation. Retrieved from https://docs.gatesfoundation.org/documents/SSWG%20Final%20Report%2011%2019%2013_designed.pdf.

Reporting of Adverse Event Reports. *The role of the medical representative*. (n.d.). Retrieved from http://www.abpi.org.uk/our-work/library/guidelines/documents/adverse-drug-reactions.pdf.

Safety Monitoring of Medicinal Products. (2002). *The importance of pharmacovigilance*. Geneva: World Health Organization.

Santosh, K. C., Tragulpiankit, P., Gorsanan, P., Edwards, I. R., & Alam, K. (2013). Strengthening pharmacovigilance programme in Nepal. *Nepal Journal of Epidemiology*, *3*, 230–235.

Shalviri, G. (n.d.). *Pharmacovigilance activities in Iran experience in managing medication errors*. Retrieved from http://capm.ma/Doc/Workshop/RAPV/Pharmacovigilance%20Activities%20in%20Iran.pdf.

Shalviri, G., Valadkhani, M., & Dinarvand, R. (2009). Ten years pharmacovigilance activities in Iran. *Iranian Journal of Public Health*, *38*(Suppl. 1), 162–166.

Shetti, S., Kumar, C. D., Sriwastava, N. K., & Sharma, I. P. (2011). Pharmacovigilance of herbal medicines: Current state and future directions. *Pharmacognosy Magazine*, *7*, 69–73.

Stoev, S., Kalaidjiev, K., Lebanova, H., & Getov, I. (2015). Review of regulatory requirements for the safety monitoring of food supplements and OTC Medicines, containing caffeine and/or taurine extracts derived from plants. *International Journal of Nutrition and Food Sciences*, *4*, 30–34.

Suwankesawong, W. *Pharmacovigilance in Thailand*. Retrieved from https://www.genome.gov/multimedia/slides/sjs_ten2015/12_sewankesawong.pdf.

Talbot, J. C. C., & Nilsson, B. S. (1998). Pharmacovigilance in the pharmaceutical industry. *British Journal of Clinical Pharmacology*, *45*, 427–431.

Uppsala Monitoring Centre (n.d.-a). *Being a member of the WHO programme for international drug monitoring*. Retrieved from http://who-umc.org/graphics/28121.pdf.

Uppsala Reports (2015). Retrieved from http://www.who-umc.org/graphics/28537.pdf.

Uppsala Reports. (2001). Retrieved from http://www.who-umc.org/graphics/24393.pdf.

Uppsala Reports. (2002). Uppsala Monitoring Centre. Retrieved from http://www.who-umc.org/graphics/24388.pdf.

Uppsala Monitoring Centre. (n.d-b). Retrieved from http://www.who-umc.org/DynPage.aspx?id=98093&mn1=7347&mn2=7252&mn3=7253&mn4=7333.

Wal, P., Singh, A., Mehra, R., Rizvi, S., & Vajpayee, R. (2014). Pharmacovigilance: Need and future prospective in herbal and ayurvedic medicines. *The Pharma Innovation Journal*, *3*, 18–22.

World Health Organization, Geneva (n.d.). *General guidelines for methodologies on research and evaluation of traditional medicine*. Retrieved from http://apps.who.int/iris/bitstream/10665/66783/1/WHO_EDM_TRM_2000.1.pdf.

Yan-Min. (n.d.). *Development of ADR reporting and monitoring in China*. Retrieved from http://www.who.int/medicines/areas/quality_safety/regulation_legislation/icdra/WG-3_2Dec.pdf.

Zhang, L., Wong, L. Y., He, Y., & Wong, I. C. (2014). Pharmacovigilance in China: Current situation, successes and challenges. *Drug Safety: an International Journal of Medical Toxicology and Drug Experience*, *37*, 765–770.

CHAPTER

BEHAVIORAL ASPECTS OF PHARMACOVIGILANCE: RESEARCH METHODS CONSIDERATIONS

10

Vibhu Paudyal[1,2]

[1]University of Birmingham, Birmingham, United Kingdom; [2]Robert Gordon University, Aberdeen, United Kingdom

CHAPTER OUTLINE

INTRODUCTION

This chapter will outline key research methods that are relevant to exploring behavioral aspects of pharmacovigilance, in particular relevance to undertaking research in developing countries.

The emerging concept of pharmacovigilance captures wider aspects of safety related to the prescribing, dispensing, storing, administration, and use of medicines. In addition to the reporting and making use of the data on suspected adverse drug reactions (ADRs), the concept also includes aspects of medication errors, overuse, misuse, and occupational exposure of medicines (European Medicines Agency, 2016).

Social and Administrative Aspects of Pharmacy in Low- and Middle-Income Countries. http://dx.doi.org/10.1016/B978-0-12-811228-1.00010-8

Low-income countries share 90% of the global disease burden and are major consumers of medicines (Pirmohamed, Atuah, Dodoo, & Winstanley, 2007). Establishing safety profiles of medicines specific to diseases that are endemic to the developing world has been historically challenging due to lack of systems of effective and efficient pharmacovigilance systems or due to nonuse of currently available systems. Widespread availability of prescription medicines over the counter due to lack of effective regulations or their enforcement adds to the challenges. Poor health leads to increased susceptibility to ADRs, and hence the need for effective pharmacovigilance becomes even more important in the context of the developing world.

Lack of effective pharmacovigilance systems is often contributed by rudimentary resources, policies, and lack of political will within a nation. Where pharmacovigilance systems have been implemented including the tools to report suspected ADRs, their use is often limited. For example, underreporting of ADRs is a serious problem globally. Systematic reviews of international literature suggest that 94% of ADRs are underreported including severe and serious ADRs (Hazell & Shakir, 2006). Underreporting is contributed mostly by beliefs, attitudes, and behaviors of healthcare professionals and patients (Lopez-Gonzalez, Herdeiro, & Figueiras, 2009). Behavioral aspects of pharmacovigilance hence merit research priority in the context of local and national practices, culture, and policies.

BEHAVIORAL ASPECTS OF PHARMACOVIGILANCE

The Oxford dictionary defines behaviors as "the way in which a person behaves in response to a particular situation or stimulus" (Oxford Dictionary, 2016). Behavioral aspects in the context of pharmacovigilance relate to a person's participation, views, attitudes, and experiences in relation to the activities of pharmacovigilance. High-quality research enables exploration of behaviors and the design of effective interventions to change target behaviors, thereby allowing advancement in practice.

KEY CONSIDERATIONS

Research around behavioral aspects of pharmacovigilance could range from reviewing current research evidence; exploring current state of practice; exploring policy priorities in the local and national contexts; development, implementation, and evaluation of novel pharmacovigilance systems; and researching patient, healthcare professional, and stakeholder perspective in their participation in pharmacovigilance. The following methodological considerations are of particular use in designing research programs in developing countries to inform effective pharmacovigilance practices including identification of challenges and exploration of relevant solutions.

SYSTEMATIC REVIEWS OF CURRENT RESEARCH AND PRACTICE

Systematic review methodology has its founding in evidence-based healthcare. Evidence-based practice is the process of systematically reviewing, appraising, and using research findings to aid the delivery of optimum clinical care to patients (Rosenberg & Donald, 1995). Systematic reviews of literature aim to synthesize research evidence on a particular topic based on a focused research question.

Systematic reviews differ from traditional narrative reviews in that the former is informed by a priori protocol and uses systematic literature search process and appraisal of the available evidence and systematic quantitative or qualitative synthesis of data where appropriate.

A well-conducted systematic review in the area of pharmacovigilance, in addition to providing current evidence, also enables the researchers to identify gaps in current research.

In behavioral pharmacovigilance, systematic reviews can be used to ask important questions from the current literature providing cumulative evidence on the rate of reporting and underreporting of ADRs, factors associated with underreporting in the national and international context (Bhagavathula, Elnour, Jamshed, & Shehab, 2016), effectiveness of novel pharmacovigilance systems in patients and healthcare professional behaviors, and identifying key features of pharmacovigilance systems best suited to their adoption by healthcare professionals. The scope of the review should be determined in informing future research and practice.

Systematic reviews are best undertaken if informed by one of the established guidelines including those published by Cochrane (Cochrane Collaboration, 2011), Centre for Review and Dissemination (CRD, 2009), and Joanna Briggs Institute (JBI) (2015a, 2015b). Researchers require access to medical and pharmaceutical research literature database for retrieving the literature. Researchers are encouraged to liaise with one of the abovementioned systematic review bodies at the early stages of the review process. Cochrane collaboration offers support to the authors to undertake literature search and subsequent stages within the review process.

The reproducible research process in a systematic review is driven by comprehensive searching of literature with scientifically valid and robust literature search (MacLure, Paudyal, & Stewart, 2016). Selection of research database should be informed by relevance to the field with MEDLINE, EMBASE, CINAHL, and International Pharmaceutical Abstracts among key databases featuring relevant journal repositories in behavioral pharmacovigilance. Identification, selection of literature, and data extraction and assessment of quality are usually undertaken by two researchers working independently. Validated tools are available in assessing the quality of the literature. Critical Appraisal Skills Programme (CASP) (CASP, 2013) have produced eight tools, each specific to assessing quality of literature pertaining to specific study designs, including randomized controlled trials (RCTs) and qualitative studies. Literature using RCT designs are also subjected to assessment of bias around methodological aspects of the trial including participant selection and blinding of assessors in the research. Cochrane risk of bias assessment tool (Higgins et al., 2011) has been widely adopted for the purpose.

Researchers conducting systematic reviews on research topics related to behavioral aspects of pharmacovigilance are often likely to come across analyzing data sets that do not lend to conducting traditional quantitative synthesis. Such data sets are often suited to narrative synthesis. For example, in a systematic review investigating what factors determine pharmacists' adoption of new medicines into practice (Paudyal, Hansford, Cunningham, & Stewart, 2012), through narrative synthesis, a total of 28 potentially relevant factors that could inform pharmacists' adoption of new medicines into practice were identified, with safety of a medicine among factors of paramount importance to pharmacists. This systematic review then informed the development of a comprehensive survey instrument that allowed the researchers further explore the factors in the context of the local and national practice (Paudyal, Hansford, Cunningham, & Stewart, 2014).

Narrative synthesis hence can be a component within a systematic review. However, it is important to distinguish systematic review with a narrative review. Systematic reviews aim to answer a specific review question and follow a structured and reproducible stages described earlier.

Systematic reporting guidelines are available in ensuring that researchers report minimum relevant items within a report of a systematic review. The preferred items for reporting systematic reviews and meta-analysis (PRISMA) (Moher et al., 2015) is the widely adopted tool and is best considered at the outset of the research.

UNDERTAKING REVIEW OF CURRENT POLICIES AND GUIDELINES

Review of pharmacovigilance policies and guidelines provides historical context to their development and allows researchers and stakeholders to identify gaps and inform future direction. For example, researchers may wish to compare and contrast pharmacovigilance policies and guidelines across different regions within developing countries and against those with established pharmacovigilance systems allowing common barriers of effective and efficient pharmacovigilance to be explored and to share best practices. Such reviews may allow setting up of common policy and research agenda through collaborative partnership across different countries.

Pharmacovigilance policies and guidelines often exist as gray literature. Gray literature may be available online and can often be resourced through search engines and government or local health bodies, hospitals, or primary care trusts webpages. Particularly, in the context of developing countries, repositories are often challenging to source with only paper copies available, which require formal and informal sources of retrieval.

Unlike established guidelines for undertaking systematic reviews of primary research literature, methodology guidance around policy and guideline review is scarce. JBI provides a useful guidance on undertaking policy reviews and defines such reviews under "scoping review methodology" (JBI, 2015a, 2015b). Chronological or thematic order of presentations is often used to synthesize data. We conducted a chronological review of UK Health Policies related to enhancing community pharmacists' management of minor ailments (Paudyal, Hansford, Cunningham, & Stewart, 2011). We were interested in reviewing how various factors including safety of medicines have been considered in enhancing patient access to newly reclassified over-the-counter medicines through pharmacy that were previously available only under prescription. Moscou, Kohler, and MaGahan (2016) recently conducted a scoping review in Brazil to identify effective strategies to promote pharmacovigilance. By undertaking review of policies, gray literature, and research literature within the same scoping review, the authors identified gaps and disparities in pharmacovigilance regulations and coordination between regions and across private and public sector healthcare institutions. Such reviews of policies are useful when supplemented with perspectives of key stakeholders (Maigetter, Pollock, Kadam, Ward, & Weiss, 2015).

EXPLORATORY RESEARCH ON BEHAVIORS OF HEALTHCARE PROFESSIONALS, PATIENTS, AND STAKEHOLDERS

Exploratory studies on behavioral pharmacovigilance are best facilitated using in-depth qualitative methods such as focus groups, in-depth interview, and case studies or through quantitative approaches such as surveys.

Creswell describes qualitative method as "an approach for exploring and understanding the meaning individuals or groups ascribe to a social or human problem" (Creswell, 2013). Qualitative methods, being exploratory in nature, are particularly useful when there is little knowledge (for example, of local context) on what aspects are likely to be influencing the behaviors under study, for example in reporting suspected ADRs. Research using qualitative methods typically provides answers to what, why, and how questions (Ritchie and Lewis, 2003). The written reports of qualitative research usually include the voices of participants, referred to as "quotes," along with description and interpretation of problems from the researchers' perspectives.

In-depth interviews conducted on a one-to-one basis with participants by the researchers either face to face or through the use of telephone provide ideal opportunities for researchers to explore participant views, experiences, and behaviors. However, focus groups, a method by which data are collected through group interaction led by a researcher (Morgan, 1996), also facilitate personal disclosures by allowing participants to react to and build on the responses of other group members (Wilkinson, 2004, pp. 177–199).

Sample sizes in qualitative studies are generally small and mainly determined by the "diminishing" returns of new information achieved, also called "data saturation" approach. A method used in recent literature to determine sample size is qualitative research is by using Francis et al.'s 10+3 approach (Francis et al. 2010). In this method, an initial sample size of 10 is selected, considering this number is adequate to the number of stratification variables in this study, e.g., professional groups and age. If saturation of data sets is not achieved (as evident during ongoing analysis of the data), further interviews are then conducted in cohorts of additional three (+3) until saturation is achieved.

Participants in a qualitative study when discussing sensitive aspects, such as detection and reporting of suspected ADRs and medication errors, may, in retrospect, be reluctant to publish of all their anonymized quotes in an interview or focus group setting. In such instance, it may be useful for the researchers to offer "member checking" of the transcripts. In this process, participants can opt out on the publication of any quote that they would fear would adversely impact on themselves (Barbour, 2001). However, it is worth considering that this is an iterative process and requires considerable time commitment from both researchers and participants. There are also potential issues with recall bias.

Various methods of analyzing qualitative data sets are reported and used in the literature. Framework approach is one of such approach used extensively in behavioral pharmacovigilance research. Ritchie and Lewis define the framework method as a "matrix-based analytic method" where data are categorized into a matrix system based on emergent themes and categories (Ritchie and Lewis, 2003). The analytical process begins during transcribing by listening/relistening and reading/rereading the transcript so that the researcher becomes immersed in the data. Key themes after coding of transcripts, which describe the data, are listed in columns while each participant is assigned a space in each row below. The construction of the initial thematic framework is guided by the research aims and objectives and questions introduced to participants from the topic guides. These are then followed by any new themes emerging during the analysis process. This approach of qualitative data analysis is usually facilitated through Computer-Assisted Qualitative Data Analysis Software (CAQDAS) such as QSR NVivo8.

Surveys are a systematic and mostly quantitative approach to gathering information on behavioral pharmacovigilance. The design and administration of survey instrument such as questionnaire requires health services research grounding with adequate considerations given to every stages of the research process as in a qualitative study. In a UK study of nonmedical prescribers' activity, participation, and knowledge around yellow card reporting, we designed an online questionnaire based on any previous literature and researcher knowledge (Stewart et al., 2013). Depending on the scope of the research enquiry, researchers may use descriptive analysis of the data sets. Where association between participant demography and behaviors are investigated, inferential statistics are often used including the use of multivariate analytical methods. However, it is worth noting that surveys conducted without longitudinal follow-up provide cross-sectional data and hence it is difficult to ascertain the direction of correlation between participant characteristics and their behaviors.

Mixed-method exploratory studies allow diverse data sets to be gathered in answering a research question. Qualitative and quantitative research are undertaken within one research study both for complementary purposes (where one phase assists the development of other phase) and for the integration of the findings (where findings from two research phases are combined). Such combination is also often called triangulation (Creswell, 2013). When used for complementary purposes, the quantitative stage within a mixed method study offers the opportunity to test hypotheses generated through the qualitative stage, or where the qualitative can aid the identification of variables allowing scale construction and interpretation of relationships between variables such as for survey design (Brannen, 1992, pp. 3–38). This includes using focus groups and interview data to aid the development of questionnaire content.

USING ROUTINELY COLLECTED DATA

Analyzing routinely collected data provides a great resource to understand patient, healthcare professionals' behaviors, and participation in pharmacovigilance. Routinely collected data, such as the reports of the suspected ADR reports submitted to the UK Medicines and Healthcare Regulatory Agency (MHRA), can be used in undertaking research in behavioral pharmacovigilance. The primary purpose of such reports is to generate Drug Analysis Prints by the MHRA in documenting all suspected ADRs on a particular medicine. However, researchers may get insight into healthcare professionals and patient behaviors by investigating the patterns of reports across different healthcare professionals and the quality and quantity of the reported data to thereof identify any educational or training needs. A good level of activity and participation in pharmacovigilance by healthcare professionals and patients does not always indicate good practice. For example, healthcare practitioners and patients may lack knowledge on what should be reported and when. In addition, high level of underreporting means that data sets are often limited in their scope.

CONSENSUS METHODS FOR POLICY AND GUIDELINE DEVELOPMENT

Consensus methods allow researchers to identify current issues and agree on the best practice and policy of pharmacovigilance to be established by gathering the views of experts. The WHO strengthening pharmacovigilance system encourages researchers in developing countries to use consensus methods to review the scope of existing pharmacovigilance activities and to identify priorities and roles the stakeholders should play to establish a functioning pharmacovigilance system (WHO, 2009).

Consensus methods often use priori statements allowing the participants to express their extent of agreement on the current state of practice and future directions. This is then followed by the process to resolve any disagreement (Jones & Hunter, 1995). The later stage may take several attempts with items that do not invite majority agreement dismissed from the consensus building exercise in the subsequent later stages. The statements that are used in a consensus exercise are best derived from a priori research with relevant research participants, for example using qualitative interviews and focus groups (see above).

Such statements are often presented in their entirety allowing views of the participants in their natural language and are often powerful in engaging the consensus group participants in the research exercise. Consensus process are conducted either as (1) a nominal group method allowing participants to undergo the research process in a face-to-face group setting or (2) the Delphi process whereby consensus process is undertaken through either mailed questionnaire or electronic methods such as emails or web links. The first stage in the consensus method is to identify stakeholders as research participants that are relevant to formulating the implementation of the policies and guidelines that the exercise is seeking to develop.

Persistent engagement of the participants is required when running consensus research. Low responses at the outset or during later stages of the consensus exercise may compromise on the impact of the outcome.

DEVELOPMENT, IMPLEMENTATION, AND EVALUATION OF INTERVENTIONS

Promoting participation in pharmacovigilance by healthcare professionals and patients often requires "complex" behavioral change interventions. Researchers may benefit by using UK Medical Research Council (MRC) framework (MRC, 2006), which lists the essential stages in developing, pilot/feasibility testing, evaluating, reporting, and implementing a complex intervention. Complexity of an intervention is defined by its "difficulty" of implementation, diversity of both population to which it is targeted and its associated outcomes (MRC, 2006).

The exploratory research processes described above, for example, the in-depth qualitative and survey methods, systematic review of literature, and consensus methods, provide scientific and robust foundational knowledge in exploring and identifying what intervention is needed and its essential elements. For example, in identifying the type of interventions that are needed for pharmacists to promote ADR reporting in their clinical practice, researchers may undertake exploratory qualitative research and identify the behavioral determinants and associated barriers and facilitators of reporting suspected ADRs. The results of such enquiry may, in turn, inform the behaviors to be targeted, nature of behavioral intervention, and elements of the planned interventions.

USE OF THEORY

Theory allows researchers to define the problem in behavioral terms. It allows structured and holistic approach in identifying a particular behavior that is important to target through interventions. Interventions are known to be more successful if the interventions are designed based on theories of behavior change (Cane, O'Connor, & Michie, 2015). Given the plethora of theories that have their grounding in health psychology and sociology, making a selection about a particular theory in a research study may provide challenges to the researchers. Frameworks of theories have been recently developed and are being utilized by international researchers in behavioral aspect of clinical practice including pharmacy practice (Stewart & Klein, 2015).

Behavior change wheel (BCW) model provides a framework in relation to designing interventions that are most likely to be effective. BCW recognizes that behavior (B) is an interactive system consisting of "capability (C)," "opportunity (O)," and "motivation (M)," often expressed as COM-B (Michie, Atkins, & West, 2014). Different components of interventions could be designed to target on specific components of COM.

A variant of the BCW is the theoretical domains framework (TDF) and further divides the COM into 14 different domains (Michie et al., 2014). These include knowledge; skills; memory, attention, and decision processes; behavioral regulation; social/professional role and identify; beliefs about capabilities; optimism; beliefs about consequences; intentions; goals and reinforcement; emotion, environmental contexts, and resources; and social influences. Researchers can apply the TDF to investigate determinants of a particular behavior or to explore issues around implementation of a particular behavior change interventions (Atkins et al., 2016). For example, during the exploratory stages of the research associated with developing an intervention, the framework can be applied either all or part of the research stages including formulation of research instrument, such as survey or topic guide/interview schedule for qualitative study; to draw a framework for undertaking qualitative data analysis; or to interpret the results. In researching behavioral determinants of healthcare professional reporting of medication errors in the United Arab Emirates, researchers used TDF to map the determinants of the behavior, i.e., medication error reporting to different domains of the framework (Alqubaisi, Tonna, Strath, & Stewart, 2016).

We have successfully applied TDF across a wide range of behavioral pharmacy research including patient and healthcare professional perspective of the multicompartmental device use, aspects of medicines adherence in diverse population including the homeless and the offshore workers, and pharmacists' management of homeless patients.

Behavior change technique taxonomy has also been developed (BCTTv1), which enables researchers to design the ingredients of a particular behavioral intervention (Michie et al., 2011).

RIGOR IN BEHAVIORAL PHARMACOVIGILANCE RESEARCH

Rigor refers to the quality of being extremely thorough and careful in conducting any research study. Research conducted without sufficient consideration of rigor is often labeled as being "no different than fictional journalism" (Tobin & Begley, 2004). Aspects of trustworthiness and internal and external validity of research need careful consideration.

Aspects of validity that covers most of the applied research methods in behavioral pharmacovigilance can be maintained by ensuring that the research tools are designed based on background literature and any primary/feasibility study data that the researchers would have already collected, expertise of the research team, use of theory, and subjecting the research instruments (e.g., topic guide, questionnaire) to review by an expert panel independent of the research team and through piloting of the research instruments to a small number of research participants. The assessment is mainly around whether the questions within the questionnaire appear to be relevant, reasonable, unambiguous, and clear. The content and wording of the research instruments should be carefully selected to avoid ambiguity.

Validity refers to whether the findings are correct or the extent to which findings represent reality (Slevin & Sines, 1999). Creswell's validity framework (Creswell, 2012) and Paterson's reactivity framework (Paterson, 1994) are useful in considering internal validity of research. These include the need to clarify researcher bias; engagement and observation in the field; peer review of the study materials (including international peer review where relevant and possible); and reactivity, which relates to how the research participants and the researcher respond to each other during the research process, particularly in a qualitative study. For example, lack of trust of participants with the researcher could undermine the nature of the data shared with the researcher. Behavioral pharmacovigilance research could be particularly sensitive to this issue as cultural practices may deter participants from reporting true practices where there is lack of adequate trust.

Reliability can be defined as the degree to which findings are independent of accidental circumstances of the research (Paterson, 1994). This requires the researcher to reassure the readers that similar results would have been produced if the research were to be repeated using same or similar methods (Peräkylä, 2004). Reliability is sought both in terms of the consistency or replicability of the original data as well external reliability, as well as whether the interpretations obtained from the analysis would be reproduced if performed by an independent analyst. For example, in systematic reviews and qualitative methods, it is imperative that an independent researcher should be used in various stages of the research. Trustworthiness in qualitative data comes from ensuring credibility such as by ensuring that participant responses to researchers' questions come with all honesty (Shenton, 2004).

It is important to have careful consideration of the transferability (applies to qualitative research and relates to whether findings could be applied to another similar context of practice) and generalizability (applies to quantitative data and relates to whether findings could be generalized to wider population beyond the sample of research participants) of the research data. While making suggestions about whether research data apply to other settings, it is helpful for the readers if as much details about the study setting and cultural context are provided alongside other information. For example, a system designed to improve pharmacovigilance practice and demonstrated to improve the reporting process in one country and setting may not always be transferable to another setting and country, given the differences in culture and practice. In borrowing a system or standard operating procedures that have been evaluated in other settings and countries, it is important for the researchers and stakeholders to be careful of the disparity that exist across the settings.

ACHIEVEMENTS

The WHO is actively promoting establishment of national and local pharmacovigilance programs. For example, regional and national drug safety monitoring and medicines information systems have been established, which enables to build on the capacity on medicines information and safety. Such establishment has enabled identification of pharmacovigilance issues specific to the local and national population (WHO, 2009). International consortiums are being established in enabling greater use of technology in the reporting and management of data related to pharmacovigilance in specific or wider therapeutic areas (Pal, Olsson, & Brown, 2015). Where national and local pharmacovigilance centers do not exist, academic centers are experimenting novel methods of surveillance, including the use of mobile phones in reporting ADRs (Baron, Goutard, Nguon, & Tarantola, 2013). Adoption of the new systems and technologies should be supported by behavioral pharmacovigilance research. It is important that perspectives of potential adopters are considered in establishing successful pharmacovigilance systems. Research should be embedded as part of development, feasibility, and establishment of novel pharmacovigilance systems and changing behaviors of healthcare professionals and patients. International collaboration on pharmacovigilance research needs to be promoted.

CHALLENGES

Lack of research expertise, resources, and opportunities for multidisciplinary collaborations are key challenges to undertaking behavioral pharmacovigilance research in the developing world. Despite the majority burden of diseases, only 10% of the healthcare research funding is consumed within developing world. This limits advancement in the knowledge and practice around medicines safety. Behavioral research is also often discouraged and is limited by lack of interests from stakeholders with regard to misconceptions about the impact such research may have on practice and policy.

Promoting rigor in the conduct of research is essential to impact on practice and policy. Quality is essential so that the outcome of the research can be adopted.

Lack of expertise in research methodology can be a major barrier to overcome. Researchers in the developing countries may also face challenges in accessing current literature in planning and undertaking behavioral pharmacovigilance research. However, a growing number of open access journals are providing researchers with free access to scientific literature.

RECOMMENDATIONS: THE WAY FORWARD

International collaboration around behavioral pharmacovigilance research in developing countries can positively impact on the extent and quality of behavioral pharmacovigilance research. Particularly, such collaborations can provide researchers in the developing countries with access and support around research methods from international experts in the field. There are multiple examples of successful collaborative partnership in both research and implementation of novel pharmacovigilance systems. Collaborative research training partnerships are also essential in enhancing research skills.

Behavioral pharmacovigilance should also be incorporated in pharmacy and clinical education. Patients are not allowed to yet directly report on suspected ADRs in many parts of the world. Future research programs should incorporate patient perspectives on pharmacovigilance.

CONCLUSIONS

Establishment of effective pharmacovigilance in the developing world requires understanding and where necessary impacting on patients and healthcare professionals' behaviors. Exploratory and evaluative research requires health services research grounding. Such research may range from reviewing current evidence and policies, establishing consensus on future practice and policies, and exploring patient and healthcare professional behaviors. These in turn may inform the development, implementation, and evaluation of successful interventions to positively impact on pharmacovigilance practices in developing countries.

LESSONS LEARNED

- Promoting effective and efficient pharmacovigilance practice requires understanding and where necessary impacting the behaviors of the healthcare professionals, patients, policy makers, and wider stakeholders.

- Undertaking research into behavioral aspects of pharmacovigilance requires researcher awareness with the choice of appropriate research methods linked to the research enquiry.
- A well-conducted research study grounded in the current literature and theory can enable behaviors to be identified and addressed through appropriate interventions.
- International collaborations can enhance sharing of research knowledge and expertise on behavioral pharmacovigilance, thereby impacting practice, policy, and future research.

REFERENCES

Alqubaisi, M., Tonna, A., Strath, A., & Stewart, D. (2016). Exploring behavioral determinants relating to health professional reporting of medication errors: A qualitative study using the theoretical domains framework. *European Journal of Clinical Pharmacology*, *11*, 1–9.

Atkins, L., Hunkeler, E. M., Jensen, C. D., Michie, S., Lee, J. K., Doubeni, C. A., … Corley, D. A. (March 31, 2016). Factors influencing variation in physician adenoma detection rates: A theory-based approach for performance improvement. *Gastrointestinal Endoscopy*, *83*(3), 617–626.

Barbour, R. S. (2001). Checklists for improving rigour in qualitative research: A case of the tail wagging the dog? *BMJ: British Medical Journal*, *322*(7294), 1115–1117.

Baron, S., Goutard, F., Nguon, K., & Tarantola, A. (2013). Use of a text message-based pharmacovigilance tool in Cambodia: Pilot study. *Journal of Medical Internet Research*, *15*(4), e68.

Bhagavathula, A. S., Elnour, A. A., Jamshed, S. Q., & Shehab, A. (2016). Health professionals' knowledge, attitudes and practices about pharmacovigilance in India: A systematic review and meta-analysis. *PLos One*, *11*(3), e0152221.

Brannen, J. (1992). Combining qualitative and quantitative approaches: An overview. In J. Brannen (Ed.), *Mixing methods: Qualitative and quantitative research* (pp. 3–38). Hants: Ashgate Publishing Company.

Cane, J., O'Connor, D., & Michie, S. (2015). Validation of the theoretical domains framework for use in behavior change and implementation research. *Implementation Science*, *7*(1), 1.

Centre for Review and Dissemination (CRD). (2009). *CRD's guidance for undertaking reviews in healthcare* [Internet]. Retrieved from http://www.york.ac.uk/media/crd/Systematic_Reviews.pdf.

Cochrane Collaboration. (2011). *Cochrane handbook for systematic reviews of interventions* [Internet]. Retrieved from http://handbook.cochrane.org.

Creswell, J. W. (2012). *Qualitative inquiry and research design: Choosing among five traditions* (California: Thousand Oaks).

Creswell, J. W. (2013). *Research design: Qualitative, quantitative, and mixed methods approaches*. London: Sage Publications.

Critical Appraisal Skills Programme. (2013). *CASP tools and Checklists* [Internet]. Retrieved from http://www.casp-uk.net/casp-tools-checklists.

European Medicines Agency. (2016). *Pharmacovigilance*. Retrieved from http://www.ema.europa.eu/ema/index.jsp?curl=pages/special_topics/general/general_content_000570.jsp.

Francis, J. J., Johnston, M., Robertson, C., Glidewell, L., Entwistle, V., Eccles, M., & Grimshaw, J. M. (December 1, 2010). What is an adequate sample size? Operationalising data saturation for theory-based interview studies. *Psychology and Health*, *25*(10), 1229–1245.

Hazell, L., & Shakir, S. A. (2006). Under-reporting of adverse drug reactions: A systematic review. *Drug Safety*, *29*, 385–396.

Higgins, J. P., Altman, D. G., Gøtzsche, P. C., Jüni, P., Moher, D., Oxman, A. D., … Sterne, J. A. (2011). The Cochrane Collaboration's tool for assessing risk of bias in randomised trials. *BMJ: British Medical Journal*, *18*(343), d5928.

Joanna Briggs Institute (JBI). (2015a). *Systematic review resource Package* [Internet]. Retrieved from http:// joannabriggs.org/assets/docs/jbc/operations/can-synthesise/CAN_SYNTHSISE_Resource-V4.pdf.

Joanna Briggs Institute (JBI). (2015b). *The Joanna Briggs Institute Reviewers' Manual 2015- methodology for JBI scoping reviews* [Internet]. Retrieved from http://joannabriggs.org/assets/docs/sumari/Reviewers-Manual_Methodology-for-JBI-Scoping-Reviews_2015_v2.pdf.

Jones, J., & Hunter, D. (1995). Consensus methods for medical and health services research. *BMJ: British Medical Journal, 311*(7001), 376.

Lopez-Gonzalez, E., Herdeiro, M. T., & Figueiras, A. (2009). Determinants of under-reporting of adverse drug reactions. *Drug Safety, 32*(1), 19–31.

MacLure, K., Paudyal, V., & Stewart, D. (2016). Reviewing the literature, how systematic is systematic? *International Journal of Clinical Pharmacy, 38*(3), 685–694.

Maigetter, K., Pollock, A. M., Kadam, A., Ward, K., & Weiss, M. G. (2015). Pharmacovigilance in India, Uganda and South Africa with reference to WHO's minimum requirements. *International Journal of Health Policy and Management, 4*(5), 295.

Medical Research Council (MRC) [Internet] 2006. Developing and evaluating complex interventions: new guidance [Internet]. [United Kingdom]: Retrieved from https://www.mrc.ac.uk/documents/pdf/complex-interventions-guidance/.

Michie, S., Ashford, S., Sniehotta, F. F., Dombrowski, S. U., Bishop, A., & French, D. P. (2011). A refined taxonomy of behavior change techniques to help people change their physical activity and healthy eating behaviors: The CALO-re taxonomy. *Psychology & Health, 26*(11), 1479–1498.

Michie, S., Atkins, L., & West, R. (2014). *The behavior change wheel: A guide to designing interventions*. Great Britain: Silver Black Publishing.

Moher, D., Shamseer, L., Clarke, M., Ghersi, D., Liberati, A., Petticrew, M., … Stewart, L. A. (2015). Preferred reporting items for systematic review and meta-analysis protocols (PRISMA-P) 2015 statement. *Systematic Reviews, 4*(1), 1.

Morgan, D. L. (1996). Focus groups. *Annual Review of Sociology, 22*(1), 129–152.

Moscou, K., Kohler, J. C., & MaGahan, A. (2016). Governance and pharmacovigilance in Brazil: A scoping review. *Journal of Pharmaceutical Policy and Practice, 8*(9), 1.

Oxford Dictionary [Internet]. (2016). Retrieved from http://www.oed.com.

Pal, S. N., Olsson, S., & Brown, E. G. (2015). The monitoring medicines project: A multinational pharmacovigilance and public health project. *Drug Safety, 38*, 319. http://dx.doi.org/10.1007/s40264.

Paterson, B. L. (1994). A framework to identify reactivity in qualitative research. *Western Journal of Nursing Research, 16*(3), 301–316.

Paudyal, V., Hansford, D., Cunningham, S., & Stewart, D. (2011). Pharmacy assisted patient self care of minor ailments: A chronological review of UK health policy documents and key events 1997–2010. *Health Policy, 101*(3), 253–259.

Paudyal, V., Hansford, D., Cunningham, S., & Stewart, D. (2012). Community pharmacists' adoption of medicines reclassified from prescription-only status: A systematic review of factors associated with decision making. *Pharmacoepidemiology and Drug Safety, 21*(4), 396–406.

Paudyal, V., Hansford, D., Cunningham, S., & Stewart, D. (2014). Pharmacists' adoption into practice of newly reclassified medicines from diverse therapeutic areas in Scotland: A quantitative study of factors associated with decision-making. *Research in Social and Administrative Pharmacy, 10*(1), 88–105.

Peräkylä, A. (2004). Reliability and validity in research based on naturally occurring social interaction. In D. Silverman (Ed.), *Qualitative research: Theory, method and practice* (2nd ed.) (pp. 283–304). London: SAGE publications.

Pirmohamed, M., Atuah, K. N., Dodoo, A. N. O., & Winstanley, P. (2007). Pharmacovigilance in developing countries. *BMJ: British Medical Journal, 335*(7618), 462.

Ritchie, J., & Lewis, J. (Eds.). (2003). *Qualitative research practice, a guide for social science students and researchers*. London: SAGE publications.

Rosenberg, W., & Donald, A. (1995). Evidence based medicine: An approach to clinical problem-solving. *BMJ: British Medical Journal, 310*(6987), 1122.

Shenton, A. K. (2004). Strategies for ensuring trustworthiness in qualitative research projects. *Education for Information, 22*(2), 63–75.

Slevin, E., & Sines, D. (1999). Enhancing the truthfulness, consistency and transferability of a qualitative study: Utilising a manifold of approaches. *Nurse Researcher, 7*, 79–97.

Stewart, D., & Klein, S. (2015). The use of theory in research. *International Journal of Clinical Pharmacy, 28*, 1–5.

Stewart, D., MacLure, K., Paudyal, V., Hughes, C., Courtenay, M., & McLay, J. (2013). Non-medical prescribers and pharmacovigilance: Participation, competence and future needs. *International Journal of Clinical Pharmacy, 35*(2), 268–274.

Tobin, G. A., & Begley, C. M. (2004). Methodological rigour within a qualitative framework. *Journal of Advanced Nursing, 48*(4), 388–396.

Wilkinson, S. (2004). Focus group research. In D. Silverman (Ed.), *Qualitative research: Theory, method and practice* (2nd ed.) (pp. 177–199). London: SAGE publications.

World Health Organization (WHO). (2009). *Supporting pharmacovigilance in developing countries the systems perspective* [Internet]. Retrieved from http://apps.who.int/medicinedocs/documents/s18813en/s18813en.pdf.

CHAPTER

KNOWLEDGE, ATTITUDE, AND PRACTICE OF PHARMACOVIGILANCE IN DEVELOPING COUNTRIES

11

Dixon Thomas[1], Seeba Zachariah[2]

[1]Gulf Medical University, Ajman, United Arab Emirates; [2]Gulf Medical University/Thumbay Hospital, Ajman, United Arab Emirates

CHAPTER OUTLINE

INTRODUCTION

This chapter discusses the knowledge, attitude, and practice (KAP) of pharmacovigilance (Pv) among different stakeholders. All the discussions were focused on economically developing countries and economically rich countries with developing Pv systems.

The 2010s have witnessed a trend in KAP studies related to Pv among health professionals in developing countries, especially in Asia and Africa. In many developed countries, Pv is a culture within the healthcare system. Social and administrative pharmacists work in close contact with consumers, healthcare professionals, healthcare agencies, regulators, and other administrators. It is important to discuss the KAP of Pv from a societal perspective (Fig. 11.1).

Knowledge is the understanding of any given topic. ***Attitude*** is the emotional, motivational, perceptive and cognitive beliefs that positively or negatively influence the behavior or practice of an individual. An attitude will change on the basis of internal or external cues. Individuals evaluate information as favorable or unfavorable. ***Practice*** is the observable action of a healthcare professional in observing, assessing, reporting, and taking further healthcare actions (CommGAP, 2010; UNICEF & ILO, 2011).

Social and Administrative Aspects of Pharmacy in Low- and Middle-Income Countries. http://dx.doi.org/10.1016/B978-0-12-811228-1.00011-X

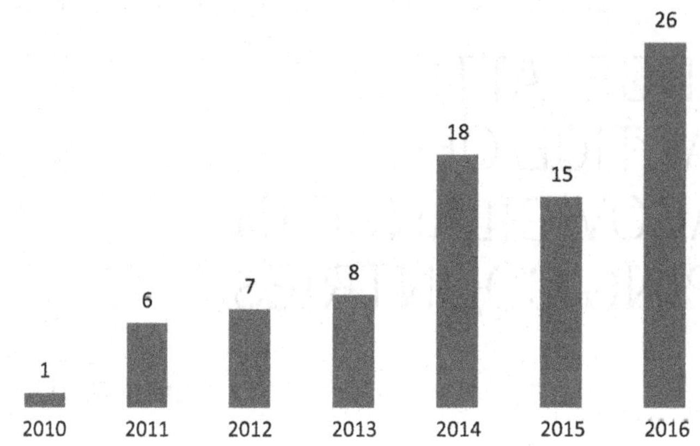

FIGURE 11.1

Trend in published Pv KAP studies from developing countries. *KAP*, knowledge, attitude, and practice; *Pv*, pharmacovigilance.

Based on Google and PubMed search in December 2016.

Knowledge and attitudes can influence practice. They are hierarchical in a sense that knowledge influences the development of attitude, and attitude influences practice. Knowledge and attitude can be reinforced with practice. It is also possible that new knowledge and attitude can develop through practical experiences. A positive attitude improves practice, and appropriate knowledge grooms a positive attitude. Even if a professional has good knowledge, it may not improve their practice if their attitude is negative (Abubakar, Ismail, Rahman, & Haque, 2015).

The KAP of Pv in developing countries needs improvement. The relevant professionals have poor to moderate knowledge, a positive attitude, and poor practice.

The gap from knowledge and attitude to practice is high in Pv (Kamtane & Jayawardhani, 2012). In an Indian hospital survey, 64.4% of professionals observed adverse drug reactions (ADRs) in their patients, but only 22.8% ever reported any of these reactions (Gupta, Nayak, Shivaranjani, & Vidyarthi, 2015). Another survey reported that 50.2% of the respondents observed ADRs, but only 8.1% actually reported them to the Pv center. Their average attitude was greater than 70%. The respondents even felt that it was important to report ADRs, irrespective of the seriousness of the reaction (Siddeshwara, Santoshkumar, & Vardhamane, 2016). The gap from Pv knowledge and attitude to practice is therefore significant.

A systematic review collected 28 studies from India, of which 18 were processed for meta-analysis (Bhagavathula, Elnour, Jamshed, & Shehab, 2016). The review was conducted from January 2011 to July 2015. The study findings revealed that the following:

- 55.6% of the professionals were unaware of the Pv Program of India (PvPI);
- 31.9% thought all drugs that were legally available on the market were safe;
- 28.7% were not interested in reporting any ADRs; and
- 74.5% never reported any ADRs to the national program.

The number of developing countries that became members of the WHO Program for International Drug Monitoring (PIDM) has increased. The Uppsala Monitoring Centre (UMC) is the WHO

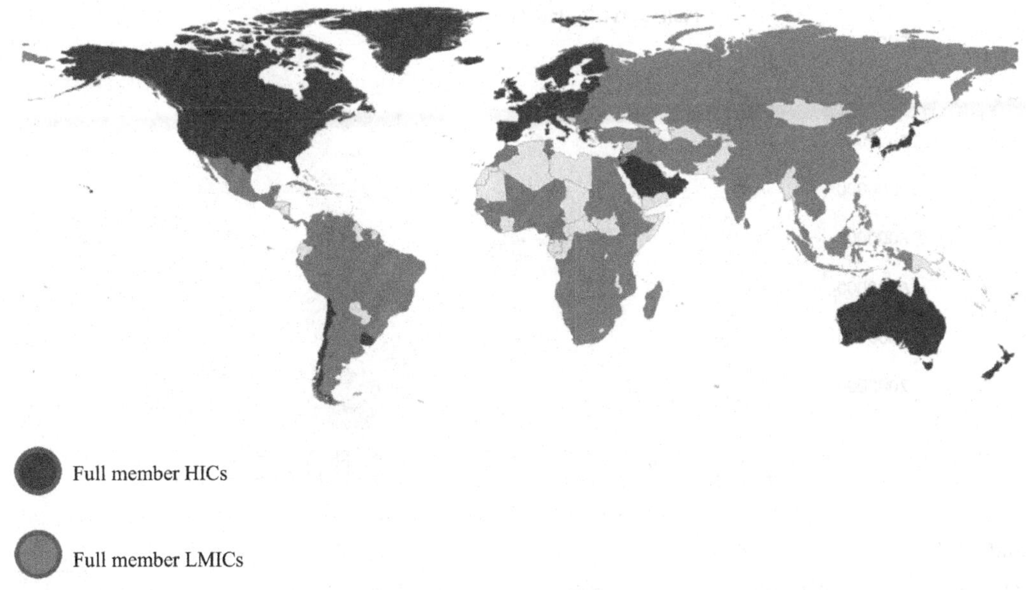

FIGURE 11.2

Countries in the WHO Program for International Drug Monitoring (PIDM). *HICs,* high-income countries; *LMICs,* low- and middle-income countries.

Adapted with permission from the Uppsala Monitoring Centre.

collaborating center for the PIDM. The UMC does not have a definition for "developing country," and the UMC often uses the low- and middle-income countries (LMIC) definition by the World Bank as a proxy. The grouping of nations into LMIC or high-income countries (HIC) is updated once yearly and no prior history is saved, and thus a country that is classed as an LMIC today might have been an HIC when it initiated Pv activities and vice versa. As of October 2016, the current number of associate members is 28, and the majority of them are LMICs (UMC, 2016b) (Fig. 11.2).

Most of the Individual Case Safety Reports (ICSRs) that have been submitted to the WHO VigiBase came from HICs (UMC, 2016a). The trend is the opposite in KAP studies, most of which have been published from LMICs. This gap shows the struggle in developing countries to implement efficient Pv systems. Most developing countries are members or associate members of the WHO PIDM. Key features of Pv operations in developing countries were identified as having the following:

- Coordination by drug regulatory agencies,
- A limited budget allocated for Pv,
- Support from funding agencies from developed countries, especially for Africa,
- Relatively better-established Pv in some national public health programs, and
- Insufficient regional or peripheral centers to support national centers.

Most of the centers were also involved in other activities such as drug information, rational drug use, poison information, etc. (Olsson, Pal, Stergachis, & Couper, 2010) (Fig. 11.3).

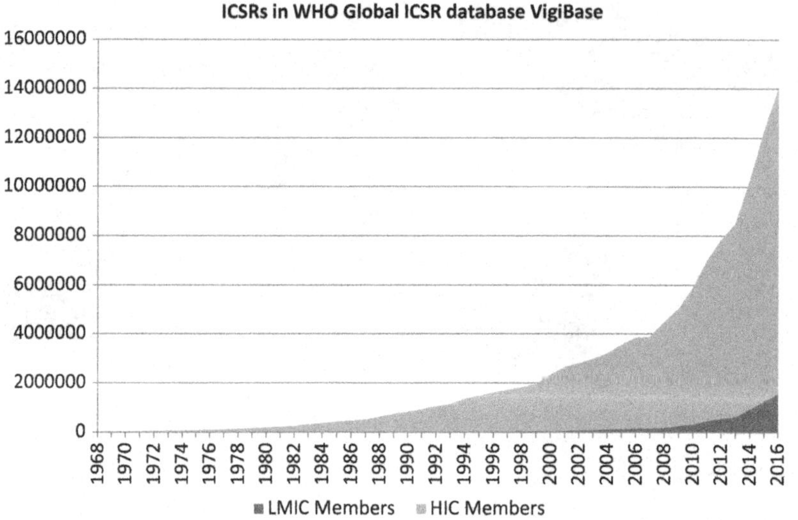

FIGURE 11.3

Most Individual Case Safety Reports (ICSRs) in VigiBase come from high-income countries.

Adapted with permission from Uppsala Monitoring Centre.

Even with relatively better enforced health regulations, the KAP of healthcare professionals in the Arab region was found to be insufficient (Suyagh, Farah, & Farha, 2014). All this background information required a thorough review of Pv KAPs among different healthcare stakeholders. A further assessment of the progress and present challenges will enable us to recommend solutions to improve the Pv KAP of developing countries.

PV KAP AMONG HEALTHCARE PROFESSIONALS

KAP studies of Pv among healthcare professionals, which have been published from developing countries have been increasing since 2010.

A study from Nepal stated that the Pv KAPs of doctors, nurses, and pharmacists in one hospital were not found to be much different among each type of professional. The overall KAPs were poor and needed improvement. A full 62.3% of the respondents did not report any ADRs (Palaian, Ibrahim, & Mishra, 2011).

There were few studies that included the Pv of doctors, pharmacists, and nurses together. It was surprising to observe that many multiprofessional studies usually called the study population "healthcare professionals" but excluded pharmacists; e.g.,

- An Indian Pv survey included doctors, medical residents, and nurses but not pharmacists (Abidi, Ahmad, Gupta, Rizvi, & Sing, 2014).
- Another Indian survey mentioned "various medical fraternities" in the title and healthcare professionals in the abstract, but it only included medical students, residents, and nurses. However, that study did mention the need for Pv training among doctors, nurses, and pharmacists in their conclusion (Ponmari, Sivaraman, Aruna, Subashree, & Jawahar, 2015).

- Another Indian study mentioned healthcare providers in the title and healthcare professionals in the abstract, but it included doctors, nurses, and dental practitioners only (Torwane, Hongal, Gouraha, Saxena, & Chavan, 2015).
- A Yemeni study mentioned healthcare professionals in the title and abstract, but it included only doctors and nurses (Alshakka et al., 2016).
- Two more studies that addressed KAPs among healthcare professionals included doctors only (Hardeep, Bajaj & Rakesh, 2013; Karelia & Piparava, 2014).

The reasons for this trend could be as follows:

- The majority of healthcare professionals in the hospitals are nurses and doctors.
- There is underrecognition of pharmacists as healthcare professionals.
- Pharmacists are not performing structured patient assessments, limiting their chances to identify ADRs. In most of the hospitals, pharmacist duties end at dispensing medication.

Few studies that frame healthcare professionals as the study population have included pharmacists along with doctors and nurses (Bharadwaj, Budania, Mondal, Yadav, & Sharma, 2016; Gupta et al., 2015).

A systematic review of doctors from 10 countries was published in 2014, with 32 studies from 2004 to 2014. The reviewed studies consisted of 19 from India, 4 from Nigeria, 2 from Romania, and 1 each from Pakistan, Malaysia, the UAE, and some European countries. The KAPs in the reported ADRs were found to be poor among doctors, but educational interventions were effective at improving their results (Abubakar, Simbak, & Haque, 2014; Chandrakapure, Giri, Khan, Mateenuddin, & Faheem, 2015). In many hospitals, prescribers demonstrated positive attitudes toward Pv services, but they had less knowledge and poor practices (Kulkarni et al., 2013; Vora & Barvaliya, 2014).

Poor practice could be due to a lack of awareness about the ADR reporting process and to inconveniences. Many doctors perceived ADR reporting as an important responsibility (Desai, Iyer, Panchal, Shah, & Dikshit, 2011). Not knowing where and how to report an ADR was the major problem reported by clinicians; 77% of the clinicians in an Indian hospital observed ADRs, but only 15% of them reported any at all. Awareness of a functional Pv center in the hospital was also found to be poor (Kiran, Shivashankaramurthy, Bhooma, & Dinakar, 2014). Hospitals with highly active Pv services showed satisfactory knowledge and attitudes among clinicians, but they were still neglectful in terms of Pv practice (Bisht, Singh, & Dhasmana, 2014).

A study from an Egyptian hospital demonstrated the difference between general practitioners (GP) and specialists. GPs were less aware of the national Pv center and they reported fewer ADRs compared to specialists. The overall Pv KAPs of physicians were found to be substantial yet unsatisfactory (Kamal, Kamel, & Mahfouz, 2014).

The findings were not so different for dental practitioners. Dentists did report few ADRs, even though many ADRs were observed in regular practice (Torwane et al., 2015).

Year IV and V medical students from Malaysia and Nigeria were surveyed in 2015 to assess their Pv KAPs. Nigerian medical students had relatively better knowledge and practice in Pv than their Malaysian peers. Their attitudes were not significantly different. The relationship between knowledge and practice was positive but weak. The study team observed that the whole study population needed improvement in their KAPs (Abubakar et al., 2015).

Some studies showed very poor knowledge of Pv among undergraduate medical students. Even though most of the medical residents had heard the term "Pv," only a few knew how to practice it (Vora, Paliwal, Doshi, Barvaliya, & Tripathi, 2012). They had positive attitudes but were poor in their practice

(Meher, Joshua, Asha, & Mukherji, 2015). For the majority of medical residents, those who observed ADRs were not reporting them to the Pv center in the hospital or their national center (Pimpalkhute, Jaiswal, Sontakke, Bajait, & Gaikwad, 2012).

A high level of Pv knowledge among medical students was observed right after they took a Pv course (Deepak & Nagaral, 2014). This finding could be interpreted as the effectiveness of course instruction. The efficient delivery of educational interventions can improve KAP in medical students (Nadendla, Gangisetty, Goka, RamaRao, & Nadendla, 2015). KAP in a practical sense is more appropriate if measured at the end of their education or residency. Students who were about to become practitioners were accepting that ADR reporting was their responsibility (Bansode, Zad, Sawa, & Dudhal, 2015; Reddy, Varma, & Reddy, 2014).

Studies showed improved Pv KAP among medical students with higher education. It is still justifiable to educate undergraduate medical students to report ADRs because they could implement it in their general practice (Hema, Bhuvana & Sangeetha, 2012; Parthiban, Nileshraj, Mangaiarkkarasi, & Meher, 2015).

A Tanzanian study described poor Pv KAP among drug dispensers. Among all the dispensers, 52% were nurse assistants. Pharmacy dispensers had significantly higher knowledge and practice in reporting ADRs. However, most of the dispensers had a positive attitude toward reporting ADRs (Shimwela, 2011).

Pv knowledge and practices among community pharmacists in India were found to be low. Participant attitude scores were higher than their knowledge and practice, which explained that they could improve if knowledge and practice skills are facilitated (Rathod & Panchal, 2014). Similarly, a study from Jordan described inadequate knowledge and extremely low practice among pharmacists, while their attitude toward PV was positive (Suyagh et al., 2014).

Studies in Pv KAP among pharmacy students were few. An Iranian study described moderate knowledge and attitudes in pharmacy students. Among them, 63% had a chance to observe ADRs, but only 5% attempted to report these findings to the body of concern (Isfahani et al., 2013). A Pakistani study observed promising Pv attitudes in pharmacy students (Shakeel et al., 2014).

A Yemeni study compared nurses and doctors in relation to their Pv KAPs. Nurses had better knowledge and attitudes toward Pv in their teaching hospital. Both nurses and physicians regarded Pv as an important part of healthcare education and practice (Alshakka et al., 2016). An Iranian study focusing on nurses found that their knowledge and practice were not satisfactory. Ninety-one percent of nurses never reported any ADRs. The nurses had a positive attitude about reporting ADRs but they preferred to report to a doctor, pharmacist, or the hospital ADR reporting center rather than to the national reporting system directly (Hanafi, Torkamandi, Hayatshahi, Gholami, & Javadi, 2012).

Prefinal and final year nursing students in an Indian institution were moderately aware of Pv practices, and their attitude was positive with respect to Pv improvements (Sivadasan & Sellappan, 2015).

ACHIEVEMENTS

There are reports to show improved Pv KAP among healthcare professionals. The major reason for this improvement is repeated educational interventions (Bharadwaj et al., 2016). Attitudes and practices are difficult to change. Educational interventions generally focused on improving knowledge of how to report ADRs (Hema, Bhuvana, & Sangeetha, 2012). Educational interventions are shown to have a high impact on knowledge, relatively less impact on attitude, and even less impact on practice. Many factors influence emotional, motivational, perceptive and cognitive beliefs. In most cases, it is true that the professionals perceive themselves as being responsible for the development of ADRs, and they are afraid to report these observations. Because they were aware of Pv, all the health professionals knew ADRs were part of a clinical practice, and they might report high attitudes when their attitudes are actually negative.

Most of the Pv KAP studies involved cross-sectional surveys. The surveys themselves were shown to improve KAP levels on the survey subject. In an Indian hospital study, two similar Pv surveys were conducted with a gap of 1 year and the awareness of the healthcare professionals was much higher in the second survey. All the participants responded yes to having access to ADR reporting forms (Palanisamy, Kumaran, & Rajasekaran, 2013).

Longitudinal studies involving educational interventions improved related knowledge and attitudes (Abubakar et al., 2014). Studies explaining the perceptions of healthcare professionals at pre- and post-educational intervention improved participant KAP (Bagewadi, Venkatadri, & Nayaka, 2015; Chandrakapure et al., 2015). Providing educational materials a few days before the training was well appreciated. Microsoft PowerPoint presentations were rated higher than the blackboard and overhead projector for training (Bagewadi, Rekha, & Anandh, 2015). The outcomes of educational interventions were positive. The participants knew where to report, how to report, and why it is important to report an ADR better than those who did not attend. A study from Bangladesh reinforced the need for training and clinician assistance in improving Pv awareness and practice (Nahar, Karim, Paul, & Khan, 2011). Even though the ADR identification was higher in the trained group, its reporting was not much different from that of the nontrained group (Bisht et al., 2014). This finding indicates that the gap is in the administration of the healthcare system. The retention of knowledge is better if it is applied in practice. Attitudes keep improving with rational practice. If the healthcare system is not functioning properly, then ADR reporting could be inconvenient. The focus is on the need to expand from the KAP of healthcare professionals to national healthcare delivery.

Even though further improvements are required, the practice of Pv in structured national health programs is expected to be relatively higher (Denekew & Adisse, 2014). Many of the professionals who were training under active programs were aware of the national Pv system (Hardeep et al., 2013). In the absence of a clearly defined governmental program, public hospital drug prescribers have demonstrated low knowledge and practice of Pv (Kulkarni et al., 2013). This trend explains the need for more hands-on training within a structured program. Those who are attending regular continuing education programs were found to have better Pv KAP. Capacity building and improved logistics could result in better Pv KAP (Okechukwu, Odinduka, Ele, & Okonta, 2013).

Improving the Pv system is a key focus of the health sector. Governmental agencies lead the development of Pv systems with the support of national and international funds. Theoretically, the Pv KAP in public hospitals is generally higher than that of the private sector (Karelia & Piparava, 2014).

Practitioners in teaching hospitals, even if private, are more oriented towards Pv through the academic environment. Most healthcare professionals recognize the importance of reporting ADRs (Abidi et al., 2014; Desai et al., 2011). The presence of clinical pharmacists on the healthcare team shall improve the Pv awareness of other healthcare professionals (Palanisamy et al., 2013).

To develop a better Pv system, it is necessary to create a framework relating people, functions, structures, expected outcomes, and impacts. A framework for developing countries was set up by Strengthening Pharmaceutical Systems (SPS) and USAID (Strengthening Pharmaceutical Systems Program & USAID, 2009). SPS program USAID (funded) strives to build capacity within developing countries. Major supports have been provided for HIV/AIDS, tuberculosis, and malaria. Successful models from developed countries will not be copied directly. Countries need to systematically plan and build Pv systems that are suitable locally and matched globally. Appropriate technological and financial support is required to achieve long-term goals (SPS. Strengthening Pharmaceutical Systems & USAID, 2009).

Some of the public health programs that have financial and technical support from global health initiatives have implemented active medicine surveillance. There are funding mechanisms available for countries to strengthen their Pv systems, such as the Global Fund to Fight AIDS, Tuberculosis and Malaria, the US President's Emergency Plan for AIDS Relief (PEPFAR), the US President's Malaria Initiative (PMI), the Affordable Medicines Facility-malaria (AMFm), and the Global Alliance for Vaccines and Immunization (GAVI). Various technical agencies, including the WHO, UMC, the USAID-funded SPS, the United States Pharmacopeia/Promoting the Quality of Medicines (USP/PQM) programs, and Medicines for Malaria Venture, provide support to build or improve Pv systems (Strengthening Pharmaceutical Systems (SPS) Program, 2011).

Studies have also reported that healthcare professionals expect better information technology support to ease their use of the Pv system. The ADR reporting system should be easy to operate and easily accessible, in the same way as VigiBase and VigiAccess (Rishi, Patel, & Bhandari, 2012; UMC, n.d.-b). Take and Tell is a useful app that was produced by the UMC to encourage consumers to take their medicines as prescribed and report any adverse events to their doctors (UMC, n.d.-a).

The increased participation of developing countries in the WHO PIDM has improved Pv practices globally. The first African countries to join the WHO Program were Morocco and South Africa, both joining in 2002. The expansion was most dramatic after 2005, which was attributable to the establishment of WHO collaborating centers in Ghana and Morocco. These two centers trained and supported these African countries in Pv. More than 95% of the global population is covered by the WHO Pv network at present (UMC., 2016b) (Figs. 11.4 and 11.5).

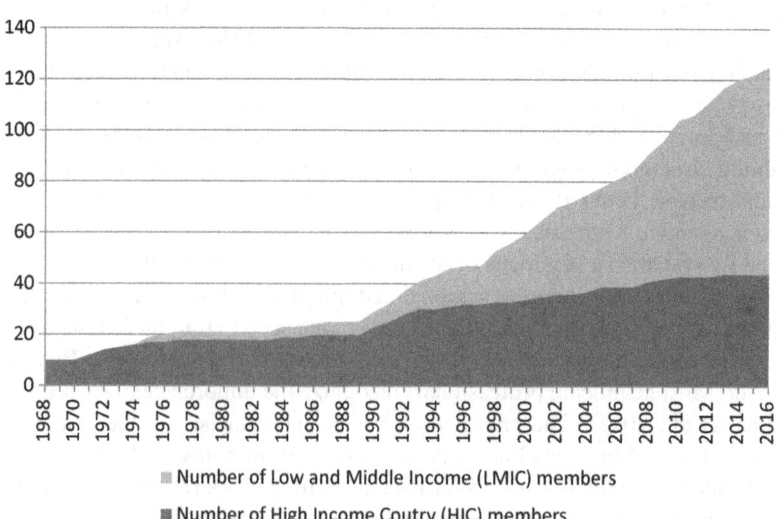

FIGURE 11.4

New member countries in the WHO Program for International Drug Monitoring, over time.

Adapted with permission from the Uppsala Monitoring Centre.

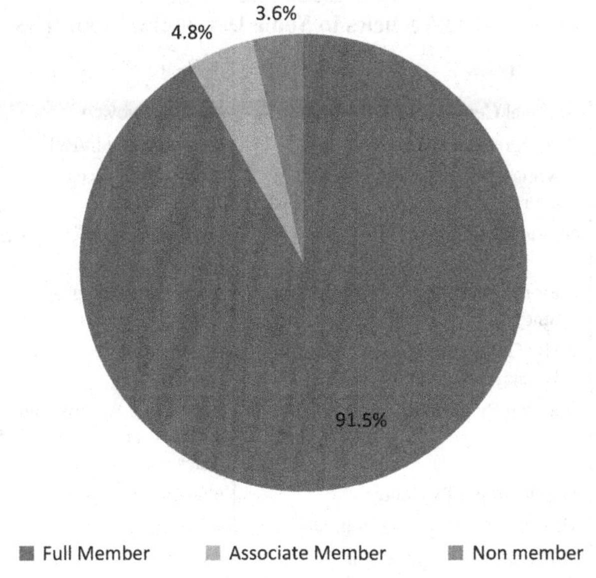

FIGURE 11.5

Percentage of global population coverage by the WHO pharmacovigilance network.

Adapted with permission from Uppsala Monitoring Centre.

Developing countries and some of the economically developed countries in the Arab region face problems in establishing state-of-the-art Pv systems. In 2014, Good Pharmacovigilance Practice for Arab Countries (GVP-Arab) was created to harmonize the Pv practices and regulations among the Arab countries. In addition to each country's regulations, the guidelines were expected to improve Pv practices in the region (Saad et al., 2014).

Building a better Pv system has been recognized as a key strategy for developing an efficient healthcare system in developing countries (Jha, Rathore, Shankar, Gyawali, & Hassali, 2015). Pv systems are under development in many developing countries (Table 11.1). The Pv system should fit within a robust healthcare system, and the healthcare system should perform better in the presence of efficient Pv systems. Toll-free numbers and emails provided by national regulators will improve ADR reporting.

CHALLENGES

The lag times have decreased between the introduction of a new drug to the United States or European market and to that of many developing countries. Accessibility to healthcare and the lifestyle, nutrition, and genetic makeup of people in developing counties are not necessarily the same as those in developed countries. It is essential to improve local effectiveness and the safety of medicines through better Pv systems (Ghosh, Bhatia, & Bhattacharya, 2012). Even though pharmaceutical companies produce and market medicines, their contributions to Pv in developing countries are insufficient. Strong policy reforms are required for pharmaceutical companies to improve their Pv support (Moscou, Kohler, & Lexchin, 2013).

Table 11.1 Pharmacovigilance (Pv) Agencies in Some Developing Countries

S. No.	Country	Pv Agencies	Website
1	China	National Center for ADR Monitoring	www.cdr.gov.cn
2	India	Pv Program of India	www.ipc.gov.in/PvPI
3	Egypt	Egyptian Pharmaceutical Vigilance Center	www.ePvc.gov.eg
4	Nigeria	National Pv Center	www.nafdac.gov.ng/index.php/about-nafdac/faqs/PV
5	Malaysia	National Pharmaceutical Regulatory Agency	www.npra.moh.gov.my
6	Africa	WHO Collaborating Center for Advocacy and Training in Pv	www.who-Pvafrica.org
7	Philippines	National Pv Center	www.fda.gov.ph/issuances/276-pharml/pharml-administrative-order/153551-administrative-order-no-2011-0009
8	Thailand	Thai National Pv Center	www.fda.moph.go.th/eng/index.stm
9	Nepal	Ministry of Health and Population	www.dda.gov.np
10	Bangladesh	Ministry of Health and Family Welfare	www.mohfw.gov.bd
11	Jordan	Jordan Food and Drug Administration	www.jfda.jo
12	Brazil	National Health Surveillance Agency	portal.anvisa.gov.br/contact-us
13	South Africa	Medicines Control Council	www.mccza.com

Consumers are in need of considerable assistance by healthcare professionals to understand the side effects of medicines. A Nigerian study observed that the patients had basic knowledge about the side effects of antiretroviral therapy (ART). ADR reporting by patients to the national system has not yet appeared to be practical (Herbert & Augustyn, 2013). Physicians were positive about ADR reporting by consumers as per a Yemeni study (Alshakka et al., 2016). An Indian study reported that 60% of the doctors favored ADR reporting by consumers (Rishi et al., 2012). Regulators from many developing countries encourage consumer reporting within their Pv systems (Jha et al., 2014) (Wilson & Amma, 2015).

From consumer and provider perspectives, the following healthcare issues reduce Pv activities:

- There were proportionally fewer healthcare professionals in the developing countries in relation to the patient load. Consumer access to these professionals was limited. When a side effect occurred, the patient generally stopped taking the medicines or went to another healthcare professional. The system of consumer–provider communication by phone is absent.
- Healthcare professionals fear to admit an ADR to a consumer. They usually pretend that the side effect is just another symptom of the disease. Many factors are involved in this refusal to accept ADRs as follows:
  - Lost reputation, which decreases further consultations.
  - Lack of trust in the integrity of the authorities; the hospital or the state authorities punish professionals to avoid agitation from the consumers.
  - Lack of confidentiality; pitfalls in the system result in unauthorized access to patient information.

- Practicing Pv involves the extra expense of lost time in practice and logistics. In the absence of funding, many professionals are discouraged from reporting ADRs.
- Accessibility to ADR reporting forms, lack of training on where and how to report, language barriers in countries with multiple languages, no response from the Pv centers to a report, lack of access to the national ADR database, etc., all decrease reporting.
- The self-medication of consumers, significant presence of traditional systems of medicines with unidentified components in medicines, the availability of prescription-only medicines without prescription, nonadherence, etc. all make it extremely difficult to confirm ADRs (Olsson, Pal, & Dodoo, 2015).

The practice of traditional or alternative systems of medicine is common in most developing countries. It is a common practice in traditional medicine to claim that their medicines are free of ADRs. In a sense, this claim gives professional security to the practitioners so they can interpret any adverse event as being unrelated to the treatment. It is essential to strictly regulate traditional medicines and establish Pv systems that are suitable to mixed practices (Wal, Singh, Mehra, Rizvi, & Vajpayee, 2014).

Many studies of developing countries found a lack of quality medicines, along with ADRs and medication errors, but most of these issues remain underreported in regular practice. In developing countries, along with many deficiencies, Pv is perceived as proof of the flaws in the system. Thus, Pv is feared in developing countries.

A review from Brazil identified gaps in regional disparities in the monitoring and assessment of drug safety. Capacity building is needed for Pv in public health programs. Healthcare policies should be transparent and accountable. There should be an ongoing system to update the policy, law, and regulation (Moscou, Kohler, & MaGahan, 2016).

It is not always the case that healthcare professionals in public health programs have better Pv KAP. Many public health programs are poorly implemented in developing countries. An Ethiopian study assessed professionals at the ART clinics of 9 public hospitals and 27 health centers. Their awareness of the national Pv program was reported to be moderate (Denekew & Adisse, 2014). A survey in the national ART program of South Africa stated satisfactory levels of knowledge and positive attitude toward reporting ADRs, even though only a few ever reported any ADRs (Herbert & Augustyn, 2013). A Nigerian study found that knowledge of the national Pv program was moderate, and nearly one-tenth of healthcare professionals actually report any ADRs (Okechukwu et al., 2013). An Iranian study reported extremely low ADR reporting in a teaching hospital, even though knowledge about the national PV system was moderate. The study mentioned many problems relating to a lack of training and limited accessibility to the PV system (Khalili, Mohebbi, Hendoiee, Keshtkar, & Dashti-Khavidaki, 2012).

The Pv of 46 sub-Saharan African (SSA) countries was studied by SPS in 2011. The capacity for regulating health products in these SSA countries was inadequate. The lack of relevant policy and regulations in the SSA region reflected fundamental limitations for enforcing medicine safety monitoring (Strengthening Pharmaceutical Systems (SPS) Program, 2011).

Interviews of government officials and KAP studies on professionals suggest that Pv practice is inadequate because of (Maigetter, Pollock, Kadam, Ward, & Weiss, 2015) the following:

- Inconvenient systems
- Lack of sufficient funding
- Limited number of trained staff
- Inadequate training programs and
- Unclear roles and poor coordination of activities

RECOMMENDATIONS: THE WAY FORWARD

We are optimistic about the ongoing improvements in Pv KAP in developing countries. The signs of these improvements are increased numbers of related publications and increased participation in the WHO program for international monitoring. The key difference between developed and developing countries is the presence of an efficient healthcare system. Pv is not a stand-alone system. The Pv system is an add-on to the national/institutional healthcare system. The practices of Pv will only improve if it is part of an efficient healthcare system. Knowledge and attitude shall not result in proportional practice if opportunities for practice are not facilitated. Knowledge will not be retained if it is not practiced. A lack of practice degrades the positive attitudes that were developed. Educational interventions will continue in healthcare professional education and in continuing professional development. Many professionals will have good attitudes about Pv but will be afraid of reporting ADRs. Educational interventions could decrease feelings of guilt, and they will aid in improving practice. These interventions will be conducted as follows:

- First, there will be interactive sessions to fill gaps in knowledge because healthcare professionals already have some level of knowledge.
- Second, there will be a focus on motivating professionals to remove incorrect perceptions.
- Third, workshops with hands-on training will be provided to increase practical skills and orient practitioners to reporting locations.

Large numbers of Pv KAP studies are symptoms of a developmental stage. Once Pv systems are well established, KAP studies will lose their relevance as is currently the case in developed countries. Pv is a trend in developing countries, and once it is well established, it will become a culture. Allowing consumer reporting is a sign of encouraging patient-centeredness in healthcare. Increasing patient-centeredness will demand more patient safety practices. The efficient implementation of locally relevant healthcare policies will provide a strong basis for Pv systems. Administrations should mandate and implement the following strategies to improve Pv KAP:

- Facilitate online/post/call modes for reporting ADRs free of charge,
- Conduct campaigns to encourage consumer reporting of side effects,
- Encourage pharmaceutical companies to participate in the Pv system through financial and technological contributions,
- Ensure the services of Pv specialists, such as clinical pharmacists, in all major healthcare institutions,
- Establish minimum performance criteria for public health programs to continue receiving funds,
- Set minimum continuing professional education credits to renew practice licenses,
- Provide professional credit points for good standing/recognition for ADR reporting as a reward for the consultation time lost,
- Secure legal immunity for reporting ADRs, and
- Develop a healthcare system to incorporate Pv programs efficiently.

The Pv KAP among healthcare professionals in developing countries will improve only if the healthcare system is suitable for practicing Pv.

CONCLUSIONS

In summary, healthcare professionals in developing countries were found to have poor to moderate knowledge, positive attitudes, and poor practices of Pv. Their primary gap was in the practice of Pv. The Pv continuing education program is a trend in developing countries. These educational interventions will improve KAPs of Pv. Patient-centeredness could also improve, the need for Pv. Major issues in the capacity building of Pv in developing countries are technological and financial. A strong base for an efficient healthcare system is essential to incorporate successful Pv models.

LESSONS LEARNED

- Healthcare professionals in developing countries have poor to moderate knowledge, positive attitudes, and poor practice of Pv.
- Interventions in professional health education and continuing education could improve Pv KAP, especially the knowledge component.
- Patient-centeredness in practice will require Pv systems for patient safety.
- Capacity building is required for the developing countries to efficiently implement and monitor a healthcare system before adding a Pv system.
- Establishing national Pv systems aligned with the WHO Pv system should harmonize the Pv practices.

REFERENCES

Abidi, A., Ahmad, A., Gupta, S., Rizvi, D., & Sing, S. (2014). Evaluation of knowledge, attitude and practice of pharmacovigilance and adverse drug reaction reporting among the prescribers and nurses in a tertiary care teaching hospital of northern India. *World Journal of Pharmaceutical Research*, *3*(6), 771–786.

Abubakar, A., Ismail, S., Rahman, N., & Haque, M. (2015). Comparative study on drug safety surveillance between medical students of Malaysia and Nigeria. *Therapeutic and Clincial Risk Management*, *11*, 1015–1025.

Abubakar, A. R., Simbak, N. B., & Haque, M. (2014). A systematic review of knowledge, attitude and practice on adverse drug reactions and pharmacovigilance among doctors. *Journal of Applied Pharmaceutical Science*, *4*(10), 117–127. http://doi.org/10.7324/JAPS.2014.40121.

Alshakka, M., Bassalim, H., Alsakkaf, K., Mokhtar, M., Alshagga, M., Al-Dubai, S., … Shanker, P. (2016). Knowledge and perception towards pharmacovigilance among healthcare professionals in tertiary care teaching hospital in Aden, Yemen. *Journal of Pharmacy Practice and Community Medicine*, *2*(1), 21–28.

Bagewadi, H., Rekha, M., & Anandh, J. (2015). A comparative evaluation of different teaching aids among fourth term medical students to improve the knowledge, attitude and perceptions about pharmacovigilance: An experimental study. *International Journal of Pharmacological Research*, *5*(4), 91–97. http://doi.org/10.7439/ijpr.

Bagewadi, H. G., Venkatadri, T. V., & Nayaka, S. R. (2015). Impact of educational intervention on knowledge, attitude, perceptions of pharmacovigilance and adverse drug reactions in fifth term medical students and their feed back. *International Journal of Research in Pharmacology & Pharmacotherapeutics*, *4*(2), 164–174.

Bansode, A. A., Zad, V., Sawa, S., & Dudhal, K. (2015). Awareness about pharmacovigilance among resident doctors in a tertiary care hospital. *Journal of Evolution of Medical and Dental Sciences*, *4*(2), 207–210. http://doi.org/10.14260/jemds/2015/33.

Bhagavathula, A. S., Elnour, A. A., Jamshed, S. Q., & Shehab, A. (2016). Health professionals' knowledge, attitudes and practices about pharmacovigilance in India: A systematic review and meta-analysis. *PLoS One, 11*(3), e0152221. http://doi.org/10.1371/journal.pone.0152221.

Bharadwaj, V., Budania, N., Mondal, A., Yadav, V., & Sharma, P. (2016). A survey to assess the awareness of adverse drug reactions and pharmacovigilance practices among healthcare professionals in a tertiary care hospital. *International Journal of Medical Research Professionals*, *2*(1), 134–137.

Bisht, M., Singh, S., & Dhasmana, D. C. (2014). Effect of educational intervention on adverse drug reporting by physicians: A cross-sectional study. *ISRN Pharmacology, 2014*, ID259476. http://doi.org/10.1155/2014/259476.

Chandrakapure, A., Giri, S., Khan, I., Mateenuddin, M., & Faheem, M. (2015). Pharmacovigilance: A study to evaluate knowledge, attitude, and practices of and impact of educational intervention among doctors in teaching hospital, in rural area of Jalna, India. *International Journal of Basic and Clinical Pharmacology*, *4*(3), 427–431. http://doi.org/10.18203/2319-2003.ijbcp20150008.

CommGAP. (2010). *Theories of behavior change*. World Bank Washington DC: The World Bank. http://doi.org/10.4236/health.2013.53A078.

Deepak, P., & Nagaral, J. V. (2014). Awareness of pharmacovigilance among medical students. *International Journal of Recent Trends in Science and Technology*, *13*(2), 262–265.

Denekew, A., & Adisse, M. (2014). *Knowledge, attitude and practice of adverse drug reaction reporting and affecting factors among health care providers working in ART clinics of public health facilities in Addis Ababa city, Ethiopia.*

Desai, C. K., Iyer, G., Panchal, J., Shah, S., & Dikshit, R. K. (2011). An evaluation of knowledge, attitude, and practice of adverse drug reaction reporting among prescribers at a tertiary care hospital. *Perspectives in Clinical Research*, *2*(4), 129–136. http://doi.org/10.4103/2229-3485.86883.

Ghosh, R., Bhatia, M. S., & Bhattacharya, S. K. (2012). Pharmacovigilance : Masterkey to drug safety monitoring and its status in India. *Delhi Psychiatry Journal*, *15*(2), 412–415.

Gupta, S., Nayak, R., Shivaranjani, R., & Vidyarthi, S. (2015). A questionnaire study on the knowledge, attitude, and the practice of pharmacovigilance among the healthcare professionals in a teaching hospital in South India. *Perspectives in Clinical Research*, *6*(1), 45–52. http://doi.org/10.4103/2229.

Hanafi, S., Torkamandi, H., Hayatshahi, A., Gholami, K., & Javadi, M. (2012). Knowledge, attitudes and practice of nurse regarding adverse drug reaction reporting. *Iranian Journal of Nursing and Midwifery Research*, *17*(1), 21–25. Retrieved from http://www.pubmedcentral.nih.gov/articlerender.fcgi?artid=3590690&tool=pmcentrez&rendertype=abstract.

Hardeep, Bajaj, J. K., & Rakesh, K. (2013). A survey on the knowledge, attitude and the practice of pharmacovigilance among the health care professionals in a teaching hospital in northern India. *Journal of Clinical and Diagnostic Research : JCDR*, *7*(1), 97–99. http://doi.org/10.7860/JCDR/2012/4883.2680.

Hema, N. G., Bhuvana, K. B., & Sangeetha (2012). Pharmacovigilance: The extent of awareness among the final year students, interns and postgraduates in a government teaching hospital. *Journal of Clinical and Diagnostic Research*, *6*(7 Suppl.), 1248–1253.

Herbert, J. W., & Augustyn, J. (2013). *Exploring the knowledge, perceptions and attitudes of the side effects of antiretroviral drugs amongst staff and HIV patients at public healthcare institutions in the Frances Baard District of the Northern Cape South Africa, 2012.*

Isfahani, M. E., Mousavi, S., Rakhshan, A., Assarian, M., Kuti, L., & Eslami, K. (2013). Adverse drug Reactions : Knowledge, attitude and practice of pharmacy students. *Journal of Pharmaceutical Care*, *1*(4), 145–148.

Jha, N., Rathore, D. S., Shankar, P. R., Gyawali, S., & Hassali, M. A. (2015). Strengthening adverse drug reaction reporting in Nepal. *The journal is Asian Journal of Medical Sciences*, *6*(4), 9–13. http://doi.org/10.3126/ajms.v6i4.11659.

Jha, N., Rathore, D. S., Shankar, P. R., Thapa, B. B., Bhuju, G., & Alshakka, M. (2014). Need for involving consumers in Nepal's pharmacovigilance system. *Australasian Medical Journal*, *7*(4), 191–195. http://doi.org/10.4066/AMJ.2014.2011.

Kamal, N. N., Kamel, E. G., & Mahfouz, E. M. (2014). Adverse drug reactions reporting, knowledge, attitude and practice of physicians towards it in El Minia University hospitals. *International Public Health Forum, 1*(4), 13–17.

Kamtane, R. A., & Jayawardhani, V. (2012). Knowledge, attitude and perception of physicians towards adverse drug reaction (ADR) reporting: A pharmacoepidemiological study. *Asian Journal of Pharmaceutical and Clinical Research, 5*(Suppl. 3), 210–214.

Karelia, B. N., & Piparava, K. G. (2014). Knowledge, attitude and practice of pharmacovigilance among private healthcare professionals of Rajkot city. *IJBCP International Journal of Basic & Clinical Pharmacology, 3*(1), 50–53. http://doi.org/10.5455/2319-2003.ijbcp20140202.

Khalili, H., Mohebbi, N., Hendoiee, N., Keshtkar, A.-A., & Dashti-Khavidaki, S. (2012). Improvement of knowledge, attitude and perception of healthcare workers about ADR, a pre- and post-clinical pharmacists' interventional study. *BMJ Open, 2*, e000367. http://doi.org/10.1136/bmjopen-2011-000367.

Kiran, L. J., Shivashankaramurthy, K. G., Bhooma, S., & Kr, D. (2014). Adverse drug reaction reporting among clinicians in a teaching hospital in South Karnataka. *Scholars Journal of Applied Medical Sciences, 2*(1D), 399–403.

Kulkarni, M., Baig, M., Chandaliya, K., Doifode, S., Razvi, S., & Sidhu, N. (2013). Knowledge, attitude and of among of government medical college and hospital, Aurangabad (Maharashtra). *International Journal of Pharmacology and Therapeutics, 3*(3), 10–18.

Maigetter, K., Pollock, A. M., Kadam, A., Ward, K., & Weiss, M. G. (2015). Pharmacovigilance in India, Uganda and South Africa with reference to WHO's minimum requirements. *International Journal of Health Policy and Management, 4*(5), 295–305. http://doi.org/10.15171/ijhpm.2015.55.

Meher, B. R., Joshua, N., Asha, B., & Mukherji, D. (2015). A questionnaire based study to assess knowledge, attitude and practice of pharmacovigilance among undergraduate medical students in a Tertiary Care Teaching Hospital of South India. *Perspectives in Clinical Research, 6*(4), 217–221. http://doi.org/. http://dx.doi.org/10.4103/2229-3485.167102.

Moscou, K., Kohler, J. C., & Lexchin, J. (2013). Drug safety and Corporate governance. *Global Health Governance, VII*(1), 56–79. Retrieved from http://pharmacy.utoronto.ca/sites/default/files/upload/faculty-staff/faculty/kohler/GHGFall2013Issue.pdf.

Moscou, K., Kohler, J. C., & MaGahan, A. (2016). Governance and pharmacovigilance in Brazil: A scoping review. *Journal of Pharmaceutical Policy and Practice, 9*(3), 1–15. http://doi.org/10.1186/s40545-016-0053-y.

Nadendla, S., Gangisetty, S., Goka, P., RamaRao, N., & Nadendla, R. (2015). Assessment of knowledge attitude practice on pharmacovigilance and ADR reporting among medical interns in tertiary care hospital. *European Journal of Biomedical and Pharmaceutical Sciences, 2*(7), 204–209.

Nahar, N., Karim, A., Paul, P., & Khan, T. (2011). Response of reporting adverse drug reactions among medical practitioners. *Bangladesh Medical Journal, 40*(2), 13–18.

Okechukwu, R., Odinduka, S., Ele, G., & Okonta, M. (2013). Awareness, attitude, and practice of pharmacovigilance among health care professionals in Nigeria: Survey in a teaching hospital. *Journal of Clinical and Diagnostic Research, 2*(3), 99–108. http://doi.org/10.7860/JCDR/2012/4883.2680.

Olsson, S., Pal, S. N., & Dodoo, A. (2015). Pharmacovigilance in resource-limited countries. *Expert Review of Clinical Pharmacology, 8*(4), 449–460. http://doi.org/10.1586/17512433.2015.1053391.

Olsson, S., Pal, S. N., Stergachis, A., & Couper, M. (2010). Pharmacovigilance activities in 55 low- and middle-income countries. *Drug Safety, 33*(8), 689–703. http://doi.org/10.2165/11536390-000000000-00000.

Palaian, S., Ibrahim, M. I., & Mishra, P. (2011). Health professionals' knowledge, attitude and practices towards pharmacovigilance in Nepal. *Pharmacy Practice, 9*(4), 228–235. http://doi.org/10.4321/S1886-36552011000400008.

Palanisamy, S., Kumaran, K., & Rajasekaran, A. (2013). A study on assessment of knowledge about adverse drug reactions. *Der Pharmacia Lettre, 5*(1), 41–52. Retrieved from http://scholarsresearchlibrary.com/dpl-vol5-iss1/DPL-2013-5-1-41-52.pdf.

Parthiban, G., Nileshraj, G., Mangaiarkkarasi, A., & Meher, A. (2015). A study on knowledge, attitude and awareness among medical students in a teaching hosptial, Puducherry. *Indian Journal of Basic and Applied Medical Research*, *5*(1), 198–203. http://doi.org/10.18410/jebmh/2015/1006.

Pimpalkhute, S. A., Jaiswal, K. M., Sontakke, S. D., Bajait, C. S., & Gaikwad, A. (2012). Evaluation of awareness about pharmacovigilance and adverse drug reaction monitoring in resident doctors of a tertiary care teaching hospital. *Indian Journal of Medical Sciences*, *66*(3–4), 55–61. http://doi.org/10.4103/0019-5359.110902.

Ponmari, S. J., Sivaraman, M., Aruna, T., Subashree, V., & Jawahar, S. (2015). Knowledge and awareness of pharmacovigilance among various medical fraternities. *Asian Journal of Pharmacology and Toxicology*, *3*(10), 45–48.

Rathod, K., & Panchal, A. (2014). Knowledge, attitude and practice of community pharmacists of Gujarat towards adverse drug reactions. *International Archives of Integrated Medicine*, *1*(1), 18–25.

Reddy, P., Varma, S. K., & Reddy, S. (2014). Knowledge, attitude and practice of ADR reporting among clinical residents: A rural medical college survey. *Journal of Drug Discovery and Therapeutics*, *2*(14), 8–13.

Rishi, R. K., Patel, R. K., & Bhandari, A. (2012). Opinion of physicians towards adverse drug reactions reporting results of pilot study. *Journal of Community Nutrition & Health*, *1*(1), 25–29.

Saad, A., Rostom, H., Bawaresh, N., Alharbi, A., Alharf, A., Aljasser, N., … Braiki, F. (2014). *Guideline on good pharmacovigilance practices (GVP) for Arab Countries*. The League of Arab State. Retrieved from http://www.jfda.jo/Download/JPC/TheGoodPharmacovigilancePracticev2.pdf.

Shakeel, S., Iffat, W., Anjum, F., Bushra, R., Ibrahim, S., & Shafiq, S. (2014). Emerging need of Pharmacovigilance : Perspectives of future pharmacist in Pakistan. *International Journal of Pharmacy Teaching & Practices*, *5*(2), 966–971.

Shimwela, G. (2011). *Adverse drug reaction reporting* (Knowledge, Attitude and Practices of Community Pharmacy Dispensers in Dar Es Salaam, Tanzania).

Siddeshwara, M., Santoshkumar, J., & Vardhamane, S. (2016). Knowledge, attitude and practice of adverse drug reactions reporting among healthcare professionals. *International Journal of Pharmacological Research*, *6*(1), 18–22. http://doi.org/10.7439/ijpr.

Sivadasan, S., & Sellappan, M. (2015). A study on the awareness and attitude towards pharmacovigilance and adverse drug reaction reporting among nursing students in a private university, Malaysia. *International Journal of Current Pharmaceutical Research*, *7*(1), 84–89.

SPS. Strengthening Pharmaceutical Systems, & USAID. (December 2009). *Indicator-Based pharmacovigilance assessment tool : Manual for conducting assessments in developing countries*, 126.

Strengthening Pharmaceutical Systems Program, & USAID. (2009). *Supporting pharmacovigilance in developing countries the systems perspective*. Retrieved from http://apps.who.int/medicinedocs/en/d/Js18813en/.

Strengthening Pharmaceutical Systems (SPS) Program. (2011). *Safety of medicines in Sub-Saharan Africa* Assessment of Pharmacovigilance Systems and their Performance. Retrieved from http://apps.who.int/medicinedocs/en/d/Js19152en/.

Suyagh, M., Farah, D., & Farha, A. (2014). Pharmacist's knowledge, practice and attitudes toward pharmacovigilance and adverse drug reactions reporting process. *Saudi Pharmaceutical Journal*, *23*, 147–153. http://doi.org/10.1016/j.jsps.2014.07.001.

Torwane, N. A., Hongal, S., Gouraha, A., Saxena, E., & Chavan, K. (2015). Awareness related to reporting of adverse drug reactions among health caregivers : A cross-sectional questionnaire survey. *The Journal of National Accreditation Board for Hospitals & Healthcare Providers*, *2*(1), 23–29.

UMC. n.d.-a. Take & Tell. Uppsala Monitoring Center. Retrieved from http://www.takeandtell.org/.

UMC. n.d.-b. VigiBase. Uppsala Monitoring Center. Retrieved from http://www.who-umc.org/DynPage.aspx?id=98082&mn1=7347&mn2=7252&mn3=7322&mn4=7326.

UMC. (2016a). *Guideline for using VigiBase data in studies*. Uppsala Monitoring Center. Retrieved from http://www.who-umc.org/graphics/28461.pdf.

UMC. (2016b). *WHO Programme members*. Uppsala Monitoring Center. Retrieved from http://www.who-umc.org/DynPage.aspx?id=100653&mn1=7347&mn2=7252&mn3=7322&mn4=7442.

UNICEF, & ILO. (2011). *Knowledge, attitudes, practices and expectations (KAPE) study on child labor in Bangladesh*. Bangladesh: UNICEF. Retrieved from https://www.unicef.org/bangladesh/KAPE_Study_on_Child_Labor.pdf.

Vora, M. B., & Barvaliya, M. (2014). Knowledge, attitude and practices towards pharmacovigilance and adverse drug reactions in health care professional of tertiary care hospital, Bhavnagar. *International Journal of Pharma Sciences and Research*, *5*(11), 820–826.

Vora, M., Paliwal, N., Doshi, V., Barvaliya, M., & Tripathi, C. (2012). Knowledge of adverse drug reactions and pharmacovigilance activity among the undergraduate medical students of Gujarat. *International Journal of Pharmaceutical Sciences and Research*, *3*(5), 1511–1515.

Wal, P., Singh, A., Mehra, R., Rizvi, S., & Vajpayee, R. (2014). Pharmacovigilance : Need and future prospective in herbal and ayurvedic medicines. *The Pharma Innovation Journal*, *3*(7), 18–22.

Wilson, V., & Amma, V. (2015). Prospects of consumer-initiated adverse drug reaction reporting in cardiovascular pharmacovigilance. *Journal of the Practice of Cardiovascular Sciences*, *1*(1), 54–57. http://doi.org/10.4103/2395-5414.157570.

SECTION

5

GENERIC MEDICINES USE IN LOW- AND MIDDLE-INCOME COUNTRIES

CHAPTER

12

OVERCOMING CHALLENGES OF GENERIC MEDICINES UTILIZATION IN LOW- AND MIDDLE-INCOME COUNTRIES: LESSONS LEARNED FROM INTERNATIONAL EXPERIENCES

Mohamed Azmi Hassali[1], **Zhi Yen Wong**[2]

[1]*Universiti Sains Malaysia, Minden, Malaysia;* [2]*Hospital Teluk Intan, Teluk Intan, Malaysia*

CHAPTER OUTLINE

INTRODUCTION

Generic medicines are those products produced by manufacturer other than an innovator company after the original patent has expired. Nevertheless, the definition of generic medicines may vary between countries and organizations. For example, the United States Food and Drug Administration (USFDA) defines generic medicine as a drug product that is identical/bioequivalent to brand-/reference-listed drug product in dosage form, strength, route of administration, quality, and performance characteristics, and intended use (U.S. Food and Drug Administration, 2012b), whereas the World Health Organization (WHO) defines generic medicines as pharmaceutical products, usually intended to be interchangeable with the innovator product, that is manufactured without license from innovator

Social and Administrative Aspects of Pharmacy in Low- and Middle-Income Countries. http://dx.doi.org/10.1016/B978-0-12-811228-1.00012-1

company and marketed after the expiry of patent or other exclusivity rights (World Health Organization, 2012a). The European Medicines Agency (EMA) defines generic medicine as a medicine that is developed to be the same as a medicine that has already been authorized (the "reference medicine") (European Medicines Agency, 2011). A generic medicine contains the same active substance(s) as the reference medicine, and it is used at the same dose(s) to treat the same disease(s) as the reference medicine. However, the name of the medicine, its appearance (such as color or shape), and its packaging can be different from those of the reference medicine (European Medicines Agency, 2011).

Despite the differences in definitions of generic medicines, one fundamental principle underpinning the safe and effective use of generic medicine is the concept of bioequivalence. Generic products are considered to be bioequivalent only if their rate and extent of absorption do not show a significant difference from the reference product (Hassali, Wong, et al., 2014; King & Kanavos, 2002). As per FDA, the regulatory limits applied in many countries are that 90% confidence intervals for the ratios (generic product: brand innovator product) of the areas under the plasma drug concentration versus time curves and the maximum plasma drug concentrations must fall between 80% and 125%, which is also known as the "−20%/+25% rule" (Center for Drug Evaluation and Research Food and Drug Administration, 2003). Based on this standard, the maximum allowable variation in bioavailability for two different products can only be ±10% (McLachlan, Pearce, & Ramzan, 2004). However, in real practice, studies showed that the mean differences in bioavailability between the brand innovator and generic equivalents approved under this standard rarely differ by more than 5% (Nightingale & Morrison, 1987).

ROLE OF GENERIC MEDICINES IN LMICS HEALTHCARE SYSTEM

The major challenge faced by many healthcare providers and policy makers in the world is the ever escalating healthcare costs (Borger et al., 2006; Steinwachs, 2002). Within this context, the cost of pharmaceuticals constitutes the second largest cost in healthcare provision after the staffing costs (Marchildon & DiMatteo, 2011). Rise in disease prevalence, an increase in population risk factors, changes in clinical thresholds for treatment, and the emergence of new medical treatments has contributed to the escalating pharmaceutical expenditure (Thorpe, 2005, 2006). Together with financial and economic crisis, policy makers face challenges to ensure access to affordable medicines with limited healthcare budgets and competing demands for scarce resources.

In developing countries, the government faces considerable challenges in financing healthcare for their populations as pharmaceuticals account for 20%–60% of healthcare expenditure as compared to 18% in Organisation for Economic Co-operation and Development (OECD) countries (Cameron, Ewen, Ross-Degnan, Ball, & Laing, 2008). To worsen the condition, most of the population in developing countries purchases medicines through out-of-pocket money (Cameron et al., 2008; World Health Organization, 2004b). As a result, medicines are unaffordable for majority of this population. In fact, more than 2 billion people in low- and middle-income countries (LMICs) lack adequate access to essential medicines (Leisinger, Garabedian, & Wagner, 2012; World Health Organization, 2004a).

In this challenging scenario of healthcare provision, greater use of generic medicine was encouraged as it was one of the effective mechanisms to curb the escalating healthcare cost, especially pharmaceutical expenditure (Haas, Phillips, Gerstenberger, & Seger, 2005; Kanavos, 2007; Karim, Pillai, Ziqubu-Page, Cassimjee, & Morar, 1996; King & Kanavos, 2002). In fact, generic medicines are 20–80% cheaper than brand innovator products (Dylst, Vulto, Godman, & Simoens, 2013; Simoens &

Coster, 2006; Vogler, 2012). In low-income countries (LICs), the price difference between innovator medicines and their branded or unbranded generic equivalents can be huge. The review of the WHO/HAI pricing studies reported that the "percentage difference in price between originator brands and lowest-priced generics (brand premium) in the private sector was over 300% in lower-middle-income countries and low-income countries, whereas in upper-middle-income countries it was substantially lower (152%), and in India it was only 6%" (World Health Organization, 2011).

Generic medicine is cheaper because generic manufacturers bypass the expenses and time required to demonstrate the drug's efficacy and safety through extensive clinical trials which is usually used in the development of the brand innovator drugs (Stoppler, 2009; U.S. Food and Drug Administration, 2012a). Besides, generic medicines are cheaper as the generic manufacturers do not pay for the expensive marketing and advertising (Stoppler, 2009; U.S. Food and Drug Administration, 2012a). Moreover, that price competition from multiple generic companies will eventually results the price to go lower (Stoppler, 2009; U.S. Food and Drug Administration, 2012a).

Money saved by using generic medicines could be used to finance the procurement of newer, more effective medications required to treat diseases that currently lack of adequate pharmaceutical treatment (Ess, Schneeweiss, & Szucs, 2003; King & Kanavos, 2002; McGavock, 1997, 2001). In addition, the extra budget saved by encouraging greater use of generic medicines can be used by policy makers or government to finance the research and development and reimbursement of newer, expensive innovative medicines (Simoens & Coster, 2006). Besides, competition forces from the entry of generic medicines will encourage the development of innovative medicines and price reduction for the off-patent original drugs by originator companies (Dylst, Vulto, Godman et al., 2013). Previous literature has reported that entry of one additional generic medicine lower the price of innovator medicines by an average of 4–7% (Bergman & Rudholm, 2003; Dylst & Simoens, 2010). Moreover, another benefit of generic medicines besides cost containment is promoting patient adherence to the medications (Kesselheim, Fischer, & Avorn, 2006; Kesselheim et al., 2010).

ACHIEVEMENTS

Previous literature reported that the total generic medicines market share in some LMICs was greater than that of many European countries (Dylst & Simoens, 2010; Kaplan, Wirtz, & Stephens, 2013). In 2001, generic medicines (i.e., branded generic and unbranded generic) constitute between 70% and 80% of the volume market share in the private sector of the studied LMICs, which was greater than that of most European countries (Dylst & Simoens, 2010; Kaplan et al., 2013).

This might be due to the existence of some pro-generic policies and strategies in LMICs that address prescribing and dispensing practices such as financial incentive to encourage generic dispensing, generic prescribing (Cameron, Mantel-Teeuwisse, Leufkens, & Laing, 2012; Kaplan, Ritz, Vitello, & Wirtz, 2012). There are also examples of regressive markup schemes from countries such as Iran, Lebanon, Syria, South Africa, and Tunisia (Cameron et al., 2012).

In addition, national generic substitution policies are in place in many LMICs (e.g., Argentina, Bolivia, Chile, Colombia, Ecuador, Jamaica, Mexico, Peru, South Africa, and Uruguay) (Faden, Vialle-Valentin, Ross-Degnan, & Wagner, 2011; Gossell-Williams, 2007; Homedes & Ugalde, 2005). In fact, a WHO survey in 2007 found that generic substitution was allowed in 75% of LMICs (Cameron et al., 2012; World Health Organization, 2009).

Moreover, LMICs play an important role in manufacturing generic medicines, especially in the case of China and India. Of the 312 medicines on the WHO List of prequalified medicines at the end of 2012, 231 (74%) were generic, of which 200 (87%) were manufactured in India (World Health Organization, 2012b). This might be due to lower production costs in India and China (Bumpas & Betsch, 2009). For example, developing, testing, manufacturing, and marketing a generic medicine in India generally costs 20–40% of what it costs in the Western countries (Bumpas & Betsch, 2009). In addition, lower labor, infrastructure, transportation and equipment costs, fewer environmental regulations, larger manufacturing scale, lower market entry barriers have caused the manufacturing of active pharmaceutical ingredient slowly been shifting from the historical leaders in Western countries to manufacturers in India and China (Bumpas & Betsch, 2009).

CHALLENGES

SUPPLY-SIDE CHALLENGES

Given few achievements of LMICs in encouraging the generic medicine uses, there are few challenges to be overcome to further encourage greater uptake of generic medicines in the health systems. One of the barriers is the intellectual property/access to medicines narrative, with complex issues involving the link between multinational pharmaceutical company patents and delay of generic medicine approvals (Kaplan & Wirtz, 2014). Weak patent examination and granting procedures that allow the patenting of noninventive aspects is common in LMICs (Kaplan et al., 2012). Intellectual property protection serves to encourage innovation and to aid the dissemination of knowledge (Simoens, 2013). However, it may also inhibit market access of generic medicines in some cases. Previous studies reported that innovator companies used patent clustering (acquisition of multiple patents surrounding the basic patents of the drug products) and follow-on patenting (otherwise called patent "ever-greening" or "secondary patents") to deter the entry of generic medicines (Fatokun, Ibrahim, & Hassali, 2013). However, in a study conducted in 2004 to investigate the relationship between patents and access to essential medicines reported that in 65 studied LMICs, overall patent incidence is low (1.4%) and concentrated in larger markets (Attaran, 2004). Thus, there are no patent barriers to accessing generic essential medicines. This might be due to the lack of pharmaceutical patenting laws or a functioning patent office in LMICs. An inventor's initiative to patent (for medicines or otherwise) is greatest where there are more consumers having more disposable income. Previous study reported that patent laws are only used more frequently in developing countries having larger populations, richer per capita national income (Attaran, 2004).

Another common barrier to generic medicines in LMICs is delay of generic medicine approvals. There are many factors responsible for the lengthy approval. For example, redundancy across steps since there was no leveraging of the technical reviews already performed by competent bodies, inefficiencies in the regulatory processes themselves, failure of manufacturers to meet the international standards required and capability challenges, lack of qualified staff, and few available resources lead to increased complexity and long product approval timelines (Ahonkhai, Martins, Portet, Lumpkin, & Hartman, 2016; World Health Organization, 2010).

Moreover, large multinational manufacturers usually did not prioritize early registration of generic medicines and introduction of their products into LICs due to low commercial potential in LMICs. In addition, unlike high-income countries (HICs), varying legal requirements in LMICs limit the ability of manufacturers to submit a single dossier concurrently to those countries (Ahonkhai et al., 2016). In HICs, the regulation of pharmaceutical products is relatively uniform. For example, the International Conference on Harmonisation of Technical Requirements for Registration of Pharmaceuticals for Human Use (ICH) is usually followed by HICs. ICH is a collaboration initiated in 1990 between the US, EU, and Japan aimed at adhering to a uniform set of scientific and technical standards (Ahonkhai et al., 2016). As a result, low commercial potential and the enormous resources required to prepare unique submissions for each country and response to questions from each individual national regulatory authorities (NRA) may cause further delay of registration of generic medicines (Ahonkhai et al., 2016). Furthermore, generic medicines distributed in HICs were missing important clinical data relevant to the target LMIC population. A recent study of generic product dossiers submitted to WHO prequalification found that most contained significant deficiencies, either in safety or quality data (Ahonkhai et al., 2016; World Health Organization, 2010).

Even though the total generic medicines market share in some LMICs was greater than that of many European countries (Dylst & Simoens, 2010; Kaplan et al., 2013), the branded generic medicine market share is much higher than unbranded generics in private sector of many LMICs, as compared to HICs. This scenario was most notably in countries in the region of Middle East plus South Africa and Asia (Kaplan et al., 2013). Branded generics are generic medicines that are sold under a brand/trade name instead of the nonproprietary name (for example: Uphamol as a trade name instead of paracetamol, the nonproprietary name) (Kaplan & Wirtz, 2014). Even though, there is little information on the price differences between unbranded generic medicines and branded generic medicines, previous study conducted by WHO and Health Action International had reported that branded generics can be priced at the same price as the innovator medicines or more expensive than international nonproprietary name (INN) generics (Kaplan & Wirtz, 2014; World Health Organization, 2011).

In terms of manufacturing generic medicines, besides the case of China and India, previous literature reported that there were a limited number of companies that are capable of manufacturing high-quality generic medicine and can provide a complete registration dossier for use outside their home markets (Hall et al., 2007).

In many LMICs, governments try to control prices for the benefit of consumers who pay out of pocket by setting the maximum retail prices as in South Africa and China (Gray, 2009; Nguyen, Knight, Roughead, Brooks, & Mant, 2015). This mechanism actually serves as a barrier for further price competition as there were no additional price reductions beyond those imposed by the regulation (Dylst & Simoens, 2010). Other LMICs may vary in the degree of pharmaceutical price control or price regulation. Some counties practice "free market" principles where medicine prices are not subject to regulations. Examples of these countries are Indonesia, Malaysia, and Ukraine (Cameron et al., 2012), while in countries such as Jordan, Lebanon, and Morocco, prices are regulated using a variety of methods (Cameron et al., 2012). In South Africa, price controls are applied to medicine at different stages in the supply chain (Cameron et al., 2012), while in Pakistan only selected medicines are subject to price controls (Cameron et al., 2012).

DEMAND-SIDE CHALLENGES

Generics substitution is an act of switching from an innovator medicine to an equivalent generic medicine (Alrasheedy, Hassali, Aljadhey, Ibrahim, & Al-Tamimi, 2013; Hassali, Thambyappa, Saleem, Haq, & Aljadhey, 2012; Hassali & Wong, 2015). In many European countries, generics substitution has been implemented to improve the utilization of generics (Dylst, Vulto, & Simoens, 2013). However, the implementation of the generic substitution differs from country to country (Dylst, Vulto et al., 2013). It can be mandatory in some countries (e.g., Finland, France, Germany, Norway, Spain, and Sweden), prohibited in some countries (e.g., primary care in the United Kingdom), and only indicative/voluntary in the other countries (e.g., Czech Republic, Denmark, Hungary, Italy, Latvia, the Netherlands, Poland, Japan, and Portugal) (Dylst, Vulto et al., 2013). Literature reported that medicine price reduction of 10–15% can be achieved via mandatory generics substitution as seen in Sweden and Finland (Dylst, Vulto et al., 2013). Even though previous study reported that generic substitution was allowed in 75% of LMICs (Cameron et al., 2012; World Health Organization, 2009), effective implementation in resource-constrained settings is likely to be challenging. Besides, there are still some LMICs (e.g., Malaysia, Thailand, Vietnam) that do not have a generics policy or have not positioned their generics policy as an integral part of their medicines policy (Nguyen, Hassali, & McLachlan, 2013). In addition, lack of clarity in legal regulations might prevent effective generics substitution (Kaplan et al., 2012). For example, Malaysia had formulated a generics substitution policy as part of its National Medicines Policy in 2007. However, to date, there is still a lack of implementation and enforcement through legislation (Wong et al., 2014).

Another barrier is lack of generic substitution opportunities at the community pharmacies due to weak separation of prescribing and dispensing in LMICs. At present, in some LMICs, dispensing of prescription medicines still follows a traditional "dispensing doctors" system in which medical practitioners still dispense medicines as a part of their professional practice. By separating the prescribing and dispensing of medicines, it is believed that the process will also reduce the overuse and misuse of medicines, improve the quality of the consumption of prescription drugs, and enhance the patients' right to know about medications (Saleem & Hassali, 2016). The efforts of separation roles between two professions remained unsuccessful due to strong opposition and criticism from physicians, who make a large percentage of their earnings from the sale of medicines (Saleem & Hassali, 2016). Therefore, prescribing behavior of dispensing physicians is strongly influenced by the "price–gap profit," which prefers to dispense innovator medicines that are more profitable (Iizuka & Kubo, 2011).

Facilitating the dispensing of generic medicines by pharmacists can only work if their remuneration system is adjusted so that the dispensing of generic medicines is financially neutral or attractive compared with the dispensing of innovator medicines (Dylst, Vulto et al., 2013). Experience from Italy and Spain reported that percentage per prescription remuneration system is not suitable as it is financially more attractive for pharmacists to dispense a more expensive originator medicine than a less expensive generic medicine (Dylst, Vulto et al., 2013; Simoens, 2013). In other words, pharmacists are being penalized for dispensing generic medicines. As with other HICs, the existence of pro-generic policies in LMICs is a positive step toward promoting generic medicine use. However, in a number of LMICs, practising such policy tools is limited. Previous literature reported that financial incentives for private pharmacies to encourage generic dispensing was practiced only in 30% and 27% of low- and middle-income countries, respectively, and mandatory generic prescribing in the private sector was only in 22% and 28% of low- and middle-income countries, respectively (Cameron et al., 2012).

Moreover, there is still a significant proportion of doctors, pharmacists, and lay people hold negative perceptions of generic medicines (Colgan et al., 2015), and the situation is worse in less mature healthcare system (Toverud, Hartmann, & Håkonsen, 2015). In LMICs, generics were usually being viewed to have a lower or uncertain efficacy and as being inferior in quality on the basis of negative experiences, attitudes, and perceptions (Chua, Hassali, Shafie, & Awaisu, 2010; Fabiano et al., 2012; Gossell-Williams, 2007; Hassali, Wong, et al., 2014; Jamshed, Hassali, Ibrahim, & Babar, 2011; Paraponaris et al., 2004; Shrank et al., 2011; Theodorou et al., 2009; Toverud et al., 2015; Tsiantou, Zavras, Kousoulakou, Geitona, & Kyriopoulos, 2009). Bioequivalence forms the basis of generics substitution (Alrasheedy et al., 2013; Hassali & Wong, 2015). In fact, concerns about bioequivalence and interchangeability of generics were the main factors affecting healthcare stakeholders', i.e., physicians, pharmacists, and patients, attitudes toward generics substitution (Dylst, Vulto et al., 2013). In addition, both physicians and pharmacists in LMICs were highly concerned about the manufacturing sources of generic drugs and the companies' trustworthiness (Babar & Awaisu, 2008; Chong, Hassali, Bahari, & Shafie, 2011; Chua et al., 2010; Gill, Helkkula, Cobelli, & White, 2010; Grover et al., 2011; Toverud et al., 2015).

Moreover, concern should be placed on substandard and counterfeit medicines especially in countries that lack stringent regulation as it can decrease prescribers' and patients' confidence in generics as a whole (Cameron et al., 2012).

RECOMMENDATIONS: THE WAY FORWARD

SUPPLY-SIDE RECOMMENDATIONS

As in HICs, NRAs in LMICs have responsibility to make sure the safety, efficacy, and quality of medicines delivered to their populations, and this lead to requirement of local registration of medicines (Ahonkhai et al., 2016). However, the mandatory individual review by multiple countries, each with its own regulatory authority, processes leads to increased complexity and delay of generic medicine approvals (Ahonkhai et al., 2016). NRAs often repeated assessments of quality, safety, and efficacy already performed by other NRAs, such as dossier review, product sample testing, and manufacturing site inspections (Ahonkhai et al., 2016). Redundant assessments should be a great concern as LMICs usually have the greatest burden of disease and also have the most resource limited NRAs. Lesson can be learned from the European Union where authorization of generic medicines can be done through Mutual Recognition Procedure (MRP) (Dunne, Shannon, Dunne, & Cullen, 2013). The MRP is based on the principle of mutual recognition, by EU member states, of their respective national marketing authorizations. Any national marketing authorization granted by an EU member state's national authority can be used to support an application for its mutual recognition by other member states (Dunne et al., 2013). This approach allows appropriate reliance on what is already known about a drug, thereby saving time and resources and avoiding unnecessary evaluation of data that have already been considered in the marketing authorization procedure in other member's national authority. Such dependence on the work products of trusted counterpart NRAs to inform one's own regulatory decision making is already being implemented by few regulatory authorities (Ahonkhai et al., 2016). For example, the various GMP reliance programs by countries, which are members of Pharmaceutical Inspection Cooperation Scheme (PIC/S) (Ahonkhai et al., 2016). Cooperative activities such as these should be further expanded to LMICs. Examples of potential LMIC trading and regulatory partners are ASEAN and COMESA.

In addition, with MRP, development of uniform standards among neighboring countries with closely tied economic interests provides one promising solution (Ahonkhai et al., 2016). The continent's regulatory systems can be improved by moving from a country-focused approach to simplified approaches through regional collaboration and harmonization of regulatory standards as seen in HICs (Ahonkhai et al., 2016). As a result, this reduces the cost and effort of generic pharmaceutical companies in preparing submission for each individual NRA as generic pharmaceutical companies can only submit a single dossier concurrently to LMICs who have MRP.

Moreover, large multinational manufacturers should place adequate emphasis on early registration of generic medicines and introduction of their products into LICs as LMICs are becoming an increasingly important market given that pharmaceutical expenditures increase faster in LMICs than in HICs (Nguyen et al., 2015; World Health Organization, 2011).

Besides, the LMICs can work in collaboration with international bodies before granting/extending patent to the innovator companies. Moreover, policies that could improve the availability of generics such as "Bolar" provisions, fast-track approval of generics, reduced fees for market authorization applications of generic medicines (Kaplan & Laing, 2003; Kaplan et al., 2012) should be encouraged. In the United States, the Drug Price Competition and Patent Term Restoration Act 1984 (i.e., the Hatch–Waxman Act) speeds the availability of generics by protecting the first generic by a market exclusivity period of 6 months (Kaplan et al., 2012). However, there is lack of such pro-generic supply-side policy in LMICs.

In terms of medicine price, one potential way forward for LMICs to consider is implementing reference pricing. A reference pricing system sets a common reimbursement price (the reference price) for a group of interchangeable medicines (the reference group) (Simoens, 2013). Reference groups can be defined by active substance, pharmacological class, therapeutic class, or a combination of these (Simoens, 2013). Definition of reference group is important as reallocation of demand may occur if reference group is defined by active substance. Physicians may shift their prescribing patterns away from generic medicines in the reference pricing system toward innovator medicines with a similar therapeutic indication outside the reference pricing system (Simoens & Coster, 2006). Examples can be seen for some active substances in Italy, the Netherlands, and Spain (Dylst, Vulto, & Simoens, 2011; Simoens, 2013). The introduction of substitution/interchangeable lists and therapeutic guidelines may reduce such prescription shift. Such changing prescribing practice does not occur when reference groups are defined by therapeutic class (Simoens, 2013).

Reference pricing is important to stimulate the demand for generic medicines because patients have to pay an additional copayment if they consumed innovator medicines, which are usually priced above the level of the reference price (Wong, Alrasheedy, Hassali, & Saleem, 2016). Establishment of the appropriate reference price is important. For example, establishing the reference price at the level of the most expensive generic medicines as seen in Portugal should be avoided (Barros, Machado, & Simões, 2011; Simoens, 2009) to avoid generic companies to set the medicine prices around the maximum level that is allowed (Simoens, 2009). As a result, it does not stimulate price competition among companies and reduce the medicines prices below the level of the reference price (Simoens, 2009). In Europe, reference price usually set at the level of the lowest priced medicine (e.g., Bulgaria, Czech Republic, Finland, Hungary, Italy, Latvia, Poland, Spain, and Turkey) or the lowest priced generic medicine (e.g., Austria, Bulgaria, France, and Latvia) (Simoens, 2013). Such an approach may help to promote price competition between companies if there are sufficient incentives to support generic medicine use. Nevertheless, caution should be taken to prevent fierce competition as too low generic medicine prices may remove the incentive for entry of generic manufacturers to the market (Malkawi, 2009).

DEMAND-SIDE RECOMMENDATIONS

There is a need to have clear generic substitution policy to allow pharmacist to perform generic substitution. The generic substitution reinforced with financial incentives for pharmacist to dispense generic medicines can be a good alternative to further increase utilization of generic medicines.

This is important especially in the case of LMICs, where physicians and pharmacists who benefit from the sale of higher-cost medicines (e.g., when margins are set as a percentage of the price) may also encourage the perception that "low price = low quality" where generics are perceived to be less effective and/or unsafe than innovator medicines (Cameron et al., 2012). One way to reduce resistance from prescribers and "compensate" their loss is by introducing financial incentives to stimulate the prescribing of generic medicines by physicians (Dylst, Vulto et al., 2013). As an example, prescription fee increment was introduced in 2002 in Japan where an additional 20 yen was given to both physicians for writing a prescription containing a generic drug and to pharmacist for filling such a prescription (Jakovljevic, Nakazono, & Ogura, 2014a). In France, the government has introduced the CAPI scheme. This is a voluntary pay for performance scheme, whereby physicians received additional payment for increasing their prescribing of generic medicines versus innovator medicines and achieving certain targets for specific drug classes (e.g., antibiotics, proton-pump inhibitors, statins, antihypertensive drugs, and antidepressants) (Dylst, Vulto et al., 2013).

In addition, fee for performance payment system (as compared to when margins are set as a percentage of the price) is more suitable where pharmacists are rewarded dependent on the level of service (Dylst, Vulto et al., 2013). This fee for performance payment encourages generic substitution or generic dispensing as the pharmacists' decision is not affected by price of medicines dispensed. Examples of countries using the fee for performance system are the Netherlands, Slovenia, and the UK (Dylst, Vulto et al., 2013).

A functioning and reliable medicines regulatory authority is important in ensuring the quality of generics (Kaplan et al., 2012). Formulation or implementation of generics medicines policy in LMICs will be difficult unless stakeholders believe generic medicines are quality medicines (Kaplan et al., 2012). Therefore, communication between medicines regulatory authorities in LMICs and healthcare professionals and medicine consumers is important to increase awareness of generics regulatory approval requirements and improve confidence in generics (Hassali, Alrasheedy et al., 2014). In addition, generic manufacturers in LMICs can play an active role in providing information about generic medicines. As an example, generic companies in Japan publish detailed drug monographs of the generic products at their own websites. In addition, a "Generic Drug Information Provision System" was initiated at the website of the Japan Society of Generic Medicines to provide the most up-to-date detailed information on generic medicines to healthcare professionals on demand (Jakovljevic, Nakazono, & Ogura, 2014b; Wong et al., 2016).

Moreover, evidenced-based guidelines could be useful to assist healthcare professionals to appropriately perform generics substitution. Examples of such guidelines are the Orange Book in the United States, the British National Formulary (BNF) in the UK, the Schedule of Pharmaceutical Benefits in Australia, and the list of interchangeable medicines in Finland and Sweden (Hassali, Alrasheedy et al., 2014).

CONCLUSIONS

This chapter has drawn attention to achievements and challenges to generic medicine utilization in LMICs. In light of international experience, there does not seem to be a single approach toward developing generic medicine policy in LMICs. To boost the generic utilization in LMICs health system, there is a need to have a coherent generic medicine policy addressing both supply- and demand-side measures. In fact, the experience from Europe indicates that a country needs to implement a coherent generic medicines policy that consists of both supply and demand policies to develop its generic medicines market (Simoens, 2010).

LESSONS LEARNED

- Greater use of generic medicine should be encouraged to ensure sustainability of healthcare system in LMICs as pharmaceuticals in these countries account for 20%–60% of healthcare expenditure.
- Supply-side challenges in LMICs include (1) intellectual property/access to medicines narrative, with complex issues involving the link between multinational pharmaceutical company patents and delay of generic medicine approvals, (2) weak patent examination and granting procedures that allow the patenting of noninventive aspects, (3) lack of clarity in the legal regulation of substitution can inhibit efficient substitution, and (4) price regulation that sets maximum retail price.
- Demand-side challenges in LMICs include (1) lack of clarity in the legal regulation of substitution can inhibit efficient substitution, (2) rules permitting physicians to dispense medicines can result in lower utilization rate of generic medicines, (3) low markups for the dispensing of generic medicines create incentives not to prescribe generics, (4) concerns about quality, safety, and efficacy of generic medicines among healthcare stakeholders.
- To boost the generic utilization in LMICs health system, there is a need to have a coherent generic medicine policy addressing both supply- and demand-side measures.

REFERENCES

Ahonkhai, V., Martins, S. F., Portet, A., Lumpkin, M., & Hartman, D. (2016). Speeding access to vaccines and medicines in low-and middle-income countries: A case for change and a framework for optimized product market authorization. *PLoS One*, *11*(11), e0166515.

Alrasheedy, A. A., Hassali, M. A., Aljadhey, H., Ibrahim, M. I. M., & Al-Tamimi, S. K. (2013). Is there a need for a formulary of clinically interchangeable medicines to guide generic substitution in Saudi Arabia? *Journal of Young Pharmacists*, *5*(2), 73–75.

Attaran, A. (2004). How do patents and economic policies affect access to essential medicines in developing countries? *Health Affairs*, *23*(3), 155–166.

Babar, Z. U. D., & Awaisu, A. (2008). Evaluating community pharmacists' perceptions and practices on generic medicines: A pilot study from peninsular Malaysia. *Journal of Generic Medicines*, *5*(4), 315–330.

Barros, P. P., Machado, S. R., & Simões, J. A. (2011). Portugal health system review. *Health Systems in Transition*, *13*(4), 1–156.

Bergman, M. A., & Rudholm, N. (2003). The relative importance of actual and potential competition: Empirical evidence from the pharmaceuticals market. *Journal of Industrial Economics*, *51*(4), 455–467.

Borger, C., Smith, S., Truffer, C., Keehan, S., Sisko, A., Poisal, J., & Clemens, M. K. (2006). Health spending projections through 2015: Changes on the horizon. *Health Affairs*, *25*(2), w61–w73.

Bumpas, J., & Betsch, E. (2009). *Health, Nutrition and Population (HNP) Discussion Paper. Exploratory study on active pharmaceutical ingredient manufacturing for essential medicines*. Retrieved from http://siteresources.worldbank.org/HEALTHNUTRITIONANDPOPULATION/Resources/281627-1095698140167/APIExploratoryStudy.pdf.

Cameron, A., Ewen, M., Ross-Degnan, D., Ball, D., & Laing, R. (2008). Medicine prices, availability, and affordability in 36 developing and middle-income countries: A secondary analysis. *The Lancet, 373*, 240–249.

Cameron, A., Mantel-Teeuwisse, A. K., Leufkens, H. G., & Laing, R. O. (2012). Switching from originator brand medicines to generic equivalents in selected developing countries: How much could be saved? *Value in Health, 15*(5), 664–673.

Center for Drug Evaluation and Research Food and Drug Administration. (2003). *Guidance for industry. Bioavailability and bioequivalence studies for orally administered drug products-general considerations*. Retrieved from http://www.fda.gov/downloads/Drugs/GuidanceComplianceRegulatoryInformation/Guidances/ucm070124.pdf.

Chong, C. P., Hassali, M. A., Bahari, M. B., & Shafie, A. A. (2011). Exploring community pharmacists' views on generic medicines: A nationwide study from Malaysia. *International Journal of Clinical Pharmacy, 33*(1), 124–131.

Chua, G. N., Hassali, M. A., Shafie, A. A., & Awaisu, A. (2010). A survey exploring knowledge and perceptions of general practitioners towards the use of generic medicines in the northen state of Malaysia. *Health Policy, 95*(2), 229–235.

Colgan, S., Faasse, K., Martin, L. R., Stephens, M. H., Grey, A., & Petrie, K. J. (2015). Perceptions of generic medication in the general population, doctors and pharmacists: A systematic review. *BMJ Open, 5*(12), e008915.

Dunne, S., Shannon, B., Dunne, C., & Cullen, W. (2013). A review of the differences and similarities between generic drugs and their originator counterparts, including economic benefits associated with usage of generic medicines, using Ireland as a case study. *BMC Pharmacology and Toxicology, 14*(1), 1.

Dylst, P., & Simoens, S. (2010). Generic medicine pricing policies in Europe: Current status and impact. *Pharmaceuticals, 3*(3), 471–481.

Dylst, P., Vulto, A., Godman, B., & Simoens, S. (2013). Generic medicines: Solutions for a sustainable drug market? *Applied Health Economics and Health Policy, 11*(5), 437–443.

Dylst, P., Vulto, A., & Simoens, S. (2011). The impact of reference-pricing systems in Europe: A literature review and case studies. *Expert Review of Pharmacoeconomics & Outcomes Research, 11*(6), 729–737.

Dylst, P., Vulto, A., & Simoens, S. (2013). Demand-side policies to encourage the use of generic medicines: An overview. *Expert Review of Pharmacoeconomics & Outcomes Research, 13*(1), 59–72.

Ess, S. M., Schneeweiss, S., & Szucs, T. D. (2003). European healthcare policies for controlling drug expenditure. *Pharmacoeconomics, 21*(2), 89–103.

European Medicines Agency. (2011). *Questions and answers on generic medicines*. Retrieved from http://www.emea.europa.eu/docs/en_GB/document_library/Medicine_QA/2009/11/WC500012382.pdf.

Fabiano, V., Mameli, C., Cattaneo, D., Delle Fave, A., Preziosa, A., Mele, G., … Zuccotti, G. V. (2012). Perceptions and patterns of use of generic drugs among Italian Family Pediatricians: First round results of a web survey. *Health Policy, 104*(3), 247–252.

Faden, L., Vialle-Valentin, C., Ross-Degnan, D., & Wagner, A. (2011). Active pharmaceutical management strategies of health insurance systems to improve cost-effective use of medicines in low-and middle-income countries: A systematic review of current evidence. *Health Policy, 100*(2), 134–143.

Fatokun, O., Ibrahim, M. I. M., & Hassali, M. A. (2013). Factors determining the post-patent entry of generic medicines in Malaysia: A survey of the Malaysian generic pharmaceutical industry. *Journal of Generic Medicines, 10*(1), 22–33.

Gill, L., Helkkula, A., Cobelli, N., & White, L. (2010). How do customers and pharmacists experience generic substitution? *International Journal of Pharmaceutical and Healthcare Marketing, 4*(4), 375–395.

Gossell-Williams, M. (2007). Generic substitutions: A 2005 survey of the acceptance and perceptions of physicians in Jamaica. *West Indian Medical Journal, 56*(5), 458–463.

Gray, A. L. (2009). Medicine pricing interventions–the South African experience. *Southern Med Review, 2*(2), 15–19.

Grover, P., Stewart, J., Hogg, M., Short, L., Seo, H. G., & Rew, A. (2011). Evaluating pharmacists' views, knowledge, and perception regarding generic medicines in New Zealand. *Research in Social and Administrative Pharmacy*, *7*(3), 294–305.

Haas, J. S., Phillips, K. A., Gerstenberger, E. P., & Seger, A. C. (2005). Potential savings from substituting generic drugs for brand-name drugs: Medical expenditure panel survey, 1997–2000. *Annals of Internal Medicine*, *142*(11), 891–897.

Hall, P. E., Oehler, J., Woo, P., Zardo, H., Chinery, L., Singh, J. S., … Essah, N. M. (2007). A study of the capability of manufacturers of generic hormonal contraceptives in lower-and middle-income countries. *Contraception*, *75*(4), 311–317.

Hassali, M. A., Alrasheedy, A. A., McLachlan, A., Nguyen, T. A., Al-Tamimi, S. K., Ibrahim, M. I. M., & Aljadhey, H. (2014). The experiences of implementing generic medicines policy in eight countries: A review and recommendations for a successful promotion of generic medicines use. *Saudi Pharmaceutical Journal*, *22*(6), 491–503. http://dx.doi.org/10.1016/j.jsps.2013.12.017.

Hassali, M. A., Thambyappa, J., Saleem, F., Haq, N. U., & Aljadhey, H. (2012). Generic substitution in Malaysia: Recommendations from a systematic review. *Journal of Applied Pharmaceutical Science*, *02*(08), 159–164.

Hassali, M. A., & Wong, Z. Y. (2015). Challenges of developing generics substitution policies in low- and middle-income countries (LMICs). *Generics and Biosimilars Initiative Journal*, *4*(3), 1–2.

Hassali, M. A., Wong, Z. Y., Alrasheedy, A. A., Saleem, F., Yahaya, A. H. M., & Aljadhey, H. (2014). Perspectives of physicians practicing in low and middle income countries towards generic medicines: A narrative review. *Health Policy*, *117*(2014), 297–310. http://dx.doi.org/10.1016/j.healthpol.2014.07.014.

Homedes, N., & Ugalde, A. (2005). Multisource drug policies in Latin America: Survey of 10 countries. *Bulletin of the World Health Organization*, *83*(1), 64–70.

Iizuka, T., & Kubo, K. (2011). The generic drug market in Japan: Will it finally take off? *Health Economics, Policy, and Law*, *6*(3), 369–389. http://dx.doi.org/10.1017/s1744133110000332.

Jakovljevic, M. B., Nakazono, S., & Ogura, S. (2014a). Contemporary generic market in Japan–key conditions to successful evolution. *Expert Review of Pharmacoeconomics & Outcomes Research*, *14*(2), 181–194. http://dx.doi.org/10.1586/14737167.2014.881254.

Jakovljevic, M. B., Nakazono, S., & Ogura, S. (2014b). Contemporary generic market in Japan - key conditions to successful evolution. *Expert Review of Pharmacoeconomics & Outcomes Research*, *14*(2), 181–194. http://dx.doi.org/10.1586/14737167.2014.881254.

Jamshed, S. Q., Hassali, M. A., Ibrahim, M. I., & Babar, Z. (2011). Knowledge attitude and perception of dispensing doctors regarding generic medicines in Karachi, Pakistan: A qualitative study. *Journal of the Pakistan Medical Association*, *61*(1), 80–83.

Kanavos, P. (2007). Do generics offer significant savings to the UK National Health Service? *Current Medical Research and Opinion*, *23*(1), 105–116.

Kaplan, W. A., & Laing, R. (2003). Paying for pharmaceutical registration in developing countries. *Health Policy and Planning*, *18*(3), 237–248.

Kaplan, W. A., Ritz, L. S., Vitello, M., & Wirtz, V. J. (2012). Policies to promote use of generic medicines in low and middle income countries: A review of published literature, 2000–2010. *Health Policy*, *106*(3), 211–224.

Kaplan, W. A., & Wirtz, V. J. (2014). A research agenda to promote affordable and quality assured medicines. *Journal of Pharmaceutical Policy and Practice*, *7*(1), 1.

Kaplan, W. A., Wirtz, V. J., & Stephens, P. (2013). The market dynamics of generic medicines in the private sector of 19 low and middle income countries between 2001 and 2011: A descriptive time series analysis. *PLoS One*, *8*(9), e74399.

Karim, S. A., Pillai, G., Ziqubu-Page, T., Cassimjee, M., & Morar, M. (1996). Potential savings from generic prescribing and generic substitution in South Africa. *Health Policy and Planning*, *11*(2), 198–202.

Kesselheim, A. S., Fischer, M. A., & Avorn, J. (2006). Extensions of intellectual property rights and delayed adoption of generic drugs: Effects on medicaid spending. *Health Affairs*, *25*(6), 1637–1647.

Kesselheim, A. S., Stedman, M. R., Bubrick, E. J., Gagne, J. J., Misono, A. S., Lee, J. L., ... Shrank, W. H. (2010). Seizure outcomes following use of generic vs. brand-name antiepileptic drugs: A systematic review and meta-analysis. *Drugs*, *70*(5), 605–621.

King, D. R., & Kanavos, P. (2002). Encouraging the use of generic medicines: Implications for transition economies. *Croatian Medical Journal*, *43*(4), 462–469.

Leisinger, K. M., Garabedian, L. F., & Wagner, A. K. (2012). Improving access to medicines in low and middle income countries: Corporate responsibilities in context. *Southern Med Review*, *5*(2), 3–8.

Malkawi, B. H. (2009). Patent protection and the pharmaceutical industry in Japan. *Asián Journal of WTO and International Health Law and Policy*, *4*, 93–127.

Marchildon, G., & DiMatteo, L. (2011). *Health care cost drivers: The facts*. Retrieved from https://secure.cihi.ca/free_products/health_care_cost_drivers_the_facts_en.pdf.

McGavock, H. (2001). Generic substitution: Issues relating to the Australian experience. *Pharmacoepidemiology and Drug Safety*, *10*(6), 555–556.

McGavock, H. (1997). Strategies to improve the cost effectiveness of general practitioner prescribing: An international perspective. *Pharmacoeconomics*, *12*(3), 307–311.

McLachlan, A. J., Pearce, G. A., & Ramzan, I. (2004). Bioequivalence: How, why and what does it really mean? *Journal of Pharmacy Practice and Research*, *34*(3), 195–200.

Nguyen, T. A., Hassali, M. A., & McLachlan, A. (2013). Generic medicines policies in the Asia Pacific region: Ways forward. *WHO South-East Asia Journal of Public Health*, *2*(1), 72–74.

Nguyen, T. A., Knight, R., Roughead, E. E., Brooks, G., & Mant, A. (2015). Policy options for pharmaceutical pricing and purchasing: Issues for low-and middle-income countries. *Health Policy and Planning*, *30*(2), 267–280.

Nightingale, S. L., & Morrison, J. C. (1987). Generic drugs and the prescribing physician. *Journal of the American Medical Association*, *258*(9), 1200–1204.

Paraponaris, A., Verger, P., Desquins, B., Villani, P., Bouvenot, G., Rochaix, L., ... Paca, P. M. (2004). Delivering generics without regulatory incentives? Empirical evidence from French general practitioners about willingness to prescribe international non-proprietary names. *Health Policy*, *70*(1), 23–32.

Saleem, F., & Hassali, M. A. (2016). The true picture of dispensing separation in Malaysia. *Research in Social and Administrative Pharmacy*, *12*(1), 173–174.

Shrank, W. H., Liberman, J. N., Fischer, M. A., Girdish, C., Brennan, T. A., & Choudhry, N. K. (2011). Physician perceptions about generic drugs. *Annals of Pharmacotherapy*, *45*(1), 31–38.

Simoens, S. (2009). The Portuguese generic medicines market: A policy analysis. *Pharmacy Practice*, *7*(2), 74–80.

Simoens, S. (2010). Creating sustainable European health-care systems through the increased use of generic medicines: A policy analysis. *Journal of Generic Medicines*, *7*(2), 131–137. http://dx.doi.org/10.1057/jgm.2010.8.

Simoens, S. (2013). Sustainable provision of generic medicines in Europe. *Report for the European Generic Medicines Association*. Retrieved from http://www.generikusegyesulet.hu/contents/uploads/documents/document_1371468848_620.pdf.

Simoens, S., & Coster, S. D. (2006). Sustaining generic medicines markets in Europe. *Journal of Generic Medicines*, *3*(4), 257–268.

Steinwachs, D. M. (2002). Pharmacy benefit plans and prescription drug spending. *Journal of the American Medical Association*, *288*(14), 1773–1774.

Stoppler, M. (September 28, 2009). *Generic drugs, are they as good as brand names?*. Retrieved from http://www.medicinenet.com/script/main/art.asp?articlekey=46204.

Theodorou, M., Tsiantou, V., Pavlakis, A., Maniadakis, N., Fragoulakis, V., Pavi, E., & Kyriopoulos, J. (2009). Factors influencing prescribing behaviour of physicians in Greece and Cyprus: Results from a questionnaire based survey. *BMC Health Services Research*, *9*(1), 150.

Thorpe, K. E. (2005). The rise in health care spending and what to do about it. *Health Affairs*, *24*(6), 1436–1445.

Thorpe, K. E. (2006). Factors accounting for the rise in health-care spending in the United States: The role of rising disease prevalence and treatment intensity. *Public Health, 120*(11), 1002–1007.

Toverud, E.-L., Hartmann, K., & Håkonsen, H. (2015). A systematic review of physicians' and pharmacists' perspectives on generic drug use: What are the global challenges? *Applied Health Economics and Health Policy, 13*(1), 35–45.

Tsiantou, V., Zavras, D., Kousoulakou, H., Geitona, M., & Kyriopoulos, J. (2009). Generic medicnes: Greek physicians' perceptions and prescribing practices. *Journal of Clinical Pharmacy and Therapeutics, 34*(5), 547–554.

U.S. Food and Drug Administration. (2012a). *Facts about generic drugs*. Retrieved from http://www.fda.gov/Drugs/ResourcesForYou/Consumers/BuyingUsingMedicineSafely/UnderstandingGenericDrugs/ucm167991.htm#_ftnref2.

U.S. Food and Drug Administration. (2009a). *What are generic drugs?*. Retrieved from http://www.fda.gov/Drugs/ResourcesForYou/Consumers/BuyingUsingMedicineSafely/UnderstandingGenericDrugs/ucm144456.htm.

Vogler, S. (2012). The impact of pharmaceutical pricing and reimbursement policies on generics uptake: Implementation of policy options on generics in 29 European countries—an overview. *Generics and Biosimilars Initiative Journal, 1*(2), 93–100.

Wong, Z. Y., Alrasheedy, A. A., Hassali, M. A., & Saleem, F. (2016). Generic medicines in Malaysian health care system: Opportunities and challenges. *Research in Social and Administrative Pharmacy*. http://dx.doi.org/10.1016/j.sapharm.2016.04.002.

Wong, Z. Y., Hassali, M. A., Alrasheedy, A. A., Saleem, F., Yahaya, A. H. M., & Aljadhey, H. (2014). Malaysian generic pharmaceutical industries: Perspective from healthcare stakeholders. *Journal of Pharmaceutical Health Services Research, 5*(4), 193–203. http://dx.doi.org/10.1111/jphs.12072.

World Health Organization. (2004a). *Access to essential medicines the world medicines situation 2004*. Geneva: World Health Organization.

World Health Organization. (2004b). *Equitable access to essential medicines: A framework for collective action*. Geneva, Switzerland: World Health Organization.

World Health Organization. (2009). *Country pharmaceutical situations: Fact book on WHO level 1 indicators 2007*. Geneva, Switzerland: World Health Organization.

World Health Organization. (2010). *Assessment of medicines regulatory systems in Sub-Saharan African countries* An overview of findings from 26 assessment reports. Retrieved from http://apps.who.int/medicinedocs/en/d/Js17577en/.

World Health Organization. (2011). *The world medicines situation*. Retrieved from http://apps.who.int/medicinedocs/documents/s20054en/s20054en.pdf.

World Health Organization. (2012a). *Generic drugs*. Retrieved from http://www.who.int/trade/glossary/story034/en/index.html.

World Health Organization. (2012b). *WHO Prequalification of medicines programme: Annual report 2012 globalizing quality*. Retrieved from http://apps.who.int/prequal/info_general/documents/WHO_PQP_Annual_report_2012web.pdf.

CHAPTER

13 ASSESSMENT OF POLICIES, DETERMINANTS, AND CHARACTERISTICS OF GENERIC MEDICINES ENTRY INTO THE PHARMACEUTICAL MARKETS

Omotayo Fatokun

UCSI University, Kuala Lumpur, Malaysia

CHAPTER OUTLINE

Social and Administrative Aspects of Pharmacy in Low- and Middle-Income Countries. http://dx.doi.org/10.1016/B978-0-12-811228-1.00013-3

INTRODUCTION

The availability and use of generic medicines provide opportunities for the containment of pharmaceutical costs. This is especially important in developing countries where spending on medicines is mostly out of pocket. However, to derive the maximum benefit from a generic medicine, its prompt market entry following patent expiration on the innovator product is crucial (Sheppard, 2010). A generic medicine is a pharmaceutical product, usually intended to be interchangeable with the innovator product, which is usually manufactured without a license from the innovator company and marketed after the expiry of patent or other exclusivity rights (World Health Organization, 2011); an innovator product is generally that which was authorized first for marketing on the basis of documentation of efficacy, safety, and quality (WHO, 2011). A number of interrelated factors influence the dimensions and dynamics of postpatent entry of generic medicines in the pharmaceutical industry. These factors, which are discussed in this chapter, with primary focus on developing countries, include the prevailing pharmaceutical policy and regulatory environment, the existence and strength of entry barriers, and the level of competition in the pharmaceutical market.

POLICIES RELATING TO GENERIC MEDICINES ENTRY

The policies relating to generic medicines are highly diverse in nature with various policy measures implemented to meet the overall objectives of drug affordability and accessibility, including promoting the domestic industry (González, Fitzgerald, & Rovira, 2008). Generic medicines policy measures are generally classified into two domains: the supply-side and the demand-side domains (King & Kanavos, 2002; Nguyen, Kaplan, & Laing, 2008). The supply-driven policy domain is directly associated with the market entry and penetration of generic medicines and comprises patents, regulation and registration, price competition, pricing, and reimbursement. The demand-driven policy domains are prescribing policies, sales and dispensing policies, labeling and promotional activities, public education, and quality assurance. The demand-side policy measures incentivize generic uptake, thereby helping to create a conducive market environment for generic production, and thus indirectly encourage generic entry. These policy domains can be further categorized into different specific policy components as indicated in Table 13.1.

Although many of these policy measures are in place in developing countries, they are much less robust compared with developed countries, and the degree of their implementation in encouraging generic entry and uptake in developing countries is less impressive (Kaplan, Ritz, Vitello, & Wirtz, 2012).

DETERMINANTS OF GENERIC MEDICINES ENTRY

The phenomenon of pharmaceutical patent expiration and the entry of generic medicines is primarily characterized by two types of pharmaceutical firms: innovator firms and generic firms (European Commission, 2009). Innovator firms are the pioneers in the pharmaceutical market. They invest and engage in research and development into new pharmaceuticals (new chemical entities) and market them around the world, following marketing approval. Theoretically, once the patent protection on the

Table 13.1 Domains and Components of Policies Relating to Generic Medicines

Policy Domains		Policy Components				
Supply side	Patents	Regulatory exception	Exemption from patentability	Compulsory licensing	Patent term extension	Patent administration system
	Regulation and registration	Data exclusivity	Patent linkage	Differential registration fees	Generics approval time	Transparency of approval process
	Pharmaceutical pricing policies	Free pricing	Direct price regulation	Indirect price regulation		
	Reimbursement policies	Reimbursable positive list in generic names				
	Price competition	Generic price competition				
Demand side	Sales and dispensing policies	Generic substitution	Public availability of generic equivalents catalog	Drugs in national formulary available as multisource products	Incentives for generic dispensing	
	Quality assurance	Bioequivalence requirements	Good manufacturing practice (GMP) inspections	Postmarketing surveillance	Pharmacovigilance activities	
	Prescribing policies	Generic names prescribing	Incentives for generic prescribing			
	Labeling and promotional activities	Inclusion of generic names in promotional materials	Use of international nonproprietary name (INN) in institutional procurement			
	Public education	Programs and campaigns on generic medicines	Training medical and pharmacy students in INNs			

Based on De Joncheere, K., Rietveld, A. H., Huttin, C. (2002). Experiences with generics. International Journal of Risk & Safety in Medicine, 15, *101–109; Kaplan, W. A., Ritz, L. S., Vitello, M., & Wirtz, V. J. (2012). Policies to promote use of generic medicines in low and middle income countries: A review of published literature, 2000–2010.* Health Policy, 106, *211–224; Kanavos, P., Costa-Font, J., & Seeley, E. (2008). Competition in off-patent drug markets: Issues, regulation and evidence.* Economic Policy, 23, *499–544; King, D., & Kanavos, P. (2002). Encouraging the use of generic medicines: Implications for transition economics.* Croatian Medical Journal, 43, *462–469; Nguyen, A., Kaplan, W. A., & Laing, R. (2008).* Policy options for promoting the use of generic medicines in developing and transitional countries: A review paper. *Geneva: World Health Organization.*

innovator product has expired, generic firms can enter the market with a medicine that is chemically equivalent and bioequivalent to the innovator product. Although the entry process is multifaceted and varied, in general, it is comprised of four stages, namely, predevelopment, development, marketing authorization, and market launch (Prasnikar & Skerlj, 2006). However, the eventual market entry of generic medicine is determined by several variables, which may either promote or impede the entry process.

DRIVERS OF GENERIC ENTRY

Although several factors may promote generic medicines entry, both directly and indirectly, the following factors represent the most relevant in the context of developing countries.

Market Size of Innovator Medicines

A major driver of generic medicines entry into the pharmaceutical market is the prepatent expiration sales revenue of the innovator products. This is because the preexpiration innovator revenue serves as an attraction to generic manufacturers to invest in the production of a new generic version in anticipation of profits that might be derived from the new generic drug (Reiffen & Ward, 2005). Although much evidence of this has been demonstrated extensively in the large markets of the developed countries of North America and Europe, it is also an important factor in the emerging markets of the developing countries, particularly among those with significant generic manufacturing capacity, such as India, China, and Brazil (Chaudhuri, 2016; Fiuza & Caballero, 2015; Rao, 2008). For instance, the high price of innovator medicines and associated revenue has encouraged many generic companies in India to enter the market with their lower-priced generics on patent expiration of the innovator product and then to grow market share in the patent-expired product (Chaudhuri, 2016). A study of generic markets in 10 countries, including Brazil and Mexico also indicates that the probability of generic entry is positively related to market size of the innovator products in almost all countries (Danzon & Furukawa, 2011). Even in smaller markets in developing countries, the market size of innovator products is a key factor in driving generic entry, particularly in those operating a national health system that is largely financed by public funding (Fatokun, Ibrahim, & Hassali, 2013a) or through a national insurance health scheme (Liu & Cheng, 2012).

Regulatory Exception Provision

The implementation of regulatory exception provision in national patent legislation is an important driver of generic entry. Under the World Trade Organization's Agreement on Trade-Related Aspects of Intellectual Property Rights (TRIPS), generic medicines manufacturers are allowed the use of a patented innovator's pharmaceutical product for the development of a generic equivalent and filing for regulatory approval prior to the expiration of the patent on the innovator patented product (United Nations Conference on Trade and Development and International Centre for Trade and Sustainable Development UNCTAD-ICTSD, 2005), thereby enabling prompt entry of generic medicines as soon as the patent expires. The regulatory exception provision was first introduced in the US pharmaceutical legislation. Subsequently, a number of countries in both developed and developing countries have incorporated the provision in their domestic patent laws, although less widespread among the developing countries (Garrison, 2006; Musungu & Oh, 2006). Without the regulatory exception, innovator manufacturers are effectively granted extension of their patent period for the length of time it would take a generic manufacturer to develop a generic equivalent of an innovator products and filing for regulatory approval. Therefore, regulatory exception provision is a vital mechanism in facilitating the production of and accelerating market entry of generic medicines on patent expiry (UNCTAD-ICTSD, 2005), although its effectiveness in ensuring prompt entry of generic medicines in developing countries may be constrained by trade policies (Correa, 2016a) and lack of coherence in generic policies implementation (Fatokun, Ibrahim, & Hassali, 2013b).

Abbreviated Generic Approval Process

As for innovator medicines, generic medicines must obtain regulatory approval before they can be marketed. However, because the safety and efficacy of the active ingredient in generic medicines have already been established through the earlier application by the innovator firm, drug regulatory authorities in most countries, including developing countries, usually do not require the conduct and submission of clinical trials data by the generic drug manufacturers to receive approval for marketing. The generic drug manufacturers, however, need to prove that their product exhibits pharmaceutical equivalence and bioequivalence to the innovator product and also submit chemistry and manufacturing quality data (WHO, 2011). The elimination of clinical trials for generic products approval reduces the cost of generic medicines development, thus promoting the prompt entry of generics to the market.

Fast-Track Generic Approval

The administrative procedure to shorten the approval time for generic medicines in many developing countries may facilitate prompt entry of generic medicines. Approval time is defined as the amount of time taken to register a pharmaceutical product, from the time an application is submitted to the time when the final decision is reached (Ratanawijitrasin & Wondemagegnehu, 2002). Although the approval times vary among drug products, generally, the process of generic registration is simpler and faster than that for new chemical entities. For instance, Ratanawijitrasin and Wondemagegnehu (2002) found that, in practice, the average time taken to register a product containing a new chemical entity range from 6 to 19 months, whereas it takes 2–18 months for generic drugs. For example, in Brazil, registration of generic medicines was reported to occur between 6 and 8 months, compared with 8–14 months for innovator products; in Colombia, generics registration time was 3 months, whereas it takes 6 months to register an innovator product (Homedes & Ugalde, 2005). Generally, the faster a generic product application is reviewed and granted marketing authorization, the faster the generic product is expected to enter the market. However, the effectiveness of fast-track procedures in ensuring a quality review of generic medicines registration applications and eventual market entry may be affected by the available expertise and resources at the disposal of the regulatory authorities. For instance, the implementation of fast-track approval for the registration of generic medicines in South Africa in 2005 was found to result in backlog of application because of inadequate human resources and operational constraints (Leng, 2015).

Differential Registration Fee

Differential registration fee is an administrative or legislative policy instrument of charging lower fees for the registration of generic medicines compared with new chemical entities. The justification is that regulatory review process for generic medicines is much quicker and simpler than that for new chemical entities and thus involves lower administrative costs (Kaplan & Laing, 2003). A number of countries, especially developing countries, have implemented differential registration fees in their drug registration process. For instance, Homedes and Ugalde (2005) reported that, in Argentina, the innovator products registration fees was US$ 1000 compared with US$ 333 for generic drugs, and in Chile, the innovator product registration fee was US$ 1300 and US$ 800 for generic drugs. Differential registration fee has been seen as a policy instrument to encourage generic manufacturers to file for market approval, thereby encouraging market entry of generic medicines (De Joncheere, Rietveld, & Huttin, 2002).

Existing Technical Capabilities

Another important factor that drives generic entry decisions is the compatibility of the new generic medicines with the generic firm existing technical capabilities and resources. According to the literature, a firm's existing technical capabilities and product specialization predict the firm's market entry with a new product because the cost of entry will be reduced (Nerkar & Roberts, 2004; Scott-Morton, 1999). Therefore, a generic manufacturer may only decide to develop and introduce a new generic drug within a certain therapeutic class or in certain dosage form that is compatible with their existing technical capability, as they would benefit from economies of scale or scope in production (Scott-Morton, 1999). This factor is especially relevant in developing countries with small pharmaceutical markets (Attridge & Preker, 2005). For instance, in Malaysia, generic drug manufacturers ranked compatibility of the new generic medicine with a company product portfolio second, among the factors influencing decisions for generic development and market entry (Fatokun et al., 2013a).

BARRIERS TO GENERIC ENTRY

The existence and strength of entry barriers is one of the most important determinants for a firm to enter a given market. Several sources of barriers to generic medicines entry in developing countries have been identified. A majority of these barriers, which are discussed in the following sections, arise from the drug regulatory approval process, the patent system, and the strategic behaviors of the innovators.

Data Exclusivity

Data exclusivity (DE) refers to a practice whereby, for a specified period of time, drug regulatory authorities are not allowed to rely on the innovator's safety and efficacy data to register a generic version of an innovative drug product (WHO, 2006). In other words, the innovator drug product is granted a nonpatent exclusivity for the fixed period during which generic medicines cannot be registered and enter the market, otherwise generic producers would have to submit their own safety and efficacy data (Timmermans, 2005; WHO, 2006). This requirement diminishes the likelihood of speedy marketing of generic medicines, as conducting clinical trials to prove safety and efficacy are time-consuming and expensive and would present substantial barriers for the market entry of small producers of generic products (Roffe & Spennemann, 2006). The approach and scope of DE vary among countries. For example, DE may apply to only new chemical entities or both new chemical entities and new uses of already-approved drugs, and the period of exclusivity differs among countries (Roffe & Spennemann, 2006). In developing countries, DE has been incorporated into some national legislations and regulations (Cerón & Godoy, 2009; Fatokun, Hassali, & Ibrahim, 2015). Other developing countries have adopted DE in bilateral or regional trade agreements signed with developed countries, particularly the United States (Roffe & Spennemann, 2006), with exclusivity periods up to 5 years for new chemical entities and in some cases, with 3 years for new clinical information or new uses for previously approved drug products (Roffe & Spennemann, 2006). Examples of developing countries with DE include Vietnam, Jordan, Singapore, Chile, Morocco, Bahrain, Dominican Republic, Costa Rica, El Salvador, Guatemala, Honduras, and Nicaragua (Cerón & Godoy, 2009; Roffe & Spennemann, 2006). Others include China, Thailand (Chakrabarti, 2014), and Malaysia (Fatokun et al., 2015). Although, the effect of DE on generic entry is yet to be extensively assessed in developing countries, available studies suggest that generic entry is restricted, with implication for generic competition. For example, DE provisions of the US-Jordan Free Trade Agreement (FTA) was found to delay generic competition in Jordan for 79%of medicines newly launched by 21 multinational pharmaceutical companies between 2002 and mid-2006, which otherwise would have been available in generic version (Malpani, 2009). Another study of the effect of the US-Central America Free Trade Agreement (US-CAFTA) found that DE provisions in the FTA restrict the entry of generic medicines and competition in Guatemala (Shaffer & Brenner, 2009).

Patent Linkage

Patent linkage is the practice whereby the marketing approval for a generic medicine is linked to the patent status of the innovator reference product. As a result, drug regulatory authorities are not able to grant marketing authorization for a generic medicine until either the expiration of all patents covering the drug product or the determination that the patents is not being infringed, or the patents are invalid or unenforceable (Correa, 2006b). This practice has a strong potential negative impact on generic entry because of the proliferation of multiple patents on a single product in the pharmaceutical industry (Correa, 2011). Patent linkage implementation varies from country to country. In developing countries, the patent linkage practice is found either as part of the legislative framework or as part of trade agreements. Examples of countries with patent linkage include Singapore, Chile, Morocco, Bahrain, Dominican Republic, Costa Rica, El Salvador, Guatemala, Honduras, Nicaragua (Cerón & Godoy, 2009; Roffe & Spennemann, 2006), and China (Bhardwaj, Raju, & Padmavati, 2013). The actual effect of patent linkage on generic entry has not been fully studied in developing countries. However, findings from developed countries showed that generic entry is severely delayed, as innovator firms file multiple patents on their product to prevent registration of generic version of the product (Bouchard, Hawkins, Clark, & Sawani, 2010). Available analysis in developing countries similarly indicates that patent linkage can potentially delay generic entry and competition (Correa, 2006b; Timmermans, 2005).

Patent Term Extension

Under the TRIPS agreement, the minimum period of patent protection is 20 years from the date of patent application (UNCTAD-ICTSD, 2005). However, some national legislations and trade policies under various bilateral and regional trade agreements have provided for extension of pharmaceutical patent term beyond the TRIPS mandated period of 20 years, consequently extending the date of generic entry. In the developing countries, patent term extension provision is commonly found as part of bilateral or regional free trade agreements, with varying number of years of extension. For instance, the US-Singapore FTA and US-Chile FTA provided for an extension of patent term for up to 5 years (Jorge, 2004); however, no maximum period is provided for most of the other US FTAs (Correa, 2006b). The reason for the patent term extension has been to compensate the patent holder for delay in the patent office or time required by national drug regulatory authorities for product marketing approval (Correa, 2006b). However, it has been argued that such extensions would allow patent holders to enjoy a monopoly beyond the 20-year period and further delay generic entry (Gopakumar & Smith, 2010).

Patent Administration System

The operation of a country's patent administration system, with respect to the competence and efficiency in the examination of pharmaceutical patent claims and the possibility of generic producers in determining patent expiration dates, has implications for generic market entry (Correa, 2006a; Nguyen et al., 2008). Many patent offices in developing countries lack adequate human resources and technical competence and expertise for a quality assessment of pharmaceutical patents (Correa, 2006a; Drahos, 2007). As such, a patent may be granted to a pharmaceutical claim that would otherwise not have been if a rigorous examination was carried out, thereby creating a barrier to market entry of generics. Besides, generic producers, especially in developing countries, generally do not possess the substantial technical and financial resources needed to challenge wrongly granted patents or defend against infringement claims (Correa, 2006a). Thus, once patents are granted, they may be particularly difficult to invalidate in developing countries (Sampat & Shadlen, 2015). Additionally, some patent offices in developing countries do not have efficient information systems to obtain full and accurate information on patented products (Correa, 2011). Although a growing number of developing countries' national patent offices are providing searchable databases, identifying patents related to specific medicines is still a challenge (Correa, 2011; Sampat & Shadlen, 2015). Together, these factors make it difficult for generic manufacturers in developing countries to plan for entry as soon as patent expires, thereby delaying the entry of generic medicines.

Innovators' Entry Deterrence Behaviors

Because the market entry and uptake of generic medicines ultimately lead to erosion of the market share of the innovator products, various entry-deterrence strategies are typically deployed by the innovator firms to deter or delay generic entry, particularly toward the end of the patent protection on the innovator product. The patent system, which is meant to reward the innovation and provide incentive for continued research and development into new pharmaceuticals, has been noted to be used extensively by the innovator firms to delay generic entry (Correa, 2011). A variety of patent-related strategies that may have the effects of delaying or blocking generic entry have been identified in the literature. Chief among them is patent *evergreening*, a strategy by which pharmaceutical companies apply for patents over derivatives, formulations, dosage forms, isomers, polymorphs, salts or new medical uses, etc., of known drugs to extend their exclusive rights beyond the expiry of the primary or original patent (Correa, 2016b; Rathod, 2010), thus resulting in several secondary patents and creating patent clusters (Abud, Hall, & Helmers, 2015; Sampat & Shadlen, 2015). As such, even when the primary patent has expired, the generic version still finds it difficult to enter the market as the innovator may claim legal infringement on any of the multiple patents surrounding the primary patent. This patenting strategy is pervasive in developed and developing countries alike. For example, a study of patenting trends in five developing countries—Argentina, Brazil, Colombia, India, and South Africa—reports of a significant proliferation of secondary pharmaceutical patents in those countries (Correa, 2011). Similar findings have been reported in Thailand and Philippines (Rathod, 2010). Another study in Chile found that, for each primary patent of an active drug ingredient, there are four secondary patents (Abud et al., 2015). In Malaysia, a study among generic producers also found patent clustering by innovator as the foremost barrier to generic entry (Fatokun et al., 2013a). Overall, innovator patent-related behavior, particularly the proliferation of secondary patents, delays generic entry, as it creates ambiguities on the patent status of the innovator product, thus making the generic manufacturers uncertain of when to produce and enter the market or else risk costly patent ligations. Other entry-deterrence strategies that have been reported, although less commonly used in developing countries, include the market introduction of innovator-own generics and cross-licensing of innovators' generics (Fiuza & Caballero, 2015).

Weak Demand-Side Policies

To enhance a sustainable postpatent entry of generic medicines and the efficiency of the generic industry, an optimal mix of both supply-side and demand-side policies is important. In developing countries, however, the demand-side policies that incentivize generic uptake through generic prescription, dispensing, and consumption are weak (Kaplan et al., 2012). In most developing countries, generic awareness and acceptance is low, and there is a general lack of confidence in generic prescribing by physicians. Similarly, a legal framework that supports generic substitution by pharmacists is either nonexistent or inadequately implemented (Hassali & Wong, 2015). The absence of a robust and adequate demand-side policy environment for generic uptake discourages generic production and market entry.

CHARACTERISTICS OF POSTPATENT ENTRY OF GENERIC MEDICINES

The features characterizing generic entry in the pharmaceutical market, with potential impact on price-lowering competition, include the time to entry and number of generic entrants following patent expiration on the innovator products and the effect of generic entry and competition on drug prices.

TIME TO GENERIC ENTRY

Prompt entry of generic medicines following patent expiration accelerates the onset of price-lowering competition in the pharmaceutical market and helps reduce the overall pharmaceutical costs. Ideally, the entry of generic medicines a day following the expiration of the basic patent of the innovator products should be possible, as innovator firms are expected to have recouped their investments on research and development during the period of the basic patent (European Commission, 2009). In practice, however, an immediate generic entry is very difficult because of the existence of several barriers discussed in earlier sections. A number of studies in developed markets have examined the time lag between patent expiration and the first generic entry and have reported considerable delays (European Commission, 2009; Hudson, 2000). Although literature on the characteristics of generic entry in developing countries is limited, findings from available studies reflected those obtained in developed countries. For instance, a study in Brazil indicated a median time to generic entry of 4 years after the patent expiration on the primary patents (Otterson & Pereira, 2013). Another study in Malaysia reported an average time to entry of 397 days, which was found to be significantly delayed beyond the day following basic patent expiration of the innovator product (Fatokun, Ibrahim, & Hassali, 2013c). Delayed generic entry thus erodes the opportunities that could be derived from the immediate availability of generic medicines in the pharmaceutical market.

NUMBER OF GENERIC ENTRANTS

Evidence from both developed and developing countries showed that the entry of generic medicines following patent expiration of innovator products is characterized by a sequential and nonlinear entry, whereby the number of generic entrants steadily increases during the first few years following patent expiration and then decline some years later (Danzon & Furukawa, 2011; Kanavos, Costa-Font, & Seeley, 2008; Reiffen & Ward, 2005). The initial sequential entry is attributable to the differing marketing approval times for potential generic entrants and strategic entry by generic producers, whereas the subsequent decline in the number of entrants over time is due to competition in the generic market, whereby the entry of new generic entrants leads to increased competition and subsequent decline in product prices and market size, thus resulting in decline of attractiveness of further entry (Ching, 2010; Kanavos et al., 2008). The number of generic entrants following patent expiration across countries is quite variable and comparability may be difficult due to differences in market structure and regulatory policies. However, postpatent generic entry rate in most developing countries seems less impressive compared with developed countries (Danzon & Furukawa, 2011; Scott-Morton & Kyle, 2012). For instance, Danzon and Furukawa (2011), in a study of the performance of generic markets in 10 countries (the United States, the United Kingdom, Germany, France, Spain, Italy, Japan, Canada, Brazil, and Mexico) over the period 1998–2009, reported a postpatent entry of one to two generic equivalents per innovator product for Brazil and Mexico compared with a range of four to nine for the rest of the study countries.

EFFECT OF GENERIC ENTRY ON DRUG PRICES

The effect of generic entry on drug prices is important in the containment of pharmaceutical costs. A large number of economic studies in developed countries have shown that generic entry reduces the prices of generic versions and the overall price of a patent-expired active ingredient drug product (multisource products), as more generics enter the market (Frank & Salkever, 1997; Reiffen & Ward, 2005). However, findings from the literature are mixed on the effect of generic entry on innovators brand prices (Congressional Budget Office, 2010). In the developing countries, some data on generic competition and drug prices have also been reported. For example, a study of commonly used drugs for chronic diseases in South Africa found that the differential cost between brand and generic equivalents increases with increasing number of generic equivalents off-patent drugs, although the observed increase was not significant (Nicolosi & Gray, 2009). Yet another study of off-patent cardiovascular drugs in South Africa found no observable decrease in drug prices with increasing number of generics (Bangalee & Suleman, 2016), suggesting that any price-lowering effect of generic competition in South Africa may not be realized across all therapeutic groups. Although a similar study in Malaysia revealed evidence of a price-lowering effect of generic competition among patent-expired active ingredient drug products in Malaysia, the effect was not observable across all drug brands (Fatokun, Ibrahim, & Hassali, 2011). Another study of price and quantity changes in relation to the evolution of market structure, from patent implementation to expiry and entry of new producers of commonly used drugs in Morocco and Tunisia, found that the generic prices and the generic–innovator brand price ratio decreases as the number of generic entrants increase (Driouchi & Zouag, 2012). However, compared with most developed countries, price-lowering effects of generic entry in developing countries are generally low (Danzon & Furukawa, 2011). Overall, although some degree of generic competition is seen in pharmaceutical markets in developing countries, the effect of generic entry in lowering overall drug price appears minimal.

ACHIEVEMENTS

The increasing recognition of the benefits of generic medicines in containing the rising pharmaceutical costs and in ensuring access to affordable medicines in developing countries has led to the formulation of various policies that may foster the postpatent entry of generic medicines into the pharmaceutical markets in developing countries. Additionally, driven by the potential economic returns and for the sustainability of the generic industry, the generic firms in developing countries, like their counterparts in developed countries, have demonstrated the willingness to introduce new generic medicines into the market following patent expiration on innovator products. Although the extent of postpatent entry of generic medicines and competition in developing countries is limited, some degree of price-lowering effect of generic availability is observable, a situation that is of crucial importance to the reduction of the overall pharmaceutical costs. In general, competition-induced price-lowering effect of generic medicines can be achieved in developing countries, provided there are sufficient numbers of generic entrants on patent expiration of innovator products.

CHALLENGES

Despite the willingness of the generic industry to develop and introduce a new generic medicine, there exist a number of challenges that hinder the entry of generic medicines into the pharmaceutical markets in developing countries. Although both the supply-side and the demand-side generic policies are in place in developing countries, they are less robust, they seem less coherent, and there are potential gaps between policy intent and implementation, leading to a constrained generic entry in the pharmaceutical markets. Besides, the proliferation of trade-related agreements and policies in developing countries, with provisions such as DE, patent linkage, and patent term extension, poses considerable challenges to generic entry. Additionally, the deployment of various entry-deterrence strategies by the innovator firms, particularly the use of secondary patents, creates ambiguities on the patent status of the innovator product, thus making the generic manufacturers uncertain of when to produce and enter the market. These situations delay the entry of generic medicine, resulting in low generic availability and competition.

RECOMMENDATIONS: THE WAY FORWARD

To maximize the potential benefits from generic medicines and to enhance the competitiveness of the generic industry in the developing countries, it is recommended that greater coherence between intellectual property rights and health policies be ensured. This can minimize possible conflict between the government goals of providing incentive for pharmaceutical development and the government efforts toward ensuring medicines accessibility, affordability, and containment of pharmaceutical costs. The patent administration system should be enhanced and there should be strict adherence to the patentability criteria of novelty, inventive step, and usefulness in the examination and grant of pharmaceutical patents. This can help address the problem of erroneously granting patents and also prevent the granting of multiple patents on a single active pharmaceutical substance. Increased and sustained generic medicines education and awareness of health professional and the public in developing countries is needed to foster generic prescribing, dispensing, and consumption, thereby creating an enabling environment for generic production and market entry following patent expiration on innovator products.

CONCLUSIONS

A variety of policies and regulatory measures relating to generic medicines are in place in developing countries. The postpatent entry of generic medicines in developing countries is majorly determined by the prevailing regulatory policies and intellectual property rights, prepatent market size of the innovator products, generic firm's characteristics, and the existence and the degree of the entry-deterrence strategies by innovators, majority of which are derived from the patent system. In the event of entry, the pattern of generic entry is similar to what is obtained in developed countries, but in most developing countries, the time to generic entry is delayed and the number of generic entrants is limited. Competition in off-patent pharmaceutical markets in the developing countries could lower the overall drug prices, provided prompt and sufficient market entry of generic medicines occur following patent expiration on the innovator product.

LESSONS LEARNED

- A variety of policies and regulatory measures relating to generic medicines entry are in place in developing countries.
- Entry decisions by developing generic medicines producers are driven by factors consistent with the entry model of the generic pharmaceutical industry, which is the development of a generic equivalent of an economically successful innovator product, at minimal costs, and market it as soon as the innovator product patent expires.
- The proliferation of trade-related agreements and policies with provisions such as DE, patent linkage, and patent term extension pose considerable challenges to generic entry in developing countries.
- The deployment entry-deterrence strategies by the innovator firms, particularly the use of secondary patents, deter generic entry to the pharmaceutical markets.
- Generic entry in developing countries is characterized by sequential entry, but the speed of entry and number of entrants following patent expiration is limited, potentially resulting in minimal effects on drug prices.

REFERENCES

Abud, M. J., Hall, B., & Helmers, C. (2015). An empirical analysis of primary and secondary pharmaceutical patents in Chile. *PLoS One*, *10*, e0124257. http://dx.doi.org/10.1371/journal.pone.0124257.

Attridge, C. J., & Preker, A. S. (2005). *Improving access to medicines in developing countries: Application of new institutional economics to the analysis of manufacturing and distribution issues*. Washington, DC: World Bank.

Bangalee, V., & Suleman, F. (2016). Has the increase in the availability of generic drugs lowered the price of cardiovascular drugs in South Africa? *Health SA Gesondheid*, *21*, 60–66.

Bhardwaj, R., Raju, K. D., & Padmavati, M. (2013). The impact of patent linkage on marketing of generic drugs. *Journal of Intellectual Property Rights*, *18*, 316–322.

Bouchard, R. A., Hawkins, R. W., Clark, H. R., & Sawani, J. (2010). Empirical analysis of drug approval-drug patenting linkage for high value pharmaceuticals. *Northwestern Journal of Technology and Intellectual Property*, *8*, 174–227. Retrieved from http://scholarlycommons.law.northwestern.edu/njtip/vol8/iss2/2/.

Cerón, A., & Godoy, A. S. (2009). Intellectual property and access to medicines: An analysis of legislation in Central America. *Bulletin of the World Health Organization*, *87*, 787–793.

Chakrabarti, G. (2014). Need of data exclusivity: Impact on access to medicine. *Journal of Intellectual Property Rights*, *19*, 325–336.

Chaudhuri, S. (2016). Can foreign firms promote local production of pharmaceuticals in Africa? In M. Mackintosh, G. Banda, W. Wamae, & P. Tibandebage (Eds.), *Making medicines in Africa: The political economy of industrializing for local health* (pp. 103–121). Basingstoke, England: Palgrave Macmillan.

Ching, A. T. (2010). Consumer learning and heterogeneity: Dynamics of demand for prescription drugs. *International Journal of Industrial Organization*, *28*, 619–638.

Congressional Budget Office. (2010). *Effects of using generic drugs on medicare's prescription drug spending*. Washington, DC: Congressional Budget Office. Retrieved fromhttps://www.cbo.gov/sites/default/files/cbofiles/ftpdocs/118xx/doc11838/09-15-prescriptiondrugs.pdf.

Correa, C. (2006a). *Guidelines for the examination of pharmaceutical patents: Developing a public health perspective- a working paper*. Geneva: World Health Organization (International Centre for Trade and Sustainable Development and United Nations Conference on Trade and Development).

Correa, C. M. (2006b). Implications of bilateral free trade agreements on access to medicines. *Bulletin of the World Health Organization*, *84*, 399–404.

Correa, C. M. (2011). *Pharmaceutical innovation, incremental patenting and compulsory licensing*. Geneva: South Centre. Retrieved from http://apps.who.int/medicinedocs/documents/s21395en/s21395en.pdf.

Correa, C. M. (2016a). *The bolar exception: Legislative models and drafting options*. Geneva: South Centre. Retrieved from https://www.southcentre.int/wp-content/uploads/2016/03/RP66_The-Bolar-Exception_EN1.pdf.

Correa, C. M. (2016b). *Guidelines for the examination of patent applications relating to pharmaceuticals*. New York, NY: United Nations Development Programme. Retrieved from http://www.undp.org/content/undp/en/home/librarypage/hiv-aids/guidelines-for-the-examination-of-patent-applications-relating-t.html.

Danzon, P. M., & Furukawa, M. F. (2011). *Cross-national evidence on generic pharmaceuticals: Pharmacy vs. physician-driven markets*. NBER Working Paper No. 17226. Retrieved from http://www.nber.org/papers/w17226.

De Joncheere, K., Rietveld, A. H., & Huttin, C. (2002). Experiences with generics. *International Journal of Risk & Safety in Medicine*, *15*, 101–109.

Drahos, P. (2007). *"Trust me": Patent offices in developing countries*. Canberra, Australia: Australian National University. Retrieved from https://www.anu.edu.au/fellows/pdrahos/pdfs/2007Drahostrustmessrn.pdf.

Driouchi, A., & Zouag, N. (2012). Pharmaceutical patents and prices of generics in Morocco and neighbouring economies. *Journal of World Intellectual Property*, *15*, 103–132.

European Commission. (2009). *Pharmaceutical sector inquiry final report*. Retrieved from http://ec.europa.eu/competition/sectors/pharmaceuticals/inquiry/staff_working_paper_part1.pdf.

Fatokun, O., Hassali, M. A., & Ibrahim, M. I. (2015). Characterizing pharmaceuticals on data exclusivity in Malaysia. *Journal of Intellectual Property Rights*, *20*, 223–229.

Fatokun, O., Ibrahim, M. I., & Hassali, M. A. (2011). Generic competition and drug prices in the Malaysian off-patent pharmaceutical market. *Journal of Applied Pharmaceutical Science*, *1*, 33–37.

Fatokun, O., Ibrahim, M. I., & Hassali, M. A. (2013a). Factors determining the post-patent entry of generic medicines in Malaysia: A survey of the Malaysian generic pharmaceutical industry. *Journal of Generic Medicines*, *10*, 22–33.

Fatokun, O., Ibrahim, M. I., & Hassali, M. A. (2013b). Generic industry's perceptions of generic medicines policies and practices in Malaysia. *Journal of Pharmacy Research, 7*, 80–84.

Fatokun, O., Ibrahim, M. I., & Hassali, M. A. (2013c). Time to entry of generic medicines in Malaysia: Implications for pharmaceutical cost containment. *Journal of Pharmaceutical Health Services Research, 4*, 203–210.

Fiuza, E. P., & Caballero, B. (2015). Estimations of generic drug entry in Brazil using count versus ordered models. *Brasília: Institute for Applied Economic Research*. Retrieved from http://www.ipea.gov.br/portal/images/stories/PDFs/TDs/ingles/dp_186.pdf.

Frank, R., & Salkever, D. (1997). Generic entry and the pricing of pharmaceuticals. *Journal of Economics and Management Strategy, 6*, 75–90.

Garrison, C. (2006). *Exceptions to patent rights in developing countries*. Geneva: International Centre for Trade and Sustainable Development (ICTSD) and United Nations Conference on Trade and Development (UNCTAD). Retrieved from https://iprsonline.org/resources/docs/Garrison%20-%20Patent%20Exceptions%20DC%20-%20Blue%2017.pdf.

González, C. P., Fitzgerald, J. F., & Rovira, J. (2008). Generics in Latin America: Trends and regulation. *Journal of Generic Medicines, 6*, 43–56.

Gopakumar, K., & Smith, S. R. (2010). IPR provisions in FTAs: Implications for access to medicines. In World Health Organization (Ed.), *Intellectual property and access to medicines: Papers and perspectives* (pp. 141–149). New Delhi: World Health Organization.

Hassali, M. A., & Wong, Z. Y. (2015). Challenges of developing generics substitution policies in low-and middle-income countries (LMICs). *Generics and Biosimilars Initiative Journal, 4*, 171–172. http://dx.doi.org/10.5639/gabij.2015.0404.038.

Homedes, N., & Ugalde, A. (2005). Multisource drug policies in Latin America: Survey of 10 countries. *Bulletin of the World Health Organization, 83*, 64–70.

Hudson, J. (2000). Generic take-up in the pharmaceutical market following patent expiry: A multi-country study. *International Review of Law and Economics, 20*, 205–221.

Jorge, M. F. (2004). TRIPS-plus provisions in trade agreements and their potential adverse effects on public health. *Journal of Generic Medicines, 1*, 199–211.

Kanavos, P., Costa-Font, J., & Seeley, E. (2008). Competition in off-patent drug markets: Issues, regulation and evidence. *Economic Policy, 23*, 499–544.

Kaplan, W. A., & Laing, R. (2003). Paying for pharmaceutical registration in developing countries. *Health Policy and Planning, 18*, 237–248.

Kaplan, W. A., Ritz, L. S., Vitello, M., & Wirtz, V. J. (2012). Policies to promote use of generic medicines in low and middle income countries: A review of published literature, 2000–2010. *Health Policy, 106*, 211–224.

King, D., & Kanavos, P. (2002). Encouraging the use of generic medicines: Implications for transition economics. *Croatian Medical Journal, 43*, 462–469.

Leng, H. M. (2015). Pro-generics policies and the backlog in medicines registration in South Africa: Implications for access to essential and affordable medicines. *Generics and Biosimilars Initiative Journal, 4*, 58–63. http://dx.doi.org/10.5639/gabij.2015.0402.014.

Liu, Y. M., & Cheng, J. S. (2012). Determinants of generic entry in the regulated Taiwanese prescription drug market. *Health Policy, 108*, 228–235.

Malpani, R. (2009). All costs, no benefits: How the US-Jordan free trade agreement affects access to medicines. *Journal of Generic Medicines, 6*, 206–217.

Musungu, S. F., & Oh, C. (2006). *The use of flexibilities in TRIPS by developing countries: Can they promote access to medicines?* Geneva: South Centre.

Nerkar, A., & Roberts, P. W. (2004). Technological and product-market experience and the success of new product introductions in the pharmaceutical industry. *Strategic Management Journal, 25*, 779–799.

Nguyen, A., Kaplan, W. A., & Laing, R. (2008). *Policy options for promoting the use of generic medicines in developing and transitional countries: A review paper*. Geneva: World Health Organization.

Nicolosi, E., & Gray, A. (2009). Potential cost savings from generic medicines -protecting the prescribed minimum benefits. *South African Family Practice*, *51*, 59–63.

Otterson, J., & Pereira, D. G. (2013). *Entry and competition in the Brazilian generic drug market*. Retrieved from http://www.webmeets.com/files/papers/earie/2013/346/EntryAnalysis2.pdf.

Prasnikar, J., & Skerlj, T. (2006). New product development process and time-to-market in the generic pharmaceutical industry. *Industrial Marketing Management*, *35*, 690–702.

Rao, P. M. (2008). The emergence of the pharmaceutical industry in the developing world and its implications for multinational enterprise strategies. *International Journal of Pharmaceutical and Healthcare Marketing*, 2, 103–116.

Ratanawijitrasin, S., & Wondemagegnehu, E. (2002). *Effective drug regulation. A multicountry study*. Geneva: World Health Organization.

Rathod, S. K. (2010). Ever-greening: A status check in selected countries. *Journal of Generic Medicines*, *7*, 227–242.

Reiffen, D., & Ward, M. R. (2005). Generic drug industry dynamics. *Review of Economics and Statistics*, *87*, 37–49.

Roffe, P., & Spennemann, C. (2006). The impact of FTAs on public health policies and TRIPS flexibilities. *International Journal of Intellectual Property Management*, *1*, 75–93.

Sampat, B. N., & Shadlen, K. C. (2015). TRIPS implementation and secondary pharmaceutical patenting in Brazil and India. *Studies in Comparative International Development*, *50*, 228–257.

Scott-Morton, F. M. (1999). Entry decisions in the generic pharmaceutical industry. *The RAND Journal of Economics*, *30*, 421–440.

Scott-Morton, F., & Kyle, M. (2012). Markets for pharmaceutical products. In M. V. Pauly, T. G. Mcguire, & P. P. Barros (Eds.), *Handbook of health economics* (Vol. II) (pp. 763–823). Oxford: Elsevier.

Shaffer, E. R., & Brenner, J. E. (2009). A trade agreement's impact on access to generic drugs. *Health Affairs*, *28*, 957–968.

Sheppard, A. (2010). *Generic medicines: Essential contributors to the long-term health of society*. London: IMS Health. Retrieved from http://www.medicinesforeurope.com/wp-content/uploads/2016/03/IMS_Generic_Medicines_Essential_contributors.pdf.

Timmermans, K. (2005). Intertwining regimes: Trade, intellectual property and regulatory requirements for pharmaceuticals. *The Journal of World Intellectual Property*, *8*, 67–74.

United Nations Conference on Trade and Development and International Centre for Trade and Sustainable Development (UNCTAD-ICTSD). (2005). *Resource book on TRIPS and development: An authoritative and practical guide to the TRIPS agreement*. New York: Cambridge University Press.

World Health Organization. (2006). *Data exclusivity and other "TRIPS-PLUS" measures. WHO Briefing Note: Access to medicines*. Retrieved from http://www.searo.who.int/entity/intellectual_property/data-exclusively-and-others-measures-briefing-note-on-access-to-medicines-who-2006.pdf.

World Health Organization. (2011). *Marketing authorization of pharmaceutical products with special reference to multisource (generic) products: A manual for national medicines regulatory authorities* (2nd ed.). Geneva: World Health Organization.

SECTION 6

RATIONAL AND RESPONSIBLE MEDICINE USE IN LOW- AND MIDDLE-INCOME COUNTRIES

CHAPTER

14

MISCONCEPTIONS AND MISUSE OF MEDICINES IN DEVELOPING COUNTRIES

Pathiyil Ravi Shankar

American International Medical University, Gros Islet, Saint Lucia

CHAPTER OUTLINE

INTRODUCTION

Problems have been noted with the use of medicines by prescribers, dispensers, consumers, and other individuals, all over the world. Although fewer studies have been conducted regarding medicine use in developing countries, available evidence seems to show that problems with medicine use may be more common in developing countries. The authors of a study published in 2001 mention that developing countries waste a large amount of their scarce healthcare resources on medicines of doubtful therapeutic value (Homedes, Ugalde, & Chaumont, 2001). Physician's instructions are often not followed by patients, and self-medication is common. Complementary and alternative medicines (CAMs) are widely used along with western, allopathic medicines in developing nations (Mathez-Stiefel, Vandebroek, & Rist, 2012; Shaikh & Hatcher, 2005; Shankar, Partha, & Shenoy, 2002). CAMs are widely regarded by populations as safe and having little or no adverse effects and more in tune with the traditional belief systems and cultural values of the population. Adverse drug reactions (ADRs) have, however, been reported with complementary medicines in the literature (Niang et al., 2015; Stickel & Shouval, 2015). There have been reports of interactions between prescribed allopathic medicines and complementary remedies (Calitz et al., 2014).

Social and Administrative Aspects of Pharmacy in Low- and Middle-Income Countries. http://dx.doi.org/10.1016/B978-0-12-811228-1.00014-5

The author will examine the situation with regard to the rational and responsible use of medicines in developing nations in this chapter. The objectives of this chapter are as follows:

1. To provide an overview of the medicine use situation in developing countries
2. To highlight misconceptions about and the improper use of medicines by prescribers and consumers in developing countries
3. To mention a selection of successful interventions to promote the rational use of medicines (RUM)
4. To enumerate challenges in promoting the RUM
5. To put forward recommendations to improve the use of medicines in developing countries

THE MEDICINE USE SITUATION IN DEVELOPING COUNTRIES

As mentioned in the introduction, problems have been noted with the use of medicines in both developed and developing nations. As the focus of this book is on developing countries, in this section a selection of studies dealing with medicine use in developing nations will be examined.

Medicines are stored in households to treat future illnesses and chronic diseases among family members. These medicines may also be used by neighbors and extended family members. Studies have shown that often medicines are improperly stored and households were not aware about the proper indications and use of these medications. A study conducted among urban households in Iran found that medicines were widely stored in households, and medicines acting on the central nervous system, antiinfectives, and gastrointestinal medications were commonly stored (Zargarzadeh, Tavakoli, & Hassanzadeh, 2005). According to the authors, the real wastage of medicines was around 40% in these households. A similar situation was noted in Saudi Arabia and other Gulf countries according to a study published in 2003 (Abou-Auda, 2003). Families had spent approximately USD 150 million on medicines that were never consumed in the Gulf region, which was a cause for concern.

Self-medication is commonly observed in developing countries, and consumers often lack adequate knowledge about the medicines they use to self-medicate. Self-medication is using drugs that have not been prescribed, recommended, or controlled by a licensed healthcare practitioner. According to the results of a study conducted in Chile, 75% of consumers surveyed in community pharmacies self-medicate and nonsteroidal antiinflammatory drugs were the most common drug group used (Fuentes Albarrán & Villa Zapata, 2008). Most consumers used medicines without a proper knowledge of the medicines' benefits, treatment effects, and duration. In a study conducted in the Pokhara valley, western Nepal self-medication and nondoctor prescribing were commonly noted (Shankar et al., 2002). Paracetamol and antimicrobials were commonly used, and herbal remedies were often used along with allopathic medicines. Medicines, especially antimicrobials, were not taken for the proper duration of time.

The availability, accessibility, and prescribing patterns of medicines were studied in the Islamic Republic of Iran (Cheraghali et al., 2004). The stock-out duration for essential medicines in health facilities was less than 1 month on an average, and the prescription of antibiotics and injectables was very high (58% and 41%, respectively). Table 14.1 highlights some of the major medicine use problems in developing countries.

To sum up, medicines are often stored in households, but the general public lacks information about their proper use. Self-medication is common and allopathic medicines are often used together with CAM remedies.

Table 14.1 Major Medicine Use Problems in Developing Nations

Major Medicine Use Problems	Studies Cited in This Chapter
Widespread storage of medicines in household medicine cabinets; improper knowledge about medicines	Zargarzadeh et al. (2005) and Abou-Auda (2003)
Problems with self-medication	Fuentes Albarrán and Villa Zapata (2008), Shankar et al. (2002), Okumura et al. (2002), Saradamma et al. (2000), Yusuff and Omarusehe (2011), Ocan et al. (2015), Ocan et al. (2014), and Mesko et al., 2003
Problems with medicine prescribing and dispensing at health facilities	Cheraghali et al. (2004), Fadare et al. (2015), Kamuhabwa and Silumbe (2013), Fenta et al. (2013), Siddiqi et al. (2002), Adebayo and Hussain (2009), Hazra et al. (2000), Ghimire et al. (2009), Alam et al. (2006), Shankar et al. (2006), and Shankar et al. (2003)
Deficiencies in knowledge, attitude, and practice regarding adverse drug reactions of medicines	Jose et al. (2011, 2013, 2014)
Improper use of antibiotics	Md Rezal et al. (2015)
Misconceptions about generic medicines	Basak and Sathyanarayana (2012)
Use of complementary and alternative medicine remedies concurrently with allopathic medicines	O'Connell et al. (2012) and Metta et al., 2014
Dispensing doctors	Trap and Hansen (2002a), Trap and Hansen (2002b), Lim et al. (2009), Shafie et al. (2012) and Tiong et al. (2016)
Inappropriate drug donations	van Dijk et al. (2011)

MISCONCEPTIONS ABOUT MEDICINES AMONG PRESCRIBERS, DISPENSERS, AND CONSUMERS

Because of various reasons, misconceptions about medicines exist among prescribers, dispensers, and consumers in developing nations. In this section, some of these misconceptions will be examined using a selection of studies from the literature with a focus on generic medicines, attitudes toward CAMs, self-medication practices, and knowledge and attitudes toward ADRs.

A cross-sectional study was conducted in Oman to study the knowledge, beliefs, and behaviors of an Omani population with regard to ADRs of medicines (Jose, Jimmy, Al-Mamari, Al-Hadrami, & Al-Zadjali, 2015). Nearly half of the participants believed that ADRs occur only with high doses of allopathic medicines and over 30% were of the opinion that they did not occur with traditional and over-the-counter (OTC) medicines. Participants obtained knowledge about medicines from various sources with doctors being the most widely used source. Another study examined knowledge, belief, and behavior toward antibiotic use in an Omani population (Jose, Jimmy, Alsabahi, & Al Sabei, 2013). The authors observed a moderate knowledge and behavior score while the belief scores of the participants were low. Antibiotics were frequently used by the public, and inappropriate beliefs and behaviors were noted, which according to the authors may reflect inadequate knowledge.

The knowledge, beliefs, and behavior of the Malaysian general population with regard to the adverse effects of medicines were studied (Jose, Chong, Lynn, Jye, & Jimmy, 2011). Knowledge of the respondents was moderate and was influenced by educational level and previous experience of ADRs. Respondents underestimated the risk potential of complementary medicines and OTC medicines. A cross-sectional study conducted in Oman assessed the knowledge, attitude, and behavior about ADRs among community pharmacists (CPs) (Jose, Jimmy, Al-Ghailani, & Al Majali, 2014). The results showed that CPs responded incorrectly to some important and practical questions regarding ADR reporting. A systematic review of the literature published in 2015 examined physicians' knowledge, perceptions, and behavior toward antibiotic prescribing (Md Rezal et al., 2015). The authors concluded that physicians still demonstrated inadequate knowledge and misconceptions about antibiotic prescribing. Patients' expectations, duration and severity of the infection, uncertainty about diagnosis, fear of losing patients, and the influence of pharmaceutical promotion were mentioned as important factors influencing the use of antibiotics.

Generic medicines have been highlighted as an important measure to reduce costs and improve medicine use. Studies, however, have revealed apprehensions and misconceptions about generic medicines among various stakeholders involved in medicine use. Knowledge and perception regarding generic medicines was studied among CPs and drug retailers in Tamil Nadu, India (Basak & Sathyanarayana, 2012). About 30% of the respondents did not know what generic medicines were, and about the same percentage were of the opinion that they were inferior to branded medicines. Pharmacists with a higher level of education had better knowledge and the majority did not support generic substitution.

Community beliefs about diseases and medicine can influence their treatment seeking behavior and concordance with therapy. A study conducted in Cambodia showed that the population initially treated malaria at home using home remedies and traditional medicines (O'Connell et al., 2012). A cocktail of medicines from trusted providers was regarded as more effective and cheaper compared with prepackaged medicines. The authors concluded that cultural beliefs, practical factors, and episode-related issues influence malaria treatment. An exploratory, qualitative study of consumers' perceptions regarding modern medicines was conducted in Penang, Malaysia (Babar et al., 2012). Many respondents were able to correctly mention the major characteristics of modern medicines. They had doubts about the safety, quality, and efficacy of modern medicines. Many stated that they would stop taking the medicines once they started feeling better and mentioned that color was a strong determinant of the safety and characteristics of a medicine. In southeastern Tanzania, respondents self-treated malaria at home using both local herbs and western medicines (Metta, Haisma, Kessy, Hutter, & Bailey, 2014). Self-medication with a pain killer was the initial response followed by the use of local herbs. The easy availability of facilities for diagnosis and treatment of malaria motivated self-treatment using monotherapy. The recommended combination of artemether–lumefantrine was less used because of doubts about ADRs and effectiveness.

In this section, misconceptions about medicines in developing countries were discussed. There were problems noted with regard to ADRs, and a large percentage of respondents believed CAM remedies did not cause ADRs. Misconceptions regarding antibiotics were also noted. Respondents had doubts about generic medicines and did not regard them as equivalent to brand name medicines. Consumers in many studies continued to have doubts about modern medicines.

IMPROPER USE OF MEDICINES BY PRESCRIBERS IN DEVELOPING COUNTRIES

Many studies have evaluated the prescribing practices of doctors and other prescribers at various levels of healthcare in developing nations. Problems were observed in most studies and some of these are mentioned below.

Drug utilization was noted to be generally good during a study conducted at selected health facilities in the Oromia region of Ethiopia (Kebede, Kebebe Borga, & Mulisa Bobasa, 2015). Majority of the prescribers studied had access to up-to-date drug information, considered cost of the drugs while prescribing, and followed the standard treatment guidelines (STGs) of Ethiopia. Certain deviations from rational prescribing were, however, noted by the investigators. In Nigeria, drug prescribing pattern among under-fives was studied (Fadare, Olatunya, Oluwayemi, & Ogundare, 2015). Antibiotics were overprescribed, injections overused, and majority of medicines prescribed using brand names. Antimalarial drug prescribing practices were studied at public health facilities in Dar es Salaam, Tanzania (Kamuhabwa & Silumbe, 2013). Many prescriptions contained antimalarial medicines, which have been declared ineffective for malaria treatment in Tanzania, and antibiotics and analgesics were used unnecessarily with antimalarials.

Prescribing of antibacterial drugs according to different categories of prescribers was studied in Bahir Dar, Ethiopia (Fenta, Belay, & Mekonnen, 2013). Antibacterial drugs were prescribed in a significant number of patient encounters, but there was no significant difference in antibacterial prescribing according to the duration of training and categories of prescribers. The prescribing practices of prescribers in the private and public health sectors were compared in the Attock district of Pakistan (Siddiqi et al., 2002). Most prescribing indicators were worse in the private sector. The mean number of drugs was 4.1 for the private sector compared with 2.7 for the public sector. Injection use was much higher in the private sector, and oral rehydration salts were prescribed less frequently in the private sector. Another study of drug prescribing practices in a Nigerian military hospital revealed a number of problems (Adebayo & Hussain, 2009). The average number of drugs per encounter was higher than that noted in other African studies, and only about 44% of drugs were prescribed using generic names, which was low. A large number of patients were prescribed antibiotics and injections.

In certain countries, doctors not only prescribe medicines but also dispense the prescribed medicines to their patients. The issue of "dispensing doctors" has received a lot of attention, and studies carried out suggest that lack of separation of prescribing and dispensing may lead to irrational use of medicines. In Zimbabwe, the rationality of cotrimoxazole prescribing by dispensing and nondispensing doctors was studied (Trap & Hansen, 2002a). There was no significant difference between the two groups of prescribers with regard to the rationality of prescribing cotrimoxazole. Both groups had prescribed the drug for diagnoses and symptoms where the use could not be justified. The same authors compared the treatment of upper respiratory infections among dispensing and nondispensing doctors (Trap & Hansen, 2002b). Dispensing doctors prescribed a greater number of medicines and more injections and used more analgesics. The authors concluded that symptomatic treatment with a drug for each symptom was commonly practiced especially by dispensing doctors. Antibiotics were overprescribed, and drugs were often used in subtherapeutic doses. A systematic review of the literature comparing the practices of prescribing and nonprescribing doctors was published in 2009 (Lim, Emery, Lewis, & Sunderland, 2009). Twenty-one published papers were included in the review, and the authors concluded that dispensing doctors prescribed more medicines and more commonly prescribed using brand names. Patient convenience was mentioned as a major reason why doctors dispensed, but the dispensing role should be balanced against scarce medical resources being utilized for dispensing.

Prescribing activities at outpatient facilities maintained by a nongovernmental organization (NGO) in West Bengal, India, were studied (Hazra, Tripathi, & Alam, 2000). An average of 3.2 drugs were prescribed per patient and only about 46% of drugs were prescribed using generic names. Antibiotics and irrational fixed-dose combinations were frequently used. Free or subsidized health camps are often organized by the government and NGOs in developing nations. There are not many published studies in the literature examining the quality of prescribing and dispensing during these camps. Drug prescribing patterns were studied during a free health camp organized in western Nepal (Thapa, Thapa, Parajuli-Baral, & Khan, 2015). The number of drugs prescribed was 1.6, and 21.4% of the medicines were antibiotics. Over 90% of medicines were prescribed using generic names. Drug donations to developing countries may be carried out due to various reasons. The literature shows that a number of drug donations were inappropriate, and in 1999, the World Health Organization (WHO) published the "Guidelines for drug donations." A study published in 2011 found problems with drug donations in many emergency situations (van Dijk, Dinant, & Jacobs, 2011). Donations were regarded as inappropriate if there were essential medicines in excessive quantities, mixed unused drugs, and drug dumping (large quantities of useless drugs). These inappropriate donations may promote the irrational use of medicines.

Another study conducted in a teaching hospital in Nepal revealed problems in medicine use (Ghimire, Nepal, Bhandari, Nepal, & Palaian, 2009). Only 13% of medicines were prescribed using generic names and only about 33% of medicines were prescribed from the essential medicines list of Nepal. A similar situation was noted in another study conducted in the same hospital (Alam et al., 2006). Prescribing patterns among inpatients in a teaching hospital in western Nepal were studied (Shankar, Upadhyay, Subish, Dubey, & Mishra, 2006). The mean number of medicines prescribed per admission was 4.5; nearly 50% were prescribed by the parenteral route, and antibiotics were prescribed in nearly 70% of admissions. In the intensive treatment unit of a teaching hospital, about half of the patients received an antimicrobial and over 84% of the antimicrobials were prescribed without obtaining bacteriological evidence of infection (Shankar, Partha, Shenoy, & Brahmadathan, 2003).

Improper use of medicines by prescribers was discussed in this section. Polypharmacy, overuse of antibiotics and injections, and prescribing using brand names were some of the problems. Problems were also noticed in antimalarial treatment. Lack of separation between prescribing and dispensing and "dispensing doctors" are present in some countries. Inappropriate drug donations may contribute to irrational use, and prescribing in both primary health facilities and tertiary care hospitals was studied.

MISUSE OF MEDICINES BY CONSUMERS IN DEVELOPING COUNTRIES

Various medicine use problems have been noted among consumers in developing nations. Problems with the use of antibiotics, analgesics, and potential interactions from concomitant use of allopathic and CAM remedies have been observed. Self-medication carried out responsibly for certain self-limiting illnesses has been recommended as saving resources and improving self-care. But inappropriate self-medication carries a number of risks including adverse effects, drug interactions, and the development of antimicrobial resistance (AMR). In this section a selection of published studies dealing with the use of medicines by consumers and self-medication practices from developing nations will be examined.

In 2002 about 40–60% of the Vietnamese population were dependent on self-medication. A sample of women with at least one child younger than 5 years of age were interviewed in their homes about their medication practices (Okumura, Wakai, & Umenai, 2002). About 25% of households stocked medicines for future illness, and self-medication increased when the mother kept medicines at home. The authors mention that mothers used antibiotics as if those drugs were panaceas. Self-medication with antibiotics is common in developing countries according to the scientific literature. The magnitude of self-medication with antibiotics and factors influencing this practice was studied in Kerala, South India (Saradamma, Higginbotham, & Nichter, 2000). About 69% of households had a family member using a pharmaceutical product during the 2-week recall period, and antibiotics formed almost 11% of the consumed medicines. The authors concluded that about 4 persons of 1000 used antibiotics without a prescription in the state during a 2-week period. Families with better education, higher incomes, and higher status occupations were less likely to use antibiotics without a prescription. Determinants of self-medication practices were studied among pregnant women in Ibadan, Nigeria (Yusuff & Omarusehe, 2011). Both allopathic and herbal medicines were used as the first response to ill health by a significant majority of the respondents. The most frequent source of medicines was medicine stores, and mothers-in-law and relatives were most frequently cited sources of advice. Only 32% of respondents could identify medicines, which could be potentially harmful during pregnancy.

A systematic review and meta-analysis of household antimicrobial self-medication examining its burden, risk factors, and outcomes in developing countries was recently published (Ocan et al., 2015). The overall prevalence of self-medication with antimicrobials was 38.8%, and common symptoms managed were respiratory, fever, and gastrointestinal problems. Level of education, age, gender, history of successful antimicrobial use, severity of illness, and income were determinants of self-medication. A cross-sectional survey of teachers was conducted in Yemen, Saudi Arabia, and Uzbekistan to study antibiotic use and knowledge (Belkina et al., 2014). According to the authors, the prevalence of non-prescription antibiotic use ranged from 48% in Saudi Arabia to 78% in Yemen and Uzbekistan. Cough and influenza were the most common reasons for the use of antibiotics, and nearly half the respondents discontinued antibiotics once they started feeling better. Patterns and predictors of self-medication in northern Uganda were recently studied (Ocan et al., 2014). Over 75% of the respondents were practicing antimicrobial self-medication, and drug use was initiated mainly by self-medication and by medicine shop attendants. Risks associated with self-medication, including wastage of money, drug resistance, and masking symptoms of an underlying disease, were reported by 76% of respondents. Care for perinatal illness was studied in rural Nepal (Mesko et al., 2003). Women usually sought care within the household, and self-medication was common. Patients usually consulted traditional healers, and there was delay in seeking care from the allopathic healthcare system.

In this section the misuse of medicines by consumers was examined. Inappropriate self-medication and lack of adequate knowledge about medicines remain major problems. Self-medication with antibiotics is especially dangerous. Teachers can play an important role in promoting RUM. Low knowledge, attitude, and practice (KAP) scores among teachers were noted in some studies, but the scores improved following an educational intervention.

ACHIEVEMENTS: SUCCESSFUL INTERVENTIONS TO PROMOTE THE RATIONAL USE OF MEDICINES

Healthcare practitioners, health administrators, and health policy makers have recognized the importance of promoting RUM to reduce medicine and healthcare costs, decrease adverse drug events and reactions, and reduce the development of AMR. In this section a selection of successful interventions to reduce misuse and promote RUM in developing countries will be mentioned. Table 14.2 provides a selection of successful interventions, which have been carried out to improve the use of medicines.

A study published in 2015 mentions some of the measures adopted to promote the quality use of medicines in Malaysia and highlights the need for strengthening these initiatives (Mohd-Tahir, Paraidathathu, & Li, 2015). The authors mention that Malaysia has adopted some of the concepts of rational medicine use such as adopting a national essential medicines list (NEML) and promoting generic medicines in their health policy. A more equitable and rational distribution of healthcare resources and a more progressive and sustainable system of healthcare financing were recommended. The authors conclude that Malaysia has achieved good population health outcomes using fewer resources since independence. The impact of essential medicine lists (EMLs), STGs, and prescriber restrictions on improving the RUM in Papua New Guinea was studied (Joshua, Passmore, & Sunderland, 2016). All drugs mentioned in the STGs for the treatment of the chronic diseases studied were mentioned in the medical and dental catalog, which serves as the EML for the country. Many medicines recommended in the STGs had prescriber restrictions, which limited access to those living in the remote and rural areas of the country.

Growing costs of medicines put increasing strain on resources in both developed and developing countries. Caps (maximum numbers of prescriptions or medicines that are reimbursed), fixed copayments (patients pay a fixed amount per prescription or medicine), coinsurance (patients pay a percentage of the price), ceilings (patients pay the full price or part of the cost up to a ceiling, after which medicines are free or are available at reduced cost), and tier copayments (differential copayments usually assigned to generic and brand medicines) are different strategies used to reduce medicine

Table 14.2 Successful Interventions to Improve the Use of Medicines

Intervention	Country/Region	Group Involved/Describing the Interventions
Adopting national essential medicines list, promoting generic medicines	Malaysia	Mohd-Tahir and coworkers
Essential medicine lists, standard treatment guidelines, prescriber restrictions	Papua New Guinea	Joshua and coworkers
Caps, fixed copayments, coinsurance, ceilings, tier copayments		Luiza and coworkers
Accredited drug dispensing outlets	Tanzania	Valimba and coworkers
Improving antibiotic prescribing in children	Resource limited settings	Le Doare and coworkers
Removing economic incentives for overprescribing	China	Chen and coworkers
Educational sessions for medical students on RUM	Brazil	Patricio and coworkers
Prescribing skills assessment for newly graduated doctor	United Kingdom	Selvaskandan and Baheerathan
Educating medical students to use essential medicines rationally	Nepal	Shankar and coworkers
Focused training to informal drug sellers	Nepal	Kafle and coworkers
Improving knowledge, attitude, and practice of school teachers about medicines	Nepal	Jha and coworkers

consumption and resource utilization. A recent systematic review examined the impact of these policies (Luiza et al., 2015). The reviewers concluded that cap and copayment policies may reduce medicine use and the expenditure on medicines for health insurers. However, they also found that these could reduce the use of medicines in life-threatening conditions and in chronic diseases. In Tanzania, a public–private partnership launched the accredited drug dispensing outlet program to improve medicine access and use and pharmaceutical care services in rural areas (Valimba et al., 2014). Posters, sensitizing providers on issues related to AMR, training, and onsite support were provided. The authors concluded that the intervention significantly improved community medicine use and could possibly reduce AMR. A recent article examined initiatives for improving antibiotic prescribing for children in resource-poor settings (Le Doare, Barker, Irwin, & Sharland, 2015). The authors highlight WHO initiatives such as "Make medicines child size," and the model list of medicines and the model formulary for children as significant steps forward.

Economic reasons, for example, greater profit from greater prescribing of medicines, can be an important reason for irrational prescribing. For example, in Malaysia, private medical practitioners were able to dispense medicines diluting the role of CPs because of overlapping roles (Shafie, Hassali, Azhar, & See, 2012). An article published in 2016 examines the two-tier system operating in Malaysia at present and highlights how separation of prescribing and dispensing has only been implemented in government hospitals (Tiong, Mai, Gan, Johnson, & Mak, 2016). The authors conclude that the absence of this separation in the private sector has led to possible profit-oriented practices in both medical and pharmacy sectors and may hinder rational and cost-effective service delivery. In China, before the implementation of a new round of healthcare reforms, healthcare providers could obtain a markup of 10% or more by prescribing and selling medicines (Chen et al., 2014). Chen et al. studied prescribing patterns before and after the economic incentive was removed. They found no significant difference in prescribing indicators overall, but differences were noted for certain specific diseases.

The focus of this section was on interventions to promote RUM. At a national level, NEML, STGs, and use of generic medicines are important. Increasing cost of medicines puts increasing strain on resources, and measures have been taken to address this problem. In developing countries, the nonformal sector meets a large percentage of medicine needs and a system of training and accreditation of informal drug sellers has shown promise. Removing economic incentives for prescribing has also been carried out.

ROLE OF EDUCATION IN IMPROVING THE USE OF MEDICINES

Education directed at health professions students, healthcare practitioners, patients, and the general public can play an important role in promoting RUM. Using medicines rationally and cost-effectively is gaining increasing recognition in the undergraduate medical curriculum, and many courses have been developed based on the WHO publications "Guide to good prescribing" and "Teacher's guide to good prescribing.". At a medical school in Brazil, a module on RUM is being conducted for medical students (Patrício, Alves, Arenales, & Queluz, 2012). The authors concluded that students liked the teaching methodology employed and the opportunity provided to reflect on various factors involved in the prescribing process. However, former students, who were now working as doctors in training or in practice, thought that senior medical staff were often not in favor of RUM concepts, and they were not always allowed to implement the lessons they had learned.

The British Pharmacological Society has been involved in developing an online prescribing skills assessment for students who have completed their medical training in the United Kingdom (Selvaskandan & Baheerathan, 2014). At a medical school in Nepal, 10 basic competencies for undergraduate pharmacology education have been identified (Shankar, 2011). These are mostly related to rational prescribing and educating patients to use medicines rationally.

The WHO office for South-East Asia has published a book dealing with the role of education in the RUM (WHO SEARO, 2006). The book examines the role of public education, education for health professionals, and education for policy makers. Education for the general public can be provided through street plays, use of various media, and patient information leaflets. Examples of community-oriented programs and programs targeting special groups such as women, women's groups, and mothers are provided in the book. In developing nations, nonpharmacists play an important role in dispensing and selling medicines. In Nepal, focused training was provided to drug sellers concentrating on treating upper respiratory infections, diarrhea in children, and anemia during pregnancy (Kafle et al., 2013). The authors concluded that training intervention as well as training followed by practice feedback was effective in improving the management of common illnesses and pregnancy by private drug sellers.

School teachers occupy an important position as educated individuals in many communities and can play an important role in promoting RUM. In Lalitpur district of Nepal, KAP of school teachers about medicines was studied before and after an educational intervention (Jha, Bajracharya, & Shankar, 2013). A combination of methods including brainstorming sessions, presentations, interactive discussions using posters, and distribution of medicine information leaflets was successful in improving the knowledge and attitude of teachers. An overview of systematic reviews of interventions to promote the safe and effective use of medicines by consumers was recently published (Ryan et al., 2014). The reviews assessed diverse interventions ranging from support for behavioral change, risk minimization, and skills acquisition. Medicines self-monitoring and self-management programs appear generally effective to improve medicines use, concordance with treatment, adverse events, and clinical outcomes. Interventions involving pharmacists in medicine management and provision of pharmaceutical care were recommended as requiring further study. Strategies providing only education or information were not effective in improving medicines adherence/concordance and clinical outcomes but may improve knowledge, which is important for promoting informed medicine choices by consumers. In an article Ryan & Hill (2016) examined interventions, which can best support consumers to use medicines rationally. They identified a relatively small number of interventions as effective and mention self-monitoring and self-management programs, simplified dosing regimens, and pharmacist-delivered medication review. The individual's context and preferences should be considered while designing interventions.

The WHO book on education about RUM also mentions different methods, which can be used to educate policy makers, political leaders, bureaucrats, and planners. Among these are using mass media, inviting policy makers to various programs and events related to RUM, instituting a special day to promote RUM, and having ready a brief presentation about the topic and fact sheets ready for distribution.

In this section the role of education in promoting RUM was discussed. For health professions students, courses based on the WHO publication "Guide to good prescribing" are becoming increasingly common. Prescribing skills of newly graduated doctors are being assessed in some countries. Education of the public and of policy makers and politicians is important. School teachers can play an important role in educating school children and the general public. Pharmacists have an important role in educating patients about their medicines.

Table 14.3 Important Challenges in Promoting the Rational Use of Medicines in Developing Countries

Challenges
High cost of new medicines especially antimicrobials, anti-HIV medicines, and medicines for diabetes and cancer
Access to medicines for HIV, cancer, and TB
Adoption of stronger intellectual property rights
Aggressive pharmaceutical promotion
Misperceptions about generic medicines
Improper use of antibiotics
Problems with self-medication

CHALLENGES IN PROMOTING THE RATIONAL USE OF MEDICINES

Some of these challenges have been mentioned in preceding sections. Newer medicines are usually priced at a premium, and even developed nations are struggling to finance access for their populations to these medicines. Only few of these new medicines can be considered as "innovative," and the requested reimbursement prices for new medicines are high especially for oncology, orphan diseases, diabetes, and other diseases (Godman et al., 2015). The selection process of oncology medicines in low- and middle-income countries (LMICs) was recently studied (Bazargani, de Boer, Schellens, Leufkens, & Mantel-Teeuwisse, 2014). The overall median number of oncology medicines on NEMLs was 16, and the authors concluded that the list may reflect inadequacies and inequalities in access to oncology medicines at least in the public sector of LMICs. Access to antiretroviral medicines remains a challenge; however, the situation has improved recently including the development of newer medicines and simpler, affordable treatment regimens (Ford & Calmy, 2010). Table 14.3 mentions important challenges with regard to promoting the RUM in developing countries.

Achievements and challenges with regard to RUM were examined in an article published in 2010 (Thawani, 2010). The author mentions that RUM in a country is influenced by the national medicine policies. The author mentions that adoption of stronger intellectual property rights may hamper access to medicines.

RECOMMENDATIONS: THE WAY FORWARD

Promoting and maintaining RUM is a journey and not a destination. There are many challenges to be addressed and overcome while promoting RUM. Promoting RUM in developing countries may be more challenging than in developed nations due to a variety of reasons. However, promoting RUM is extremely important because these countries waste a large amount of scarce resources on medicines of doubtful value. Although data on medicine utilization in the developing world are less compared with developed nations, an increasing number of studies are being conducted on this subject and are being published. Bibliographic journal sources such as African Journals Online (AJOL, www.ajol.info) and Nepal Journals Online (NepJOL, www.nepjol.info) have helped in ensuring access to full texts of published articles. Increasingly many universities and other organizations in the developing world are creating online sites and portals for readers to access their dissertations and publications.

Table 14.4 Recommendations to Improve the Use of Medicines

Recommendations
Access to scientific studies dealing with medicine use in developing nations
Conferences and workshops to share information and promote RUM
Training "informal" medicine prescribers and dispensers
Educating the public about RUM
Educating key community leaders and stakeholders about RUM
Strengthening "marginalized" community groups and educating and empowering them
Educating healthcare professionals and health science students about RUM
Understanding and responding to pharmaceutical promotion
Ensuring and strengthening access to objective sources of medicine information
Prescribing restrictions for antimicrobials

The HINARI initiative established by the WHO in association with major publishers and other agencies provides either free or low cost access to journals, textbooks, and other publications to researchers in developing countries. All universities, schools, and colleges in eligible countries should utilize the "rich" resources provided by the portal. International conferences on improving the use of medicines bring together researchers and other stakeholders from a number of nations. Various studies dealing with the RUM in developing nations can be collated together and analyzed, and recommendations can be provided if possible to practitioners. Table 14.4 mentions recommendations to improve the use of medicines.

In developing nations a number of individuals who are not formally trained in modern western healthcare are involved in prescribing and dispensing medicines. Traditional medicine practitioners, persons who have little training in healthcare, and compounders may be among these individuals. Training programs for these individuals may be useful in promoting RUM. Also in developing countries, self-medication by individuals and/or use of medicines based on advice from family members and other community members is common. Providing education to the public about RUM is important. Ensuring that the educational material and sessions is tailored to the level of the respondents is important. Although the percentage is decreasing, even today, a large number of individuals are illiterate or have only a basic level of education. Educational sessions for these individuals should use more of visual material and provide a simplified but correct view of complex concepts. In addition, women play an important role in medicine use by households and in treatment of children. Because of social, religious, and community norms, women may be more reluctant to attend training sessions, and the possibility of conducting special sessions for them utilizing female resource persons can be considered.

In developing countries, doctors, pharmacists, and nurses are regarded by patients as the most authoritative and reliable sources of medicine information. Health professionals should be educated about RUM, prescribing, dispensing, and counseling patients about their disease and the use of medicines. They should be aware about objective, unbiased sources of medicine information and about presenting information in a simple manner to patients. Communities may sometimes have inaccurate beliefs about disease and medicines, which may have to be corrected using a nonconfrontational approach. Involving local community members may facilitate this process. The pharmaceutical industry has a strong influence on prescribing and dispensing, and health professionals should be taught during their education to understand and respond to pharmaceutical promotion in an appropriate manner. Hospitals and clinics should regulate access of health professionals to pharmaceutical sales representatives, and if possible, academic detailing sessions can be conducted.

Many developing countries utilize paramedical personnel to provide healthcare in primary care settings. These personnel should undergo periodic training, and the conditions which they can treat and the medicines they can prescribe should be clearly described. To reduce the risk of AMR, countries and regions have placed restrictions on the antimicrobials, which can be prescribed by different categories of prescribers with newer, reserve antimicrobials requiring approval from an infectious disease specialist.

CONCLUSIONS

Problems with the RUM have been noted in both developed and developing nations. Because of various reasons, these problems may be more pressing in developing countries. In this chapter a selection of studies examining the medicine use situation in developing nations were examined. Improper storage of medicines in household medicine cabinets and their irrational use are an important medicine use problem. Self-medication is common.

Using studies from the literature, misconceptions about medicines among prescribers, dispensers, and consumers were examined with a special emphasis on generic medicines, CAM, self-medication, and ADRs. Following this the misuse of medicines by prescribers was explored, and although some studies mentioned that the use of medicines was generally good, problems were noted in other studies. Overuse of antibiotics and injections, polypharmacy, and prescribing using brand names were the major problems. With regard to the use of medicines by consumers, problems were noted with the use of antibiotics, analgesics, and potential interactions resulting from the concomitant use of allopathic and complementary medicines. AMR is an important consequence of improper use of these medicines by consumers.

A selection of interventions, which have been carried out to promote RUM, were examined. Education plays an important role in promoting proper use of medicines, and educational initiatives directed at health science students, healthcare professionals, the general public, and politicians and policy makers were highlighted. In the last part of the chapter, recommendations to promote RUM in developing countries were put forward.

LESSONS LEARNED

- Irrational use of medicines continues to be an important problem in developing nations.
- Prescribers, dispensers, and consumers all have an important role to play in promoting the RUM.
- Polypharmacy, overuse of antibiotics and injections, prescribing using brand names, and concomitant use of allopathic and complementary remedies are among the major medicine use problems.
- There have been many successful interventions in developing nations to promote the RUM.
- Education of healthcare professionals, general public, special groups, policy makers, and politicians is important to ensure medicines are used properly.

REFERENCES

Abou-Auda, H. S. (2003). An economic assessment of the extent of medication use and wastage among families in Saudi Arabia and Arabian Gulf countries. *Clinical Therapeutics*, *25*, 1276–1292.

Adebayo, E. T., & Hussain, N. A. (2009). A baseline study of drug prescribing practices in a Nigerian military hospital. *Nigerian Journal of Clinical Practice*, *12*, 268–272.

Alam, K., Mishra, P., Prabhu, M., Shankar, P. R., Palaian, S., Bhandari, R. B., & Bista, D. (2006). A study on rational drug prescribing and dispensing in outpatients in a tertiary care teaching hospital of Western Nepal. *Kathmandu University Medical Journal*, *4*, 436–443.

Babar, Z. U., Hassali, M. A., Shyong, T. L., Hin, T. K., Cien, C. S., Bin, L. S., & Singh, J. K. (2012). An evaluation of consumers' perceptions regarding "modern medicines" in Penang, Malaysia. *Journal of Young Pharmacists*, *4*, 108–113.

Basak, S. C., & Sathyanarayana, D. (2012). Exploring knowledge and perceptions of generic medicines among drug retailers and community pharmacists. *Indian Journal of Pharmaceutical Sciences*, *74*, 571–575.

Bazargani, Y. T., de Boer, A., Schellens, J. H., Leufkens, H. G., & Mantel-Teeuwisse, A. K. (2014). Selection of oncology medicines in low- and middle-income countries. *Annals of Oncology*, *25*, 270–276.

Belkina, T., Al Warafi, A., Hussein Eltom, E., Tadjieva, N., Kubena, A., & Vlcek, J. (2014). Antibiotic use and knowledge in the community of Yemen, Saudi Arabia, and Uzbekistan. *Journal of Infection in Developing Countries*, *8*, 424–429.

Calitz, C., Steenekamp, J. H., Steyn, J. D., Gouws, C., Viljoen, J. M., & Hamman, J. H. (2014). Impact of traditional African medicine on drug metabolism and transport. *Expert Opinion on Drug Metabolism & Toxicology*, *10*, 991–1003.

Chen, M., Wang, L., Chen, W., Zhang, L., Jiang, H., & Mao, W. (2014). Does economic incentive matter for rational use of medicine? China's experience from the essential medicines program. *Pharmacoeconomics*, *32*, 245–255.

Cheraghali, A. M., Nikfar, S., Behmanesh, Y., Rahimi, V., Habibipour, F., Tirdad, R., … Bahrami, A. (2004). Evaluation of availability, accessibility and prescribing pattern of medicines in the Islamic Republic of Iran. *Eastern Mediterranean Health Journal*, *10*, 406–415.

Fadare, J., Olatunya, O., Oluwayemi, O., & Ogundare, O. (2015). Drug prescribing pattern for under-fives in a paediatric clinic in South-Western Nigeria. *Ethiopian Journal of Health Sciences*, *25*, 73–78.

Fenta, A., Belay, M., & Mekonnen, E. (2013). Assessment of antibacterial drug exposure patterns of patient encounters seen by different categories of prescribers at health institutions in Bahir Dar, Ethiopia. *Ethiopian Medical Journal*, *51*, 33–39.

Ford, N., & Calmy, A. (2010). Improving first-line antiretroviral therapy in resource-limited settings. *Current Opinion in HIV and AIDS*, *5*, 38–47.

Fuentes Albarrán, K., & Villa Zapata, L. (2008). Analysis and quantification of self-medication patterns of customers in community pharmacies in Southern Chile. *Pharmacy World & Science*, *30*, 863–868.

Ghimire, S., Nepal, S., Bhandari, S., Nepal, P., & Palaian, S. (2009). A prospective surveillance of drug prescribing and dispensing in a teaching hospital in western Nepal. *JPMA. the Journal of the Pakistan Medical Association*, *59*, 726–731.

Godman, B., Malmström, R. E., Diogene, E., Gray, A., Jayathissa, S., Timoney, A., Acurcio, F., … Gustafsson, L. L. (2015). Are new models needed to optimize the utilization of new medicines to sustain healthcare systems? *Expert Review of Clinical Pharmacology*, *8*, 77–94.

Hazra, A., Tripathi, S. K., & Alam, M. S. (2000). Prescribing and dispensing activities at the health facilities of a non-governmental organization. *National Medical Journal of India*, *13*, 177–182.

Homedes, N., Ugalde, A., & Chaumont, C. (2001). Scientific evaluations of interventions to improve the adequate use of pharmaceuticals in third world countries. *Public Health Reviews*, *29*, 207–230.

Jha, N., Bajracharya, O., & Shankar, P. R. (2013). Knowledge, attitude and practice towards medicines among school teachers in Lalitpur district, Nepal before and after an educational intervention. *BMC Public Health, 13*, 652.

Jose, J., Chong, D., Lynn, T. S., Jye, G. E., & Jimmy, B. (2011). A survey on the knowledge, beliefs and behaviour of a general adult population in Malaysia with respect to the adverse effects of medicines. *The International Journal of Pharmacy Practice*, *19*, 246–252.

Jose, J., Jimmy, B., Al-Ghailani, A. S., & Al Majali, M. A. (2014). A cross sectional pilot study on assessing the knowledge, attitude and behavior of community pharmacists to adverse drug reaction related aspects in the Sultanate of Oman. *Saudi Pharmaceutical Journal*, *22*, 162–169.

Jose, J., Jimmy, B., Al-Mamari, M. N., Al-Hadrami, T. S., & Al-Zadjali, H. M. (2015). Knowledge, beliefs and behaviours regarding the adverse effects of medicines in an Omani population: Cross-sectional survey. *Sultan Qaboos University Medical Journal*, *15*, e250–e256.

Jose, J., Jimmy, B., Alsabahi, A. G., & Al Sabei, G. A. (2013). A study assessing public knowledge, belief and behavior of antibiotic use in an Omani population. *Oman Medical Journal*, *28*, 324–330.

Joshua, I. B., Passmore, P. R., & Sunderland, B. V. (2016). An evaluation of the Essential Medicines List, Standard Treatment Guidelines and prescribing restrictions, as an integrated strategy to enhance quality, efficacy and safety of and improve access to essential medicines in Papua New Guinea. *Health Policy and Planning*, *31*, 538–546.

Kafle, K. K., Karkee, S. B., Shrestha, N., Prasad, R. R., Bhuju, G. B., Das, P. L., & Ross-Degnan, D. (2013). Improving private drug sellers' practices for managing common health problems in Nepal. *Journal of Nepal Health Research Council*, *11*, 198–204.

Kamuhabwa, A. A., & Silumbe, R. (2013). Knowledge among drug dispensers and antimalarial drug prescribing practices in public health facilities in Dar es Salaam. *Drug, Healthcare and Patient Safety*, *5*, 181–189.

Kebede, M., Kebebe Borga, D., & Mulisa Bobasa, E. (2015). Drug utilization in selected health facilities of south west Shoa Zone, Oromia region, Ethiopia. *Drug, Healthcare and Patient Safety*, *7*, 121–127.

Le Doare, K., Barker, C. I., Irwin, A., & Sharland, M. (2015). Improving antibiotic prescribing for children in the resource-poor setting. *British Journal of Clinical Pharmacology*, *79*, 446–455.

Lim, D., Emery, J., Lewis, J., & Sunderland, V. B. (2009). A systematic review of the literature comparing the practices of dispensing and non-dispensing doctors. *Health Policy*, *92*, 1–9.

Luiza, V. L., Chaves, L. A., Silva, R. M., Emmerick, I. C., Chaves, G. C., Fonseca de Araújo, S. C., & Oxman, A. D. (2015). Pharmaceutical policies: Effects of cap and co-payment on rational use of medicines. *The Cochrane Database of Systematic Reviews*, *5*, CD007017.

Mathez-Stiefel, S. L., Vandebroek, I., & Rist, S. (2012). Can Andean medicine coexist with biomedical healthcare? A comparison of two rural communities in Peru and Bolivia. *Journal of Ethnobiology and Ethnomedicine*, *8*, 26.

Md Rezal, R. S., Hassali, M. A., Alrasheedy, A. A., Saleem, F., Md Yusof, F. A., & Godman, B. (2015). Physicians' knowledge, perceptions and behaviour towards antibiotic prescribing: A systematic review of the literature. *Expert Review of Anti-infective Therapy*, *13*, 665–680.

Mesko, N., Osrin, D., Tamang, S., Shrestha, B. P., Manandhar, D. S., Manandhar, M., … Costello, A. M. (2003). Care for perinatal illness in rural Nepal: A descriptive study with cross-sectional and qualitative components. *BMC International Health and Human Rights*, *3*, 3.

Metta, E., Haisma, H., Kessy, F., Hutter, I., & Bailey, A. (2014). "We have become doctors for ourselves": Motives for malaria self-care among adults in southeastern Tanzania. *Malaria Journal*, *13*, 249.

Mohd-Tahir, N. A., Paraidathathu, T., & Li, S. C. (2015). Quality use of medicine in a developing economy: Measures to overcome challenges in the Malaysian healthcare system. *SAGE Open Medicine*, *3* 2050312115596864.

Niang, S. O., Tine, Y., Diatta, B. A., Diallo, M., Fall, M., Seck, N. B., & Kane, A. (2015). Negative cutaneous effects of medicinal plants in Senegal. *British Journal of Dermatology*, *173*(Suppl. 2), 26–29.

O'Connell, K. A., Samandari, G., Phok, S., Phou, M., Dysoley, L., Yeung, S., … Littrell, M. (2012). "Souls of the ancestor that knock us out" and other tales. A qualitative study to identify demand-side factors influencing malaria case management in Cambodia. *Malaria Journal*, *11*, 335. http://dx.doi.org/10.1186/1475-2875-11-335.

Ocan, M., Bwanga, F., Bbosa, G. S., Bagenda, D., Waako, P., Ogwal-Okeng, J., & Obua, C. (2014). Patterns and predictors of self-medication in northern Uganda. *PLoS One*, *9*, e92323.

Ocan, M., Obuku, E. A., Bwanga, F., Akena, D., Richard, S., Ogwal-Okeng, J., & Obua, C. (2015). Household antimicrobial self-medication: A systematic review and meta-analysis of the burden, risk factors and outcomes in developing countries. *BMC Public Health*, *15*, 742.

Okumura, J., Wakai, S., & Umenai, T. (2002). Drug utilisation and self-medication in rural communities in Vietnam. *Social Science & Medicine*, *54*, 1875–1886.

Patrício, K. P., Alves, N. A., Arenales, N. G., & Queluz, T. T. (2012). Teaching the rational use of medicines to medical students: A qualitative research. *BMC Medical Education*, *12*, 56.

Ryan, R., & Hill, S. (2016). Making rational choices about how best to support consumers' use of medicines: A perspective review. *Therapeutic Advances in Drug Safety*, *7*, 159–164.

Ryan, R., Santesso, N., Lowe, D., Hill, S., Grimshaw, J., Prictor, M., … Taylor, M. (2014). Interventions to improve safe and effective medicines use by consumers: An overview of systematic reviews. *Cochrane Database of Systematic Reviews*, *29*, CD007768.

Saradamma, R. D., Higginbotham, N., & Nichter, M. (2000). Social factors influencing the acquisition of antibiotics without prescription in Kerala State, south India. *Social Science & Medicine*, *50*, 891–903.

Selvaskandan, H., & Baheerathan, A. (2014). .The prescribing skills assessment. *The Clinical Teacher*, *11*, 58–59.

Shafie, A. A., Hassali, M. A., Azhar, S., & See, O. G. (2012). Separation of prescribing and dispensing in Malaysia: A summary of arguments. *Research in Social and Administrative Pharmacy*, *8*, 258–262.

Shaikh, B. T., & Hatcher, J. (2005). Complementary and alternative medicine in Pakistan: Prospects and limitations. *Evidence-based Complementary and Alternative Medicine*, *2*, 139–142.

Shankar, P. R. (2011). Ten basic competencies for undergraduate pharmacology education at KIST Medical College, Lalitpur, Nepal. *Australasian Medical Journal*, *4*, 677–682.

Shankar, P. R., Partha, P., & Shenoy, N. (2002). Self-medication and non-doctor prescribing practices in Pokhara valley, western Nepal: A questionnaire-based study. *BMC Family Practice*, *3*, 17.

Shankar, P. R., Partha, P., Shenoy, N., & Brahmadathan, K. N. (2003). Investigation of antimicrobial use pattern in the intensive treatment unit of a teaching hospital in western Nepal. *American Journal of Infection Control*, *31*, 410–414.

Shankar, P. R., Upadhyay, D. K., Subish, P., Dubey, A. K., & Mishra, P. (2006). Prescribing patterns among paediatric inpatients in a teaching hospital in western Nepal. *Singapore Medical Journal*, *47*, 261–265.

Siddiqi, S., Hamid, S., Rafique, G., Chaudhry, S. A., Ali, N., Shahab, S., & Sauerborn, R. (2002). Prescription practices of public and private health care providers in Attock District of Pakistan. *The International Journal of Health Planning and Management*, *17*, 23–40.

Stickel, F., & Shouval, D. (2015). Hepatotoxicity of herbal and dietary supplements: An update. *Archives of Toxicology*, *89*, 851–865.

Thapa, R. K., Thapa, P., Parajuli-Baral, K., & Khan, G. M. (2015). Disease proportions and drug prescribing pattern observed in a free health camp organized at Dhorphirdi Village Development Committee of Western Nepal. *BMC Research Notes*, *8*, 494.

Thawani, V. (2010). Rational use of medicines: Achievements and challenges. *Indian Journal of Pharmacology*, *42*, 63–64.

Tiong, J. J., Mai, C. W., Gan, P. W., Johnson, J., & Mak, V. S. (2016). Separation of prescribing and dispensing in Malaysia: The history and challenges. *International Journal of Pharmacy Practice*, *24*, 302–305.

Trap, B., & Hansen, E. H. (2002a). Cotrimoxazole prescribing by dispensing and non-dispensing doctors: Do they differ in rationality? *Tropical Medicine and International Health*, *7*, 878–885.

Trap, B., & Hansen, E. H. (2002b). Treatment of upper respiratory tract infections–a comparative study of dispensing and non-dispensing doctors. *Journal of Clinical Pharmacy and Therapeutics*, *27*, 289–298.

Valimba, R., Liana, J., Joshi, M. P., Rutta, E., Embrey, M., Bundala, M., & Kibassa, B. (2014). Engaging the private sector to improve antimicrobial use in the community: Experience from accredited drug dispensing outlets in Tanzania. *Journal of Pharmaceutical Policy and Practice*, *7*, 11.

van Dijk, D. P., Dinant, G., & Jacobs, J. A. (2011). Inappropriate drug donations: What has happened since the 1999 WHO guidelines? *Education for Health (Abingdon)*, *24*, 462.

World Health Organization Regional Office for South-East Asia. (2006). *The role of education in the rational use of medicines. SEARO technical publication series no. 45*. Available from http://apps.who.int/medicinedocs/documents/s16792e/s16792e.pdf.

Yusuff, K. B., & Omarusehe, L. D. (2011). Determinants of self-medication practices among pregnant women in Ibadan, Nigeria. *International Journal of Clinical Pharmacy*, *33*, 868–875.

Zargarzadeh, A. H., Tavakoli, N., & Hassanzadeh, A. (2005). A survey on the extent of medication storage and wastage in urban Iranian households. *Clinical Therapeutics*, *27*, 970–978.

CHAPTER

STRENGTHS AND WEAKNESSES OF PHARMACEUTICAL POLICY IN RELATION TO RATIONAL AND RESPONSIBLE MEDICINES USE

15

Tuan A. Nguyen, Elizabeth E. Roughead

University of South Australia, Adelaide, SA, Australia

CHAPTER OUTLINE

INTRODUCTION

Medicines are key healthcare technologies that play an important role in improving public health outcomes. However, the use of medicines is not without risks. Problems with medicines, also known as medication incidents, are the most common safety issues in healthcare. In the 1985 World Health Organization (WHO) Nairobi Conference of Experts on the Rational Use of Drugs, "rational use of medicines" was defined as "patients receive medications appropriate to their clinical needs, in doses that meet their own individual requirements, for an adequate period of time, and at the lowest cost to them and their community" (WHO, 1985). Irrational use of medicines occurs when one or more of these conditions are not met (Holloway & van Dijk, 2011).

To complement the 1985 WHO's definition of rational use of medicines, a new term "responsible use of medicines" has been developed. It implies that "the activities, capabilities and existing resources of health system stakeholders are aligned to ensure patients receive the right medicines at the right time,

Social and Administrative Aspects of Pharmacy in Low- and Middle-Income Countries. http://dx.doi.org/10.1016/B978-0-12-811228-1.00015-7

use them appropriately, and benefit from them" (WHO, 2012). This emphasizes the importance of stakeholder responsibility and engagement in the context of finite resources to promote the appropriate use of medicines according to their potential benefit for the health of the patients. The opposite of responsible use is referred to as suboptimal use (WHO, 2012).

The rational use of medicines is also known as quality use of medicines (QUMs). In Australia, this is defined as

- "*Judicious selection of management options* This means consideration of the place of medicines in treating illness and maintaining health, recognising that for the management of many disorders nondrug therapies may be the best option;
- *Appropriate choice of medicines, where a medicine is considered necessary* This means that, when medicines are required, selecting the best option from the range available taking into account the individual, the clinical condition, risks, benefits, dosage, length of treatment, co-morbidities, other therapies and monitoring considerations. Appropriate selection also requires a consideration of costs, both human and economic. These costs should be considered both for the individual, the community and the health system as a whole; and
- *Safe and effective use* This means ensuring best possible outcomes of therapy by monitoring outcomes, minimising misuse, over-use and under-use, as well as improving the ability of all individuals to take appropriate actions to solve medication-related problems, e.g. adverse effects and managing multiple medications" (Commonwealth Department of Health and Ageing, 2002).

The Australian definition provides a wider context for considering QUMs, by highlighting the place of nondrug therapies in management as part of its definition.

The medical therapeutic view of the rational use of medicines or QUMs might be different from the consumers' perspective of rational, which is based on the interpretation of the value of using a medicine for daily life and influenced by cultural perceptions and economic conditions (le Grand et al., 1999). The former view is critical in designing pharmaceutical policy, whereas the latter perspective dictates the context in which the policy is implemented. Both perspectives need to be considered for a full understanding of medicine use and successful policy implementation (le Grand et al., 1999). This chapter aims to provide an overview of existing literature on international experience in improving medicine use. It begins with a review of problems commonly associated with medicine use and factors contributing to the problems with medicine use. A section follows on how to assess medicine use. The chapter continues with identification of national policies and strategies intended to improve the use of medicines. The effect of these strategies on QUMs is then reviewed, highlighting the achievements and challenges in this area. The chapter ends with a conclusion and recommendations for the way forward.

THE MEDICINE USE PROBLEM

A prerequisite to QUMs is ensuring that medicines are available and affordable to the patient and the community. The lack of availability and affordability of medicines is common. According to the WHO, one-third of the world's population still lacks regular access to essential medicines with the figure increasing to 50% in the poorest countries of Africa and Asia (World Health Organization, 2011). Where accessible, problems with medicine use are still common, with estimates that more than 50% of all medicines are prescribed, dispensed, or sold inappropriately by health-care providers (WHO, 2002).

In turn, about 50% of all patients fail to take their medicines correctly (Sabaté, 2003; WHO, 2002). The main problems with medicine use include the following:

- Need for additional therapy
- Use of unnecessary medicine
- Use of wrong or inappropriate medicine
- Use of too much medicine
- Use of too little medicine
- Adverse drug reactions (ADRs) present
- Compliance problems (Hepler & Strand, 1990)

Problems with medicine use can lead to health and economic consequences. Lack of access to medicines means that patients often go without treatment. Suboptimal use of medicines can result in limited efficacy of the therapy, poorer health outcomes as well as ADRs and increased harms (Hardon & le Grand, 1993). ADRs are estimated to be responsible for 6.5% of all acute hospital admissions and at least 5000 deaths annually in England (Pirmohamed et al., 2004), and one of the leading causes of death in the United States (Lazarou, Pomeranz, & Corey, 1998). In Australia, 230,000 hospital admissions each year are estimated to be due to problems with medicine use (Roughead, Semple, & Rosenfeld, 2013). In many developing countries, the widespread overuse and suboptimal dosage of antibiotics leads to increased antibiotic resistance (Hossain, Glass, & Khan, 1982; Kunin, 1985). Other examples include increased drug dependence due to overuse of painkillers (Legrand, Sringernyuang, & Streefland, 1993) and tranquilizers (Hardon & le Grand, 1993) and increased risk of infection and transmission of bloodborne diseases due to nonsterile injections (e.g., abscesses, hepatitis, and HIV/AIDS) (Reeler, 1990; WHO, 2002; Wyatt, 1984).

Suboptimal use of medicines has a significant impact on household and national health budgets. In Australia, hospital admissions alone due to medicine use problems cost approximately AUD 1.2 billion per year (Roughead et al., 2013). The figure for the United Kingdom is estimated to be £770 million (Frontier Economics, 2014) and in the United States USD 3.5 billion (Aspden Wolcott, Lyle Bootman, & Cronenwett, 2007). Inappropriate use of medicines also wastes scare financial resources (le Grand et al., 1999; WHO, 2002). In the public sector in sub-Saharan Africa, it is estimated that inappropriate prescribing wastes up to 50%–70% of medicine expenditure (Barnett, Creese, & Ayivor, 1980; Foster, 1991; World Bank, 1994). The waste of limited resources results in increased costs of medicines, medicine shortages, and loss of patient confidence in the health system, which in turn can lead to reduced access to other essential medicines and reduced patient attendance rates (WHO, 2001, 2002; World Bank, 1994).

FACTORS CONTRIBUTING TO PROBLEMS WITH MEDICINE USE

Problems with medicine use are not due to any one factor, but usually the result of multiple factors, some relating to the health-care system including those to the pharmaceutical system more specifically, while others may be physician- and health professional–related factors or patient-related factors (Holloway, 2011; Radyowijati & Haak, 2003; Rowe de Savigny, Lanata, & Victora, 2005).

System factors affecting medicine use may include the pharmaceutical policies, laws, and regulations, the scheduling of medicines, the costs of medicines, the availability of formularies and guidelines, availability of medicines of appropriate safety, efficacy and quality, practice organization, and the availability of services supporting appropriate medicine use, as well as pharmaceutical company promotion (Lipton & Bird, 1993; Sutters, 1990).

The physician- and health professional–related factors may include diagnostic and therapeutic knowledge and skills, communication skills, availability of qualified staff, access to independent medicines information, access to continuing medical education and supervision (Holloway, 2011), skills in stock management, and perverse systems incentives (for example, prescribing for private gain rather than on the basis of clinical need) (Nguyen, 2011).

With regard to the patient-related factors, patient or family beliefs and influences can negatively influence use of medicines (Lipton & Bird, 1993). For example, patients from a particular background may be unwilling to take some medicines. Patients may demand medicines that they believe to have better efficacy than those that are prescribed. Preference for or aversion to injections or other dosage forms of medicine can influence medicine use in some cultures (Falkenberg et al., 2000). Lack of adherence to the treatment by patients is another reason for suboptimal use of medicines (Sabaté, 2003).

ASSESSING THE MEDICINE USE PROBLEM

To address suboptimal use of medicines, problems with medicine use need to be identified and quantified. Important questions to be answered include the type of problems with medicine use that exist, the extent of the problems, and the reasons why the problems exist (WHO, 2002). Of similar importance is the question whether medicine use improves following interventions. Answering these questions will support the development, implementation, and evaluation of policy supporting QUMs.

Measuring the type and extent of suboptimal use of medicines can include an assessment of the amount of medicine procured, sold, prescribed, supplied, or used. The unit of measurement can include counts of stock, prescriptions written or dispensed, as well as costs or volume. Where individual patient-level data are available, measures may include counts of people receiving the medicines and counts of people starting new medicines. Volume measures that have been developed include the defined daily dose per 1000 population per day, which is recommended by the WHO and the less commonly used measure of prescribed daily dose per 1000 population per day (Roughead et al., 2015).

A number of tools have been developed for assessing the use of medicines. Tools using aggregate data include ABC analysis; drug utilization 90%; vital, essential, nonessential analysis; time series trends; and segmented regression analysis (Roughead et al., 2015). Tools using individual patient data include prevalence and incidence counts, the duration index, the Lorenz curve, waiting time distributions, prescription sequence symmetry analysis, and patient adherence measures such as the medication possession ratio (Roughead et al., 2015) and WHO medicine use indicators (WHO, 1993). Using the tools to identify problems regarding the use of specific medicines or the treatment of specific conditions is referred to as drug use evaluation or drug utilization review (DUR) (WHO, 2002). A comprehensive account of these tools can be found in WHO (2003) and Roughead et al. (2015).

The quantitative methods mentioned above are effective in monitoring medicine use. However, they are not sufficient to answer questions of why the problem exists or how to address the problems. For these types of questions, qualitative methods are needed. Well-established qualitative methods are available, which include in-depth interviews, focus group discussions, or observation (Patton, 1990).

The International Network for Rational Use of Drugs has developed a manual of applied qualitative methods for use in designing interventions to improve medicine use (Arhinful et al., 1996). Guidelines to use qualitative methods to investigate medicine use in communities have also been developed by the WHO (1992).

In many developed countries, reliable computerized administrative data on medicine use are available, including data from insurance claims or electronic medical records. Analyzing these data over time can provide an effective way of regularly monitoring the use of medicines to identify potential problems and to evaluate the effect of any intervention. Administrative data may not be available in developing countries (Holloway & van Dijk, 2011). Procurement, sales, and commercial medicine utilization data (e.g., IMS Health data) or community and household survey data are alternative sources of medicine use data.

To support developing countries, the WHO has created a database of medicine use in developing and transitional countries based on published studies (Holloway et al., 2013; WHO, 2009). It is recommended that individual countries establish mechanisms to monitor medicine use so that information is available to identify problems, develop intervention strategies, and evaluate the effect of these strategies on medicine use (Laing, Hogerzeil, & Ross-Degnan, 2001). Experiences from developing countries have shown the feasibility and benefit of regularly monitoring medicine use in improving the use of medicines (Santoso, 1995).

INDIRECT POLICIES AND STRATEGIES TO IMPROVE MEDICINE USE WITHIN THE CONTEXT OF THE PHARMACEUTICAL SYSTEM

To improve medicine use, governments in many countries have policies and strategies in place to ensure the availability, accessibility, and quality use of affordable medicines that have reasonable quality, efficacy, and safety (Ratanawijitrasin, Soumerai, & Weerasuriya, 2001). QUMs is dependent on the availability of affordable essential medicines. Policies to improve the use of medicines therefore need to be considered within the broader context of other activities to strengthen the pharmaceutical sector, optimally under the umbrella of a national medicines policy (NMP) (WHO, 1988). The WHO recommends individual countries develop their own locally appropriate NMP, primarily focused on improved access, quality, and rational use of medicines (Nguyen, Hassali, & McLachlan, 2013).

A major strategy of WHO to support the pharmaceutical sector is the concept of essential medicines (Laing et al., 2001). In 1977, the WHO introduced their first Model List of Essential Medicines of 204 pharmaceutical formulations involving 186 core medicines (Greene, 2011; WHO, 2017). The list provides an indicative guide of what medicines are needed and is periodically updated to meet the changing global public health need, with the current version identifying 409 active substances (WHO, 2015). The medicines included on the list are not necessarily essential for all countries but do provide a guide for what countries may require and can be used to guide purchasing decisions. Countries can adapt the list to create their own national list taking into account their country-specific context including epidemiological features, human and financial resources, and the existing health system (Antezana & Seuba, 2009). The advantage of creating a limited list of medicines, which is relevant to the priority health needs of the country, is that it enables government authorities to optimize pharmaceutical production, distribution, and procurement to improve availability and reduce costs, thus improving access (Antezana & Seuba, 2009). It also makes it easier for prescribers and patients to familiarize themselves with a limited list of medicines and to create standard treatment guidelines for the listed medicines (WHO, 2004).

A comprehensive review relevant to developing countries of policies to support pharmaceutical pricing and purchasing for improving access to medicine has been published elsewhere (Nguyen et al., 2014). Many of the pricing and purchasing policies provide support, to some extent, for rational and responsible use of medicines (Almarsdottir & Traulsen, 2005) and are often referred to as **financial strategies**. Cost-sharing and reimbursement mechanisms (e.g., reference price systems or index price systems) that require patients to pay part of the costs of their medicines (e.g., copayment, brand premium, or therapeutic premium) can assist to moderate demand for medicines that have little or marginal benefit to the patients (Nguyen et al., 2014). However, if copayments are too high, they may lead to lack of use of necessary medicines and therefore be counterproductive. Generic substitution where expensive innovator brands are substituted by cheaper generic products can also lead to financial savings. The use of FDA-approved generic medicines instead of more expensive innovator brand products saved the US healthcare system about USD 1.07 trillion in the period between 2002 and 2011 with USD 192.8 billion in savings achieved in 2011 alone (GPhA, 2012).

Another financial strategy is capitation-based budgeting, where global financial ceilings on healthcare expenditure at regional or individual general practitioner levels are set. This may assist to improve prescribers' rational and responsible use of medicines by limiting the use of overly expensive medicines where cheaper alternatives are available (Ess, Schneerweiss, & Szucs, 2003; Rietveld & Haaijer-Ruskamp, 2002). However, where budgets are capped too low, this mechanism can be counterproductive by reducing the use of necessary medicines.

Financial strategies targeting pharmaceutical companies include managed entry schemes such as price–volume agreements, which set a predetermined budget for reimbursement based on a sales forecast of country need. Any sales beyond the estimated need may indicate that the medicine has been used in populations less likely to benefit or that there is overuse of the medicine in the targeted population. In this case, the company is required to pay a rebate (Nguyen et al., 2014). This type of policy is intended to reduce the likelihood of marketing of the medicines to groups outside of the subsidized or agreed indication.

Assessing the effectiveness of **financial strategies** in pharmaceutical pricing and purchasing policies, Cochrane reviews have found that cap and copayment policies decrease overall medicine use (Austvoll-Dahlgren et al., 2008) as do reference pricing policies (Aaserud et al., 2006). However, a reduction in the use of medicines may have adverse effects on health where appropriate use of medicines is ceased, thus increasing the use of healthcare services and overall expenditures. It was posited that these adverse effects might be overcome if exemptions were built into systems to ensure that patients receive essential medical care.

DIRECT POLICIES AND STRATEGIES FOR IMPROVING THE USE OF MEDICINES

As previously described, problems with medicine use are not the fault of any one group or person, but because of a variety of factors that include systems-related factors, health professional–related factors, and patient-related factors. Thus improving the use of medicines requires activities that target all of the relevant factors. This is sometimes described as a systems approach to improving healthcare. Reviews have been published on national policies and strategies to improve the use of medicines (Bloom, 2005; Figueiras, Sastre, & Gestal-Otero, 2001; Holloway, 2011; le Grand et al., 1999; Ostini et al., 2009; Pearson et al., 2003; Ratanawijitrasin et al., 2001; Sketris, Langille Ingram, & Lummis, 2009). These strategies are often categorized into educational, managerial, and regulatory strategies (Quick, Laing, & Rossdegnan, 1991, WHO, 2001). The educational strategies are designed to target health professional–related and patient-related factors, whereas managerial and regulatory strategies aim to address organizational issues relevant to health professional–related and patient-related factors as well as systems-related factors.

Educational strategies use information and persuasion to influence the knowledge, attitudes, and practices of healthcare practitioners and consumers (Quick et al., 1991). They include continuing education and academic detailing to health professionals or health promotion and education about medicines for patients.

Managerial strategies aim to structure the healthcare environment (Almarsdottir & Traulsen, 2005) to support the decision-making process of health professionals and patients about medicines (Quick et al., 1991). Managerial strategies include clinical guidelines, essential medicines lists, dispensing standards, drug and therapeutics committees, audit and feedback to prescribers, and computerized clinical decision support systems (Quick et al., 1991; WHO, 2001, 2002). Financial strategies such as financial incentives for prescribers, dispensers, and patients are also sometimes categorized as managerial strategies (Quick et al., 1991).

Regulatory strategies include laws and regulations to ensure the availability of safe and effective medicines on the market. Health technology assessment is used to ensure critical evaluation of medicines before registering or subsidizing the medicines (WHO, 2001). Other regulatory strategies include monitoring and regulating medicine promotion, regulating medicine information, licensing health professionals and medicine outlets, scheduling medicines so that they are only available with a prescription or require consultation or justifications (Quick et al., 1991; WHO, 2001, 2002). Some financial strategies to restrict the reimbursement or subsidization of medicines to specific indications or specific brands or products can also be categorized as regulatory strategies.

ACHIEVEMENTS

There is a considerable body of literature on the effect of different strategies on the use of medicines, most of which has been undertaken in developed countries. A number of reviews have assessed the effectiveness of different **educational strategies** (Bloom, 2005; Figueiras et al., 2001; Grol & Grimshaw, 2003; Lu et al., 2008; Ostini et al., 2009; Pearson et al., 2003; Sketris et al., 2009). Educational outreach by key opinion leaders and academic detailing involving a trained educator visiting prescribers' practice settings to deliver key messages are among the most effective educational strategies to change prescribing behavior (Cantillon & Jones, 1999; Grol & Grimshaw, 2003); however, they are quite costly (Sketris et al., 2009). Small group participatory meetings, especially at practice sites, are more effective than traditional lectures. Large didactic educational meetings or passive distribution of educational materials alone often result in very small or no effect on changing prescribing practice (Holloway, 2011).

The effectiveness of varying **managerial and regulatory strategies** has also been reviewed (Francke et al., 2008; Grimshaw et al., 2004; Grol & Grimshaw, 2003; Jamtvedt et al., 2006; Lu et al.,

2008; Ostini et al., 2009; Parrino, 2005; Pearson et al., 2003; Sketris et al., 2009). Although clinical guidelines recommend the best practices available, different guideline implementation strategies have different effects on adherence to guidelines. In general, a combination of multiple strategies is more effective than single interventions (Francke et al., 2008; Sketris et al., 2009; Wensing, van der Weijden, & Grol, 1998), especially in developing countries where the intervention may also require building infrastructure that is otherwise lacking (Holloway, 2011).

Audit and feedback including DUR result in small to moderate effects (Jamtvedt et al., 2006; Grimshaw et al., 2004; Ostini et al., 2009; Sketris et al., 2009). The improvement is greater when baseline adherence to the standard practice is low (Jamtvedt et al., 2006) or the audit is performed concurrently with an intervention (Sketris et al., 2009). Feedback to prescribers by clinical pharmacists after conducting medicine reviews has also been shown to result in improved prescribing practice (Kaur et al., 2009).

Computerized clinical decision support systems has been shown to improve the initiation and monitoring of pharmaceutical therapy, especially in institutional settings and when decision support was initiated automatically by the system rather than user initiation (Pearson et al., 2009). Authorization systems with structured order entry, formulary restriction, and mandatory consultation have been found effective in improving antibiotic prescribing patterns in clinical practice (Parrino, 2005).

A Cochrane review also confirmed that the restrictions on reimbursement policies can have a positive effect on prescribing practices (Green et al., 2010). Implementing restrictions to coverage and reimbursement of more expensive medicines can result in cheaper alternatives being used without increasing the use of other health services. Similarly, relaxing reimbursement rules for medicines used for secondary prevention can result in increased appropriate use of these medicines, thus improving patients' health outcomes and saving costs (Green et al., 2010). Prescribing restrictions, however, should be carefully evaluated for instances of the effect of the restriction and for instances of inappropriate therapeutic shift, as in some instances restrictions can lead to increased use of less appropriate medicines.

Given the diversity and complexity of determinants of medicine use that include health system, professional, and patient factors (Davis, 1997; Nguyen, 2011; Sketris et al., 2009), a national coordinated approach using national policies to improve the use of medicines is recommended (WHO, 2002; WHO, 2007). Australia was among the first of the few developed countries to have developed a national strategy for QUM, a strategy that sits firmly within the framework of their NMP (Australian Government Department of Health and Ageing, 2002). The Australian strategy for QUMs is underpinned by behavioral, health promotion and public health theories as well as evidence of the effectiveness of individual strategies for improving medicine use. The Australian strategy identifies the need to implement multiple strategies simultaneously targeting all stakeholders whose activities influence medicine use, including health professionals, consumers, government, industry, and media, as well as targeting the systems and organizational factors influencing medicines use. Indicators to monitor the implementation and evaluation of the national strategy for QUMs were developed, and in the second report of Australia's national indicators, the impact indicators showed increasing uptake of QUM services and activities over time. Indicators monitoring the overall effect of the policy demonstrated improvements in medication use and health outcomes (Australian Government Department of Health and Ageing, 2003). Other examples of the success of specific national policies include the Korean policy prohibiting dispensing by general practitioners, which led to a 7.5% reduction in antibiotic use for viral illness episodes (Park et al., 2005), and the Swedish Strategic Programme Against Antibiotic Resistance, which was associated with a 20% and 30% reduction in antibiotic use in adults and children, respectively, in the period 1995–2004 (Molstad et al., 2008).

Because evidence from developed countries might not be able to be extrapolated to the poorer resource settings of developing countries, efforts have been made to evaluate the effects of the strategies to improve the use of medicines in developing countries' contexts (Holloway & Henry, 2014; Holloway et al., 2013; le Grand et al., 1999; Ratanawijitrasin et al., 2001; Ross-Degnan et al., 1997; Siddiqi, Newell, & Robinson, 2005; WHO, 2009). The findings are similar to those found in developed countries. Indirect policies using financial strategies such as user fees led to reduced use of medicines, including the essential ones (Gilson, 1997), highlighting the need for these policies to be targeted to nonessential medicines. Policies directly aimed at improving the use of medicines such as a combination of educational components with other measures in a multifaceted intervention package have been shown to result in larger effects than single interventions (Holloway et al., 2013; WHO, 2009). Audit and feedback, particularly when combined with other measures, was also effective in the developing country setting (Siddiqi et al., 2005). The WHO essential medicines concept has been associated with improved use of medicines in developing countries (Holloway & Henry, 2014). Similar to developed countries the use of simple measures alone, such as the use of printed materials alone or NMPs without associated interventions, had little or no positive impact (Holloway et al., 2013; WHO, 2009).

CHALLENGES

Although collectively the evidence shows that the strategies described for improving the use of medicines are generally effective, many of the evaluated interventions to improve medicine use in healthcare have had mixed results (Gilbert et al., 2011; Gilbert et al., 2013; Grimshaw et al., 2001; Grimshaw et al., 2003; Hartikainen et al., 2014; Roughead et al., 2013; Saha et al., 2012). One reason that strategies are less likely to be successful is the lack of application of theoretical behavioral frameworks to the planning and delivery of the intervention (Eccles et al., 2005). There are many theories from behavioral science (Bandura, 1986, 1989; Prochaska & Di Clemente, 1986; Prochaska & Velicer, 1997; Prochaska et al., 1994), communication science (Declercq et al., 2013; Snowdon, Galanos, & Vaswani, 2011a, 2011b), social marketing (Snowdon et al., 2006; Snowdon et al., 2011a, 2011b), and community development and organizational change (Berwick, 2003; Green & Kreuter, 1992, 1995; Michie, van Stralen, & West, 2011; Pan et al., 2014; Winett, 1995; Winett, King, & Altman, 1989) that can be used to inform the development, implementation, and evaluation of interventions. Their application to intervention planning for QUMs and program evaluation has been described elsewhere (Roughead & Gilbert, 2016), as has their application to enhancing uptake of evidence about medicines (Roughead, 2006). Key features of the frameworks highlight the need for engaging all groups whose activities influence medicine use at all stages of the intervention planning, implementation, and evaluation; the need for multiple interventions to change behaviors so that awareness, knowledge, skills, and appropriate behaviors are learned; and the need for repetition and reinforcement of messages and opportunities to practice new behaviors so that behaviors are maintained. The theories also identify the requirement to attend to systems factors, which enable or hinder a program's success.

The effectiveness of a policy or intervention is determined by the quality of its content and how well it is implemented (Holloway et al., 2013; Ratanawijitrasin et al., 2001). Evidence has been shown that interventions or policies with similar content can produce different outcomes (Ratanawijitrasin et al.,

2001). Existing literature on intervention research in QUMs has rarely described the details of the policy setting within which the research occurred, whether the intervention was designed taking into account the determinants of inappropriate use, the theoretical framework underpinning the intervention, and how well the intervention was implemented (WHO, 2009; Holloway et al., 2013). This creates difficulty in determining whether the failure of an intervention was due to the design of the intervention or the way the intervention was implemented. Lack of proper implementation of effective intervention might have the same consequence as implementation of an ineffective intervention (Holloway, 2011). Evaluation encompassing process, impact, and outcome measures (Donabedian, 1987, 1988) is recommended to ensure both the quality of implementation and the effectiveness of the intervention are assessed.

Although there is increasing high-quality intervention research to improve the use of medicines occurring in developing countries over time, overall the scope of work is still limited (Ross-Degnan et al., 1997). Much remains to be studied and understood about the types of problems that occur, the settings in which they occur, and the factors underpinning those problems. Many interventions and activities to improve medicine use have not been evaluated (Ross-Degnan et al., 1997). For those strategies that have been tested, the median intervention effect size has been found to be small (WHO, 2009; Holloway et al., 2013), most interventions have been small scale, and very few have been scaled up and coordinated nationally (MSH, 2011). Although single, isolated interventions might work in developed countries (Grimshaw et al., 2004) perhaps supported by existing health infrastructure (e.g., supervisory systems), they may not have the same effect in the poorer resource settings of developing countries (Holloway, 2011) and therefore require testing in the developing country setting. For interventions that have been scaled up as national policies, the evidence regarding the effectiveness of the national policies is inconclusive (Ratanawijitrasin et al., 2001).

The complexity of pharmaceutical policies themselves can contribute to difficulty in evaluating the effects. Ratanawijitrasin et al. (2001) have identified several characteristics of NMPs that might create challenges for policy evaluation. These include the national scale (i.e., application to entire population leads to a lack of any nonexposed comparison groups), the use of multicomponent interventions, assumptions of multistage causal relationship (e.g., the assumption that regulating prescription only medicines will first lead to controlled availability of medicines and the controlled availability of medicine will then result in better use of medicines), and an evolving policy environment (Ratanawijitrasin et al., 2001).

Based on expert opinion and best evidence available, the WHO recommends a number of national policies and strategies to promote QUMs (WHO, 2012; WHO, 2002). They include a mandated multidisciplinary national body to coordinate medicine use policies, standard treatment guidelines, essential medicine list, drugs and therapeutics committees, obligatory continuing in-service medical education for doctors, or public education about medicines (WHO, 2012). However, the WHO survey in 2007 showed that uptake of WHO's recommendations was low, with more than half of WHO Member States not implementing basic recommended policies such as updating their standard treatment guidelines in the previous 2 years (WHO, 2010). A number of reasons for the low uptake of WHO's policy recommendations were identified, including lack of institutionalization support promoting appropriate use of medicines, lack of investment, the fragmentation of the health system, and lack of relevant research to address QUMs needs (Holloway, 2011; Holloway & van Dijk, 2011).

RECOMMENDATIONS: THE WAY FORWARD

The evidence base and behavioral theoretical frameworks both find that multifaceted interventions targeting the groups whose activities influence medicine use undertaken within supportive policy environments are required to improve the use of medicines. The best mix of strategies within country- or program-specific settings is, however, not known, and there is even more limited evidence of the best mix of strategies in the developing country context. Furthermore, problems with medicine use may be country specific or area specific; therefore interventions need to be implemented to address local issues. Given the existing evidence base, there is significant opportunity within developing countries to undertake rigorous evaluation of interventions that are underpinned by behavioral theoretical frameworks within the context of the developing policy environment. Consideration should be given to adapting evidence-based strategies to meet the local contextual environment and needs. In addition, the scope of policy interventions for evaluation needs to be expanded to areas where evidence is lacking and where new opportunities for intervention have arisen, such as use of social and electronic media and integration of traditional medicines within the QUMs conceptualization. Given the national scale of policy interventions that makes it difficult to choose nonexposed comparison groups, interrupted time series analysis is recommended to be the standard design for rigorous policy evaluations. Cost-effectiveness evaluation of policy interventions is also needed.

CONCLUSIONS

The determinants of inappropriate use of medicines are much more than just lack of knowledge. National policy interventions should be developed based on the country's context within which problems with medicines use occur. A national situation analysis of the pharmaceutical sector and health system is recommended as a first step, which takes into account the government, consumers', and health professionals' perspectives to identify and prioritize problems for policy and intervention development. Monitoring the implementation and policy evaluation through strategic research and routine data collection should be a building block for this work within the framework of a NMP and broader national health policies.

LESSONS LEARNED

- Multifaceted policy interventions based on country-specific medicine use problems are necessary to address the multideterminants of inappropriate use of medicines.
- Strategies to improve the use of medicines should be underpinned by a theoretical model for behavior change, include active stakeholder engagement, and be targeted to identified problems with medicine use, with opportunities over time for repetition and reinforcement.
- Routine data collection, monitoring and documentation of the implementation, and adequate evaluation of policies to improve the use of medicines should be a building block to support improvements in medicine use within the broader framework of the NMP and national health policies.

REFERENCES

Aaserud, M., et al. (2006). Pharmaceutical policies: Effects of reference pricing, other pricing, and purchasing policies. *Cochrane Database of Systematic Reviews* (2).

Almarsdottir, A. B., & Traulsen, J. M. (2005). Rational use of medicines - an important issue in pharmaceutical policy. *Pharmacy World & Science*, *27*(2), 76–80.

Antezana, F., & Seuba, X. (2009). *Thirty years of essential medicines: The challenge*. Barcelona, Spain: Farmamundi.

Arhinful, D. K., et al. (1996). *How to use applied qualitative methods to design drug use interventions*. Available from http://www.inrud.org/documents/upload/How_to_Use_Applied_Qualitative_Methods.pdf.

Aspden, P., Wolcott, Julie A., Lyle Bootman, J., & Cronenwett, Linda R. (2007). *Preventing medication Errors: Quality chasm series*. Washington, DC: The National Academic Press.

Australian Government Department of Health, Ageing. (2002). *The national strategy for quality use of medicines*. Canberra, Australia: Commonwealth of Australia.

Australian Government Department of Health, Ageing. (2003). *Measurement of the quality use of medicines component of the Australia's National Medicines Policy – second report of the national indicators*. Available from http://www.health.gov.au/internet/main/publishing.nsf/content/ddd3943c4fe07e3dca257bf000211e3b/$file/qumnmp.pdf.

Austvoll-Dahlgren, A., et al. (2008). Pharmaceutical policies: Effects of cap and co-payment on rational drug use. *Cochrane Database of Systematic Reviews* (1), CD007017.

Bandura, A. (1986). *Social foundations of thought and action: A social cognitive theory.* , Englewood Cliffs, New Jersey: Prentice-Hall, Inc.

Bandura, A. (1989). Human agency in social cognitive theory. *American Psychological*, *44*, 1175–1184.

Barnett, A., Creese, A. L., & Ayivor, E. C. K. (1980). The economics of pharmaceutical policy in Ghana. *International Journal of Health Services*, *10*(3), 479–499.

Berwick, D. M. (2003). Disseminating innovations in health care. *JAMA*, *289*(15), 1969–1975.

Bloom, B. S. (2005). Effects of continuing medical education on improving physician clinical care and patient health: A review of systematic reviews. *International Journal of Technology Assessment in Health Care*, *21*(3), 380–385.

Cantillon, P., & Jones, R. (1999). Does continuing medical education in general practice make a difference? *BMJ: British Medical Journal*, *318*, 1276–1279.

Commonwealth Department of Health, Ageing. (2002). *The national strategy for quality use of medicines*. Canberra: Commonwealth Department of Health and Ageing.

Davis, P. (1997). *Managing medicines: Public policy and therapeutic drugs.* , Buckingham: Open University Press.

Declercq, T., et al. (2013). Withdrawal versus continuation of chronic antipsychotic drugs for behavioural and psychological symptoms in older people with dementia. *The Cochrane Database of Systematic Reviews [Electronic Resource]*, *3*, CD007726.

Donabedian, A. (1987). Some basic issues in evaluating the quality of health care. *NLN Publications* (21–2194), 3–28.

Donabedian, A. (1988). The quality of care. How can it be assessed? *JAMA*, *260*(12), 1743–1748.

Eccles, M., et al. (2005). Changing the behavior of healthcare professionals: The use of theory in promoting the uptake of research findings. *Journal of Clinical Epidemiology*, *58*(2), 107–112.

Ess, S. M., Schneerweiss, S., & Szucs, T. D. (2003). European healthcare policies for controlling drug expenditure. *Pharmacoeconomics*, *21*(2), 89–103.

Falkenberg, T., et al. (2000). Pharmaceutical sector in transition-a cross sectional study in Vietnam. *The Southeast Asian Journal of Tropical Medicine and Public Health*, *31*(3), 590–597.

Figueiras, A., Sastre, I., & Gestal-Otero, J. J. (2001). Effectiveness of educational interventions on the improvement of drug prescription in primary care: A critical literature review. *Journal of Evaluation in Clinical Practice*, *7*(2), 223–241.

Foster, S. (1991). Supply and use of essential drugs in Sub-Saharan Africa – some issues and possible solutions. *Social Science & Medicine*, *32*(11), 1201–1218.

Francke, A. L., et al. (2008). Factors influencing the implementation of clinical guidelines for health care professionals: A systematic meta-review. *BMC Medical Informatics and Decision Making*, *8*, 38.

Frontier Economics. (2014). *Exploring the costs of unsafe care in the NHS*. London: Frontier Economics Ltd.

Gilbert, A. L., et al. (2011). Ageing well: Improving the management of patients with multiple chronic health problems. *Australasian Journal on Ageing* (30 Suppl. 2), 32–37.

Gilbert, A., et al. (2013). *Multiple chronic health conditions in older people: Implications for health policy planning, practitioners and patients*. Adelaide: University of South Australia.

Gilson, L. (1997). The lessons of user fee experience in Africa. *Health Policy and Planning*, *12*(4), 273–285.

GPhA. (2012). *Generic drug savings in the U.S.* Washington, DC: Generic Pharmaceutical Association.

Greene, J. A. (2011). Making medicines essential: The emergent centrality of pharmaceuticals in global health. *Biosocieties*, *6*(1), 10–33.

Green, C. J., et al. (2010). Pharmaceutical policies: Effects of restrictions on reimbursement. *The Cochrane Database of Systematic Reviews [Electronic Resource]* (8), CD008654.

Green, L. W., & Kreuter, M. W. (1992). CDC's planned approach to community health as an application of PRECEDE and an inspiration for PROCEED. *Health Education Journal*, *23*, 140–147.

Green, L. W., & Kreuter, M. W. (1995). *Health program planning, an educational and ecological approach* (4th ed.). , New York: McGraw Hill.

Grimshaw, J. M., et al. (2001). Changing provider behavior: An overview of systematic reviews of interventions. *Medical Care*, *39*(8 Suppl. 2), II2–45.

Grimshaw, J., et al. (2003). Systematic reviews of the effectiveness of quality improvement strategies and programmes. *Quality & Safety in Health Care*, *12*(4), 298–303.

Grimshaw, J. M., et al. (2004). Effectiveness and efficiency of guideline dissemination and implementation strategies. *Health Technology Assessment*, *8*(6), iii–iv 1–72.

Grol, R., & Grimshaw, J. (2003). From best evidence to best practice: Effective implementation of change in patients' care. *Lancet*, *362*, 1225–1230.

Hardon, A., & le Grand, A. (1993). Pharmaceuticals in Communities: Practices, public health consequences and intervention strategies. *Bulletins of the Royal Tropical Institute* (Vol. 330). Amsterdam, The Netherlands: Royal Tropical Institute.

Hartikainen, S., et al. (2014). Incidence of antipsychotic use in relation to diagnosis of Alzheimer's disease among community dwelling persons: Nationwide population based study. *Pharmacoepidemiology and Drug Safety*, *23*(S1), 342.

Hepler, C. D., & Strand, L. M. (1990). Opportunities and responsibilities in pharmaceutical care. *American Journal of Hospital Pharmacy*, *47*(3), 533–543.

Holloway, K. A. (2011). Combating inappropriate use of medicines. *Expert Review of Clinical Pharmacology*, *4*(3), 335–348.

Holloway, K. A., et al. (2013). Have we improved use of medicines in developing and transitional countries and do we know how to? Two decades of evidence. *Tropical Medicine & International Health: TM & IH*, *18*(6), 656–664.

Holloway, K. A., & Henry, D. (2014). WHO essential medicines policies and use in developing and transitional Countries: An analysis of reported policy implementation and medicines use surveys. *PLoS Medicine*, *11*(9).

Holloway, K., & van Dijk, L. (2011). Rational use of medicines. In *The world medicines situation 2011*. Geneva: World Health Organization.

Hossain, M. M., Glass, R. I., & Khan, M. R. (1982). Antibiotic use in a rural-community in Bangladesh. *International Journal of Epidemiology*, *11*(4), 402–405.

Jamtvedt, G., et al. (2006). Audit and feedback: Effects on professional practice and health care outcomes. *The Cochrane Database of Systematic Reviews [Electronic Resource]* (2), CD000259.

Kaur, S., et al. (2009). Interventions that can reduce inappropriate prescribing in the elderly: A systematic review. *Drugs & Aging*, *26*(12), 1013–1028.

Kunin, C. M. (1985). The responsibility of the infectious-disease community for the optimal use of antimicrobial agents. *Journal of Infectious Diseases*, *151*(3), 388–398.

Laing, R., Hogerzeil, H., & Ross-Degnan, D. (2001). Ten recommendations to improve use of medicines in developing countries. *Health Policy and Planning*, *16*(1), 13–20.

Lazarou, J., Pomeranz, B. H., & Corey, P. N. (1998). Incidence of adverse drug reactions in hospitalized patients: A meta-analysis of prospective studies. *JAMA: The Journal of the American Medical Association*, *279*(15), 1200–1205.

le Grand, A., Hogerzeil, H. V., & Haaijer-Ruskamp, F. M. (1999). Intervention research in rational use of drugs: A review. *Health Policy Plan*, *14*(2), 89–102.

Legrand, A., Sringernyuang, L., & Streefland, P. H. (1993). Enhancing appropriate drug-use - the contribution of herbal medicine promotion – a case-study in Rural Thailand. *Social Science & Medicine*, *36*(8), 1023–1035.

Lipton, H., & Bird, J. (1993). Drug utilization review in ambulatory settings: State of the science and directions for outcomes research. *Medical Care*, *31*, 1069–1082.

Lu, C. Y., et al. (2008). Interventions designed to improve the quality and efficiency of medication use in managed care: A critical review of the literature - 2001–2007. *BMC Health Services Research*, *8*, 75.

Michie, S., van Stralen, M. M., & West, R. (2011). The behaviour change wheel: A new method for characterising and designing behaviour change interventions. *Implement Sci*, *6*, 42.

Molstad, S., et al. (2008). Sustained reduction of antibiotic use and low bacterial resistance: 10-year follow-up of the Swedish Strama programme. *Lancet Infectious Diseases*, *8*(2), 125–132.

MSH. (2011). *International conferences on improving use of medicines (ICIUM 2011, ICIUM 2004 and ICIUM 1997)*. Available from http://icium.msh.org/index.htm.

Nguyen, T. A. (2011). *Medicine prices and pricing policies in Vietnam* (p. 248). Sydney, Australia: School of Public Health and Community Medicine, The University of New South Wales.

Nguyen, T. A., et al. (2015). Policy options for pharmaceutical pricing and purchasing: Issues for low- and middle-income countries. *Health Policy and Planning*, *30*(2), 267–280.

Nguyen, T. A., Hassali, M. A., & McLachlan, A. (2013). Generic medicines policies in the Asia Pacific region: Ways forward. *WHO South-east Asia Journal of Public Health*, 2(1), 72–74.

Ostini, R., et al. (2009). Systematic review of interventions to improve prescribing. *The Annals of Pharmacotherapy*, *43*(3), 502–513.

Pan, Y. J., et al. (2014). Antipsychotic discontinuation in patients with dementia: A systematic review and meta-analysis of published randomized controlled studies. *Dementia and Geriatric Cognitive Disorders*, *37*(3–4), 125–140.

Park, S., et al. (2005). Antibiotic use following a Korean national policy to prohibit medication dispensing by physicians. *Health Policy and Planning*, *20*(5), 302–309.

Parrino, T. A. (2005). Controlled trials to improve antibiotic utilization: A systematic review of experience, 1984–2004. *Pharmacotherapy*, *25*(2), 289–298.

Patton, M. Q. (1990). *Qualitative evaluation and research methods* (2nd ed.). Newbury Park, California: Sage.

Pearson, S. A., et al. (2003). Changing medication use in managed care: A critical review of the available evidence. *The American Journal of Managed Care*, *9*(11), 715–731.

Pearson, S. A., et al. (2009). Do computerised clinical decision support systems for prescribing change practice? A systematic review of the literature (1990–2007). *BMC Health Services Research*, 9.

Pirmohamed, M., James, S., Meakin, S., Green, C., Scott, A. K., Walley, T. J., … Breckenridge, A. M. (2004). Adverse drug reactions as cause of admission to hospital: Prospective analysis of 18 820 patients. *Bmj: British Medical Journal*, *329*(7456), 15–19.

Prochaska, J. O., & Di Clemente, C. O. (1986). Towards a comprehensive model of change. In W. R. Miller, & N. Heather (Eds.), *Treating addictive behaviours: Processes of change* (pp. 3–27). New York: Plenum Press.

Prochaska, J. O., et al. (1994). Stages of change and decisional balance for 12 problem behaviours. *Health Psychol, 13*, 39–46.

Prochaska, J. O., & Velicer, W. F. (1997). The transtheoretical model of health behaviour change. *American Journal of Health Promotion, 12*(1), 38–48.

Quick, J. D., Laing, R. O., & Rossdegnan, D. G. (1991). Intervention research to promote clinically effective and economically efficient use of pharmaceuticals - the international Network for rational use of drugs. *Journal of Clinical Epidemiology, 44*, S57–S65.

Radyowijati, A., & Haak, H. (2003). Improving antibiotic use in low-income countries: An overview of evidence on determinants. *Social Science & Medicine, 57*(4), 733–744.

Ratanawijitrasin, S., Soumerai, S. B., & Weerasuriya, K. (2001). Do national medicinal drug policies and essential drug programs improve drug use?: a review of experiences in developing countries. *Social Science & Medicine, 53*(7), 831–844.

Reeler, A. V. (1990). Injections – a fatal attraction. *Social Science & Medicine, 31*(10), 1119–1125.

Rietveld, A. H., & Haaijer-Ruskamp, F. M. (2002). Policy options for cost containment of pharmaceuticals. In M. N. G. Dukes, et al. (Ed.), *Drugs and money – Prices, affordability and cost containment* (pp. 29–54). IOS Press.

Ross-Degnan, D., et al. (1997). Improving pharmaceutical use in primary care in developing countries: A critical review of experience and lack of experience. In *International conference on improving use of medicines* (Chiang Mai, Thailand).

Roughead, E. E. (2006). Enhancing early uptake of drug evidence into primary care. *Expert Review of Pharmacoeconomics & Outcomes Research, 6*, 661–671.

Roughead, E. E., et al. (2013). Bridging evidence-practice gaps: Improving use of medicines in elderly Australian veterans. *BMC Health Services Research, 13*, 514.

Roughead, L., et al. (2015). *Medicine utilisation methods to support pharmaceutical policy implementation. The first step of WHO/EMP work for improving medicine use in low and middle income countries.* World Health Organization.

Roughead, E., & Gilbert, A. (2016). Development, delivery and evaluation of implementation programs. In M. Elseviers, et al. (Ed.), *Drug utilization Research: Methods and applications.* Wiley-Blackwell.

Roughead, L., Semple, S., & Rosenfeld, E. (2013). *Literature review: Medication safety in Australia.* Available from http://www.safetyandquality.gov.au/wp-content/uploads/2014/02/Literature-Review-Medication-Safety-in-Australia-2013.pdf.

Rowe, A. K., de Savigny, D., Lanata, C. F., & Victora, C. G. (2005). How can we achieve and maintain high-quality performance of health workers in low-resource settings? *Lancet, 366*(9490), 1026–1035.

Sabaté, E. (2003). Adherence to long-term therapies. *Evidence for Action*, 2016. Available from http://www.who.int/chp/knowledge/publications/adherence_report/en/.

Saha, S., et al. (2012). Pyrrolidinediones reduce the toxicity of thiazolidinediones and modify their anti-diabetic and anti-cancer properties. *European Journal of Pharmacology, 697*(1–3), 13–23.

Santoso, B. (1995). From research to action: The Gunungkidul experience. *Essential Drugs Monitor, 1995*(20), 21–22.

Siddiqi, K., Newell, J., & Robinson, M. (2005). Getting evidence into practice: What works in developing countries? *International Journal for Quality in Health Care, 17*(5), 447–453.

Sketris, I. S., Langille Ingram, E. M., & Lummis, H. L. (2009). Strategic opportunities for effective optimal prescribing and medication management. *The Canadian Journal of Clinical Pharmacology, 16*(1), e103–e125.

Snowdon, J., et al. (2006). Duration of risperidone treatment for BPSD. *Int J Geriatr Psychiatry, 21*(7), 699–701.

Snowdon, J., Galanos, D., & Vaswani, D. (2011a). Patterns of psychotropic medication use in nursing homes: Surveys in Sydney, allowing comparisons over time and between countries. *Int Psychogeriatr, 23*(9), 1520–1525.

Snowdon, J., Galanos, D., & Vaswani, D. (2011b). A 2009 survey of psychotropic medication use in Sydney nursing homes. *The Medical Journal of Australia, 194*(5), 270–271.

Sutters, C. A. (1990). The management of a hospital formulary. *Journal of Clinical Pharmacy and Therapeutics, 15*(1), 59–76.

Wensing, M., van der Weijden, T., & Grol, R. (1998). Implementing guidelines and innovations in general practice: Which interventions are effective? *The British Journal of General Practice: the Journal of the Royal College of General Practitioners, 48*(427), 991–997.

WHO. (1985). *The rational use of drugs. Report of the conference of experts.* Geneva: World Health Organization.

WHO. (1988). *Guidelines for developing national drug policies.* Geneva: World Health Organization.

WHO. (1992). *How to investigate drug use in communities. Guidelines for social science research.* , Geneva: World Health Organization.

WHO. (1993). *How to investigate drug use in health facilities. Selected drug use indicators.* , Geneva: World Health Organization.

WHO. (2001). *How to develop and implement a national drug policy* (2nd ed.). , Geneva: World Health Organization.

WHO. (2002). Promoting rational use of medicines: Core components. In *WHO policy perspectives on medicines.* Geneva: World Health Organization.

WHO. (2003). *Drug and therapeutic committees: A practical guide.* France: World Health Organization.

WHO. (2004). *The essential medicines concept: From its beginnings until today. WHO/EDM/2004.3.* Available from http://apps.who.int/iris/bitstream/10665/69134/1/WHO_EDM_2004.3.pdf.

WHO. (2007). Progress in the rational use of medicines. In *World health Assembly Resolution, WHA60.16.* Geneva, Switzerland: World Health Organization.

WHO. (2009). *Medicines use in primary care in developing and transitional countries: Fact Book summarizing results from studies reported between 1990 and 2006. WHO/EMP/MAR/2009.3.* Geneva: World Health Organization.

WHO. (2010). *Country pharmaceutical situations: Fact book on WHO level I indicators 2007. WHO/EMP/MPC/2010.1.* Geneva, Switzerland: World Health Organization.

WHO. (2012). The persuit of responsible use of medicines: Sharing and learning from country experiences. In *Technical report prepared for the Ministers Summit on the benefits of responsible use of medicines: Setting policies for better and cost-effective health care.* Geneva: World Health Organization.

WHO. (2015). *The WHO model list of essential medicines* (19th ed.). Geneva: World Health Organization.

WHO. (2017). *Comparative table of medicines on the WHO essential medicines list from 1977-2011.* Available from http://www.who.int/selection_medicines/list/en/.

Winett, R. A. (1995). A framework for health promotion and disease prevention programs. *The American Psychologist, 50*, 341–350.

Winett, R. A., King, A. C., & Altman, D. G. (1989). *Health psychology and public health: An integrative approach.* New York: Pergamon Press.

World Bank. (1994). *Better health in Africa. Experiences and lessons learned.* Washington DC: The World Bank.

World Health Organization. (2011). In H. V. Hogerzeil, & Z. Mirza (Eds.), *The World Medicines Situation: Access to essential medicines as part of the right to health* (p. 14). Geneva: World Health Organization.

Wyatt, H. V. (1984). The popularity of injections in the third-world – origins and consequences for poliomyelitis. *Social Science & Medicine, 19*(9), 911–915.

CHAPTER

RATIONAL AND RESPONSIBLE MEDICINES USE

16

Arjun Poudel, Lisa M. Nissen
Queensland University of Technology, Brisbane, QLD, Australia

CHAPTER OUTLINE

Social and Administrative Aspects of Pharmacy in Low- and Middle-Income Countries. http://dx.doi.org/10.1016/B978-0-12-811228-1.00016-9

INTRODUCTION

Global health spending is growing, having increased from 2% in 2012 to 2.8% in 2013 alone (Morris & Yoritomo, 2015). The growing prevalence of chronic diseases, new technological advances in treatment options, evolving market expansion, and increasing aging population drive health spending, which is projected to accelerate, increasing an average of 5.2% a year in 2014–18 (Morris & Yoritomo, 2015). However, the significant progress in health over recent decades has been profoundly unequal. Health provision varies across the world and is challenging particularly to the developing countries because of the associated costs and other various cultural, political, and socioeconomic conditions (Smith, 2015). This gives rise to health inequalities within countries. A global stewardship initiated by the World Health Organization (WHO) and the United Nations constitutes a range of strategies aimed at minimizing global burden of disease and promoting human development through the achievement of the Millennium Development Goals (MDGs). A major focus of the MDG is to reduce health inequalities and to develop a framework for health service development and public health interventions, which includes improved access and responsible use of medications (Smith, 2015).

Appropriate supply and use of medicines in the last decade has had a positive influence on health that has decreased disease burden, reduced mortality, and improved the overall quality of life (World Health Organization, 2012). However, this has also been given rise to irrational, inappropriate, and ineffective use of medications commonly observed in healthcare system all over the world, with more concerns in developing countries (World Health Organization, 2000) because of the way in which medicines are used: the WHO indicates that a third of the world's population living in developing countries lacks access to medicines and approximately 50% of all patients fail to take their medicines correctly (World Health Organization, 2011). A major step toward rational use of medicines (RUM) was initiated by WHO after the establishment of the first Model List of Essential Medicines in 1977. Later in 1989, the International Network for the Rational Use of Drugs was formed with the aim to assist multidisciplinary intervention research projects to promote more RUM (World Health Organization, 2002a). More recently, the WHO published a technical report on *the benefits of responsible use of medicines*, which explores solutions to improve patient outcomes and support sustainable and cost-effective healthcare.

This chapter will highlight the significance of rational and responsible medication use focusing on developing countries. The instances of irrational medication use and factors associated with it will be discussed with further elaboration on the challenges and strategies to improve and promote rational medication use.

DEFINITION

RATIONAL MEDICINES USE

"Safe," "rational," and "optimal" are words often used to define standards that should be achieved in prescribing. In the early 1970s, the term "appropriate prescribing" was introduced as a general concept that comprises a range of different prescribing values and practices (Parish, 1973). Later in 1985, the Conference of Experts on the Rational Use of Drugs, convened by the World Health Organization (2002b), defined rational medicine use as "The rational use of drugs requires that patients receive medicines appropriate to their clinical needs, in doses that meet their own individual requirements, for an adequate period of time, and at the lowest cost to them and their community."

More general descriptions of what constitutes rational medicine use have included: appropriate indication based on sound medical consideration; appropriate medicine based on efficacy, safety, affordability, and suitability for the patient; appropriate dosage, administration, and duration of treatment; appropriate patient selection based on no contraindications and minimal likelihood of adverse reactions; appropriate medicine information for patients; and patient adherence to the treatment.

IRRATIONAL MEDICINES USE

Irrational medicines use has been defined as the use of a particular medicine that poses greater risk of harm than benefit, especially when safer and more effective options are available for the same condition (Spinewine et al., 2007). The concept of irrational prescribing recognizes that there are no medications without any risk, whereby appropriate use of medications requires that the risks associated with its use outweigh the anticipated benefits (Beers, 1997). Irrational use also includes not prescribing suboptimal doses of medication (Gallagher, Barry, & O'Mahony, 2007). Based on the concept of risk–benefit definition of appropriateness, irrational medicines use can be defined as follows:

- overuse of a medication where there is no clear indication,
- misuse of a medication in relation to wrong drug, dose, and duration, or
- underuse of a medication where there is a clear indication.

RESPONSIBLE MEDICINES USE

The term "responsible use of medicines" implies that the activities, capabilities, and existing resources of health system stakeholders are aligned to ensure patients receive the right medicines at the right time, use them appropriately, and benefit from them (World Health Organization, 2012). This definition highlights the significance of stakeholder responsibility and addresses the challenges in resource-limited settings and also complements WHO definition of rational medicine use.

INSTANCES OF IRRATIONAL MEDICATION USE

The factors underlying the irrational use of medicines are diverse ranging from overuse, underuse, and misuse of prescription or nonprescription medicines. Studies report that more than 50% of all medications prescribed, dispensed, or sold are inappropriate (World Health Organization, 2009, 2010) and that half of all patients fail to take medications appropriately as prescribed or dispensed (Sabaté, 2003). Despite a global prevalence of irrational medicine use, leadership among countries around monitoring this issue has been limited (World Health Organization, 2006). Many developing or transitional countries with limited resources to combat these issues face a vast range of problems. For example, primary care settings in developing countries, less than 40% of patients in public sector and less than 30% of patients in private sector, are treated according to the clinical practice guidelines for common diseases (World Health Organization, 2011).

There are many factors that contribute to irrational medicine use, and these impact various levels of the medicine management pathways (e.g., direct to consumer advertising). Factors such as provision of economic incentives, promotional practices, knowledge, attitude, and practices within the community healthcare can contribute to irrational medicine use. Inappropriate prescribing can also result from a number of components of the prescribing process itself such as follows:

1. Polypharmacy: Polypharmacy indicates the prescribing practice of multiple medications that are considered clinically necessary. The minimum number of medications used to define "polypharmacy" is variable but generally ranges from 5 to 10 (Gnjidic et al., 2012). It also includes the practice of prescribing medications at a higher dose, at a greater frequency, or for a period longer than is clinically indicated.
2. Unfavorable risk–benefit ratio: Irrational prescribing occurs when the risks of an adverse event associated with a medication use outweigh the clinical benefits, where safe and more effective alternative therapy is available (Corsonello et al., 2009).
3. Prescribing medications with high risk of drug–drug or drug–disease interactions (Aronson, 2009).
4. Prescribing medications where there are no specific indication and clinical significance for a specific patient (Gallagher et al., 2007).
5. Underprescribing or underutilization of medications: Irrational prescribing occurs when there is a failure to prescribe a clinically significant medication for a patient for whom there is no valid reason not to prescribe the said medication and for whom there is no contraindication to this beneficial pharmacotherapy, e.g., if a patient is suffering from a particular disease and no medicine is prescribed to treat that particular condition, or the dose of the medication is insufficient to treat that condition effectively (Aronson, 2009).
6. Excessive use of irrational fixed dose combinations (FDCs): Although rational FDCs can be of immense help to the healthcare system, which may improve patient compliance and quality of life, irrational FDCs increase the risk of adverse drug reactions, lead to an ineffective dosages, and ultimately increase cost. In many cases their stability is doubtful, reducing the efficacy of many preparations (Poudel, Palaian, Shankar, Jayasekera, & Izham, 2008).

FACTORS UNDERLYING IRRATIONAL MEDICINES USE

Medicines use is influenced by several interrelated factors that are involved in the therapeutic process as illustrated in Fig. 16.1.

PRESCRIBER

A number of factors can influence prescribers, leading to misuse of medications during prescribing practices. Several prescription audits from developing countries have report poor prescribing practices including missing dosages on the prescription, not including duration of treatment, and using brand names extensively on their prescriptions (Aslam, Khatoon, Mehdi, Mumtaz, & Murtaza, 2016; Biswas, Jindal, Siddiquei, & Maini, 2001; Ghimire, 2009; Gopalakrishnan, Ganeshkumar, & Katta, 2013; Patel, Vaidya, Naik, & Borker, 2005; Shamna & Karthikeyan, 2011). Inadequate proper clinical training, poor supervisory system, and increased dependency on diagnostic aids rather than clinical diagnosis are among several other existing factors that exist as a gap between prescribers' knowledge and practice, which plays a significant role in promoting irrational medicines use (Yousefi, Majdzadeh, Valadkhani, & Nedjat, 2012). Moreover, prescribers' decisions are also influenced by other factors such as time

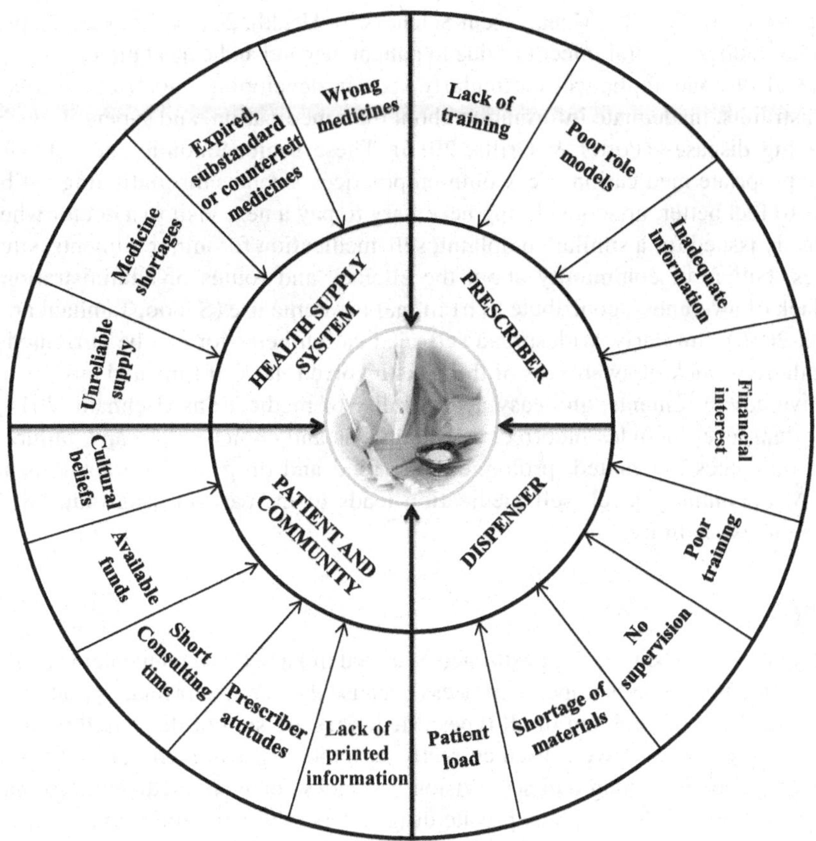

FIGURE 16.1

Factors that influence prescribing.

pressure, peer and patient pressure, and pressure form pharmaceutical companies. This may lead prescribers fail to educate and counsel patients on appropriate use of medications.

Other factors that lead to inappropriate use include time constraints, diagnostic uncertainties, and medication costs. With intentions to make higher profit, prescribers use expensive medicines; however, the cheaper alternatives are available. On the other hand, the higher cost of some medicine will restrict the use of appropriate medicine and hence patients are prescribed with less appropriate medicine (Sarkar, Chakraborty, Misra, Shukla, & Swain, 2013).

PATIENTS AND COMMUNITY

A number of factors relate to consumer influences including noncompliance, self-medication, and demand of quick relief or treatment. Patients often have a conviction that "there is a pill for every ill." This belief and expectation of patient and patient parties often demand and compel physicians to prescribe medicines irrationally (Management Sciences for Health, 2012), for example, prescribing of unnecessary antibiotics for viral infections due to patient demand and expectations.

A high level of noncompliance, particularly seen in developing countries, results because of financial constraints, inadequate information about their medication, and superstitious belief about their underlying diseases (Porter & Grills, 2016). These socioeconomic and behavioral factors result in inappropriate medication use. Common practices, such as discontinuing antibiotics once person starts to feel better, not considering necessary to pay a next visit to a doctor when prescription was already issued for a similar complaint, self-medication for minor ailments, situational use of antibiotics, beliefs of community about the efficacy and routes of administration of certain drugs, and lack of awareness, contribute to irrational medicine use (Sahoo, Tamhankar, Johansson, & Lundborg, 2010). Similarly, widespread self-medication behavior can be attributed to the lack of strict regulations, lack of awareness of the risks involved, lack of time and money, urge of self-care, extensive advertisements, and easy accessibility of medications (Bennadi, 2014). Potential risk at individual level includes incorrect self-diagnosis and choice of therapy, failure to identify any adverse outcomes associated, prolonged use, food and drug interactions, dependence, and abuse risk. At community level, self-medication leads to increase in drug-induced disease and increased public expenditure.

DISPENSER

Pharmacists and other dispensers are positioned as a final linkage between medicine and patient. The dispensers play a vital role in therapeutic process because they are the primary point of contact consulted for heath advice on problem of all types. Medicines are sold or dispensed in every consults, which might be safe and effective if used correctly but otherwise can be hazardous if sold by a dispenser who lacks timely training and supervision and lacks adequate medicine information. These types of dispensers are usually seen as private drug sellers who get regular financial incentives by dispensing irrationally. Dispensing is also influenced by the availability of dispensing materials and time taken to dispense. Studies suggest that the lack of availability of dispensing materials and short dispensing time observed in many of the country indicator surveys do affect dispensing quality (Porter & Grills, 2016; World Health Organization, 2009). For example, an average dispensing time reported by WHO in developing countries was 1 min; only half of these patients are told about the proper administration of medicine and almost 50% of medicines are dispensed without label (World Health Organization, 2011).

HEALTH SYSTEMS

Health systems in every country aim to safeguard high-quality healthcare to their citizens at an affordable cost. WHO advocates guidelines, policies, and key interventions to promote more RUM. However, not all countries (less than half of all countries) adhere to the basic policies to ensure safe and rational use of medicines such as frequent monitoring of use, regular updating of clinical guidelines, and easy access to medicine information centers (World Health Organization, 2011). Unlike developed countries where the use of medicines is regularly monitored through electronic medical record or through insurance data, developing countries lack this system and hence monitoring and implementation of interventions to improve use of medicine are often ineffective.

Literatures from developing and transitional countries report the existence of weak regulatory and health systems that directly influence irrational medicine use (Okeke et al., 2005; Porter & Grills, 2016; Sahoo et al., 2010). Health system leaders often fail to prioritize medicine in policy agenda during their healthcare reform. This lack of political–economic interests along with an inadequate regulatory framework facilitated irrational use of medications in developing countries that resulted in poor health outcomes, diminished quality of life, and other adverse events (Porter & Grills, 2016; World Health Organization, 2012).

IMPACTS OF IRRATIONAL MEDICINE USE

The irrational use of medicines is harmful at both individual and community level. It has significant adverse effects on quality of care, healthcare costs, emergence of drug resistance such as in antimicrobial therapy, drug interactions, lost resources, and eroded patient confidence due to poor health outcomes. Diminished quality of care and therapy is associated with increased morbidity and mortality, increased costs, wastage of resources that limits the availability of vital medicines, and increased risk of adverse events.

Scholarly publications demonstrate the widespread impact of overuse or misuse of medications especially in developing countries. The availability of lifesaving antibiotics in developing countries has increased standard of living in most cases; however, antibiotics are prescribed rampantly without any valid indication and for lesser period than that of recommended treatment duration (Garg, Vishwakarma, Sharma, Nehra, & Saxena, 2014). This has led to a resistant strain of deadly bacteria, which has become a major public health burden owing in part to a lack of strict regulations (Reardon, 2014). Some common example includes the development of drug-resistant malaria and tuberculosis and the emergence of resistance to anti-HIV drug. In countries where pharmacies sell antibiotics without prescription and healthcare centers receive financial incentives for prescribing, antibiotics are misused (Reardon, 2014).

Similarly, irrational use of medicines possesses huge financial burden to the patient, community, and the overall healthcare system. A study from Nepal reports more than half of total medicine expenditure accounts for irrational medicines (Holloway, Gautam, & Reeves, 2001a). A similar study from India reported 69.2% of medicine expenditure wastage in private sector and 55.4% of wastage in the public sector (Chaturvedi, Mathur, & Anand, 2012). Other nonessential pharmaceuticals such as multivitamins, tonics, and cough mixtures are prescribed excessively in developing countries (Garg et al., 2014). Expenditure on these products decreases the allocation of already limited financial resources that could otherwise be used for other vital and essential medicines such as antibiotics and vaccines. The out-of-pocket spending on irrational medicines also hampers the household expenditures in poor countries. Adverse psychosocial impact, such as the perceived notion of "pill for every ill," also favors irrational prescribing. Patients rely completely on medications, which causes an apparent increase in demand for medicines.

STRATEGIES FOR IMPROVING AND PROMOTING RATIONAL MEDICINES USE

Rational prescribing strategies can be broadly classified into targeted and system-oriented approaches.

TARGETED APPROACHES

This involves educational and managerial interventions that are targeted directly toward prescribers.

Educational Interventions

In educational interventions, information and knowledge are provided to prescribers in the form of face-to-face training, symposium, seminars, and provision of written materials. These types of intervention are the most common interventions practiced. However, these interventions without sufficient follow-up and monitoring are often not sustainable and least effective. Educational interventions only when coupled with managerial or regulatory interventions result in desired outcomes.

Sound training of doctors has a significant impact on RUM as they have a capacity to control and manage limited pharmaceutical resources by their prescription practices as well as through their guidance as leaders, supervisors, or trendsetters for other healthcare staffs. Number of educational programs and manuals to improve the teaching of pharmacotherapy has been developed based on the principles of rational prescribing. However, the teaching of RUM by incorporating and implementing into the undergraduate curricula is still a challenge in many countries. Continuing medical education after the completion of prescribers' formal education is essential to keep prescribers informed and updated about recent changes in the use of medicines. Activities such as symposium, seminar, workshops, and lectures organized for relatively large number of people are commonly used methods for continuing medical education. Printed materials such as clinical literatures and newsletters, treatment guidelines, medicine formularies, and illustrated materials (flyers, posters, and leaflets) are used to update prescriber knowledge and bring changes in prescriber behavior.

Another method includes face-to-face contact, which is found to be the most effective approach for behavior change. A study reported positive prescribing practice when visited by trained personnel to a healthcare provider in his or her own setting (O'brien et al., 2008). Face-to-face interventions involve several components, including targeted outreach educational programs, written materials, and feedback sessions. Patient or consumer educations through mass campaigns via radio, television, or other printed materials and influencing opinion leaders who can encourage young and junior doctors to prescribe rationally are other educational strategies that promote rational prescribing.

Managerial Intervention

A managerial intervention guides prescribers in decision-making process. They are guided through provisions of treatment guidelines, medication review and feedback and, supervision and monitoring. Although these types of interventions require more effort to initiate, they produce a sustainable outcome.

Effective supervision and monitoring involves prescription audit and feedback. Prescribers are made aware about their prescribing practice, and the practice is compared with the standard guidelines. There are differences in how these activities are monitored and supervised in public and private sectors. Some countries encourage hospitals to have drug and therapeutics committee (DTC) as part of accreditation requirements. DTC established in health facilities such as tertiary hospitals can act as a monitoring body that can provide feedback for rational medicine use. In private sectors, monitoring and supervision of prescription habit is always a challenge.

Aspects of pharmaceutical management such as selection, procurement, and distribution greatly influence medicine use. A drug use review tool has been developed that recognizes difficulties in the medication use process. Hence, strategies are made and implemented to improve the use of medicines.

Similarly, approaches for selection of cost-effective pharmaceuticals are used such as cost bar graphs (figure or chart showing side-by-side comparison of prices for alternative medicine), mentioning recent pharmaceutical prices in manuals and on requisition forms. The intention is not always to mandate prescribers to choose least expensive medicine but rather to inform them about the available cheaper alternative that might be relevant. Other interventions involve the development of disease-specific standard diagnostic and treatment guidelines. This indorses standard patient treatment following the protocols.

SYSTEM-ORIENTED APPROACHES

This involves economic and regulatory interventions, which focus on policies, guidelines, and regulations.

Economic Intervention

Economic interventions are designed in such a way that prescribers get motivated due to positive financial incentives. These strategies include price setting and prescription fees, changes in reimbursement methods, insurance plans, and quality-based performance contracts.

The price setting can often encourage rational use of pharmaceuticals. For example, cross-subsidization approach that aids setting of lower price than their actual costs for vital medicines and setting higher prices than their actual costs for nonessential medicines favors the use of vital medicines, which limits the use of nonessential medicines. In addition, encouraging generic prescribing rather than using brand names leads to rational use from a cost perspective. This is observed in a study from 17 developing countries, which reports 9%–89% of saving could be achieved by an individual country by switching to lowest priced generics from originator brands (Cameron, Mantel-Teeuwisse, Leufkens, & Laing, 2012).

The insurance scheme that includes pharmaceutical benefits and capitation-based reimbursement scheme by third party also influences the RUM. While flat prescription fees (covering all medicines in any amount) in developing countries has resulted in overprescribing (Holloway, Gautam, & Reeves, 2001b), prohibiting medicine sales by prescribers eliminates financial incentives for overprescribing. Hence, interventions aimed toward charging item-based fees would lead to better prescribing quality.

Regulatory Intervention

Regulatory interventions aim to impose decisions that are intended to promote rational prescribing. These interventions set policies and guidelines such as encouraging prescribers to use generic products, restrictions on prescribing and dispensing practices, and withdrawal of irrational medicines from market. These types of interventions are successful with strong monitoring and vigilance; however, they are often disliked by prescribers and consumers and may also lead to inappropriate prescribing practices.

Despite the presence of drug regulation authority and legal restrictions for medication use in most countries, lack of resources and absence of well-organized approach have restricted their effectiveness. WHO reports the presence of adequate pharmaceutical regulation in fewer than one in six member states, while two in six has no or little pharmaceutical regulatory capacity. Successful regulatory strategies are based on the extent to which consumer behavior and demand are addressed. For instance, regulations to ban certain medicines might promote black marketing of banned medicines as well as may promote (other) irrational medicines. For example, banning of a pediatric antidiarrheal medicine in Pakistan was unsuccessful because it failed to address patient demand factors (Bhutta & Balchin, 1996).

ACHIEVEMENTS

National pharmaceutical policies based on the affordability, quality, and availability of medicines play an important role in meeting healthcare needs and economic priorities especially in developing countries. In 1970s, the concept of essential medicines was introduced and promoted by WHO, which were limited to only few countries. The scenario has now improved promptly with more than 150 countries adopting national medicine policies (World Health Organization, 2007). Similarly, the concept of RUM, which was not well adopted in developing countries, had the scenario changing with more than 135 countries currently having their own therapeutic manuals and formularies that assist in promoting RUM (World Health Organization, 2007). Information on availability and pricing was virtually not available, and few countries encouraged generic substitution. Today, several countries participate in availability and pricing surveys to provide information publicly, which has eventually reduced prices because of generic substitution (Bansal & Purohit, 2013).

Progress in ensuring the accessibility, availability, and affordability of medicines across several countries has been significant within the past few years. WHO and Health Action International (HAI) have suggested several strategies and policy perspectives for RUM, which was adopted and implemented in numerous countries (World Health Organization, 2002b). Some strategies for RUM suggested in WHO policy perspective include evidence-based standard treatment guidelines (STGs) to assist prescribers in clinical decision-making of appropriate treatments for specific clinical conditions, preparing essential medicines list based on treatments of choice, establishing drugs and therapeutics committees in district and hospitals, initiating problem-based training in pharmacotherapy in undergraduate curriculum, and continuing medical education as licensure requirements, effective supervision, audit and feedback, and enforced drug regulation.

While some of the initiatives had adequate attention, much remains to be done. Despite the recent progress in relation to RUM, access to medicines remain less than optimal in many countries, especially for the poor and underprivileged (FIP Statements of Policy, 2005). Some other challenges are discussed further in this chapter.

CHALLENGES

Current health system trends around the world suggest that many poor countries will find it a big challenge to meet the health-related MDGs (United Nations Millennium Development Goals, 2000). Even countries using vibrant and cost-effective interventions to promote population health find inequalities among countries and among socioeconomic groups within them (Darmstadt et al., 2005). These interventions are delivered through health systems with a primary intention to promote, restore, and maintain health. National medicine policies often govern rational medicine use in any country, but unfortunately the need for rational medicine use is higher in developing countries that have limited financial resources and multiple pressing needs (Thawani, 2010). This leads to the limited attention of policy makers toward rational medicine use as well as shadows the necessity for sufficient resource allocation because of skewed preferences. As part of its health system strengthening approach, a number of government bodies, funding agencies, and international organizations strive to work toward promotion of rational medicine use. However, the conflicting demands and weakened collaboration between health systems often in developing and low-income countries hinder the execution and successful implementation of health promotions.

Many people lack easy access to health technologies in developing countries. These technologies range from basic ones such as lifesaving medications (antiretroviral), life-enhancing medicines (anti-asthma) to vaccines for prevention of debilitating diseases in children (Frost & Reich, 2014). A major challenge to access is cost. For a developing country, the affordability of medicine for an individual patient is a factor that limits access to care and treatment, and sustainable financing of healthcare is a major burden (KC, Poudel, & Ibrahim, 2012). Unlike in developed countries where copay systems or medical insurance covers the healthcare cost, patients in developing countries pay out of pocket for their medications. The situation is even aggravated by the practice of selling medications in higher rate (lowest priced generics found more expensive than the originator brand) with an intention to make greater profit (Thawani, 2010). The social as well as cultural perceptions of disease and medicines influenced by knowledge, background, and economic factors in developing countries also make the task of intervention on rational medicine use difficult.

Many interventional studies conducted to promote RUM often lack reproducibility and sustainability (Thawani, 2010). Successful interventions require the political willingness with consequent enactment of laws and regulations, which is often lacking in developing countries. In addition, developing countries lack adequate education and training of healthcare workers on rational medicine use, regular update of STGs, and adequate system to monitor and regulate how medicines are used. Other obstacles that have compounded the problem of irrational medicine use in developing countries include limited capacity of health systems, lack of political commitment, disputes on patents and international trade, influence of pharmaceutical industries, persistent corruption in healthcare sector, and difficulties in prescribing, dispensing, delivering, and distributing healthcare products (Frost & Reich, 2014).

RECOMMENDATIONS: THE WAY FORWARD

There is now ample evidence to suggest global irrational medicine use with alarming situation in developing countries. While much still remains to be known regarding the effectiveness and impact of various strategies, following recommendations can be suggested to promote RUM:

1. A management information center to monitor medicine use is essential along with a national body to coordinate, monitor, and implement policies on medicine use.
2. Starting and uplifting DTC at district and facility levels is essential, which brings key stakeholders together to reach common consensus on medicine use including setting up the medicines management policies, developing treatment protocols, and choosing drug formularies.
3. Setting rational use standards through STGs, essential medicine lists, and formularies is vital. Adoption of these standards with frequent monitoring will minimize inappropriate prescribing practices.
4. Implementation of problem-based learning and training in pharmacotherapy in undergraduate medical curriculum.

5. Obligatory continuing medical education for licensure of health professionals practiced in developed countries could be adopted by developing countries where few options are available for regular in-service education.
6. Adequate and reliable medicine information should be prioritized by government. In many countries the only source of medicine information for prescribers is from pharmaceutical industry. This information may be biased focusing only on positive aspects of medicine. While government invests less in medicine information for prescribers, industry makes huge expenditure. This imbalance must be addressed by making information publicly available, understandable, independent, and unbiased. Regulations should also exist to ensure that promotional materials will meet the ethical standards.
7. Adequate allocation of funding is required to ensure availability of medicines and infrastructures, and adequate manpower is required to undertake the necessary monitoring, implementation, and follow-up review of interventions. This might be achieved by limiting government supply and procurement to essential medicines only, and allocating more on training, supervision, and salary incentives.
8. Upgrading the skills and knowledge of pharmacists and drug dispensers is important, as they play significant role in medicine recommendation and retail purchase.
9. Long-term interventions on multiple levels of healthcare system are essential. Sustainable multifaceted interventions can therefore be scaled up to national level, with monitoring systems to observe the long-term impacts.

CONCLUSIONS

Irrational use of medicine continues to be a challenge and major public health concern, especially in developing countries that have limited resources. Identification of major problem and developing a coordinated action plan that effectively implements, evaluates, and monitors strategies that discourage the use of inappropriate medicines are fundamental to the success of RUM. Hence, combating irrational use of medicine requires institutionalization of an approach into the healthcare system with adequate investment in infrastructure development and capacity building. There is an urgent need of harmonization and coordination between government, funding bodies, and international organizations working to provide universal social protection and effective coverage of essential health interventions, which in the long run ensures rational and responsible medicine use.

LESSONS LEARNED

- Inappropriate use of medicines is globally rampant, and action to combat it is urgently required. Many developing or transitional countries with limited resources to combat these issues face a vast range of problems.
- Promoting RUM is a shared responsibility of all key stakeholders involved. There is a need of continuous regulation and monitoring on medicine procurement, prescription, and dispensing.
- Sustainable interventions on multiple levels of healthcare system are essential with monitoring systems to observe the long-term impacts.

REFERENCES

Aronson, J. K. (2009). Medication errors: What they are, how they happen, and how to avoid them. *QJM : Monthly Journal of the Association of Physicians*, *102*(8), 513–521.

Aslam, A., Khatoon, S., Mehdi, M., Mumtaz, S., & Murtaza, B. (2016). Evaluation of rational drug use at teaching hospitals in Punjab, Pakistan. *Journal of Pharmacy Practice and Community Medicine*, *2*(2).

Bansal, D., & Purohit, V. K. (2013). Accessibility and use of essential medicines in health care: Current progress and challenges in India. *Journal of Pharmacology & Pharmacotherapeutics*, *4*(1), 13–18.

Beers, M. H. (1997). Explicit criteria for determining potentially inappropriate medication use by the elderly: An update. *Archives of Internal Medicine*, *157*(14), 1531–1536.

Bennadi, D. (2014). Self-medication: A current challenge. *Journal of Basic and Clinical Pharmacy*, *5*(1), 19.

Bhutta, T. I., & Balchin, C. (1996). Assessing the impact of a regulatory intervention in Pakistan. *Social Science & Medicine*, *42*(8), 1195–1202.

Biswas, N. R., Jindal, S., Siddiquei, M. M., & Maini, R. (2001). Patterns of prescription and drug use in ophthalmology in a tertiary hospital in Delhi. *British Journal of Clinical Pharmacology*, *51*(3), 267–269.

Cameron, A., Mantel-Teeuwisse, A. K., Leufkens, H. G., & Laing, R. O. (2012). Switching from originator brand medicines to generic equivalents in selected developing countries: How much could be saved? *Value in Health: the Journal of the International Society for Pharmacoeconomics and Outcomes Research*, *15*(5), 664–673.

Chaturvedi, V., Mathur, A., & Anand, A. (2012). Rational drug use–As common as common sense? *Medical Journal Armed Forces India*, *68*(3), 206–208.

Corsonello, A., Pranno, L., Garasto, S., Fabietti, P., Bustacchini, S., & Lattanzio, F. (2009). Potentially inappropriate medication in elderly hospitalized patients. *Drugs & Aging*, *26*(1), 31–39.

Darmstadt, G. L., Bhutta, Z. A., Cousens, S., Adam, T., Walker, N., de Bernis, L., & Lancet Neonatal Survival Steering Team (2005). Evidence-based, cost-effective interventions: How many newborn babies can we save? *Lancet*, *365*(9463), 977–988.

FIP Statements of Policy. (2005). *International pharmaceutical federation (FIP) statement of policy on improving access to medicines in developing countries (2005, Cairo)*.

Frost, L. J., & Reich, M. (2014). *Access: How do good health technologies get to poor people in poor countries?* Bibliomotion, Inc.

Gallagher, P., Barry, P., & O'Mahony, D. (2007). Inappropriate prescribing in the elderly. *Journal of Clinical Pharmacy and Therapeutics*, *32*(2), 113–121.

Garg, M., Vishwakarma, P., Sharma, M., Nehra, R., & Saxena, K. (2014). The impact of irrational practices: A wake up call. *Journal of Pharmacology & Pharmacotherapeutics*, *5*(4), 245.

Ghimire, S. (2009). Students' Corner-A prospective surveillance of drug prescribing and dispensing in a teaching hospital in Western Nepal. *JPMA. The Journal of the Pakistan Medical Association*, *59*(10), 726.

Gnjidic, D., Hilmer, S. N., Blyth, F. M., Naganathan, V., Waite, L., Seibel, M. J., … Le Couteur, D. G. (2012). Polypharmacy cutoff and outcomes: Five or more medicines were used to identify community-dwelling older men at risk of different adverse outcomes. *Journal of Clinical Epidemiology*, *65*(9), 989–995.

Gopalakrishnan, S., Ganeshkumar, P., & Katta, A. (2013). Assessment of prescribing practices among urban and rural general practitioners in Tamil Nadu. *Indian Journal of Pharmacology*, *45*(3), 252.

Holloway, K. A., Gautam, B. R., & Reeves, B. C. (2001a). The effects of different kinds of user fee on prescribing costs in rural Nepal. *Health Policy and Planning*, *16*(4), 421–427.

Holloway, K. A., Gautam, B. R., & Reeves, B. C. (2001b). The effects of different kinds of user fees on prescribing quality in rural Nepal. *Journal of Clinical Epidemiology*, *54*(10), 1065–1071.

KC, B., Poudel, A., & Ibrahim, M. (2012). Health priorities of the Nepal government: Where are the essential medicines? *Journal of Pharmaceutical Health Services Research*, *3*(2), 125–126.

Management Sciences for Health. (2012). *MDS-3: Managing access to medicines and health technologies.* Arlington, VA: Management Sciences for Health.

Morris, M., & Yoritomo, W. (2015). *Global health care outlook: Common goals, competing priorities*. Retrieved from deloitte. com http://www2.deloitte.com/au/en/pages/life-sciences-and-healthcare/articles/global-health-care-sector-outlook.html.

Okeke, I. N., Klugman, K. P., Bhutta, Z. A., Duse, A. G., Jenkins, P., O'Brien, T. F., … Laxminarayan, R. (2005). Antimicrobial resistance in developing countries. Part II: Strategies for containment. *The Lancet Infectious Diseases*, *5*(9), 568–580.

O'brien, M., Rogers, S., Jamtvedt, G., Oxman, A., Odgaard-Jensen, J., Kristofferson, D., & Davis, D. (2008). Educational outreach visits: Effects on professional practice and health care outcomes (review). *The Cochrane Library*, *3*, 1–64.

Parish, P. A. (1973). Drug prescribing—the concern of all. *The Journal of the Royal Society for the Promotion of Health*, *93*(4), 213–217.

Patel, V., Vaidya, R., Naik, D., & Borker, P. (2005). Irrational drug use in India: A prescription survey from Goa. *Journal of Postgraduate Medicine*, *51*(1), 9.

Porter, G., & Grills, N. (2016). Medication misuse in India: A major public health issue in India. *Journal of Public Health*, *38*(2), e150–e157.

Poudel, A., Palaian, S., Shankar, P., Jayasekera, J., & Izham, M. (2008). Irrational fixed dose combinations in Nepal: Need for intervention. *Kathmandu University Medical Journal*, *6*(3), 399–405.

Reardon, S. (2014). Antibiotic resistance sweeping developing world. *Nature*, *509*(7499), 141.

Sabaté, E. (2003). *Adherence to long-term therapies: Evidence for action*. World Health Organization.

Sahoo, K. C., Tamhankar, A. J., Johansson, E., & Lundborg, C. S. (2010). Antibiotic use, resistance development and environmental factors: A qualitative study among healthcare professionals in Orissa, India. *BMC Public Health*, *10*(1), 1.

Sarkar, P., Chakraborty, K., Misra, A., Shukla, R., & Swain, S. P. (2013). Pattern of psychotropic prescription in a tertiary care center: A critical analysis. *Indian Journal of Pharmacology*, *45*(3), 270.

Shamna, M., & Karthikeyan, M. (2011). Prescription pattern of antidiabetic drugs in the outpatient departments of hospitals in Malappuram district, Kerala. *Journal of Basic and Clinical Physiology and Pharmacology*, *22*(4), 141–143.

Smith, F. (2015). Pharmacy in developing countries. *Pharmacy Practice*, *7*, 103.

Spinewine, A., Schmader, K. E., Barber, N., Hughes, C., Lapane, K. L., Swine, C., & Hanlon, J. T. (2007). Appropriate prescribing in elderly people: How well can it be measured and optimised? *Lancet*, *370*(9582), 173–184.

Thawani, V. (2010). Rational use of medicines: Achievements and challenges. *Indian Journal of Pharmacology*, *42*(2), 63.

United Nations Millennium Development Goals. (2000). *United Nations Millennium Declaration. United Nations General Assembly Resolution 55/2*. New York: United Nations. Available http://www.un.org/millennium/declaration/ares552e.pdf.

World Health Organization. (2000). *Session guides: Problems of irratonal use of drugs*. Availalbe at http://archives.who.int/PRDUC2004/RDUCD/Session_Guides/problems_of_irrational_drug_use.htm.

World Health Organization. (2002b). *Promoting rational use of medicines: Core components*. Available at http://apps.who.int/iris/handle/10665/67438.

World Health Organization. (2006). *Using indicators to measure country pharmaceutical situations: Fact book on WHO level I and level II monitoring indicators*. Available at http://www.who.int/medicines/publications/WHOTCM2006.2A.pdf.

World Health Organization. (2007). *The WHO essential medicines list (EML): 30th anniversary*. Available at http://www.who.int/medicines/events/fs/en/.

World Health Organization. (2009). *Medicines use in primary care in developing and transitional countries: Fact book summarizing results from studies reported between 1990 and 2006*. World Health Organization. Available at http://www.who.int/medicines/publications/who_emp_2009.3/en/.

World Health Organization. (2010). *Medicines: Rational use of medicines. Fact sheet no 338*. Availalbe at http://www.wiredhealthresources.net/resources/NA/WHO-FS_MedicinesRationalUse.pdf.

World Health Organization. (2011). *The world medicines situation 2011: Rational use of medicines*. Available at http://apps.who.int/medicinedocs/en/d/Js18064en/.

World Health Organization. (2012). *The pursuit of responsible use of medicines: Sharing and learning from country experiences*. Availalbe at http://www.who.int/medicines/areas/rational_use/en/.

World Health Organization. (September 2002a). *Policy perspectives on medicines: Promoting rational use of medicines: Core components*. Geneva: WHO. Available at http://apps.who.int/medicinedocs/pdf/h3011e/h3011e.pdf.

World Health Organization. WHO Policy Perspectives on Medicines. Available at http://www.who.int/medicines/publications/policyperspectives/en/.

Yousefi, N., Majdzadeh, R., Valadkhani, M., & Nedjat, S. (2012). Reasons for physicians' tendency to irrational prescription of corticosteroids. *Iranian Red Crescent Medical Journal, 14*(11), 713–718.

SECTION 7

QUALITY OF PUBLIC HEALTH PHARMACY SERVICES IN LOW- AND MIDDLE-INCOME COUNTRIES

CHAPTER

QUALITY OF PHARMACY HEALTH SERVICES

17

Saira Azhar[1], Mohamed Izham Mohamed Ibrahim[2]

[1]COMSATS, Abbottabad, Pakistan; [2]Qatar University, Doha, Qatar

CHAPTER OUTLINE

INTRODUCTION

Pharmacy health services comprise the care that the pharmacist provides to the patient, which mainly focuses on drug safety, effectiveness, and health outcomes. Pharmacy health services are defined as "*an action or set of actions undertaken in or organized by a pharmacy, delivered by a pharmacist or other health practitioner, who applies their specialized health knowledge personally or via an intermediary, with a patient/client, population or another health professional, to optimize the process of care with the aim to improve health outcomes and the value of health care*."(Joanna, Daniel, Fernando, & Shalom, 2013). Although several terms and definitions have been used to describe pharmacy health services, with a focus on the provision of services by a pharmacist, there is no collectively recognized definition in the literature that focuses on the entire scope of heath care activities, services, and programs provided by pharmacists.

Social and Administrative Aspects of Pharmacy in Low- and Middle-Income Countries. http://dx.doi.org/10.1016/B978-0-12-811228-1.00017-0

Healthcare consumers and payers are continuously searching for quality goods, i.e., health services and products. They are focusing on services and goods that are worthy value for money. All healthcare stakeholders will be satisfied if the healthcare is of high quality. In addition, higher healthcare quality will enhance the performance of the healthcare organization. Quality in healthcare is a production of cooperation between the patient and the healthcare provider in a supportive environment (Mosadeghrad, 2014).

Schuster, McGlynn, and Brook (1998) defined quality healthcare as *"providing patients with appropriate services in a technically competent manner, with good communication, shared decision making and cultural sensitivity."* According to Institute of Medicine, quality of healthcare is *"the degree to which healthcare services for individuals and population increases the likelihood of desired healthcare outcomes and is consistent with the current professional knowledge"* (Institute of Medicine, 1990). In addition, according to Lohr (1990), quality of care is a function of technical care, art of care, and technical and art interaction, i.e.,

"Quality of care = f (technical care + art of care + technical and art interaction)."

There are three components of quality healthcare: interpersonal quality, technical quality, and facilities–services quality (Donabedian, 1980).

Pharmacists play a key role in providing quality healthcare. They are experts in medicines and use their clinical expertise, together with their practical knowledge to provide patients and public the professional care. Pharmacists are highly trained health professionals. Pharmacists provide services such as dispensing, advice on treatment of minor ailments, promoting healthy living, medicines use reviews, quit smoking, pregnancy testing, vaccination, and supervising use of prescribed medicines.

Personal factors of the pharmacist and the patient and factors pertaining to the pharmacy healthcare organization, pharmacy health services system, and the broader environment affect the quality of pharmacy health services. The Quality of pharmacy health services can be enhanced by supportive: (1) visionary pharmacy leadership and proper planning; (2) pharmacy education and training; (3) availability of pharmacy resources; (4) effective management of pharmacy resources; (5) pharmacy employees and processes; and (6) pharmacist collaboration and cooperation with other healthcare providers. Ensuring and measuring the quality of pharmacy health services are important because they tell the society how the pharmacy health system is performing and leads to improved pharmacy services. Guaranteeing and assessing the quality of pharmacy health services are necessary steps in the process of improving the quality of pharmacy health services. There are several ways the quality of pharmacy health services can be measured: the structure of pharmacy health services, process, and outcome; and patient experience with the pharmacy services, pharmacy facilities, and professional pharmacists.

As a new era shifts the focus of the pharmacy profession toward patient-oriented practice, there has been a clear increase in professional diversity and a focus on the quality of healthcare services. Quality can only be improved by collaboration with physicians and other healthcare professionals (Adamcik et al., 1986; Hepler & Strand, 1990).

EVOLUTION OF PHARMACY HEALTH SERVICES

The practice of treatment and pharmacy care started long back since the era of ancient Babylon (George, 1965). Then, it went through several civilizations, e.g., the Arabs, the Chinese, and the Western eras. The pharmacy and medical practices separated in 13th century, and in about 17th century, public pharmacies were established. In the early days, pharmacist is known as chemist or apothecary. The focus was more on product compounding and dispensing. The drug research and development started in the 17th century. Pharmacy has come through many revolutions. It has served the society for around 50 centuries. The pharmacy profession has moved from product- and service-oriented to patient- and public-focused.

Pharmacy's focus began to grow again in the late 20th century. During the 1980s, a professional movement that advocates called clinical pharmacy gained momentum, influencing the pharmacists to take on a vital role in the healthcare system. Now, pharmacy health services are more focused on patients. The initial concept of pharmaceutical care hypothesized that pharmacy involves "*the responsible provision of drug therapy for the purpose of achieving definite outcomes that improve a patient's quality of life*" (Hepler & Strand, 1990). In 1997, Strand coined a new definition of pharmaceutical care as "*a practice in which the practitioner takes responsibility for a patients' drug-related needs and is held accountable for this commitment*" (Strand, 1997).

The current era has seen rapid changes in healthcare delivery and demand for quality of care. At present, the pharmacy profession is experiencing significant development and growth in terms of providing a better quality of patient-centered services. Pharmacists have adopted a patient-centered approach because of patients' poor adherence to prescribed medications and increases in health demands, along with an expanding and increasingly complex range of medicines (WHO, 2006). Pharmaceutical care came to be considered a complete philosophy and a standard for providing patient-centered care as a result of pharmacy organizations' introduction of education and training programs around the world (Farris, Fernando, & Benrimoj, 2005). In essence, the pharmacy profession transformed to become more responsible for patient care in terms of drug therapy (Rosemin, 2006). This change has positioned the pharmacist as key member of the healthcare team with additional responsibility for the outcome of medication therapy. It is therefore acknowledged that pharmacists have expertise in various fields in terms of drug knowledge in primary care clinics, hospitals, and community pharmacies around the world. In developing countries, because of the healthcare environment and system, a pharmacist can greatly contribute to the provision of primary healthcare (Jesson & Bissell, 2006). As medicine experts, pharmacists serve in various roles that differ throughout the world, from preparing and supplying medicines to involvement in patient-centered care services (Gilbert, 2001).

QUALITY OF PHARMACY HEALTH SERVICES

The World Health Organization (WHO) has played a significant role in promoting and defending the role of pharmacists around the world. The WHO has taken into account that almost all healthcare providers, including public health services, include the use of drugs. Therefore, considering the need for quality in pharmacy health services and for the safe and effective administration of drugs, the WHO has rightly acknowledged a special role for pharmacists (John & John, 2002). The concept of "The seven-star pharmacist" emerged in the same context and was coined jointly by the International Pharmaceutical Federation (FIP) and the WHO. Furthermore, the WHO addresses the future, saying that in time, pharmacists should possess specific knowledge, attitudes, skills, and behaviors that support their specific roles (WHO, 2006; Zammit, 2003). The WHO also recommends solutions for providing optimal healthcare to the general population by proposing 1 pharmacist per 2000 people. This ratio would also address the increasing need for pharmacists in public health. In addition to their responsibilities as advisors to healthcare professionals, pharmacists should contribute to policy making and be held accountable for the cost and quality of pharmacy health services provided to patients and society (Khan, 2007).

Developing countries differ from the developed world in terms of the challenges that pharmacists face in providing pharmacy services. Developing countries differ significantly from one another with respect to pharmacy practice models. Major issues that are considered impediments to effective pharmacy practice models include the unavailability of qualified and competent pharmacists, no separation of dispensing practices, and a lack of standard treatment guidelines for rational practice. Among developing countries, Nepal is facing a serious shortage of capable staff and insufficient infrastructure that is affecting the quality of the health services provided to the public (Gyawali et al., 2014). In Bangladesh, the scenario is not much different from that of neighboring countries, although prescribers agree with the new extended role of pharmacists in patient care. At the same time, a lack of government interest in the profession is a serious concern (Paul, Rahman, Biswas, Rashid, & Islam, 2014). In Pakistan, because of a lack of human resources in the health sector, healthcare facilities are still unable to fulfill the demands to provide quality health services to the nation (Azhar et al., 2009a,b). Numerous factors are responsible for the failure to achieve these goals, including a lack of pharmacy practice professionals, underprivileged pharmacy practice structures, a lack of awareness among the community, and improper governance (Bhagavathula, Sarkar, & Patel, 2014). Conditions in African countries are even worse; for example, in Ghana, there are a total of 619 pharmacists for 2.9 million people in Greater Accra and just 13 pharmacists to serve 3.3 million people in rural North Ghana (Frances, Felicity, & Rita, 2008), which is far behind the WHO recommendations (i.e., 1:2000). Uganda is facing an even more severe shortage of pharmacists than in Ghana, where pharmacies are run at Voluntary Services Overseas bases (Angela, 2003).

Furthermore, in Sri Lanka, the insufficient quality of pharmacy services in the community is mainly due to inadequate compliance with standard practice guidelines. Major concerns have been reported regarding drug quality and safety (Wijesinghe, Jayakody, & Seneviratne, 2007). In developing countries, urban populations are more prosperous than rural populations; in certain areas, the differences are huge. Therefore, health professionals choose to work in cities and become centrally concentrated in urban rather than rural areas, which limits the availability of uniform nationwide healthcare services (Smith, 2004). Another factor resulting in significant differences in health services between urban and rural areas is a lack of pharmacy human resources.

An inadequate supply of quality medicines is the most common issue in the developing world (Farris et al., 2005). Irrational use of medicine and weak control of drug sales are serious issues. A survey conducted in Ghana revealed that vendors in five chemist shops had little or no training in their respective fields; moreover, people were able to buy drugs without prescriptions from certified chemists. These factors result in drug misuse because inadequate information exists about drugs and drugs are sold according to demand.

In South Asia, pharmacists are focused on working for industry. Very few pharmacists in these countries choose hospital and clinical pharmacy as their profession (Azhar et al., 2009a,b; Mizobe & Basnet, 2006; Pagamas, Petcharat, Nattiya, & Armstrong, 2008). West Asian countries such as Kuwait and Jordan face similar situations. The quality of health services still needs to be acknowledged (Matowe, Abahussain, Al-Saffar, Bihzad, & Al-Foraih, 2006; Tahaineh, Wazaify, Albsoul, Khader, & Zaidan, 2009).

In some developing countries, physicians earn profits by prescribing and dispensing drugs. This has led to high drug costs and the extensive prescription of antibiotics in Asia, particularly in countries such as China, Malaysia, and Thailand (Abe, 1985; Yang & Bae, 2000). In these Asian countries, drug costs are very high and antibiotics prescription rates have increased because physicians avail themselves of the incentives of combining prescription and dispensing, resulting in an increased number of drug prescriptions. Under such conditions, pharmacists suffer because their main role of dispensing is taken over by the large and increasing number of physicians who dispense medication as a part of their practice (Gilbert, 2001).

PHARMACY LEADERSHIP AND PLANNING

It is mentioned earlier that quality of pharmacy health services will depend very much on several factors, one of it is effective leadership and planning. This can be at the governmental level, down to the pharmacy sector level. At the governmental level, we need good governance and strong leadership. Good governance and leadership should have the following attributes: transparent, equitable, accountable, effective, efficient, and participatory (Yap, 2015). The government should have the vision on the type, quality, and future direction of the healthcare system in the country—a healthcare system that has strong organization and good social values such as universality, accessibility, social solidarity, and robust financing systems (Leonard, Graham, & Bonacum, 2004). A good system is well planned and delivers quality services to all people regardless of the place and time. This expected quality and values include the pharmacy health services. It is the responsibility of the government to ensure well-trained, well-paid, and well-qualified pharmacy workforces are positioned at least in all government healthcare institutions.

According to American Society of Health System Pharmacists (ASHP, 2006) at the level of pharmacy, there is a need for competencies inherent in pharmacy management. Directors and managers of pharmacy organizations must realize that they should not just be managing but also be leading the organizations. *"Incremental, reactive change in the traditional role is not adequate to meet the present and future requirements of hospitals and health systems"* (ASHP, 2006).

PHARMACY EDUCATION AND TRAINING

In the recent past, pharmacy education was a burning issue for developing countries. The importance of pharmacy education and its quality has been ignored and has contributed insignificantly to the provision of health services. Along with the different subjects of pharmacy that were already well established, pharmacy practice is a new, emerging field that mainly focuses on a patient-centered approach. Although pharmacy practice is considered a main subject in pharmacy education, it is not justified without an emphasis on pharmacotherapeutics and clinical pharmacy. The shift of pharmacy curricula toward a clinical approach has been criticized as an effort to simply increase the duration of the program rather than a reflection of the current needs of society (Ghayur, 2008). In addition, the social and administrative pharmacy discipline is not well covered and taught in many countries. The courses and topics such as pharmaceutical policy, pharmaceutical economics, pharmacoepidemiology, pharmacy management, and marketing are considered not relevant or less important in the pharmacy curriculum. These areas could provide another set of knowledge and skills for preparing students to become future professional pharmacists who could provide quality pharmacy health services. We have colleges of pharmacy which are led by old professors who only recognize the subjects in pharmaceutical sciences such as pharmacognosy, pharmaceutical chemistry, pharmacology, and pharmaceutics. Little emphasis is given to clinical pharmacy, pharmacy practice, and social and administrative pharmacy disciplines. To them, pharmacy is only about basic science subjects. The colleges have either lack or no qualified educators to teach and train the students for these nonbasic science courses. They refused to change and improve the curriculum. Thus, there is a gap between the requirement in the healthcare sector and the quality and competency of pharmacy graduates. The products of the colleges then later will work in pharmacy settings that require them to deal with patients, involve in medication use process, or manage the pharmacy organizations as well as making cost-effective policies for the organizations, state, or country.

AVAILABILITY AND EFFECTIVE MANAGEMENT OF PHARMACY RESOURCES

Pharmaceutical sector in developing countries needs effective management of pharmacy resources, i.e., financial, infrastructure, and manpower. Most of the developing countries experience lack of financial resources, which negatively affect the provision of adequate infrastructure in the healthcare sector. Because of scarce resources, healthcare organizations could not ensure quality and adequate supply of medicines to the people. Especially in the governmental institutions, the salary and benefits are not attractive, and pharmacy workforce would prefer other options. According to WHO, (2012), problems facing the pharmacy workforce impend the countries' ability to achieve quality pharmacy healthcare services. Among the problems that the pharmaceutical sectors are facing include retirement of senior pharmacists, transition and replacement plan, poor human capital development and planning, demand and shortage of supply, replacement of several pharmacy activities by technology, needs for pharmacy specialists, attractive salary and benefits, skill mismatch, and migration of pharmacists to other countries.

Leaders and policy makers in developing countries must recognize, engage, align, and have forward-thinking methods for helping pharmacy organizations focus on pharmacy employees and resources to achieve quality pharmacy services.

For the pharmacy sector to establish quality pharmacy health services, leaders in pharmacy organizations need to think and strategically plan at solving this crisis by effectively planning to forecast pharmacy talent supply and demand, attract great employees, educate and upskill employees, and retain great employees.

INTERPROFESSIONAL COLLABORATION BETWEEN PHARMACISTS AND OTHER HEALTH PROFESSIONALS

Collaboration is an important element of teamwork. In developing countries, there is a need for collaboration strategies that mainly focus on teamwork. To understand collaboration, one should refer to Baggs and Schmitt (1997), who posit "*cooperatively working together includes sharing responsibilities for solving problems and making decisions to formulate and carry out plans for patient care.*" This means that all healthcare providers must take collective responsibility for providing quality patient care services.

In developing countries, collaboration in healthcare is rare. The expectations of doctors differ from their actual experience with pharmacists in terms of contributing to the quality of clinically focused pharmacy services (Azhar et al., 2015). A Cochrane report indicated that the expanded role of pharmacists improved patient outcomes (Beney, Bero, & Bond, 2000; Marrison & Wertheimer, 2001). The pharmacist serving as an advisor to physicians may help lower the costs of healthcare and drugs (Zunker & Carlson, 2000). This can increase the ability of pharmacists and physicians to work collaboratively, which results in the improved quality of patient care services.

However, increased collaboration can create interpersonal conflict (Zubin, Paul, & Caring, 2010). A few studies have shown downward trends as far as the pharmacists are concerned. For example, some pharmacists have dispensed alternative medicines instead of those prescribed by physicians and have made inappropriate comments regarding physicians' prescriptions, which confuses the patient and shatters his or her confidence in the prescriber (Paul, Ranelli, & June, 2000). However, in developed countries, studies have indicated that physicians have a very promising attitude toward the clinical pharmacists' role (Grussing, Goff, Kraus, & Mueller, 1984; Hatoum, Catizone, Hutchinson, & Purohit, 1986). In Kuwait, physicians felt comfortable with pharmacists providing pharmaceutical care services. The physicians considered pharmacists are knowledgeable about drug therapy (Matowe et al., 2006). In Thailand, pharmacists are doing a great job in hospitals; they are considered an important member of the healthcare team and are involved in promoting national drug use policy for the nation (Maneerat, Wanapa, Supatra, & Albert, 2007).

Additionally, studies have shown that newly qualified young physicians had more positive attitudes toward collaborating with pharmacists because new physicians are better socialized than older ones and are open to collaboration. Thus, age may have an effect on physicians' opinions about pharmacists (Ferris & Marilyn, 1983; Grussing et al., 1984). Health authorities in several developing countries intend to implement patient-centered care services to improve the drug use process and patient's quality of life.

In health service organizations, nurses are the largest group of professionals (WHO, 2002). Therefore, nurses have a unique and wonderful opportunity to make a difference in the lives of the population. In recent years, the role of nurses in primary care has developed rapidly, and the use of their skills and experience has been accepted (Azhar, Hassali, Ibrahim, Fahad, & Liau, 2012). It became important for pharmacists to develop collaborative relationships and use the expertise of the nurses to make significant contributions to improve patient care and try to meet the expectations of the public. A few studies have examined the relationship between nurses and pharmacists, and their focus was on supplementary prescribing. Deficiencies in knowledge and experience can be overcome by collaboration between pharmacists and nursing staff, which in turn will ensure the proper administration of drugs in the general ward (Nijjer, Gill, & Nijjer, 2008).

BARRIERS TO INTERPROFESSIONAL RELATIONSHIPS

Developing countries are not only lacking in advance technology systems for the implementation of a patient-centered approach; they are also suffering from interprofessional barriers. Healthcare professionals consider themselves part of the team, but in reality, they prefer to work independently. Several studies have focused on evaluating physicians' opinions and perceptions of and attitude toward pharmacists and have tried to explain the conflicts between healthcare professionals in understanding and accepting one another's existing or desired roles. This conflict has been reported as a major barrier in collaboration among healthcare professionals (Howard et al., 2003; While, Shah, & Nathan, 2005). Barriers to interprofessional collaboration in healthcare have also been identified (Aysegul et al., 2005; San Martin, Beaulieu, D'Amour, & Ferrada-Videla, 2005) and examined in relation to healthcare professionals' acceptance of the role of pharmacist. Most physicians reported the belief that pharmacists do not have sufficient knowledge to participate in the clinical decision-making process. Most of the physicians believed that prescribing medication was the responsibility of the physician. Moreover, the physicians thought that pharmacists should stick to dispensing because their role in clinical services is not important (Adepu & Nagavi, 2006; Spencer & Edwards, 1992; Sulick & Pathak, 1996; Tanskanen, Airaksinen, Tanskanen, & Enlund, 2000). In contrast to these findings, studies on effects of exposure to pharmacy services reported that physicians had favorable attitudes toward pharmacists practicing clinical tasks and believed that the pharmacists' recommendations had a positive effect on patients' clinical status (Haxby, Weart, & Goodman, 1988; Ritchey & Raney, 1981).

Hughes and McCann (2003) observed that physicians viewed pharmacists as businesspersons and those pharmacists thought that "*image is a big obstacle that influences the opinions of physicians towards the development of pharmacists' role.*" Furthermore, studies have found that some physicians have aggressive attitudes toward pharmacists, and pharmacy students feel that physicians are threatened by pharmacists' suggestions (Cote, Legare, & Richer, 2001). Infrequent communication with the physician and lack of opportunities to meet with physicians and discuss patients' drug therapy are major barriers to collaboration (Chen, Crampton, Krass, & Benrimoj, 2001; Reebye et al., 1999). Physicians perceived that "the pharmacist is the source of the information to the patient only for nonprescribed medications and were not comfortable giving advice on the prescribed medications," whereas pharmacists perceived themselves as advisors to physicians and wanted to contribute equally to drug therapy (D'Amour, Ferrada-Videla, Martin, & Beaulieu, 2005). These attitudes resulted in professional territorialism, which has been cited as a barrier in the development of collaborative relationships, which could hinder pharmacists providing quality pharmacy health services.

PUBLIC'S PERCEPTION ON THE QUALITY OF PHARMACY HEALTH SERVICES

The pharmacy profession has shifted from product- to patient-focused, then to public-focused, with an intense focus on patient-centered care services (Kotecki, 2002; Worley et al., 2007). The public's perception of the quality of health services is critical because it is important for categorizing and developing an effective action plan for quality improvement. Although there are certain obstacles to communication that may be due to individual and community factors (Paluck, Green, Frankish, Fielding, & Haverkamp, 2003), patient participation is very important in healthcare (Tio, LaCaze, & Cottrell, 2007). Consumers' awareness regarding pharmacy care services can only be established through the abilities of the pharmacist, and regular communication with consumers will help to improve the rational use of medicines (Nau et al., 2000). In developed countries, pharmacists provide evidence-based advice to their patients. The involvement of pharmacists in patients' drug therapy will lower the risk of adverse effects; as a result, patients will consider the pharmacist as a major source of information regarding their drug therapy (Nau et al., 2000; Silcock, Moffett, Edmondson, Waddell, & Burton, 2007; Tio et al., 2007). In contrast, the situation in developing countries is characterized by a low number of pharmacists relative to the population, especially in poor and rural areas, where trained pharmacists are rarely available (Goel, Ross-Degnan, Berman, & Soumerai, 1996; Viberg, Tomson, Mujinja, Cecilia, & Lundborg, 2007). In this instance, pharmacists seem almost nonexistence and their contributions are hardly recognized and appreciated.

ACHIEVEMENTS

Even though, in general, pharmacists are still struggling for their identity and recognition, there are several initiatives undertaken toward improving the quality of healthcare services that have shown positive progress. Compared with the past decades, the contribution of pharmacists to the population's health has significantly increased. The role of pharmacy in developing countries and its impact on the society are still being assessed. Although changes in curriculum are not enough to address all areas of concern, they should still be regarded as a considerable achievement. Pharmacy colleges in some developing countries do look into best practices and teaching models from the developed countries. In some countries, they seek for accreditation from countries that have good records of accomplishment and quality standards in pharmacy education. For pharmacy colleges that obtained international accreditation, relevant topics focusing on patient-centered care and ensuring quality of pharmacy healthcare services were incorporated into the curriculum. The pharmacy education system was designed with clear program and learning objectives, as well as systematic and structured assessments. Students were provided opportunities for experiential learning in the different pharmacy settings.

Pharmacy practitioners could be seen in international professional conferences such as FIP, International Society for Pharmacoeconomics and Outcomes Research (ISPOR), American College of Clinical Pharmacy (ACCP), and European Clinical Pharmacy Conference. They attended and are interested to learn new knowledge, getting ideas about best pharmacy practices; gain new experiences; and establish networking. On the other hand, pharmacists from developing countries also shared their success stories in practice from their home countries. Other healthcare professionals are realizing that pharmacists are active members of the healthcare team and are the most accessible health professionals. Public, to a certain extent, recognized pharmacists' contributions in patient care. Research studies conducted to document cost-effective pharmacists' interventions and initiatives in healthcare services have increased over the years. In some countries, continuing education programs are important and they need to collect certain number of points for renewing their license to practice. Only because of these few initiatives, pharmacists are being recognized in developing countries.

CHALLENGES

In the recent past, the profession faced numerous challenges in all developing counties. Among these challenges, the inadequate number of pharmacists in the healthcare system is the major obstacle to the provision of patient-centered care services. In addition, in some countries, there are struggles to produce qualified pharmacists. If there is need to focus on quality and the rational use of drugs, the pharmacist's presence in the system is mandatory. There was little focus provided to the needs for managing the medication use process. Such initiatives can reduce errors, enhance treatment outcomes, improve safety, promote health, and contain costs. In many instances, the expertise of professional pharmacist was neglected. Massive disease burdens that impact the economy are another major challenge faced by developing countries. Furthermore, political instability, war, and frequent regime changes with resulting changes in health policies have resulted in inadequate time for any health policy to be properly implemented (Khan & Heuvel, 2007). Developing countries also are in great need for pharmacy policy makers and leaders with effective vision who could provide direction and help pharmacy organizations prepare quality pharmacy healthcare services. What makes thing worse is, in most cases, countries not just lacking in leadership quality but also lack and misuse of pharmacy resources, poor planning, and lack of cooperation and collaboration with other health professionals.

RECOMMENDATIONS: THE WAY FORWARD

Good-quality pharmacy health services cannot be provided without pharmacists. Proper implementation of pharmacy healthcare policy, making the best use of resources (e.g., financial, infrastructure, and manpower), effective planning, and maintaining and improving resources for the people represent the only way forward for developing countries. The participation of competent and influential pharmacists is recommended to help ensure the appropriate use of medicines. Pharmacists must be involved in medication use process. Interprofessional relationships can be improved only with an increased number of pharmacists in hospitals and in the community (Azhar, Hassali, & Ibrahim, 2010). At present, pharmacists should embrace their role and play an active part in providing quality pharmacy services under their own domain. Doing so will increase awareness of the concept of patient-centered care in the health sector. It would require the cooperation and participation of all healthcare providers, especially pharmacists, doctors, and nurses. Only by working together can professionals understand one another's roles and responsibilities. Although the pharmacy curriculum was changed from a BPharm to a PharmD program, revamping the pharmacy curriculum is of no use if the health system and pharmacy system are not effective and efficient. It has been suggested that current pharmacy residency programs in hospitals should be more comprehensive, for example, expanding from 6 months in duration to 1 year (Jamshed, Babar, & Ibrahim, 2009). Pharmacy internships should start with doctors in the third professional year to address collaboration between these two professions at the academic level. As a result, students in their final year of PharmD programs would improve their expertise as clinical pharmacists, which would be significant from a social perspective. By working together as a healthcare team with a better understanding of each other's roles, these professionals would increase the benefits to the general public. Legal reforms (e.g., dispensing separation) are strongly recommended to achieve health objectives and increase the standards of pharmacy practice in the developing world. The implementation of all these recommendations would require the cooperation and participation of all stakeholders in the healthcare system.

CONCLUSIONS

The pharmacy profession is primarily responsible for providing quality pharmacy health services. Recently, new roles for different professions, especially the pharmacy profession, have developed in the health sector. Conventionally, the pharmacist was responsible for manufacturing and supplying medicines, but today, the role has transformed from manufacturing to patient care. The profession is still evolving, and health demands increase the pharmacist's role in patient-centered care. Pharmacist involvement is a critical, cost-effective way to manage drug therapies and will have an impact on both quality of care and cost containment. However, the quality of pharmacy health services in developing countries varies significantly, and for some countries, it is below expectation. Pharmacists in developing countries are still struggling for their identity.

LESSONS LEARNED

- Qualified pharmacy professionals take responsibility for the proper implementation of patient-centered care services in hospital, primary care, and community settings.
- Quality of pharmacy health services can be enhanced through effective pharmacy leadership and planning, pharmacy education and training, availability of pharmacy resources, effective management of pharmacy resources, pharmacy employees and processes, and pharmacist collaboration and cooperation with other healthcare providers.
- Legal reforms can be implemented to achieve health objectives and increase the standards of pharmacy health services.

REFERENCES

Abe, M. (1985). Japan's clinical physicians and their behavior. *Social Science & Medicine*, *20*, 335–340.

Adamcik, B. A., Ransford, H. E., Oppenheimer, P. R., Brown, J. F., Eagan, P. A., & Weissman, F. G. (1986). New clinical roles for pharmacists: A study of role expansion. *Social Science & Medicine*, *23*(11), 187–200.

Adepu, R., & Nagavi, B. G. (2006). General practitioners' perception about the extended role of the community pharmacist in the state of Karnataka: A study. *Indian Journal of Pharmaceutical Sciences*, *68*(1), 36–40.

Angela, F. (2003). Hospital pharmacies in Uganda. *Pharmaceutical Journal*, *10*(7), 286–287.

ASHP. (2006). *The national center for health system pharmacy leadership*. Georgetown University. Retrieved from http://www.ashpfoundation.org/pladocs/FinalReport.doc.

Aysegul, Y., Metin, A., Fevzi, A., Thomas, R., Deniz, S., Halim, I., et al. (2005). Physician–nurse attitudes toward collaboration in Istanbul's public hospitals. *International Journal of Nursing Studies*, *42*, 429–437.

Azhar, S., Hassali, M. A., & Ibrahim, M. I. (2010). Doctors' perception and expectations of the role of the pharmacist in Punjab Pakistan. *Tropical Journal of Pharmceutical Research*, *9*(3), 205–212.

Azhar, S., Hassali, M. A., Ibrahim, M. I., Fahad, S., & Liau, S. Y. (2012). A survey evaluating nurses' perception and expectations towards the role of pharmacist in Pakistan's healthcare system. *Journal of Advance Nursing*, *68*(1), 199–205.

Azhar, S., Hassali, M. A., Ibrahim, M. I., Maqsood, S., Asrul, A., Fahad, S., et al. (2009b). Evaluating the perception of doctors towards the role of pharmacist in Pakistan's healthcare system. *Malaysia Journal of Pharmacy*, *1*(7), 105.

Azhar, S., Hassali, M., Iqbal, A., Akram, M., Attique, R. M., & Murtaza, G. (2015). Qualitative assessment of the pharmacist's role in Punjab, Pakistan: Medical practitioners' views. *Tropical Journal of Pharmaceutical Research*, *14*(2), 323–327.

Azhar, S., Hassali, M. A., Izham, M. I., Maqsood, A., Imran, M., & Asrul, A. (2009a). The role of pharmacists in developing countries: The current scenario in Pakistan. *Human Resources for Health*, *7*(1), 54.

Baggs, J. G., & Schmitt, M. H. (1997). Nurses' and resident physicians' perception of the process of collaboration in an MICU. *Research in Nursing & Health*, *20*, 17–18.

Beney, J., Bero, L. A., & Bond, C. (2000). Expanding the role of out patient pharmacists: Effects on out patient utilization, cost, and patient outcomes. *Cochrane Database System Review, 3*.

Bhagavathula, A. S., Sarkar, B. R., & Patel, I. (2014). Clinical pharmacy practice in developing countries: Focus on India and Pakistan. *Arch Pharma Pract, 5*(91), 4.

Chen, T. F., Crampton, M., Krass, I., & Benrimoj, S. I. (2001). Collaboration between community pharmacists and GPs impact on interprofessional communication. *Journal of Social and Administrative Pharmacy, 18*(3), 83–90.

Cote, L., Legare, F., & Richer, M. (2001). Development of pharmacist physician relationship:perception of programm directors and trainees in the faculties of pharmacy and medicine in Quebec, Canada. *American Journal of Pharmaceutical Education, 67*(2), 1–10.

D'Amour, D., Ferrada-Videla, M., San Martin, R. L., & Beaulieu, M. D. (2005). The conceptual basis for interprofessional collaboration:core concepts and theoretical framework. *Journal of Interprofessional Care, 19*(1), 116–131.

Donabedian, A. (1980). The definition of quality and approaches to its assessment. *Explorations in quality Assessment and Monitoring* (vol 1). Ann Arbor, MI: Health Administration Press.

Farris, K. B., Fernando, F., & Benrimoj, S. I. (2005). Pharmaceutical care in community pharmacies: Practice and research from around the world. *The Annals of Pharmacotherapy, 39*.

Ferris, J., & Marilyn, R. (1983). Physicians' opinions of expanded clinical pharmacy services. *American Journal of Public Health, 73*(1).

Frances, O. D., Felicity, S., & Rita, S. (2008). Addressing the workforce crisis: The professional aspirations of pharmacy students in Ghana. *Pharmacy World & Science, 30*(5), 577–583.

George, A. B. (1965). *Great moments in pharmacy*.

Ghayur, M. N. (2008). Pharmacy education in developing Countries: Need for a change. *American Journal of Pharmaceutical Education, 72*(4).

Gilbert, L. (2001). To diagnose, prescribe and dispense: Whose right is It? the ongoing struggle between pharmacy and medicine in South Africa. *Current Sociology, 49*(3), 97–118. http://dx.doi.org/10.1177/0011392101049003007.

Goel, P., Ross-Degnan, D., Berman, P., & Soumerai, S. (1996). Retail pharmacies in developing countries: A behavior and intervention framework. *Social Science & Medicine, 42*(8), 1155–1161.

Grussing, P. G., Goff, D. A., Kraus, D. M., & Mueller, C. E. (1984). Development and validation of an instrument to measure physician attitudes towards the clinical pharmacists' role. *Drug Intelligence & Clinical Pharmacy, 18*(7), 635–640.

Gyawali, S., Rathore, D. S., Adhikari, K., Shankar, P. R., Kumar, V., & Basnet, S. (2014). Pharmacy practice and injection use in community pharmacies in Pokhara city, Western Nepal. *BMC Health Services Research, 14*(190).

Hatoum, H. T., Catizone, C., Hutchinson, R. A., & Purohit, A. (1986). An eleven-year review of pharmacy literature:documentation of the value and acceptance of clinical pharmacy. *Drug Intelligence & Clinical Pharmacy, 20*(1), 33–48.

Haxby, D. G., Weart, C. W., & Goodman, B. W. (1988). Family practice physicians' perceptions of the usefulness of drug therapy recommendations from clinical pharmacists. *American Journal of Health System Pharmacy, 45*(4), 824–827.

Hepler, C. D., & Strand, L. M. (1990). Opportunities and responsibilities in pharmaceutical care. *American Journal of Hospital Pharmacy, 47*, 533–543.

Howard, M., Trim, K., Woodward, C., Dolovich, L., Sellors, C., Kaczorowski, J., et al. (2003). Collaboration between community pharmacists and family physicians: Lessons learned from the seniors medication assessment research trail. *Journal of American Pharmacist Association, 43*(5), 566–572.

Hughes, C. M., & McCann, S. (2003). Perceived interprofessional barriers between community pharmacists and general practitioners: A qualitative assessment. *British Journal of General Practice, 53*, 600–606.

Institute of Medicine. (1990). *Medicare: A strategy for quality assurance* (Vol. 1). Washington, DC: National Academy Press.

Jamshed, S., Babar, Z. U., & Ibrahim, M. I. M. (2009). Pharm D in Pakistan: A tag or a degree? *American Journal of Pharmaceutical Education, 73*(1).

Jesson, J., & Bissell, P. (2006). Public health and pharmacy: A critical review. *Critical Public Health, 16*(2), 159–169.

Joanna, C., Daniel, S., Fernando, F., & Shalom, I. (2013). Defining professional pharmacy services in community pharmacy. *Research in Social and Administrative Pharmacy, 9*, 989–995.

John, A. D., & John, P. S. (2002). Community pharmacists' perspectives on pharmaceutical care implementation in New Zealand. *Pharmacy World & Science, 24*(6), 224–230.

Khan, R. A. (2007). Pharmacy education and healthcare. Retrieved from http://www.gcu.edu.pk/Library/NI_Feb07.htm.

Khan, M. M., & Heuvel, W. (2007). The impact of political context upon the health policy process in Pakistan. *Public Health Epidemiol, 121*, 278–286.

Kotecki, J. E. (2002). Factors related to pharmacists' over-the-counter recommendations. *Journal of Community Health, 27*(4), 291–306.

Leonard, M., Graham, S., & Bonacum, D. (2004). The human factor: The critical importance of effective teamwork and communication in providing safe care. *Quality and Safety in Health Care, 13*, 85–90.

Lohr, K. N. (1990). *Medicare: A strategy for quality assurance* (Vol. 2). Washington, DC: National Academies Press.

Maneerat, R. L., Wanapa, S., Supatra, C., & Albert, I. W. (2007). Sources of information for new drugs among physicians in Thailand. *Pharmacy World & Science, 29*, 619–627.

Marrison, A., & Wertheimer, A. L. (2001). Evaluation of studies investigating the effectiveness of pharmacists' clinical services. *American Journal of Health System Pharmacy, 58*(7), 569–577.

Matowe, L., Abahussain, E. A., Al-Saffar, N., Bihzad, S. M., & Al-Foraih, A. (2006). Physicians' perception and expectations of pharmacists' professional duties in government hospital in Kuwait. *Medical Principles and Practice, 15*(6), 185–189.

Mizobe, M., & Basnet, N. S. (2006). Comparative study on the role of pharmacist in Nepal and Japan. *Nepal. Japan International Cooperation Agency (JICA), 16*, 6.

Mosadeghrad, A. M. (2014). Factors influencing healthcare service quality. *International Journal of Health Policy Management, 3*(2), 77–89.

Nau, D. P., Ried, L. D., Lipowski, E. E., Kimberlin, C., Pendergast, J., & Spivey, M. S. (2000). Patients' perceptions of the benefits of pharmaceutical care. *Journal of the American Pharmaceutical Association, 40*(1), 36–40.

Nijjer, S., Gill, J., & Nijjer, S. (2008). Effective collaboration between doctors and pharmacists. *Pharmaceutical Journal, 15*, 179–182.

Pagamas, M., Petcharat, P., Nattiya, K., & Armstrong, E. P. (2008). Pharmacist perceptions of new competency standards. *Pharmacy Practice, 6*(3), 113–120.

Paluck, E. C., Green, L. W., Frankish, C. J., Fielding, D. W., & Haverkamp, B. (2003). Assessment of communication barriers in community pharmacies. *Evaluation Health Profession, 26*(4), 380–403.

Paul, T. R., Rahman, M. A., Biswas, M., Rashid, M., & Islam, A. (2014). Practice of hospital pharmacy in Bangladesh: Currentperspective. *Bangladesh Pharmaceutical Journal, 17*(2), 187–192.

Paul, L., Ranelli, & June, B. (2000). Physicians' perceptions of communication with and responsibilities of pharmacists. *Journal of the American Pharmacists Association, 40*(5), 1–7.

Reebye, R. N., Avery, A. J., Van Den Bosch, W. J., Aslam, M., Nijholt, A., & Van der Bij, A. (1999). Exploring community pharmacist perceptions of their professional relationships with physician in Canada and The Netherlands. *International Journal of Pharmacy Practice, 26*, 167–175.

Ritchey, F. J., & Raney, M. R. (1981). Effect of exposure on physicians' attitudes toward clinical pharmacists. *American Journal of Health System Pharmacy, 38*(10), 1459–1463.

Rosemin, K. (2006). Evaluation of pharmaceutical care opportunities within an advanced pharmacy practice experience. *American Journal of Pharmaceutical Education, 70*(3), 1–9.

San Martin, R. L., Beaulieu, M. D., D'Amour, D., & Ferrada-Videla, M. (2005). The determinants of successful collaboration: A review of theoretical and empirical studies. *Journal of Interprofessional Care, 19*, 132–147.

Schuster, M. A., McGlynn, E. A., & Brook, R. H. (1998). How good is the quality of health care in the United States? *The Milbank Quarterly*, *76*(4), 517–563.

Silcock, J., Moffett, J., Edmondson, H., Waddell, G., & Burton, A. K. (2007). Do community pharmacists have the attitudes and knowledge to support evidence based self-management of low back pain? *BMC Musculoskeletal Disorders*, *8*(1), 10.

Smith, F. (2004). Community pharmacy in Ghana: Enhancing the contribution to primary health care. *Health Policy and Planning*, *19*(4), 234–241. http://dx.doi.org/10.1093/heapol/czh028.

Spencer, J. A., & Edwards, C. (1992). Pharmacy beyond the dispensary: General practitioners' views. *BMJ: British Medical Journal*, *304*(6843), 1670–1672. http://dx.doi.org/10.1136/bmj.304.6843.1670.

Strand, L. M. (1997). Re-visioning the profession. *Journal of American Pharmacist Association*, *37*(4), 474–478.

Sulick, J. A., & Pathak, D. S. (1996). The perceived influence of clinical pharmacy services on physician prescribing behavior: A match pair comparison of pharmacist and physician. *Pharmacotherapy*, *16*(6), 1133–1141.

Tahaineh, L. M., Wazaify, M., Albsoul, A., Khader, Y., & Zaidan, M. (2009). Perception, experience, and expectations of physicians in hospital settings in Jordan regarding the role of pharmacist. *Research in Social and Administrative Pharmacy*, *5*, 63–70.

Tanskanen, P., Airaksinen, M., Tanskanen, A., & Enlund, H. (2000). Counseling patients on psychotropic medication: Physician opinions on the role of community pharmacists. *Pharmacy World & Science*, *22*(2), 59–61.

Tio, J., LaCaze, A., & Cottrell, N. (2007). Ascertaining consumer perspectives of medication information sources using a modified repertory grid technique. *Pharmacy World & Science*, *29*, 73–80.

Viberg, N., Tomson, G. R., Mujinja, P., Cecilia, & Lundborg, S. (2007). The role of the pharmacist–voices from nine African countries. *Pharmacy World & Science*, *29*, 25–33.

While, A., Shah, R., & Nathan, A. (2005). Interdisciplinary working between community pharmacists and community nurses: The view of community pharmacist. *Journal of Interprofessional Care*, *19*(2), 164–170.

WHO. (2002). *Strategic directions for strengthening nursing and midwifery services*. Retrieved from http://whqlibdoc.who.int/publications/2002/924156217X.pdf.

WHO. (2006). *New tool to enhance role of pharmacists in health care*. Retrieved from http://www.who.int/mediacentre/news/new/2006/nw05/en/index.html.

WHO. (2012). *Human resources - the 2012 FIP Global pharmacy workforce report*. Retrieved from https://www.fip.org/humanresources.

Wijesinghe, P. R., Jayakody, R. L., & Seneviratne, R. (2007). An assessment of the compliance with good pharmacy practice in an urban and rural district in Sri Lanka. *Pharmacoepidemiology and Drug Safety*, *16*(2), 197–206.

Worley, M. M., Schommer, J. C., Brown, L. M., Hadsall, R. S., Ranelli, P. L., Stratton, T. P., et al. (2007). Pharmacists' and patients' roles in the pharmacist-patient relationship: Are pharmacists and patients reading from the same relationship script? *Research in Social and Administrative Pharmacy*, *3*(1), 47–69.

Yang, B., & Bae, J. (2000). *Reforming drug distribution system in Korea: correcting the economics incentives*. New Orleans: Annual metting, Allied Social Science Association.

Yap, K. S. (2015). *What is good governance?* Retrieved from www.unescap.org/sites/default/files/good-governance.pdf.

Zammit, D. (2003). How to make ethical decisions. *The Pharmaceutical Journal*, *271*, 468.

Zubin, A., Paul, G., & Caring, M. J. (2010). Pharmacists' experience of conflict in community practice. *Research in Social and Administrative Pharmacy*, *6*, 39–48.

Zunker, R. J., & Carlson, D. L. (2000). Economics of using pharmacist as a advisers to physician in risk sharing contracts. *American Journal of Health System Pharmacy*, *57*(8), 753–755.

FURTHER READING

WHO. (1948). *Definition of health*. http://www.who.int/about/mission/en/.

CHAPTER

18 ASSESSMENT OF MEDICATION DISPENSING AND EXTENDED COMMUNITY PHARMACY SERVICES

Mohamed Izham Mohamed Ibrahim

Qatar University, Doha, Qatar

CHAPTER OUTLINE

INTRODUCTION

Pharmacists serve individual, community, and societal needs. Brodie (1981) proposed that pharmacists' basic role has to expand based on advancements in technology and knowledge. In the past, pharmacists' main purpose was to prepare medicines and to ensure their availability. However, pharmacists can now react to external forces (e.g., economic, epidemiological, demographic, and technological) that are reshaping the profession by positioning themselves within the medication use system and being in control of the process. Helper (1988) suggested that pharmacists be more knowledgeable and focus on their fundamental pharmacist–society relationship to improve public health.

Social and Administrative Aspects of Pharmacy in Low- and Middle-Income Countries. http://dx.doi.org/10.1016/B978-0-12-811228-1.00018-2

WHAT IS HEALTH, PUBLIC HEALTH, AND PRIMARY HEALTHCARE?

In 1946, WHO defined health in its constitution:

> Health is a state of complete physical, mental and social well-being, not merely the absence of disease or infirmity.
>
> **WHO (2002)**

This is the most quoted definition of health, which clearly stresses "well-being." Four decades later, WHO (1984) revised its definition as follows:

> Health is the extent to which an individual or group is able, on the one hand, to realize aspirations and satisfy needs; and, on the other hand, to change or cope with the environment. Health is, therefore, seen as a resource for everyday life, not an object of living; it is a positive concept emphasizing social and personal resources, as well as physical capacities.

In developing countries, healthcare needs are more pressing than those in developed nations. Unfortunately, for various reasons, the provision of care is inadequate, particularly in the public sector; it is even worse in the private sector.

WHO (2005) has highlighted the importance of improving, monitoring, and evaluating people's wellness and quality of life, which, as a public health concern, should be the goals in a country's national development. In 1920, Winslow defined public health as follows:

> [Public health is] the science and art of preventing disease, prolonging life and promoting health through the organized efforts and informed choices of society, organizations, public and private, communities and individuals.
>
> **(Winslow, 1920)**

Public health is an organized effort to maintain the health of the people and to prevent illness, injury, and premature death by focusing on prevention and health protection services (The Association of Faculties of Medicines of Canada, n.d.).

Another relevant community-related concept is primary healthcare. Primary healthcare was the core concept of WHO's goal in health for all, which was based on the Alma Ata declaration in 1978 (WHO, 1978). Due to high healthcare expenditures, moving some of the healthcare focus from the tertiary level to the primary level is perhaps justifiable. Primary care also aims to decrease the public's reliance on hospitals to fill drug prescriptions. According to WHO, to achieve health for all, people must be put at the center of healthcare (WHO, 2007). People-centered care is focused and organized around the health needs and expectations of people and communities rather than on disease itself (WHO, 2015).

If people and society are the core of the "health for all" mission, then where do community pharmacists belong as healthcare providers? Do the pharmacy and community pharmacists fit within the system?

In this chapter, an assessment of community pharmacy practices in developing countries is particularly interesting in terms of medication dispensing and extended pharmacy services. The chapter also seeks to examine the significant societal contributions of community pharmacists, including the challenges and gaps in practice. This chapter will also focus and discuss the expected role, function, and responsibilities of community pharmacists in developing countries. This is based on the aforementioned concepts of "health," "public health," and "primary healthcare."

EXPECTED ROLE AND FUNCTION OF COMMUNITY PHARMACISTS

A community pharmacy is a healthcare facility that provides pharmaceutical and cognitive services to a specific community. From independently owned pharmacies to corporately owned chain pharmacies, a variety of pharmacies are in operation. In some developing countries in Africa and Asia, the terms "drug outlets," "retail drug outlets," "retail drug shops," and "private pharmacies" are commonly used. Community pharmacists must strategically position themselves in the community to serve the public health. Community pharmacies can be found on main streets, in malls and supermarkets, at the heart of the most rural villages, and in the center of the most deprived communities. In some countries, many community pharmacies are opened early and closed late when other healthcare professionals are unavailable (CPNI, no date). According to WHO (1994), among healthcare providers, community pharmacists are the most accessible to the public. In practice, a pharmacy provides medications and other healthcare products and services and helps people and society make the best use of them (Wiedenmayer et al., 2006). Community pharmacists supply, dispense, and sell medications according to the law. A proper dispensing practice will interpret and evaluate a prescription; select and manipulate or compound a pharmaceutical product; and label and supply the product in an appropriate container according to legal and regulatory requirements (WHO, 1994). In addition, pharmacy activities include a pharmacist's provision of information and instructions to patients, and, under a pharmacist's supervision, practices will ensure the patient's safe and effective use of the medicines.

In some countries, pharmaceutical services go beyond these basic services. These services or functions (e.g., counseling, drug information, blood pressure monitoring, immunizations, and diabetic self-management) will require professional knowledge and skills beyond those required to dispense prescription medications (Wiedenmayer et al., 2006). These services include all those delivered by pharmacy personnel to support the delivery of pharmaceutical care. Beyond the supply of pharmaceutical products, pharmaceutical services include information, education, and communication to promote public health; the provision of drug information and counseling; regulatory services; and staff education and training (Wiedenmayer et al., 2006).

Hepler and Strand (1990) coined the term "pharmaceutical care," which they defined as "the responsible provision of drug therapy for the purpose of achieving definite outcomes that improve (or maintain) a patient's quality of life."

This collaborative process aims to prevent or identify and solve pharmaceutical and health-related problems—a continuous quality improvement process regarding the use of medicines (Wiedenmayer et al., 2006). The philosophy of pharmaceutical care promoted in the early 1990s is no longer new. Many studies, initiatives, and interventions, especially in developed countries, have been conducted to improve patient care and health outcomes. In an attempt to provide health and pharmaceutical care to patients and society, the healthcare and pharmaceutical sectors in developing countries, particularly low- and middle-income countries (LMICs), are facing challenges. These challenges include the shortage of human resources in the pharmacy workforce; inefficient health systems; the rising costs of medicines and healthcare; limited financial resources; the huge burden of disease; and changing social, epidemiological, technological, economic, and political situations (Mohamed Ibrahim, Palaian, Al-Sulaiti, & El-Shami, 2016).

In general, pharmacists play an important role in the healthcare system through the provision of medicines and information (ACCP, no date). Pharmacists are drug experts who focus on patients' health and wellness. The Competency Standards for Pharmacists in Australia (SHPA, 2003) mentioned several important functional areas that community pharmacists could assume: dispensing medication; preparing pharmaceutical products; promoting and contributing to the quality use of medication; providing primary healthcare; and supplying information and instructions related to health and medication.

THE EXTENT OF THE COMMUNITY PHARMACY'S CONTRIBUTION

What kind of value and benefits does the public really gain from community pharmacy practice? Despite the widely acknowledged potential of community pharmacies in developing countries to respond to public healthcare needs, related developments have been limited (Smith, 2004). In addition, the quality of community pharmacy practices has also been questioned. In many countries, especially in LMICs, community pharmacists have only performed the basic or traditional role (i.e., as a drug dispenser), and they have sometimes indulged in unethical practices. Studies have reported mixed findings: community pharmacies make a contribution to society, but they are also problematic (i.e., they do not meet expectations and provide low-quality services).

THE TWO SIDES OF COMMUNITY PHARMACISTS' SERVICES

In Estonia, since the restoration of independence in 1991, community pharmacies have become more patient-oriented, even though the government has not pressured pharmacies to offer extended services. In addition to dispensing, pharmacies still compound extemporaneous products and sell herbal medicines. Community pharmacists continue to perform their traditional roles (Volmer, Vendla, Vetka, Bell, & Hamilton, 2008). Prior to 2007, clinical pharmacy was never practiced in community pharmacy settings in Peru. However, the pharmaceutical care initiative has been reported to be growing and well supported by the law. Peruvian pharmacists are encouraged to take this opportunity to expand their services (Alvarez-Risco & van Mil, 2007). In China, pharmaceutical care services are underdeveloped but, with the improvement of the Chinese Pharmacist Law, they will become an important part of the pharmacist's professional role (Fang, Yang, Zhou, Jiang, & Liu, 2013).

Pharmacists in Vietnam are encouraged to expand their role—from drug sellers to client counselors, drug treatment managers, adherence counselors, and advisors on illness prevention. Pharmacies are often the first place that people visit to seek medical help, and they serve as a source of health information and services. The intervention that has empowered pharmacists to serve as client advocates and client counselors has identified a few improvements, such as knowledge, behavior, increased client satisfaction, and pharmacist–healthcare provider relationships. Pharmacists can move beyond the traditional role of selling drugs to be more effective healthcare professionals, and they need continuing professional development (CPD) (Minh, Huong, Byrkit, & Murray, 2013).

From another perspective, evidence has shown that community pharmacists perform far below public expectations. Patients have encountered several problems and challenges related to community pharmacy practice, which can be discussed according to pharmacy, pharmacist, prescription, service, and system factors.

Studies have reported that community pharmacists in developing countries, especially LMICs, do not provide quality services. A quick look at 19 developing countries (Fathelrahman, Mohamed

Ibrahim, & Wertheimer, 2016) shows that the community pharmacy practice setting is regarded as popular. Unfortunately, this practice setting also presents some concerns. For example, some countries allow nonpharmacists to operate pharmacies and to handle medicines. In some countries, the practice of community pharmacy is not well regulated, with little to no minimum standard of practice (Hussain, Mohamed Ibrahim, & Zaheer, 2012d). Many pharmacy personnel who dispense medicines are unqualified, with no college/university diploma or professional degree in pharmacy (Lenjisa, Mosisa, Woldu, & Negassa, 2015). A study in Turkish Republic of Northern Cyprus (Gokcekus, Toklu, Demirdamar, & Gumusel, 2012) reported that the pharmacy employees have no pharmacy-based training and that pharmacists believed that their employees are capable to handle the prescriptions. Studies in Qatar, Pakistan, Malaysian, and Sudan have indicated that dispensing and labeling practices and provider–patient interactions are poor (Alamin Hassan, Mohamed Ibrahim, & Hassali, 2014; Hussain & Mohamed Ibrahim, 2011; Hussain et al., 2012d; Mohamed Ibrahim et al., 2014; Mohamed Ibrahim et al., 2016; Osman, Ahmed Hassan, & Mohamed Ibrahim, 2012). In addition, a few dispensing errors have been identified (Lenjisa et al., 2015). According to Basak, Arunkumar, and Masilamani (2009), community pharmacy services in India are quite problematic, and the pharmacy's role in healthcare remains unrecognized. These authors have called for reform to meet societal needs. A study in Nigeria found that some community pharmacists often administer injections for customers—in some cases, without a prescription. The number of prescriptions that community pharmacists receive is low. They suffer from the limited availability of some resources, which has a serious impact on their practice (Adje & Oli, 2013). A review of community pharmacy practices showed that, in some countries, pharmacy outlets were run by nonpharmacists; dispensing practices were unsatisfactory; drug sellers' level of knowledge regarding diseases and medicines was poor; medicines were used irrationally; pharmacies were not meeting the government's licensing requirements; medication storage conditions were improper; and customers could hardly meet with pharmacists (Hussain, Mohamed Ibrahim, & Babar, 2012a, 2012b, 2012d; Hussain & Mohamed Ibrahim, 2012). A study on over-the-counter (OTC) counseling in Brazil (Halila, Junior, Otuki, & Correr, 2015) concluded that even though the most important factors taken into account when counseling an OTC medicine were drug's efficacy and adverse effects, but only few pharmacists knew the meaning of terms related to evidence-based health. Poudel, Subish, Mishra, Mohamed Ibrahim, and Jayasekera (2010) reported that unregistered fixed-dose combinations of pharmaceutical products (e.g., antimicrobial combinations, nonsteroidal antiinflammatory drug combinations, and antimotility combinations) have been found in Nepali healthcare facilities, including drug outlets. Regarding prescription behavior, even in rural areas of India, the proportion of brand name prescriptions was high (Aravamuthan, Arputhavanan, Subramaniam, & Chander, 2017).

Other common prescription problems include the lack of information, illegible handwriting, and various errors (e.g., prescription errors, dispensing errors, and improper labeling related to particular standards or requirements) (Hussain & Mohamed Ibrahim, 2011; Syhakhang, Stenson, Wahlström, & Tomson, 2001).

Pharmacy hours vary: typically, some pharmacies are open for approximately 10h (e.g., in Malaysia), while others offer 24-h services (e.g., in Qatar). In some countries (e.g., Nepal and Sudan), pharmacy hours and operations can be affected by the availability of reliable electrical power supply. Some countries do not have conveniently located pharmacy outlets, and customers might have to walk for hours to reach one. Some pharmacies lack proper facilities (e.g., a private room for patient counseling), space, reference resources (e.g., drug information), and/or quality medication (e.g., substandard and counterfeit and irrational fixed-dose combinations); have a poor layout, impractically arranged products, and/or disorganization issues; and/or keep and sell expired or almost expired items.

Developing countries also suffer from an insufficient number of pharmacists. In addition, for economic reasons, pharmacists prefer to work or set up their pharmacies in urban areas rather than in rural areas (Smith, 2001, 2004). In addition, some pharmacists are hard to find in pharmacies ("the invisible pharmacist"), and patients/customers have to rely on pharmacy assistants/technicians (Amin & Chewning, 2016). Most of the time, these staff have no proper professional qualifications and lack important skills and knowledge. Even worse, some community pharmacists lack particular competencies and communication skills, have no or few business skills, and do not have up-to-date knowledge. In some cases, pharmacists do not comply with regulations (e.g., selling antibiotics or psychotropic drugs without a prescription), and they often fail to assume responsibility for pharmaceutical care. In the eyes of the consumers, community pharmacists are always regarded as businesspeople rather than as healthcare professionals. Community pharmacists must strike a balance between professional and business responsibilities. Having both qualities, i.e., having a high level of professionalism and an excellent business sense, should not be so difficult. How these two aspects influence the health and well-being of individuals and society is what matters.

The services provided by community pharmacists have been reported to focus more on their distributive function (e.g., basic medication dispensing and sales), not the expected proper medication dispensing practice mentioned above (Wiedenmayer et al., 2006). Most of the time, pharmacists provide no advice/counseling; rarely interact with patients and physicians; make no referrals; lack or have few medicines due to poor planning and estimation/quantification; have no records of patients/clients or the medicines dispensed; use little to no technology; mix and prepare medications in the pharmacy rather than according to standards, for example, US or British Pharmacopeia (compounding or extemporaneous dispensing); and do not provide drug information that could help reduce medication misadventures.

In 2003, the Malaysian Pharmaceutical Society introduced its benchmarking guidelines for community pharmacies. The society sought to raise the standards of practice. Unfortunately, a study reported that the level of awareness of these guidelines was low and that only around 60% of the pharmacies complied with them (Siang, Kee, Gee, Richard, & See Hui, 2008).

The quality of the pharmacy education system has been affected. Some countries lack colleges with pharmacy degrees. Even if adequate, these colleges often lack quality curricula; the syllabi are out of date and do not cater to the present needs of the healthcare system. In addition, colleges lack staff; even if they have enough staff, they lack quality staff/faculty with appropriate qualifications or expertise. The pharmacy workforce is not carefully planned according to the country's needs. Some countries do not have pharmacy associations, which could provide professional leadership, and some even are unable to provide continuing education for pharmacy staff. Another critical problem is that there are very few policy makers and regulators who understand the system, who are committed and motivated, and who have sufficient technical know-how to solve the problems. In addition, many countries have a corrupt system and authorities; a weak and unstable government and economy; problems with bureaucracy, middlemen, profits, etc. that affect the final retail price, potentially making it too high for consumers; no or few effective price containment strategies/polices, which have resulted in unaffordable prices (Khatib et al., 2016), especially for the poor and others in need. Due to the lack of an attractive salary and benefits, pharmacists have migrated to other countries for better life and career opportunities. As such, nonpharmacists are allowed to own and operate pharmacies in developing countries.

The image of the pharmacist and the profession very much depends on customer satisfaction. A study conducted in Nigeria showed that customers experienced moderate service satisfaction. Customers were mostly dissatisfied with healthcare services that related to pharmaceutical care activities (Oparah & Kikanme, 2006). In a patient satisfaction survey conducted in the United Arab Emirates (UAE), scores were significantly lower than published data, suggesting that patients' expectations of community pharmacy services have not been met there (Hasan et al., 2013). Dhote, Mahajan, and Mishra (2013) mentioned that the rise of pharmaceutical care services must be accelerated based on the rapid changes in consumers' expectations.

WHAT CAN WE LEARN FROM OTHERS?

Best practices can be adopted and adapted according to a country's needs and conditions. Does "one size" really fit all? Is "comparing apples and oranges" difficult? Adopting 100% of one country's practices in another country is unwise. Many factors need to be considered. No country has a perfect system; however, community pharmacists in developing countries can definitely learn from at least one practice or service.

According to Brodie (1981), the traditional role of dispensing medications has been expanded. Pharmacists should be both health generalists and health specialists, which will have an impact on public health. Even the American Public Health Association (1981) supports the pharmacists' role in public health. Should community pharmacists move beyond their traditional role? Even when dispensing medicines through paper-based prescription services, pharmacists should comply with some fundamental standards. Safety issues must be considered when dispensing medications. The Pharmacy Board of Australia published guidelines for medication dispensing (i.e., guidelines for scanned and faxed prescriptions and steps to take when handling Internet or mail-order dispensing); guidelines for dispensing extemporaneous medications; guidelines when handling errors (e.g., dispensing errors); guidelines for appropriate medication labeling; guidelines for patient counseling, privacy, and confidentiality; and pharmacy technicians' functions, responsibilities, and competencies (Pharmacy Board of Australia, n.d.). In addition, for pharmacies that use electronic and computer systems, the Royal Pharmaceutical Society of Great Britain (n.d.) has provided several guidelines and principles for good dispensing and appropriate dispensing procedures (e.g., professional checking, medication substitution, and labeling). Malaysia, a developing country, has also developed *Guide to Good Dispensing Practice* (Malaysian Pharmaceutical Services Division, 2016). These guidelines aim to have both public and private facilities dispensing medications according to the law and guidelines, which may ensure that patients receive the correct medications, adherence is improved, adverse effects are minimized, and errors are avoided. The document's contents relate to processing prescriptions, preparing medications, labeling, recoding, and issuing medications to the patient. In geographical areas where no pharmacists are available, a guide about managing medicines would be a handy document indeed (Andersson & Snell, 2010).

In some countries, community pharmacists are ready to provide extended services (or cognitive pharmaceutical services). According to Cipolle, Strand, and Morley (1998), cognitive pharmaceutical services entail the pharmacist's use of specialized knowledge to help patients or health professionals and promote effective and safe drug therapy. These services are simply "clinically oriented activities intended to improve medication prescribing and use" (Farris, Kumbera, Halterman, & Fang, 2002).

Why are pharmacy practices still outdated in some countries? What are the barriers to quality community pharmacy services? Are pharmacists reluctant to move forward? The lack of time, reimbursement, recognition, cooperation with general practitioners, documentation, networking; the location of services within the pharmacy premises; the attitudes of customers and pharmacists; the pharmacy owner's involvement (or lack thereof); the daily organization of services; and customer recruitment for such services are among the barriers to the successful implementation of extended services (cognitive services) (Garrett & Martin, 2003; Gastelurrutia et al., 2009; Hopp, Sørensen, Herborg, & Roberts, 2005; Rossing, Hansen, & Krass, 2002).

In some countries, pharmacists have moved away from product-oriented services toward service-oriented and then patient-oriented services, increasingly emphasizing the patient's health outcomes (the economic, clinical, and humanistic outcomes model) (Drabinski, 2000; Kozma, Reeder, & Schulz, 1993). Outcomes refer to the consequences (results) of interventions that are made to achieve therapeutic goals. Outcomes can have economic, social/behavioral, or physiological characteristics. When community pharmacists are serving the public, in addition to health outcomes, at least four important parameters should be monitored: accessibility, availability, affordability, and acceptability. When patients benefit from the medications that they take, their health improves, which ultimately reduces costs (Wiedenmayer et al., 2006).

The scope of pharmacy practice now includes patient-centered care—with all the cognitive functions of counseling, providing drug information, and monitoring drug therapy—and the technical aspects of pharmaceutical services, including medication supply management, as well as people- or public-centered care. Community pharmacies can offer comprehensive healthcare services, including advanced and enhanced services. Such services include the rational use of medicines; medication adherence; self-management clinics for group of patients with chronic diseases (e.g., diabetes mellitus, hypertension, and asthma); medication therapy management; screening and monitoring; education for enhancing medication adherence; encouraging and educating patients to receive their recommended immunizations and those for infants; home healthcare services; partnership in palliative care teams; drive-through facilities; mail and Internet orders of medicines; rural and remote area services; mobile pharmacy; helping patients with special needs; public health and primary healthcare services (e.g., HIV/AIDS and drug abuse treatment); distributing literature and educating regarding life style change for stress reduction, proper nutrition, and exercising; collaboration with other healthcare professionals during disease outbreaks (e.g., Ebola virus disease, severe acute respiratory syndrome, middle-east respiratory syndrome, and Zika virus disease); involvement in an unwanted medicines program; health promotion (the process of enabling people to increase their control over—and to improve—their health, e.g., smoking cessation, obesity management, and diabetic self-management); drug therapy problems (defined as "[a]n undesirable event, a patient experience that involves, or is suspected to involve drug therapy, and that actually or potentially, interferes with a desired patient outcome" (Cipolle et al., 1998; Strand, Cipolle, Morley, Ramsey, & Lamsam, 1990)); and pharmaceutical public health services. Pharmaceutical public health has been defined as follows:

> The application of pharmaceutical knowledge, skills and resources to the science and art of preventing disease, prolonging life, promoting, protecting and improving health for all through the organized efforts of society.
>
> **Walker (2000)**

Pharmacists could also provide public services, such as local guidelines and treatment protocols, medication use review and evaluation, national medicine policies and essential medicine lists, pharmacovigilance, needs assessment, and pharmacoepidemiology (Wiedenmayer et al., 2006). Pharmacists should be at the front line to promote safe sex, birth control education, advice on nursing babies, and caring for elderly parents and relatives. In addition, pharmacists could work with local authorities in the direction of a cleaner and safer environment (air, water, and ground) and for safe food handling. Pharmacists should only carry in stock and sell products with proven medical value, not selling tobacco products, and not supplements and homeopathic medicines that have no clear scientific evidence of safety and effectiveness.

ACHIEVEMENTS

The literature has shown that community pharmacists in some countries have had a positive impact on public health. First, training and education programs have been able to enhance the knowledge and practices of pharmacists. Continuing education programs, especially if mandatory, also play a significant role. Second, pharmacy colleges have improved by incorporating relevant courses and topics into the syllabi for undergraduate pharmacy programs. Third, strong, motivated, and uncorrupted pharmacy authorities/regulatory agencies have been able to improve community pharmacy practices because of their concern, motivation, and effort to make necessary improvements.

CHALLENGES

To progress and gain society's acceptance, community pharmacists must acknowledge the following challenges in healthcare systems:

1. One-third of the world's population is known to lack regular access to essential medicines. For many people, the cost of medication is a major constraint. Those hardest hit are patients in developing and transitional economies, where 50% to 90% of medicines are out-of-pocket expenses (WHO, 1998). The burden falls most heavily on the poor, who are not adequately protected by current policies or by health insurance.
2. Healthcare workers, including community pharmacist, are in short supply, especially in LMICs (WHO, 2016).
3. Some countries are eager to introduce and establish a Doctor of Pharmacy (PharmD) degree in pharmacy colleges, but due to several reasons, they have failed to produce competent graduates who can apply clinical knowledge in practice or who can distance the practice from its traditional role.
4. The logistical aspects of distribution, often seen as the pharmacist's traditional role (i.e., the "count and pour, lick and stick pharmacy"), represent another challenge.
5. In terms of medication quality, studied medication samples have failed quality control tests (MSH, 2012), and substandard and counterfeit medications are highly likely to be on pharmacy shelves.
6. Another major challenge is ensuring that medicines are used as advised or instructed; more than half of all prescriptions are incorrect, and more than half of the people who are prescribed with medications fail to take them correctly. Medication adherence can be affected if the medication is unavailable or unaffordable or if the instructions given are not understood or remembered. Furthermore, a patient's confidence or trust in the pharmacist or the medications prescribed may also affect adherence.

7. Especially in economically deprived communities, self-medication with either modern or traditional medicines is becoming common practice. Individuals resort to self-medication when healthcare services become more unaffordable and inaccessible (Hughes, McElnay, & Fleming, 2001). The situation deteriorates when prescription medicines can be easily obtained over the counter. Community pharmacists could play a role in mitigating the risks of self-medication (Bennadi, 2013).

Given the list of pharmacist-, pharmacy-, and practice-related issues above, are pharmacists still needed in the community and in the healthcare system? If community pharmacists still perform the basic function of medication dispensing or if a country lacks pharmacists, could we simply have medicine vending machines (i.e., a self-service technology) across the country (Adams, 2014; Poulter, 2010)? These machines could provide customers access to OTC drugs, nondrug items, and information, thereby supporting the self-care concept (Steinfirst, Cowell, Presley, & Reifler, 1985). This technology could be argued to have an adverse effect on customers. For example, the buying and selling process lacks the "human touch," or customers leave the pharmacy without information or take medication incorrectly due to a lack of quality information. However, what is the difference when the same customers visit pharmacies with "invisible pharmacists"? Do pharmacists just count pills? If community pharmacists are hesitant or refuse to change, these vending machines will put them out of business. For countries searching for cost-cutting strategies, this technology might be a solution.

RECOMMENDATIONS: THE WAY FORWARD

To be effective healthcare team members, community pharmacists need skills and abilities that will enable them to assume many different functions. WHO introduced the concept of the "seven/eight-star pharmacist," which the International Pharmaceutical Federation (FIP) adopted in 2000 in its policy statement on Good Pharmacy Education Practice to outline the caregiver, decision-maker, communicator, manager, lifelong learner, teacher, and leader roles of the pharmacist. The pharmacist's function as a researcher has since evolved, and all these roles have been addressed in the competence standards (WHO, 1997, pp. 27–29). Community pharmacists have to make efforts to move from being drug compounders and dispensers to being pharmaceutical care providers and medication experts; their role and function should focus on patient-centered care rather than products and profits. Community pharmacists must equip themselves with adequate knowledge and skills and be responsible for ensuring that, irrespective of the medications provided and used, quality products are selected, procured, stored, distributed, dispensed, and administered to enhance patients' health and do them no harm. Relevant pharmacy authorities should provide more support, training, and development for community pharmacies to help their pharmacists deliver high-quality services. Pharmacy associations could organize programs in collaboration with pharmacy colleges and could involve regional or international experts if affordable. Nonprofit international organizations, such as WHO and Management Sciences for Health (MSH), could assist LMICs in this matter. In addition, some chain pharmacies could implement monthly programs. Community pharmacists must be involved in CPD; individual pharmacists are responsible for the systematic maintenance, development, and broadening of their knowledge, skills, and attitudes to ensure their continued competence as professionals throughout their careers. Community pharmacists (with the help of academics from pharmacy colleges, if required) must conduct research to document outcomes and impacts (e.g., accessibility, effectiveness, and positive perceptions of the experience); research must be conducted to assess the minimum standards and quality of community pharmacies and to provide evidence-based practice information. The numbers of published studies from developing countries are very low compared with those from developed countries. Managerial and educational interventions are needed to improve the practice. Community pharmacists could obtain inputs/ideas and explore the perceptions of community pharmacy staff—in addition to customers and patients—regarding aspects of service quality. These inputs could then perhaps be used to improve the services offered to customers. Some pharmacists are able to use information technology to enhance pharmacy and pharmaceutical services; pharmacists in some other countries find doing it so problematic—due to a very basic infrastructure or the lack of basic competencies, among others. Finally, WHO (Wiedenmayer et al., 2006) and other sources have provided a guide and systematic approach for delivering pharmacy patient-centered care and good pharmacy and dispensing practice.

CONCLUSIONS

Public health pharmacy interventions, patient-centered care, rational medication use, and effective medication supply management are key components of an accessible, sustainable, affordable, and equitable healthcare system that ensures the efficacy, safety, and quality of medications. The customer's (patient's) expectations are rapidly changing; customers are becoming more aware of their healthcare needs. Customers now demand better quality care and more attention to maintain or improve their overall health. Evidence has shown that challenges and gaps exist in community pharmacy practice. In developing countries, the functions of community pharmacists must be redefined and reoriented. A paradigm shift in the mind-set and practices of pharmacists is urgently needed.

LESSONS LEARNED

- Although the overall level of community pharmacy services provided in developing countries does not meet the public's expectations, gradual progress has been observed.
- The number of trained community pharmacists is inadequate; their distribution is unbalanced; and, in some countries, individuals without the professional pharmacy degrees are allowed to work in pharmacies. Thus, pharmacy authorities, policy makers, and educators must collaborate to fix these problems and make improvements.
- Due to the high prevalence of chronic diseases and the need to improve public health and well-being, community pharmacists must continue to be competent in their professional and business roles; pharmacists should expand the role in delivering wellness services (e.g., disease-oriented pharmaceutical care) that go beyond filling prescriptions.
- Many developing nations do not have effective and efficient regulations, guidelines, policies, governmental support, or electronic patient records and databases in community pharmacies to help establish and implement clinical, cognitive, and extended pharmacy services.
- Community pharmacists should establish benchmark best practices—at the very least among countries with similar economies and levels of development.

REFERENCES

ACCP. Role of a pharmacist. Retrieved from http://www.aacp.org/resources/student/pharmacyforyou/Pages/roleofapharmacist.aspx.

Adams, M. (2014). *Prescription drug vending machines now being installed on college campuses across America*. Retrieved from http://www.naturalnews.com/047701_prescription_drugs_vending_machines_college_campuses.html.

Adje, D. U., & Oli, A. N. (2013). Community pharmacy in Warri, Nigeria – a survey of practice details. *Scholars Academic Journal of Biosciences*, 2(5), 391–397.

Alamin Hassan, M. A. A., Mohamed Ibrahim, M. I., & Hassali, M. A. A. (2014). Antibiotics dispensing for URTIs by community pharmacists and general medical practitioners in Penang, Malaysia: A comparative study using simulated patients. *Journal of Clinical and Diagnostic Research*, *8*, 119–123.

Alvarez-Risco, A., & van Mil, J. M. (2007). Pharmaceutical care in community pharmacies: Practice and research in Peru. *The Annals of Pharmacotherapy*, *41*, 2032–2037.

Amin, M., & Chewning, B. (2016). Pharmacies without pharmacists: Absenteeism plagues pharmacies in developing countries. *Research in Social & Administrative Pharmacy: RSAP* Retrieved from http://dx.doi.org/10.1016/j.sapharm.2016.10.013.

Andersson, S., & Snell, B. (2010). *Where there is no pharmacists: A guide to managing medicines for all health workers*. Health Action International-Asia Pacific (HAI-AP) & Third World Network (TWN).

Aravamuthan, A., Arputhavanan, M., Subramaniam, K., & Chander, J. S. J.U. (2017). Assessment of current prescribing practices using World Health Organization core drug use and complementary indicators in selected rural community pharmacies in Southern India. *Journal of Pharmaceutical Policy and Practice*, *10*, 1. http://dx.doi.org/10.1186/s40545-016-0074.

The Association of Faculties of Medicines of Canada. (n.d.). Chapter 1 Concepts of health and illness. Public and population health. Retrieved from http://phprimer.afmc.ca/Part1-TheoryThinkingAboutHealth/ConceptsOfHealthAndIllness/PublicandPopulationHealth#PublicandPopulationHealth.

Basak, S. C., Arunkumar, A., & Masilamani, K. (2009). Community pharmacists' attitudes towards use of medicines in rural India: An analysis of current situation. *Pharmacy World & Science*, *31*, 612–618.

Bennadi, D. (2013). Self-medication: A current challenge. *Journal of Basic and Clinical Pharmacy*, *5*(1), 19–23. http://dx.doi.org/10.4103/0976-0105.128253.

Brodie, D. C. (1981). Pharmacy's societal purpose. *American Journal of Hospital Pharmacy*, *38*, 1893–1896.

Cipolle, R. J., Strand, L. M., & Morley, P. C. (1998). *Pharmaceutical care practice*. New York: McGraw Hill.

CPNI. (n.d.). Retrieved from http://www.communitypharmacyni.co.uk/what-is-community-pharmacy/.

Dhote, V., Mahajan, S. C., & Mishra, D. K. (2013). Opportunities and challenges in pharmacy profession in developing countries like India: An overview. *Journal der Pharmazie Forschung*, 2(1), 17–31.

Drabinski, A. (2000). Strategies to demonstrate the value of pharmacists' cognitive services. *Health Policy Newsletter*, *13*(4) Article 11. Retrieved from http://jdc.jefferson.edu/hpn/vol13/iss4/11.

Fang, Y., Yang, S., Zhou, S., Jiang, M., & Liu, J. (2013). Community pharmacy practice in China: Past, present and future. *International Journal of Clinical Pharmacy*, *35*(4), 520–528. http://dx.doi.org/10.1007/s11096-013-9789-5.

Farris, K. B., Kumbera, P., Halterman, T., & Fang, G. (2002). Outcomes-based pharmacist reimbursement: Reimbursing pharmacists for cognitive services (part 1 of a 2-part series). *Journal of Managed Care Pharmacy*, *5*(8), 383–393.

Fathelrahman, A., Mohamed Ibrahim, M. I., & Wertheimer, A. I. (2016). *Pharmacy practice in developing countries: Achievements and challenges* (1st ed.). Cambridge, MA: Academic Press.

Garrett, D. G., & Martin, L. A. (2003). The Asheville project: Participants' perceptions of factors contributing to the success of a patient self-management diabetes program. *Journal of the American Pharmacists Association: Japha*, *43*, 185–190.

Gastelurrutia, M. A., Benrimoj, S. I., Castrillon, C. C., de Amezua, M. J., Fernandez-Llimos, F., & Faus, M. J. (2009). Facilitators for practice change in Spanish community pharmacies. *Pharmacy World & Science*, *31*, 32–39.

Gokcekus, L., Toklu, H. Z., Demirdamar, R., & Gumusel, B. (2012). Dispensing practice in the community pharmacies in the Turkish Republic of Northern Cyprus. *International Journal of Clinical Pharmacy*, *34*(2), 312–324. http://dx.doi.org/10.1007/s11096-011-9605-z.

Halila, G. C., Junior, E. H., Otuki, M. F., & Correr, C. J. (2015). The practice of OTC counseling by community pharmacists in Parana, Brazil. *Pharmacy Practice (Granada)*, *13*(4), 597. http://dx.doi.org/10.18549/PharmPract.2015.04.597.

Hasan, S., Sulieman, H., Stewart, K., Chapman, C. B., Hasan, M. Y., & Kong, D. C. M. (2013). Assessing patient satisfaction with community pharmacy in the UAE using a newly-validated tool. *Research in Social and Administrative Pharmacy*, *9*(6), 841–850.

Helper, C. D. (1988). Unresolved issues in the future of pharmacy. *American Journal of Hospital Pharmacy*, *45*(5), 1071–1081.

Hepler, C. D., & Strand, L. M. (1990). Opportunities and Responsibilities in Pharmaceutical care. *American Journal of Hospital Pharmacy*, *47*(3), 533–543.

Hopp, T. R., Sørensen, E. W., Herborg, H., & Roberts, A. S. (2005). Implementation of cognitive pharmaceutical services (CPS) in professionally active pharmacies. *International Journal of Pharmacy Practice*, *13*, 21–31.

Hughes, C. M., McElnay, J. C., & Fleming, G. F. (2001). Benefits and risks of self-medication. *Drug Safety: An International Journal of Medical Toxicology and Drug Experience*, *24*, 1027–1037.

Hussain, A., & Mohamed Ibrahim, M. I. (2012). Management of diarrhoea cases by community pharmacies in 3 cities of Pakistan. *Eastern Mediterranean Health Journal*, *18*, 635–640.

Hussain, A., Mohamed Ibrahim, M. I., & Babar, Z. U. (2012a). Using the potentials of community pharmacies to promote rational drug use in Pakistan: An opportunity exists or lost. *JPMA. The Journal of the Pakistan Medical Association*, *62*(11), 1217–1222.

Hussain, A., & Mohamed Ibrahim, M. I. (2011). Medication counselling and dispensing practices at community pharmacies: A comparative cross sectional study from Pakistan. *International Journal of Clinical Pharmacy*, *33*, 859–867. http://dx.doi.org/10.1007/s11096-011-9554-6. Epub August 19, 2011.

Hussain, A., Mohamed Ibrahim, M. I., & Malik, M. (2012b). Assessment of disease management of acute respiratory tract infection at community pharmacies through simulated visits in Pakistan. *Latin American Journal of Pharmacy*, *31*, 1435–1440.

Hussain, A., Mohamed Ibrahim, M. I., & Zaheer, U. D. B. (2012d). Compliance with legal requirements at community pharmacies: A cross sectional study from Pakistan. *International Journal of Pharmacy Practice*, *20*(3), 183–190. http://dx.doi.org/10.1111/j.2042-7174.2011.00178.x.

Khatib, R., McKee, M., Shannon, H., Chow, C., Rangarajan, S., Teo, K., et al. (2016). Availability and affordability of cardiovascular disease medicines and their effect on use in high-income, middle-income, and low-income countries: An analysis of the PURE study data. *Lancet*, *387*, 61–69. http://dx.doi.org/10.1016/S0140-6736(15)00469-9.

Kozma, C. M., Reeder, C. E., & Schulz, R. M. (1993). Economic, clinical, and humanistic outcomes: A planning model for pharmacoeconomic research. *Clinical Therapeutics*, *15*(6), 1121–1132.

Lenjisa, J. L., Mosisa, B., Woldu, M. A., & Negassa, D. E. (2015). Analysis of dispensing practices at community pharmacy settings in Ambo Town, West Shewa, Ethiopia. *Journal of Community Medicine and Health Education*, *5*, 329. http://dx.doi.org/10.4172/2376-0214.1000329.

Management Sciences for Health (MSH). (2012). *Chapter 19 quality assurance for pharmaceuticals*. Retrieved from http://projects.msh.org/resource-center/publications/upload/MDS3-Ch19-QualityAssurance-Mar2012.pdf.

Minh, P. D., Huong, D. T., Byrkit, R., & Murray, M. (2013). Strengthening pharmacy practice in Vietnam: Findings of a training intervention study. *Tropical Medicine & International Health: TM & IH*, *18*(4), 426–434. http://dx.doi.org/10.1111/tmi.12062. Epub 2013 Jan 7.

Mohamed Ibrahim, M. I., Awaisu, A., Atwa, H., Radoui, A., Kheir, N., & Maarup, N. (2014). How do community pharmacists in Qatar respond to patients presenting with symptoms of acute respiratory tract infections? *Journal of Pharmacy Practice and Research, 44*, 62–63.

Mohamed Ibrahim, M. I., Palaian, S., Al-Sulaiti, F., & El-Shami, S. (2016). Evaluating community pharmacy practice in Qatar using simulated patient method: Acute gastroenteritis management. *Pharmacy Practice, 14*(4), 800. http://dx.doi.org/10.18549/PharmPract.2016.04.800.

Oparah, A. C., & Kikanme, L. C. (2006). Consumer satisfaction with community pharmacies in Warri, Nigeria. *Research in Social & Administrative Pharmacy: RSAP, 2*(4), 499–511.

Osman, A., Ahmed Hassan, I. S., & Mohamed Ibrahim, M. I. (2012). Are Sudanese community pharmacists capable to prescribe and demonstrate asthma inhaler devices to patrons? A mystery patient study. *Pharmacy Practice (Internet), 10*, 1–6.

Pharmaceutical Services Division, MOH. (2016). *Guide to good dispensing practice (GDsP).* Retrieved from http://www.pharmacy.gov.my/v2/en/documents/guide-good-dispensing-practice-gdsp.html.

Pharmacy Board of Australia. Guidelines for dispensing of medicines. Retrieved from http://apps.who.int/medicinedocs/en/d/Js17807en/.

Poudel, A., Subish, P., Mishra, P., Mohamed Ibrahim, M. I., & Jayasekera, J. (2010). Prevalence of fixed dose drug combinations in Nepal: A preliminary study. *Journal of Clinical and Diagnostic Research [serial Online], 4*, 2246–2252.

Poulter, S. (2010). *Medicine vending machines that dispense prescriptions 24 hours a day go on trial.* Retrieved from http://www.dailymail.co.uk/health/article-1288434/Medicine-vending-machine-dispenses-prescriptions-pharmacist-launched.html.

Rossing, C., Hansen, E. H., & Krass, I. (2002). Barriers and facilitators in pharmaceutical care: Perceptions and experiences among Danish community pharmacies. *Journal of Social and Administrative Pharmacy, 19*, 55–64.

Royal Pharmaceutical Society of Great Britain. (n.d.). Practice guidance: good dispensing guidelines – England. Retrieved from http://www.rpharms.com/practice-science-and-research-pdfs/good-dispensing-guidelines.pdf.

SHPA. (2003). *Community pharmacy role/service definition grid.* Retrieved from http://cpd.shpa.org.au/lib/pdf/communitytem.pdf.

Siang, C. S., Kee, W. W., Gee, L. H., Richard, Y., & See Hui, J. T. (2008). Implementation of the benchmarking guidelines on community pharmacies in Malaysia. *Malaysian Journal of Pharmaceutical Sciences, 6*(1), 13–31.

Smith, F. (2001). *Pharmacy practice.* Taylor & Francis.

Smith, F. (2004). Community pharmacy in Ghana: Enhancing the contribution to primary health care. *Health Policy and Planning, 19*(4), 234–241. http://dx.doi.org/10.1093/heapol/czh028.

Steinfirst, J. L., Cowell, S. A., Presley, B. A., & Reifler, C. B. (1985). Vending machines and the self-care concept. *Journal of American College Health, 34*(1), 37–39.

Strand, L. M., Cipolle, R. J., Morley, P. C., Ramsey, R., & Lamsam, G. D. (1990). Drug-related problems: Their structure and function. *DICP: The Annals of Pharmacotherapy, 24*, 1093–1097.

Syhakhang, L., Stenson, B., Wahlström, R., & Tomson, G. (2001). The quality of public and private pharmacy practices. A cross sectional study in the Savannakhet province, Lao PDR. *European Journal of Clinical Pharmacology, 57*(3), 221–227.

The American Public Health Association. (1981). Policy statements adopted by the governing council. The role of the pharmacist in public health. *American Journal of Public Health, 71*, 213–216.

Volmer, D., Vendla, K., Vetka, A., Bell, J. S., & Hamilton, D. (2008). Pharmaceutical care in community Pharmacies: Practice and research in Estonia. *The Annals of Pharmacotherapy, 42*, 1104–1111.

Walker, R. (2000). Pharmaceutical public health: The end of pharmaceutical care? *Pharmaceutical Journal, 264*, 340–341.

WHO. (1978). In *Primary health care: Report of the international Conference. Primary health care, Alma-Ata, USSR, 6–12 September, 1978, jointly sponsored by the world health organization and the United nations Children's Fund*. Geneva: World Health Organization (Health for All Series No. 1).

WHO. (1998). *Health reform and drug financing, selected topics, Health economics and drugs, DAP series no. 6, WHO/DAP/98.3*. Geneva, Switzerland: World Health Organization.

WHO. (2015). *WHO global strategy on people-centred and integrated health services*. http://apps.who.int/iris/bitstream/10665/155002/1/WHO_HIS_SDS_2015.6_eng.pdf.

WHO. (August 1997). *The role of the pharmacist in the health-care system - preparing the future pharmacist: Curricular development, report of a third WHO consultative group on the role of the pharmacist*. Vancouver, Canada. http://apps.who.int/medicinedocs/en/d/Js2214e/3.2.html.

WHO Regional Office for South-East Asia, WHO Regional Office for the Western Pacific. (2007). *People at the centre of health care: Harmonizing mind and body, people and systems*. Geneva: World Health Organization. http://www.who.int/whr/2008/overview/en/.

WHO. (1994). Retrieved from http://apps.who.int/medicinedocs/en/d/Jh2995e/1.6.2.html#Jh2995e.1.6.2.

WHO. (2002). Constitution of the World Health Organization. Geneva: World Health Organization; 1948 in Bulletin of the World Health Organization, 80 (12).

WHO. (2005). *The world health report: Make every mother and child count*.

WHO. (2016). *Global strategy on human resources for health: Workforce 2030*. Geneva http://who.int/hrh/resources/global_strategy_workforce2030_14_print.pdf.

WHO. (July 1984). In *Health promotion: A discussion document on the concept and principles: Summary report of the working group on concept and principles of health promotion, Copenhagen* (pp. 9–13). Copenhagen: WHO Regional Office for Europe.

Wiedenmayer, K., Summers, R. S., Mackie, C. A., Gous, A. G. S., Everard, M., & Tromp, D. (2006). *Developing pharmacy practice: A focus on patient care. WHO (and FIP)*. Geneva, Switzerland: Department of Medicines Policy and Standards. http://www.who.int/iris/handle/10665/69399.

Winslow, C. E. A. (1920). The untilled field of public health. Modern medicine, 2, 183. Who. The world health organization quality of life assessment (WHOQOL): Position paper from the world health organization. *Social Science & Medicine*, *41*(10), 1403–1409.

FURTHER READING

Mohamed Ibrahim, M. I., Fathelrahman, A., Wertheimer, A. I. (2016). Chapter 20: Comparative analysis and conclusion. In Fathelrahman, A. I., Mohamed Ibrahim, M. I. & Wertheimer, A. I. (Eds.), Pharmacy practice in developing countries: Achievements and challenges (pp. 449–467). Cambridge, MA: Academic Press.

www.merriam-webster.com/; (n.d.). In Merriam Webster Online, Retrieved from http://www.merriam-webster.com/dictionary/citation).

CHAPTER

19

ENHANCING QUALITY OF PATIENT-CENTERED CARE SERVICES IN DEVELOPING COUNTRIES: PHARMACEUTICAL CARE APPROACH

Dinesh K. Upadhyay, Guat See Ooi

Asian Institute of Medicine, Science and Technology University, Kedah, Malaysia

CHAPTER OUTLINE

INTRODUCTION

The number of medicines and their consumptions has increased drastically over the last few decades. New revolutions in the medicine market have brought new challenges for healthcare professionals in terms of controlling medicine quality and their rational use. Rising healthcare costs, lack of human resources in healthcare sectors, inefficient health systems, the burden of diseases, and the changing social, technological, economic, and political environment encounter in providing good healthcare facilities and patient-centered care services in developing countries (WHO, 2001; Wiedenmayer et al., 2006).

Access to assured quality medicines is a global major concern. The World Health Organization (WHO) report stated that one-third of the world's population is devoid of regular access to essential

Social and Administrative Aspects of Pharmacy in Low- and Middle-Income Countries. http://dx.doi.org/10.1016/B978-0-12-811228-1.00019-4

medicines (WHO, 2004). However, affordability of medicines is a major concern in developing countries, where 50%–90% of medicines expenditure is out of pocket. Ensuring the rational use of medicine in developing countries is another major challenge, which can be resolved by ensuring that patients receive right medication to their clinical needs, in doses that meet their own individual requirements for an adequate period, and at the lowest cost to them and their community (WHO, 1987, 2002). Even though measures have been taken to follow rational use of medicines, still they are not standardized. Patients receive prescriptions and medications; more than half of all prescriptions are incorrect and more than half of the people involved fail to take them correctly (Hogerzeil, 1995; WHO, 1985). Furthermore, global threat of antimicrobial resistance is a growing concern and a major public health problem. WHO highlighted significant antibiotic resistance in various diseases such as shigellosis, pneumonia, bacterial meningitis, gonorrhea, and hospital-acquired *Staphylococcus aureus* infections worldwide (WHO, 2005).

Barriers contributing to access medicines of good quality and their rational use demand immediate global health sector reform. Various interventional approaches, effective medicine supply, and rational use of drug ensure an accessible, sustainable, affordable, and equitable healthcare system that provides efficacious, safe, and quality medicines to patients. Pharmacists play an important role in health sector reform processes. Pharmacists have the potential to improve patients' therapeutic outcomes to achieve better quality of life (QoL) within available resources. It is important that patients must receive the correct information about their disease and medicine(s) (Aslani et al., 2012).

CONCEPT OF PHARMACEUTICAL CARE

Pharmacists should move from behind the counter and start serving the public by providing care to them instead of only dispensing pills. Pharmaceutical care (PC) is one of the dimensions of pharmacy practice (PP) (Fig. 19.1) emerged in the mid-1970s (Wiedenmayer et al., 2006). The concept of PC

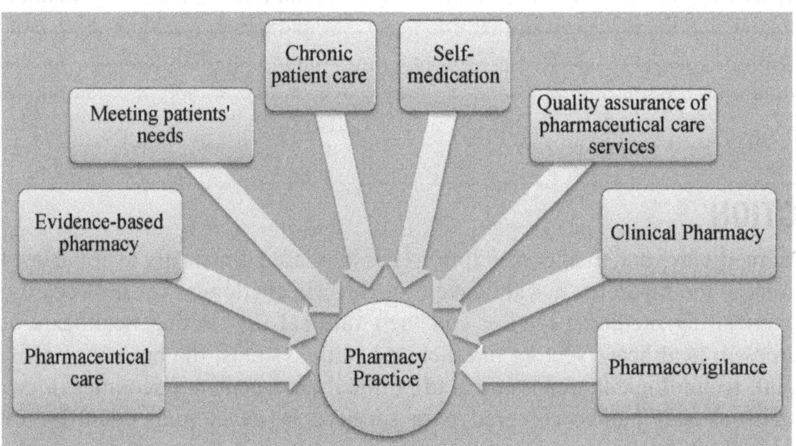

FIGURE 19.1

Dimension of pharmacy practice.

was first defined as "*the care that a given patient requires and receives which assures safe and rational drug usage*" (Mikeal et al., 1975). PC includes identifying, resolving, and preventing the issues related to drugs. It was the first integrated philosophy of PP to combine the expertise of the pharmacists in drug therapy monitoring and medication counseling to improve the patients' therapeutic outcomes and QoL.

The American Society of Hospital Pharmacy defined PC as "the direct, responsible provision of medication-related care…" (ASHP, 1993). Hepler and Strand (1990) described the concept of PC that involves direct interaction between the pharmacist and the patient, with responsible provision of drug therapy to achieve definite outcomes that improve patients' QoL and promote disease management. These outcomes are (1) cure to disease; (2) eradication or decrease of patients' symptomatology; (3) arresting or slowing disease process; or (4) preventing a disease or symptomatology (Hepler & Strand, 1990). Later, Cipolle et al. (2004) refined the philosophy of Hepler and Strand and said that "it is a patient-centered practice." The above definitions emphasized the patients' and the pharmacists' responsibility and the direct interaction to ensure good quality care to patients to achieve better health-related outcomes.

The pharmacists' role has shifted gradually from being more product-oriented to patient-focused through global PC services over the 20th century. PC deals with the way people should receive and use medications as well as providing instructions for the use of medicines. It also deals with the responsibilities, medication surveillance, counseling, and care outcomes. PC can be achieved through good communication between the different members of the healthcare team and continuity of care (Hepler & Strand, 1990; Hudson et al., 2007; Palaian et al., 2005). PC is a regime for a pharmacist to work with healthcare professionals in designing, implementing, and monitoring a therapeutic plan to produce specific outcomes for the patient. This comprises three major functions: (1) identifying potential and actual drug-related problems (DRPs), (2) resolving actual DRPs, and (3) preventing potential DRPs (Hepler & Strand, 1990). Later in 2008, a survey commissioned by the European councils concluded that "*pharmaceutical care is a quality philosophy and working method indispensable for realising the benefits of medicine use for the individual patient and at national levels.*" It emphasizes the importance of care provision in a responsible manner, in addition to functions related to medicine quality and logistics of supply (Cousins et al., 2012). Then, what does clinical pharmacy mean? Is clinical pharmacy different from PC? The American College of Clinical Pharmacy (ACCP) defined clinical pharmacy as "that area of pharmacy concerned with the science and practice of rational medication use" (ACCP, 2008). Furthermore, according to ACCP, pharmacists who involved in clinical pharmacy area "provide patient care that optimizes medication therapy and promotes health, wellness, and disease prevention." Franklin and Van Mil (2005) noted that concepts of clinical pharmacy and PC are closely related. They defined clinical pharmacy as "part of the practice of pharmacy that contributes directly to patient care and develops and promotes the rational and appropriate use of medicinal products and devices," whereas PC is defined as the person-focused care with the aim of improving the outcomes of therapy (Franklin & Van Mil, 2005). Sometimes it is confusing but what important is both concepts need to be fully understood, clearly described, and applied.

PRINCIPLES OF PHARMACEUTICAL CARE IN PRACTICES

According to the American Pharmacists Association, the goals of PC intervention are to improve health-related quality of life (HRQoL) of patients and to achieve better therapeutic outcomes with optimal economic burden on patients (APA, 1995). The way to accomplish these goals must pass through these following principles:

1. Pharmacists must have a professional and mutual relationship with the patients, which is established and maintained on caring, trust, communication, cooperation, and mutual decision-making.
2. Patients' specific medical information such as general health and activity status, medical and medication history, history of present illness, and financial situation (insured/uninsured/affordability) must be collected, organized, recorded, and kept confidential.
3. The medication therapy plan should be developed mutually with the patients after evaluating patients' specific medical information. The pharmacists must consider the psychosocial aspects of the disease, the cost, intricacies in therapy, and adherence. Information should be conveyed to the patients in very simple and understandable language. The medication therapy should be documented and conveyed to other healthcare providers if necessary.
4. The pharmacists must ensure that the patients have received all the necessary information and awareness about the disease and medication therapy to achieve better therapeutic outcomes.
5. It is the pharmacists' responsibility to monitor patients' progress, review, and even modify the therapy as necessary and appropriate. The progress and modification (if any) is accurately documented and shared with the concerned healthcare providers. The hierarchy of PC in practice is represented in Fig. 19.2 (APA, 1995).

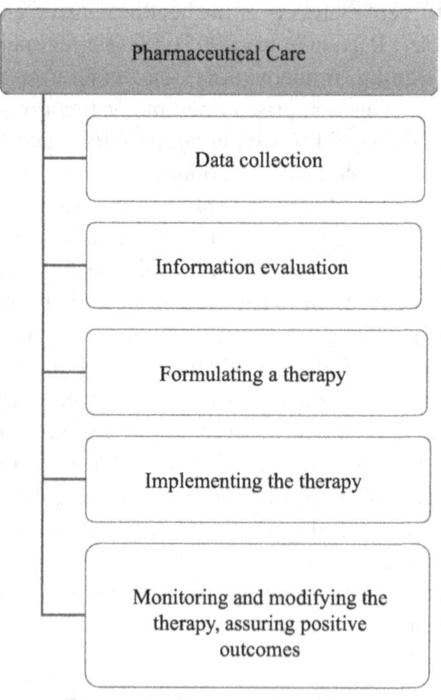

FIGURE 19.2

Hierarchy of pharmaceutical care in practice.

EVIDENCE OF THE BENEFITS OF PHARMACEUTICAL CARE INTERVENTION

A pharmacist's role in drug dispensing is well recognized and accepted as an important part of the conventional function of a pharmacist for more than two decades. The literatures from developed countries have documented the pharmacist's participation and impact in patient-centered care in hospitals and community-based pharmacy settings, which is still lacking from developing nations where pharmacists are more involved in the selling of medicines. The benefits of including a pharmacist in the healthcare team responsible for managing inpatients in a tertiary care hospital resulted in significant decrease in patients' total length of stay in hospitals and lowered their economic burden (Boyko et al., 1997). Moreover, the pharmacist's participation in ambulatory patient care benefited the patients in managing their glycated hemoglobin, low-density lipid cholesterol, and blood pressure in addition to declining adverse drug events. This was indicated as an achievement in clinical outcome because patient-centered care increased patients' knowledge about their disease, adherence to their medication, and HRQoL (Chisholm–Burns et al., 2010). Similar benefits of the pharmacist's participation in improving various markers of lipid control among hyperlipidemic patients were also summarized in another systematic review (Charrois et al., 2012). Furthermore, a 12-week study on 210 Australian community pharmacies examined a total of 6230 PC interventions provided to patients addressing their DRPs and found about 39% of PC intervention prevented or needed a physician's visit or hospital admission (Peterson et al., 2009).

Prescription errors in primary care are very common and involve greater risks of patient harm. PC interventions have prominent role in preventing prescription errors and its association with adverse drug events. Pharmacists' intervention reduced medication errors in general practices because of regular pharmacists' visits to the general practice prescriber and provided them regular feedback, educational intervention, and support related to drug prescriptions (Avery et al., 2012). The contribution of clinical pharmacists in developing an antimicrobial prescribing protocol encouraged the prescription of antimicrobials on inpatients as defined criteria in the protocol that significantly reduced the patients' duration of hospital stay, decreased the need and term of intravenous medication therapies, and resulted in the reduction in treatment failure (Al-Eidan et al., 2000). Similarly, the impact of a restrictive policy on antimicrobials used by ward pharmacists for 2 years in a tertiary university hospital contributed a significant and sustained reduction in the use and cost of restricted agents (Ansari et al., 2003). Pharmacists play an important role in understanding, reporting, and managing adverse drug reactions (ADRs) in both hospital and community pharmacies (Van Grootheest & De Jong-van den Berg, 2005).

From the above evidence, it is found that pharmacists have received good recognition in developed nations and not only involved in patient care but also contributed in developing various protocols related to drug use and managing ADRs in hospitals and community settings. However, the same is lacking in developing nations where pharmacists are still considered as drug sellers and drug dispensers.

THE NEED FOR PHARMACEUTICAL CARE IN DEVELOPING COUNTRIES

The total world population was 7.125 billion in 2013 with an annual growth rate of 1.2%, where 97% of this growth is accounted by developing countries (Haub, 2012). The WHO has recommended an allocation of 1 pharmacist per 1000 population (or 5 per 10000) in developing countries. As per FIP global pharmacy workforce report (Gall et al., 2012), Jordan has the highest ratio of pharmacists (17.5) and Burkina Faso has the lowest (0.2) ratio of pharmacists among developing countries. Ninety percent of the countries do not have enough pharmacists as recommended by WHO. Community pharmacies are the most popular area of practice (53%) followed by hospital pharmacies (26%) and pharmaceutical industries (26%) (Ibrahim, Fathelrahman, & Wertheimer, 2016).

Although developing countries are working toward good pharmacy practice (GPP) as indicated by WHO and FIP, they are still far behind in achieving these goals. Several issues such as price control, dispensing separation, counterfeit drugs, illegal practice etc. are creating gaps and barriers to GPP. The GPP guidelines released jointly by WHO and FIP are good moves for pharmacists and pharmacy organizations in developing countries to implement PC (FIP & WHO, 2011; WHO, 1996; Wiedenmayer et al., 2006). There is an immense need of PC in developing countries to resolve medication-related problems. PC models and practices are country specific and differ from each other (Farris et al., 2005). To implement and maintain the quality of PC, following basic indicators of PC can be used as a standard checklist (Table 19.1) (Cousins et al., 2012).

Table 19.1 Basic Indicators of Pharmaceutical Care

No.	Indicators	Comment
1.	Number of pharmaceutical care interventions delivered per standardized denominator, such as 1000 prescriptions dispensed or 1000 patients.	These interventions need to be formally documented and audited and are intended to improve the safe and effective use of medicines. Interventions can suggest a change in the way medicines are prescribed, dispensed, administered, or monitored. They may also confirm treatment decisions, foster patients' agreement and adherence to therapeutic plans, promote medication-related health literacy in patients, and support the joint development, agreement, and follow-up (monitoring) of treatment plans by patients and health professionals.
2.	Number of patients counseled about their medicines per standardized denominator, such as 1000 prescriptions dispensed or 1000 patients.	Formally documented and audited. Counseling comprises information given to an individual patient as part of the medication process that is adequate to ensure his/her ability to use the medication and to adapt his/her lifestyle in such a way as to have the best possible medication outcome.
3.	Number of formal written feedback responses from patients during treatment per 1000 prescriptions or 1000 patients about patients' specific medication-related literacy, concerns, life quality needs/expectations, and satisfaction.	Formally documented and audited. This feedback should be preferably encouraged at an early stage of the therapeutic plan to better implement and monitor the therapeutic plan.
4.	Number of adverse drug event reports (to include both adverse drug reactions and medication errors) per year.	Formally documented and audited and reported to recognized regional/national organizations, and there must be documented evidence of local learning and systems' improvement.

Adapted from Cousins, D., Kijlstra, N., et al. (2012). Pharmaceutical Care: Policies and practices for a safer, more responsible and cost-effective health system. Strasbourg: European Directorate for the Quality of Medicine and Healthcare (EDQM), 2012–2016, 62 pp.

CURRENT SCENARIO OF PHARMACEUTICAL CARE INTERVENTION IN DEVELOPING COUNTRIES

Several studies have been conducted in developed and developing countries to assess the impact of PC intervention among hospital inpatients and outpatients. Evidence has demonstrated an inclusion of PC services in the care of hospital inpatients resulted in improved and positive patients' health-related outcomes (Kaboli et al., 2006). Nakansha and coworkers in 2010 summarized various studies focusing on the impact of patient-centered care in community and outpatient settings. They found that most of the studies supported the pharmacists' role in medication and therapeutic management, patient counseling, and professional education to improve clinical outcomes (Nkansah et al., 2010). This section mainly focuses on studies involving PC interventions in developing countries.

In the North America region, studies from Brazil highlighted the impact of patient-centered care services in optimizing medication usage and reduction in symptoms caused by therapy, and indicated significant improvement in health condition of elderly outpatients and hypertensive patients (Junior et al., 2008; Lyra et al., 2007). A double-blind randomized controlled trial reported efficacy of patient-centered care service in improving systolic blood pressure (SBP) and diastolic blood pressure (DBP) and medication adherence of Brazilian patients with uncontrolled hypertension receiving hydrochlorothiazide therapy (De Castro et al., 2006). Another study conducted in public primary healthcare units in Brazil determined a significant improvement in pharmacotherapy adherence among elderly diabetic and hypertensive patients with positive impact on their clinical outcomes after a 36-month execution of PC program (Obreli-Neto et al., 2011). Similarly, the impact of pharmacists-supervised PC program on discharged Brazilian hypertensive patients significantly improved patients' SBP and DBP as well as the total cholesterol level (de Souza et al., 2016).

Within the South and West Africa region, a cross-sectional, operational research study described the contribution of clinical pharmacists in solving medicine-related problems and monitoring of pharmacotherapy of patients admitted in surgical and trauma intensive care unit during their ward rounds with multidisciplinary team (Bronkhorst et al., 2014). Moreover, a nonrandomized single site study from Nigeria targeting hypertensive patients in community pharmacy settings revealed significant improvement in patients' SBP and DBP and overall patients' satisfaction level because of patient-centered care services provided by pharmacists in the form of verbal counseling, providing disease and drug-related information leaflets and subsequent monitoring and reinforcement (Oparah et al., 2006). In addition, another study pointed out a significant improvement in patients' blood pressure and their physical and social domain of QoL (Aguwa et al., 2008). One more randomized controlled and 12-month follow-up study emphasized a notable improvement in overall HRQoL. In this study, an intervention group of type 2 diabetes mellitus patients was compared with a usual care group (Adibe et al., 2013). Researchers from Nigeria pointed out the effects of patient-centered care services in resolving antiretroviral drug therapy problems occurring in HIV patient's drug therapy (Nwaozuzu et al., 2013).

In the Southwest Asian region, a randomized, controlled, longitudinal prospective clinical trial, which targeted heart failure patients who were visiting a cardiology clinic in a private hospital in the United Arab Emirates (UAE), reported a vast improvement in HRQoL of patients with higher degree of adherence to their prescribed medications following patient-centered care services (Sadik et al., 2005). Another randomized controlled clinical trial on uncontrolled type 2 diabetics in diabetes clinics in Jordan highlighted the benefits of clinical pharmacists' involvement with other healthcare professionals in controlling fasting blood glucose and glycated hemoglobin (Wishah et al., 2015).

Within the Southeast Asia region, a prospective randomized controlled trial from China, which evaluated the effects of clinical pharmacists' intervention on hypertensive outpatients in hospital settings, found a noteworthy improvement in SBP and DBP of patients in intervention groups rather than controlled groups charting notable improvement in patients' medication adherence behavior to antihypertensive drugs (Zhao et al., 2012). A study from Taiwan described the involvement of clinical pharmacists in reviewing medication regimen and therapeutic recommendation to the patient with end-stage renal disease in renal transplant clinics and concluded the positive impact of patient-centered care services on physician prescriptions and patient outcomes (Wang et al., 2008). There were also few studies from Malaysia, which notified patient-centered care services and pharmacists' involvement in patient care. One study reported an active role of pharmacists in identifying different PC issues among diabetes mellitus, hypertensive, and hyperlipidemic patients and recommended some changes in disease management plan to resolve the issues related to drug use problems, ADRs, drug dosing, therapy failure, nonadherence to medication, and incorrect administration of medications (Chua et al., 2012). Similarly, impact of pharmacists' involvement through Renal Medication Therapy Adherence Clinic in managing chronic kidney disease (CKD) patients was evaluated. Patients were provided with appropriate counseling and education about their disease and medication using various pharmaceutical aids such as flip charts, drug albums, and pamphlets related to CKD, and improvement of patients' knowledge about disease and medication adherence level was noticed (Manan et al., 2016). Pharmacists were considered as an information resource for the patients with diabetes mellitus (Sulaiman et al., 2012). Patient-centered care services increased medication adherence behavior and tight glycemic control among type 2 diabetics (Chung et al., 2014). A randomized controlled study targeting postmenopausal osteoporotic women analyzed the importance of patient-centered care services in resolving drug therapy–related adverse drug events and increasing medication adherence and persistent behavior, QoL, and satisfaction level of patients (Lai et al., 2012). In addition, a pre–post quasiexperimental study targeting patients with acute coronary syndrome highlighted significant improvement in patients' physical and social components of HRQoL because of patient-centered care service provided by clinical pharmacists (Anchah et al., 2017). One survey from the Philippines described the active participation of pharmacists in dispensing, management, patients care, and public health, but they had low level of understanding the concept of PC and not much confident to perform it (Agaceta et al., 2013).

Researchers from India targeting type 2 diabetics in a private tertiary care teaching hospital and three primary healthcare centers located in urban and rural areas, respectively, also highlighted the effectiveness of PC program in improving diabetics' QoL and clinical outcomes (Arun et al., 2008; Sriram et al., 2011). Randomized clinical trial from North India emphasized a significant improvement in SBP and DBP, HRQoL, and satisfaction level of hypertensive patients because of patient-centered care services on disease management (Wal et al., 2013). Active participation of clinical pharmacists in resolving DRPs among hospitalized cardiovascular patients was notified from a prospective, observational study from South India (Movva et al., 2015). In addition, similar observation was made in another study describing a need of clinical pharmacists in healthcare teams to identify DRPs and resolve them by providing PC for better patient care (Kannan et al., 2011). A review article summarized unsatisfactory patient-centered care service in both hospital and community pharmacy settings of Pakistan because of shortage of sufficient number of qualified pharmacists and weak regulatory frameworks (Azhar et al., 2016). A greater proportion of pharmacists were unsatisfied with their participation in health awareness programs and not actively involved in patient care because of lack of time for patient counseling and poor relationship with other healthcare providers (Murtaza et al., 2015). One more study from Pakistan determined enough knowledge among pharmacists about DRPs and PC, but their active participation in reducing DRPs was little, because of lack of their acceptance by society and other healthcare professionals, lack of incentives, and occupied in managerial responsibility at retail pharmacy setups (Jamal et al., 2015). A nonclinical randomized controlled trial reported a notable increase in knowledge about hypertension and medication adherence level of Pakistani hypertensive patients with greater improvement in their HRQoL domains and blood pressure after the pharmacists-supervised intervention program (Saleem et al., 2015). Patient-centered care services to Nepali patients with CKD undergoing dialysis regarding CKD, their medications, diet, and lifestyle changes using information leaflet improved significantly their knowledge, attitude, and practice about disease management (Ghimirey et al., 2013). Additional studies from Nepal targeting newly diagnosed diabetics in a tertiary care teaching hospital reported a significant contribution of pharmacists-supervised intervention in minimizing direct healthcare cost to patients (Upadhyay et al., 2016) and at the same time improved their satisfaction level (Upadhyay et al., 2015). Another study highlighted the impact of patient-centered care services in improving knowledge and practice of inhaler technique among Nepali asthmatic patients and decreasing number of missing points leading better patient compliance and therapeutic outcome (Ansari et al., 2005). Similarly, Nepali hypertensive outpatients also improved their knowledge, attitude, and practice about disease management following pharmacist counseling in a tertiary care teaching hospital (Sushmita et al., 2010).

Although studies from developing countries documented the findings about the application of PC intervention at hospital and community pharmacy settings, pharmacists are still recognized as drug dispensers and their participation in patient care is only theoretical and practically nonexistent. Do pharmacists clearly understand the meaning of "pharmaceutical care" and able to differentiate with the concept of "clinical pharmacy"? Pharmacists in developing countries are not performing their duties in patient care because of the absence of well-defined policies at governmental and institutional levels leading to unsatisfactory PC practices and poor recognition by society and other healthcare professionals. There is an immense need of formulating new roles and responsibilities of pharmacists by healthcare policy makers at hospital and community settings, so that pharmacists can obtain professional recognition and contribute in patient care along with other healthcare professionals.

BARRIERS TO PHARMACEUTICAL CARE IMPLEMENTATION IN DEVELOPING COUNTRIES

The concept of PC is spreading over the pharmaceutical world in daily hospital and community PPs but its implementation is still in a dormant stage in developing countries. Barriers that obstruct the execution of PC in developing countries include the attitude of pharmacists, lack of pharmacists' advanced practice skills, lack of time, lack of resources, and lack of system-related constraints, as well as educational obstacles (Berenguer et al., 2004). A review article also highlighted an acute shortage of qualified pharmacists and no implementation of dispensing separation practices as major barriers for implementing PC in developing countries (Azhar et al., 2009).

In Argentina, a study reported the lack of time, lack of specific training, and lack of communication skills are perceived as barriers faced by pharmacists working in community pharmacies, hospitals, and primary care centers to implement effective PC services (Uema et al., 2008). Similarly, the lack of pharmacists and insufficient training of professionals encountered in implementing PC practice in Brazil were considered as some of the other barriers (de Castro & Correr, 2007). In addition, the positive attitude in implementing PC was shown among Nigerian pharmacists, but their knowledge, professional skills, and pharmacy layout were the main barriers highlighted (Oparah & Eferakeya, 2005).

Moreover, in Southwest Asia, the lack of time, lack of motivation, and lack of insufficient staffs were the major barriers to provide PC services by community pharmacists (Ghazal et al., 2014). Similarly, the lack of training in PC practice, lack of workplace for counseling, lack of staff, insufficient time, lack of patient demand, lack of therapeutic knowledge, and the lack of support from owners were main barriers reported by pharmacists (Al-Arifi et al., 2007). In Jordan, about 80% of the pharmacists reported the need for PC training (AbuRuz et al., 2012), whereas another study from the same country recognized lack of privacy and lack of proper educational skills as important barriers influencing PC practices (Ayoub et al., 2016). However, physicians' support toward pharmacists' role and patients' reluctance in receiving PC services were the main barriers reported from Iran (Mehralian et al., 2015).

In Southeast Asia, studies from Malaysia highlighted a shortage of community pharmacists, low pharmacists to population (1:6207) ratio, and lack of dispensing separation between doctors' clinics and pharmacies were the main hurdles in implementing effective PC in Malaysia (MOH, 2008; Sing, 2001). The pharmacy training in India focused more on the needs of pharmaceutical industry because of more demand of pharmacists in industrial sectors, leaving the PC implementation vulnerable in the lack of trained professionals (Goel et al., 1996). One survey in the Philippines addressed lack of physicians and other healthcare professional supports, whereas absence of information technology supports for data collection and documentation is also seen as an important barrier encountered in implementing PC interventions (Agaceta et al., 2013). Furthermore, shortage of time and skills, lack of information and economic incentive, and scarcity of full support from other healthcare professionals were also among the major hurdles influencing the PC practice in community pharmacies in China (Fang et al., 2011).

Studies from Northeast Africa revealed the lack of support from doctors, shortage of qualified support staff, lack of professional standards, insufficient specific training, lack of remuneration (Ibrahim & Scott, 2013), lack of pharmacists' clinical knowledge, and lack of understanding of pharmacists' new role (Mohamed et al., 2015) encountered to implementing PC practice were also among the factors.

It is concluded from the aforementioned studies that there is an immense need of developing professional relationships among healthcare professionals to achieve better patient-related outcomes. It is also required to give proper attention toward continuous pharmacy development programs and adopt suitable measures to overcome with different barriers encountered in implementing effective PC services in developing nations.

PHARMACEUTICAL CARE: CURRENT TRENDS AND CHALLENGES IN DEVELOPING COUNTRIES

In developing countries, the situation of PP is generally more product-oriented rather than patient-oriented (George et al., 2010). Pharmacists have much more to offer than what they have been providing traditionally (Hasan et al., 2012); the pharmacists' skill and knowledge in healthcare are not utilized to benefit their community. A systematic review on the quality of private pharmacy services in low- and middle-income countries concluded that the quality of professional services provided by the pharmacies are limited; however, local pharmacies played an important part in the provision of healthcare services for many people (Smith, 2009). The major challenges in the healthcare delivery system within these low- and middle-income countries included the lack of a trained health workforce and the issue of medicine supplied without a prescription. The author suggested that governments should regulate practice to promote higher standards or care, and the barriers to provision of higher quality of healthcare need to be identified and overcome (Smith, 2009).

Within the South Asia, in countries such as India and Nepal, pharmacists are trained more toward manufacturing of pharmaceuticals and limited pharmacists are involved in patient-oriented activities, especially outside healthcare institution in community setting (Azhar et al., 2009; Basak & Sathyanarayana, 2009). This is due to the high demand from the industrial sector and pharmacy curriculum in universities, which focus mainly on subjects related to the aspects of pharmaceutical production (Azhar et al., 2009). In Pakistan, the deficit of pharmacy services in hospital and community pharmacies was noticed because of isolation and lack of pharmacists' recognition as healthcare professionals by the public and other healthcare practitioners. The main reason for the lack of recognition of pharmacists was mainly due to the inadequate number of pharmacists in public health services and in community pharmacies, which lead to the absence of communication between pharmacists and other healthcare professionals and with the public. As such, pharmacists' roles are limited to drug delivery, procurement, and inventory control (Azhar et al., 2009).

In the Western Asia, findings reported that there was a lack of pharmaceutical services among the PP in the UAE (Hasan et al., 2011). Many professional healthcare services are not being offered and provided by majority of the pharmacies (Hasan et al., 2012). In the UAE, community pharmacists are generally regarded as "business person." Pharmacists were aware of the trend of patient-oriented practice, but the practice change has been slow because of barriers such as the lack of pharmacists' skills, resources, and time and low perception of the community toward the pharmacy profession; pharmacists are acknowledged as businesspeople rather than health professionals. Hasan et al. (2011) suggested that identifying factors and strategies that will bring improvement to the quality of community pharmacy services in the UAE is needed. In Saudi Arabia, community pharmacists are involved in patient counseling and providing basic drug information, such as appropriate drug usage, dosage, side effects, and so on, but they have a limited clinical role in the dispensing of medication (Al-Hassan, 2011). In addition, there was a lack in PC practice by community pharmacists in Saudi Arabia because of the concerns of community pharmacists toward their clinical knowledge, communication skills, and pharmacy layout (Al-Arifi et al., 2007). Literature suggests that community pharmacists should be trained professionally to meet the goals in promoting patient healthcare (Al-Hassan, 2011). Moreover, Alfreihi et al. (1987) reported the lack of adherence of community pharmacists to the regulations governing the dispensing of drugs. This was further supported by Bawazir, in which community pharmacists were found dispensing prescription drugs including antibiotics, cardiovascular drugs, and topical potent corticosteroids over the counter without a prescription. The studies suggested the need of strict enforcement on the regulations governing the sale of drugs and the need to introduce changes to present community PP (Bawazir, 1992).

In Malaysia, dispensing separation is not practiced, and the legal rights of private general practitioner to dispense medication in private clinics (MIDA, 2014) has limited the professional role of community pharmacists in PC delivery (Che Awang, 2008; Tarn, 2008). This has resulted in the fact that community pharmacists are generally being perceived by the community as a "sales person" or typical "assistant" providing advices on the medication (Anonymous, 2008), dispensing, and supplying a wide range of various health supplements and foods, organic products, homecare, personal hygiene products, and beauty products (Che Awang, 2008; Hassali et al., 2009; Sing, 2001). These pharmacists face challenges associated with acceptance or recognition of their professional services and the economics of providing PC (Hashim et al., 2001; Hassali et al., 2009). The phenomenon of "price war" among community pharmacies and between private clinics and community pharmacies has also brought negative impact to the profession (Hassali et al., 2010). Because of the absence of price control and regulations in Malaysia, this unhealthy business competition has been undercutting the price of pharmaceutical products and the focus of community pharmacists has been shifting from patient-oriented practice back to product-oriented to strive for survival (Hassali et al., 2010, 2013).

In Ghana, most of the community pharmacists are located in the cities leading to an unequal distribution of services across the country. Lack of enough numbers of pharmacists in many parts of the country has affected the quality of healthcare services (Smith, 2004). In South Africa, the uneven distribution of community pharmacies and pharmacists had limited their accessibility to the majority of the population. Most of the community pharmacists were located in more developed provinces, whereas very few were serving in the rural areas (Gilbert, 1998). There were only 619 pharmacists serving 2.9 million people in Africa because of serious shortage of pharmacists in the country (WHO recommendation 1:2000) (Azhar et al., 2009).

FUTURE OF PHARMACEUTICAL CARE IN DEVELOPING COUNTRIES

Despite all the mentioned challenges, a key challenge faced by the pharmacists in developing countries is whether they are ready for a change with respect to the change in PC services being provided or type of PP being delivered. Rosenthal et al. (2010) mentioned in a commentary that ultimately the traditional culture or mind-set of the pharmacists has to be renewed and changed. At present, development or further refinement, viz., benchmark, pharmacy premise benchmark, computerized pharmacy operation, appropriate and effective use of medicines, patient medication records, medicine prices control, and continuing professional development, is required (Chong et al., 2011). Efforts are much needed within the profession to understand the lack of advancement in PP.

As mentioned in the previous section, pharmacists in developing countries are facing challenges from economic and professional perspectives. The profession is at a crossroad and need to decide which path it takes to secure its future. The professional role remains to be fully defined or charted. By the introduction of PC, the roles of pharmacists have shifted toward a patient-oriented concept for achieving specific and positive patient outcomes by the provision of medicines (Hepler & Strand, 1990). Close working relationships between pharmacists and other healthcare professionals are crucial in the provision of PC (Azmi et al., 2012). Pharmacists cannot have a silo mentality. Do the physicians recognize the pharmacists' role in providing PC services and willing to give up their tasks related to medicines e.g., dispensing and counseling? Will the insurance companies recognize and accept to pay for the PC services provided by the pharmacists? A study in Eritrea reported that the physicians in Eritrea generally appreciated the role of pharmacists in patient care, supported the introduction of PC, and would accept pharmacists' recommendations about patients' medications (Awalom et al., 2013). Therefore, community pharmacists must ensure that they are well equipped and prepared in terms of updated knowledge by attending continuing professional education and willing to work with other healthcare practitioners as a team.

RECOMMENDATIONS: THE WAY FORWARD

The professional image and recognition of pharmacists as health professionals by the other healthcare professionals and public have to be improved. Pharmacy colleges should strategically plan for curriculum content that will provide the students with adequate and proper knowledge and skill when they join the pharmacy workforce. In addition, the colleges should also have faculty members who are trained, knowledgeable, and competent in the relevant areas. Pharmacists need to change their mind-set and consistently enhance their knowledge and skill. They are encouraged to take the initiative to collaborate and participate in interprofessional activities, programmes, or research, which involve the participation of various stakeholders. Pharmacists from all the division should have the ability to overcome all the barriers and to deliver quality PC to the patients.

CONCLUSIONS

PC implementation is a necessity today. Although developed countries have implemented it and been practicing it for years, gaps still exist. Even though the role of pharmacists in patient-centered care is needed and demanding, the findings and deliberations mentioned above indicated that there is still a long way to go. Developing countries face big challenges. They have several barriers, e.g., education, policy, regulation, practice, economic, technology, and sociobehavioral, which are not easy to tackle. On the other hand, pharmacists are required to implement GPPs and hence implementation of patient-centered care. They may seek technical assistance from global bodies such as WHO and FIP, who have been working on relevant models and have developed many strategies to deal with these barriers and provide services to the society.

LESSONS LEARNED

- The goal of PC is to improve effectiveness of the patients' HRQoL and promising clinical outcomes by reducing economic burden.
- The implementation of PC is essential and important for all the developing countries.
- In developing countries, pharmacists have much more to offer in terms of healthcare services than what they have been providing traditionally.
- Despite the barriers and challenges identified, the pharmacists in all developing countries have the responsibility to bring transformation to the healthcare system by the implementation of PC.
- Together with the pharmacists, all stakeholders in the country should play their role to meet the needs of the society and community in the primary healthcare system.

REFERENCES

AbuRuz, S., Al-Ghazawi, M., et al. (2012). Pharmaceutical care in a community-based practice setting in Jordan: Where are we now with our attitudes and perceived barriers? *International Journal of Pharmacy Practice*, *20*(2), 71–79.

ACCP. (2008). The definition of clinical pharmacy. *Pharmacotherapy*, *28*(6), 816–817.

Adibe, M. O., Ukwe, C. V., et al. (2013). The impact of pharmaceutical care intervention on the quality of life of nigerian patients receiving treatment for type 2 diabetes. *Value in Health Regional Issues*, *2*(2), 240–247.

Agaceta, C. C., Diano, G. T. L., et al. (2013). Current practices and perceptions on pharmaceutical care of hospital pharmacists in Metro Manila. *International Journal*, *4*(4), 821–825.

Aguwa, C. N., Ukwe, C. V., et al. (2008). Effect of pharmaceutical care programme on blood pressure and quality of life in a Nigerian pharmacy. *Pharmacy World & Science*, *30*(1), 107–110.

Al-Arifi, M. N., Al-Dhuwaili, A. A., et al. (2007). Pharmacists' understanding and attitudes towards pharmaceutical care in Saudi Arabia. *Saudi Pharmaceutical Journal*, *15*(2), 146.

Al-Eidan, F. A., McElnay, J. C., et al. (2000). Use of a treatment protocol in the management of community-acquired lower respiratory tract infection. *Journal of Antimicrobial Chemotherapy*, *45*(3), 387–394.

Al-Hassan, M. (2011). Community pharmacy practice in Saudi Arabia: An overview. *The Internet Journal of Pharmacology*, *9*(1).

Alfreihi, H., Ballal, S., et al. (1987). "Potential for drug misuse in the eastern province of Saudi Arabia.". *Annals of Saudi Medicine*, *7*(4), 301–305.

Anchah, L., Hassali, M. A., et al. (2017). Health related quality of life assessment in acute coronary syndrome patients: The effectiveness of early phase I cardiac rehabilitation. *Health and Quality of Life Outcomes*, *15*(1), 10.

Anonymous. (2008). *Dispensing role of pharmacists limited*. Retrieved from http://www.mps.org.my.2008.

Ansari, F., Gray, K., et al. (2003). Outcomes of an intervention to improve hospital antibiotic prescribing: Interrupted time series with segmented regression analysis. *Journal of Antimicrobial Chemotherapy*, *52*(5), 842–848.

Ansari, M., Rao, B., et al. (2005). Impact of pharmaceutical intervention on inhalation technique. *Kathmandu University Journal of Science, Engineering and Technology*, *1*(1).

APA. (1995). Principles of practice for pharmaceutical care. Retrieved from http://www.pharmacist.com/principles-practice-pharmaceutical-care] .

Arun, K., Murugan, R., et al. (2008). The impact of pharmaceutical care on the clinical outcome of diabetes mellitus among a rural patient population. *International Journal of Diabetes in Developing Countries*, *28*(1), 15.

ASHP. (1993). ASHP statement on pharmaceutical care. *American Journal of Hospital Pharmacy*, *50*, 1720–1723.

Aslani, P., Leucero, E., et al. (2012). *Counselling, concordance and communication: Innovative education for pharmacists* (2nd ed.). International Pharmaceutical Students' Federation (IPSF) and International Pharmaceutical Federation (FIP).

Avery, A. J., Rodgers, S., et al. (2012). A pharmacist-led information technology intervention for medication errors (PINCER): A multicentre, cluster randomised, controlled trial and cost-effectiveness analysis. *Lancet*, *379*(9823), 1310–1319.

Awalom, M. T., Kidane, M. E., et al. (2013). Physicians' views on the professional roles of pharmacists in patient care in Eritrea. *International Journal of Clinical Pharmacy*, *35*(5), 841–846.

Ayoub, N. M., Nuseir, K. Q., et al. (2016). Knowledge, attitudes and barriers towards breast cancer health education among community pharmacists. *Journal of Pharmaceutical Health Services Research*.

Azhar, S., Hassali, M. A., et al. (2009). The role of pharmacists in developing countries: The current scenario in Pakistan. *Human Resources for Health*, *7*(1), 1.

Azhar, S., Kousar, R., et al. (2016). Evolving scenario of pharmaceutical care in Pakistan and other countries: Health impact assessment in public health practice. *Acta Poloniae Pharmaceutica*, *73*, 1101.

Azmi, S., Nazri, N., et al. (2012). Extending the roles of community pharmacists: Views from general medical practitioners. *The Medical Journal of Malaysia*, *67*(6), 577–581.

Basak, S. C., & Sathyanarayana, D. (2009). Community pharmacy practice in India: Past, present and future. *South Med Rev*, *2*(1), 11–14.

Bawazir, S. (1992). Prescribing pattern at community pharmacies in Saudi Arabia. *International Pharmacy Journal*, *6*(5).

Berenguer, B., La Casa, C., et al. (2004). Pharmaceutical care: Past, present and future. *Current Pharmaceutical Design*, *10*(31), 3931–3946.

Boyko, W., Yurkowski, P. J., et al. (1997). Pharmacist influence on economic and morbidity outcomes in a tertiary care teaching hospital. *American Journal of Health-system Pharmacy*, *54*(14), 1591–1595.

Bronkhorst, E., Schellack, N., et al. (2014). The need for pharmaceutical care in an intensive care unit at a teaching hospital in South Africa. *Southern African Journal of Critical Care (Online)*, *30*(2), 41–44.

Charrois, T. L., Zolezzi, M., et al. (2012). A systematic review of the evidence for pharmacist care of patients with dyslipidemia. *Pharmacotherapy: The Journal of Human Pharmacology and Drug Therapy*, *32*(3), 222–233.

Che Awang, M. Z. (2008). *Pilot study is the best prescription*. The Star Online, Retrieved from http://www.mps.org.my/newsmaster.cfm?&menuid=37&action=view&retrieveid=2785.

Chisholm-Burns, M. A., Lee, J. K., et al. (2010). US pharmacists' effect as team members on patient care: Systematic review and meta-analyses. *Medical Care*, *48*(10), 923–933.

Chong, C. P., Hassali, M. A., et al. (2011). Generic medicine substitution practices among community pharmacists: A nationwide study from Malaysia. *Journal of Public Health*, *19*(1), 81–90.

Chua, S. S., Kok, L. C., et al. (2012). Pharmaceutical care issues identified by pharmacists in patients with diabetes, hypertension or hyperlipidaemia in primary care settings. *BMC Health Services Research*, *12*(1), 388.

Chung, W. W., Chua, S. S., et al. (2014). Effects of a pharmaceutical care model on medication adherence and glycemic control of people with type 2 diabetes. *Patient Preference and Adherence*, *8*, 1185.

Cipolle, R. J., Strand, L. M., et al. (2004). *Pharmaceutical care practice: The clinician's guide*. New York: McGraw-Hill.

Cousins, D., Kijlstra, N., et al. (2012). *Pharmaceutical Care: Policies and practices for a safer, more responsible and cost-effective health system*. Strasbourg: European Directorate for the Quality of Medicine and Healthcare (EDQM), 2012–2016. 62 pp.

de Castro, M. S., & Correr, C. J. (2007). Pharmaceutical care in community pharmacies: Practice and research in Brazil. *Annals of Pharmacotherapy*, *41*(9), 1486–1493.

de Castro, M. S., Fuchs, F. D., et al. (2006). Pharmaceutical care program for patients with uncontrolled hypertension* report of a double-blind clinical trial with ambulatory blood pressure monitoring. *American Journal of Hypertension*, *19*(5), 528–533.

de Souza Cazarim, M., de Freitas, O., et al. (2016). Impact assessment of pharmaceutical care in the management of hypertension and coronary risk factors after sischarge. *PLoS One*, *11*(6), e0155204.

Fang, Y., Yang, S., et al. (2011). Pharmacists' perception of pharmaceutical care in community pharmacy: A questionnaire survey in Northwest China. *Health & Social Care in the Community*, *19*(2), 189–197.

Farris, K. B., Fernandez-Llimos, F., et al. (2005). Pharmaceutical care in community pharmacies: Practice and research from around the world. *Annals of Pharmacotherapy*, *39*(9), 1539–1541.

FIP, & WHO. (2011). *WHO guidelines on good pharmacy practice: Standards for quality of pharmacy services*. WHO Technical Report Series (961).

Franklin, B. D., & Van Mil, J. (2005). Defining clinical pharmacy and pharmaceutical care. *International Journal of Clinical Pharmacy*, *27*(3), 137.

Gall, D., Bates, I., et al. (2012). *FIP global pharmacy workforce report 2012*.

George, P. P., Molina, J., et al. (2010). The evolving role of the community pharmacist in chronic disease management-a literature review. *Annals of the Academy of Medicine, Singapore.*, *39*(11), 861–867.

Ghazal, R., Hassan, N. A. G., et al. (2014). Barriers to the implementation of Pharmaceutical Care into the UAE community pharmacies. *IOSR Journal of Pharmacy*, *4*, 68–74.

Ghimirey, A., Sapkota, B., et al. (2013). Evaluation of pharmacist counseling in improving knowledge, attitude, and practice in chronic kidney disease patients. *SAGE Open Medicine*, *1*. http://dx.doi.org/10.1177/2050312113516111.

Gilbert, L. (1998). Community pharmacy in South Africa: A changing profession in a society in transition. *Health & Place*, *4*(3), 273–285.

Goel, P., Ross-Degnan, D., et al. (1996). Retail pharmacies in developing countries: A behavior and intervention framework. *Social Science & Medicine*, *42*(8), 1155–1161.

Hasan, S., Sulieman, H., et al. (2011). Community pharmacy in the United Arab Emirates: Characteristics and workforce issues. *International Journal of Pharmacy Practice*, *19*(6), 392–399.

Hasan, S., Sulieman, H., et al. (2012). Community pharmacy services in the United Arab Emirates. *International Journal of Pharmacy Practice*, *20*(4), 218–225.

Hashim, H., Mahmud, A., et al. (2001). Public awareness of community pharmacy and pharmacist. *Malaysian Journal of Pharmacy*, *1*(1), 22–28.

Hassali, M., Awaisu, A., et al. (2009). Professional training and roles of community pharmacists in Malaysia: Views from general medical practitioners. *Malaysian Family Physician*, *4*(2 & 3), 6.

Hassali, M., Shafie, A., et al. (2010). A qualitative study exploring the impact of the pharmaceutical price war among community pharmacies in the state of Penang, Malaysia. *Journal of Clinical and Diagnostic Research*, *4*(5), 3161–3169.

Hassali, M. A., Siang, T. C., et al. (2013). A qualitative exploration of perceptions toward pharmaceutical price war among community pharmacists in the state of Penang, Malaysia. *Journal of Medical Marketing*, *13*(1), 44–53.

Haub, C. (2012). *Fact sheet: World population trends 2012*. Retrieved from http://www.prb.org/publications/Datasheets/2012/world-population-data-sheet/fact-sheet-world-population.aspx].

Hepler, C. D., & Strand, L. M. (1990). Opportunities and responsibilities in pharmaceutical care. *American Journal of Hospital Pharmacy*, *47*(3), 533–543.

Hogerzeil, H. V. (1995). Promoting rational prescribing: An international perspective. *British Journal of Clinical Pharmacology*, *39*(1), 1–6.

Hudson, S. A., Mc Anaw, J. J., et al. (2007). The changing roles of pharmacists in society. *International e-Journal of Science, Medicine and Education*, *1*(1), 22–34.

Ibrahim, M. I. M., Fathelrahman, A. I., & Wertheimer, A. I. (2016). Comparative analysis and conclusion. In A. I. Fathelrahman, M. I. M. Ibrahim, & A. I. Wertheimer (Eds.), *Pharmacy practice in developing countries: Achievements and challenges*. Massachusetts: Academic Press.

Ibrahim, A., & Scott, J. (2013). Community pharmacists in Khartoum state, Sudan: Their current roles and perspectives on pharmaceutical care implementation. *International Journal of Clinical Pharmacy*, *35*(2), 236–243.

Jamal, I., Amin, F., et al. (2015). Pharmacist's interventions in reducing the incidences of drug related problems in any practice setting. *International Current Pharmaceutical Journal*, *4*(2), 347–352.

Junior, L., Marcellini, P. S., et al. (2008). Effect of pharmaceutical care intervention on blood pressure of elderly outpatients with hypertension. *Revista Brasileira de Ciências Farmacêuticas*, *44*(3), 451–457.

Kaboli, P. J., Hoth, A. B., et al. (2006). Clinical pharmacists and inpatient medical care: A systematic review. *Archives of Internal Medicine*, *166*(9), 955–964.

Kannan, G., Janardhan, V., et al. (2011). Pharmaceutical care in the general medicine ward of a tertiary care hospital in South India. *Journal of Pharmacy Research*, *4*(5), 1467–1469.

Lai, P., Chua, S., et al. (2012). Pharmaceutical care issues encountered by post-menopausal osteoporotic women prescribed bisphosphonates. *Journal of Clinical Pharmacy and Therapeutics*, *37*(5), 536–543.

Lyra, D. P., Rocha, C. E., et al. (2007). Influence of Pharmaceutical Care intervention and communication skills on the improvement of pharmacotherapeutic outcomes with elderly Brazilian outpatients. *Patient Education and Counseling*, *68*(2), 186–192.

Manan, W. Z. W., Wei, F. C., et al. (2016). Pharmaceutical care to improve medication knowledge among patient with chronic kidney disease. *Journal of Pharmacy & Bioallied Sciences*, *8*(3), 263.

Mehralian, G., Rangchian, M., et al. (2015). Pharmaceutical care in a community-based practice setting in Iran: Current status and future challenges. *Journal of Pharmaceutical Health Services Research*, *6*(1), 69–75.

MIDA. (2014). *Official Website of Malaysian investment development authority (MIDA)*. Retrieved from http://www.mida.gov.my/env3/index.php?page=pharmaceuticals.

Mikeal, R. L., Brown, T. R., et al. (1975). Quality of pharmaceutical care in hospitals. *American Journal of Health-system Pharmacy*, *32*(6), 567–574.

MOH. (2008). *Malaysian health statistic: Number of pharmacist and ratio Che Awang*. https://micpohling.wordpress.com/2008/03/08/malaysia-health-statistic-number-of-pharmacist-and-ratio/.

Mohamed, S. S., Mahmoud, A. A., et al. (2015). Sudanese community pharmacy practice and its readiness for change to patient care. *International Journal of Pharmacy Practice*, *23*(4), 266–273.

Movva, R., Jampani, A., et al. (2015). A prospective study of incidence of medication-related problems in general medicine ward of a tertiary care hospital. *Journal of Advanced Pharmaceutical Technology & Research*, *6*(4), 190.

Murtaza, G., Kousar, R., et al. (2015). What do the hospital pharmacists think about the quality of pharmaceutical care services in a Pakistani province? A mixed methodology study. *Biomed Research International*.

Nkansah, N., Mostovetsky, O., et al. (2010). Effect of outpatient pharmacists' non-dispensing roles on patient outcomes and prescribing patterns. *The Cochrane Database of Systematic Reviews [Electronic Resource]*, *7*(7).

Nwaozuzu, E., Okonta, J., et al. (2013). Impact of pharmaceutical care interventions on the occurrence and resolution of drug therapy problems in antiretroviral drug therapy. *International Journal of Development and Sustainability*, *2*(1), 415–429.

Obreli-Neto, P. R., Guidoni, C. M., et al. (2011). Effect of a 36-month pharmaceutical care program on pharmacotherapy adherence in elderly diabetic and hypertensive patients. *International Journal of Clinical Pharmacy*, *33*(4), 642–649.

Oparah, A. C., Adje, D. U., et al. (2006). Outcomes of pharmaceutical care intervention to hypertensive patients in a Nigerian community pharmacy. *International Journal of Pharmacy Practice*, *14*(2), 115–122.

Oparah, A. C., & Eferakeya, A. E. (2005). Attitudes of Nigerian pharmacists towards pharmaceutical care. *Pharmacy World and Science*, *27*(3), 208–214.

Palaian, S., Chhetri, A. K., et al. (2005). Role of pharmacist in counseling diabetes patients. *The Internet Journal of Pharmacology*, *4*. http://dx.doi.org/10.5580/105.

Peterson, G., Tenni, P., et al. (2009). *Documenting clinical interventions in community pharmacy: PROMISe III*. Canberra: Department of Health and Ageing.

Rosenthal, M., Austin, Z., et al. (2010). Are pharmacists the ultimate barrier to pharmacy practice change? *Canadian Pharmacists Journal/Revue des Pharmaciens du Canada*, *143*(1), 37–42.

Sadik, A., Yousif, M., et al. (2005). Pharmaceutical care of patients with heart failure. *British Journal of Clinical Pharmacology*, *60*(2), 183–193.

Saleem, F., Hassali, M. A., et al. (2015). Pharmacist intervention in improving hypertension-related knowledge, treatment medication adherence and health-related quality of life: A non-clinical randomized controlled trial. *Health Expectations*, *18*(5), 1270–1281.

Sing, W. S. (2001). Pharmacy practice in Malaysia. *Malaysian Journal of Pharmacy*, *1*(1), 3–9.

Smith, F. (2004). Community pharmacy in Ghana: Enhancing the contribution to primary health care. *Health Policy and Planning*, *19*(4), 234–241.

Smith, F. (2009). The quality of private pharmacy services in low and middle-income countries: A systematic review. *Pharmacy World & Science*, *31*(3), 351–361.

Sriram, S., Chack, L. E., et al. (2011). Impact of pharmaceutical care on quality of life in patients with type 2 diabetes mellitus. *Journal of Research in Medical Sciences*, *16*.

Sulaiman, S., Victor, S., et al. (2012). Applicability of pharmaceutical care in endocrine clinic of hospital Penang, Malaysia. *Journal of Diabetes Research and Clinical Metabolism*, *1*(1), 11.

Sushmita, S., Aarati, K., et al. (2010). Knowledge, attitude and practice outcomes: An effect of pharmacist provided counselling in hypertensive patients in a tertiary care teaching hospital in Western Nepal. *International Journal of Pharmaceutical Sciences*, *2* (2), 583–587.

Tarn, Y.-H., Hu, S., et al. (2008). Health-care systems and pharmacoeconomic research in Asia-Pacific region. *Value in Health: the Journal of the International Society for Pharmacoeconomics and Outcomes Research*, *11*, S137–S155.

Uema, S. A., Vega, E. M., et al. (2008). Barriers to pharmaceutical care in Argentina. *Pharmacy World & Science*, *30*(3), 211–215.

Upadhyay, D. K., Ibrahim, M. I. M., et al. (2015). A non-clinical randomised controlled trial to assess the impact of pharmaceutical care intervention on satisfaction level of newly diagnosed diabetes mellitus patients in a tertiary care teaching hospital in Nepal. *BMC Health Services Research, 15*(1), 57.

Upadhyay, D. K., Ibrahim, M. I. M., et al. (2016). Does pharmacist-supervised intervention through pharmaceutical care program influence direct healthcare cost burden of newly diagnosed diabetics in a tertiary care teaching hospital in Nepal: A non-clinical randomised controlled trial approach. *DARU Journal of Pharmaceutical Sciences, 24*(1), 6.

Van Grootheest, A., & De Jong-van den Berg, L. (2005). The role of hospital and community pharmacists in pharmacovigilance. *Research in Social and Administrative Pharmacy, 1*(1), 126–133.

Wal, P., Wal, A., et al. (2013). Pharmacist involvement in the patient care improves outcome in hypertension patients. *Journal of Research in Pharmacy Practice, 2*(3), 123.

Wang, H.-Y., Chan, A. L., et al. (2008). Effects of pharmaceutical care intervention by clinical pharmacists in renal transplant clinics. *Transplantation Proceedings, 40*(7), 2319–2323.

WHO. (1985). *The rational use of drugs: Report of the conference of experts*. Geneva: World Health Organization.

WHO. (1987). *The rational use of drugs: Report of the conference of experts, Nairobi, 25–29 November 1985*. Geneva: World Health Organization.

WHO. (1996). *Good pharmacy practice (GPP) in community and hospital settings*. Geneva: World Health Organization.

WHO. (2001). Globalization, TRIPS and access to pharmaceuticals. *WHO Policy Perspective on Medicines* (3).

WHO. (2002). Promoting rational use of medicines: Core components. *WHO Policy Perspective on Medicines* (5).

WHO. (2004). Equitable access to essential medicines: A framework for collective action. *WHO Policy Perspective on Medicines* (8).

WHO. (2005). Containing antimicrobial resistance. *WHO Policy Perspective on Medicines* (10).

Wiedenmayer, K., Summers, R. S., et al. (2006). *Developing pharmacy practice: A focus on patient care: Handbook. Developing pharmacy practice: A focus on patient care: Handbook: X, 87-x, 87.*

Wishah, R. A., Al-Khawaldeh, O. A., et al. (2015). Impact of pharmaceutical care interventions on glycemic control and other health-related clinical outcomes in patients with type 2 diabetes: Randomized controlled trial. *Diabetes & Metabolic Syndrome: Clinical Research & Reviews, 9*(4), 271–276.

Zhao, P.-X., Wang, C., et al. (2012). Effect of clinical pharmacists pharmaceutical care intervention to control hypertensive outpatients in China. *African Journal of Pharmacy and Pharmacology, 6*(1), 48–56.

CHAPTER 20

POLITICS AND COMPETITION BETWEEN PROFESSIONS: FUTURE SCOPE OF PHARMACY PRACTICE

Yu Fang[1], **Kangkang Yan**[1,2]
[1]Xi'an Jiaotong University, Xi'an, China; [2]Xi'an No. 3 Hospital, Xi'an, China

CHAPTER OUTLINE

THE DEFINITION FOR PHARMACY PRACTICE

The meaning of pharmacy practice is explanation, evaluation, and enforcement of medical prescriptions; distribution of medicines; drug administration; review of drug treatment; drug or drug-related research; provision of patient counseling; provision of such acts or services requiring the provision of pharmacist care in all areas of the patient, such as optimizing patient safety and quality of services (Albanese et al., 2010). Pharmaceutical care is a pioneering concept for pharmacy practices that raised in the middle of 1970s. It requires all practitioners to assume responsibility for the outcome of the

Social and Administrative Aspects of Pharmacy in Low- and Middle-Income Countries. http://dx.doi.org/10.1016/B978-0-12-811228-1.00020-0

patients' medication and includes a variety of services that were provided by pharmacists (Hepler & Strand, 1990). The concept of pharmaceutical care also includes emotional commitment to patients who need the pharmacists' sympathy, care, and trust.

In some developing countries, pharmacists have partly assumed the responsibility of pharmaceutical care gradually. Pharmacists are now primarily working in community pharmacies, clinics, hospitals, home care organizations, and medical management organizations. Other units include pharmaceutical companies, research institutes, government agencies, academic research institutes, professional associations, and toxicological information centers.

THE CURRENT SITUATION OF PHARMACY PRACTICE IN DEVELOPING COUNTRIES

SCOPE OF CONTEMPORARY PHARMACY PRACTICE IN DEVELOPING COUNTRIES: ROLE, RESPONSIBILITY, AND FUNCTION OF PHARMACISTS

A few decades ago, the World Health Organization (WHO) has began to agreed that pharmacists can make a greater contribution to the provision of medical care and healthcare, which was particularly obvious in developing countries where the health resources were insufficient (WHO, 1996, 1988). Over the past two decades, the role of pharmacists in many parts of the world has shifted from drug-oriented services to patient-centered services (Anderson, 2005; Niquille, Lattmann, & Bugnon, 2010; Peterson and Kelly, 2004). Pharmacists' role now takes various forms in developing countries but mainly to promote the safe and rational use of drugs. Pharmacists are involved in drug production, regulation, quality assurance, licensing, operation, storage, information management, distribution, monitoring, patient education, etc.

The settings of pharmacy practice in developing countries mainly include community pharmacies, hospital pharmacies, pharmaceutical companies, and academic research institutes. In addition, it includes health services management, research institutes, international health organizations, and non-governmental organizations. At present, drug-centered work remains the main part of pharmacy practice, for example, dispensing drugs and devices, processing the prescription, preparing the production, and delivering the medication. However, more and more pharmacists come from back of the counter to provide pharmaceutical care for patients.

Pharmacies are available 24 h a day to facilitate access to medicines and services for most people, so patients do not have to make appointments with pharmacists. All of these make pharmacy play a very important role to help patients overcome common diseases. Self-medication of common diseases is becoming increasingly popular as more and more safe and effective medications are available from pharmacies without the need for doctor's guidance. Pharmacists have the professional knowledge of medicine, which can provide recommendations for the drug selection and rational use of medicines. Reasonable self-medication can timely relieve symptoms of disease, save time and costs, and reduce the pressure of social health resources shortage.

Medicine safety is another important issue for pharmacists in developing countries. Due to intense competition among drug manufacturing enterprise, medicines may be registered and marketed in many countries simultaneously. Therefore, adverse drug reactions (ADRs) may not always be readily identifiable and so cannot be systematically monitored. Pharmacovigilance is a structured process for monitoring and detecting ADRs in a given situation (WHO Policy Perspectives on Medicines, 2004).

Pharmacists have an important contribution to postmarketing surveillance. Once a pharmacist discovers a drug-related problem, the pharmacist should evaluate, analyze, follow up, and communicate to the health professional in the drug administration. Pharmacovigilance requires pharmacists to disseminate this drug safety information. In some cases, the drug may need to be recalled and withdrawn from the market, and this process requires the participation of pharmacists.

THE LIMITATION OF PHARMACY PRACTICE IN DEVELOPING COUNTRIES CURRENTLY

A study conducted by *Hasan* found that there are some barriers to pharmacy services, which include lack of time to provide services, lack of pharmacy staff, low acceptance of patients, lack of appropriate knowledge and skills of pharmacists, lack of financial incentives, physician underestimation of medical services, and legal and regulatory restrictions (Hasan et al., 2011, 2012). In developing countries, many pharmacists' academic qualifications are still relatively low. Pharmacists have more knowledge and ability in pharmaceutical chemistry, pharmaceutical analysis, and pharmaceutical and other pharmaceutical production-related rudiments but lack of clinical knowledge and experience. Therefore, pharmacists are unable to shift from drug-oriented pharmacy practice to patient-centered pharmacy practice. When the patients face medicine problems for self-medication, the drugstore pharmacists are unable to perform medication counseling fully. Many pharmacists have not received adequate college education; thus they do not have adequate knowledge and experience for drug counseling.

Pharmacists are often unable to assume the current level of responsibility for pharmacy care, although it is becoming the focus of pharmacy practice gradually and it is necessary for the pharmacists. As a result, they may not be able to adequately document, monitor, and review the public needs. In developing countries, due to lack of clinically relevant education and knowledge for pharmacists, pharmacists are not able to provide excellent pharmaceutical care for patients.

Furthermore, clinical pharmacists need specialized knowledge of therapies, a good understanding of the disease process, and also knowledge of medicine. In addition, clinical pharmacists need strong communication skills, drug monitoring skills, the ability to provide drug information, and the ability to evaluate and explain physical and laboratory results (Hepler, 2004). These capacities are lacking among the pharmacists in developing countries.

THE CURRENT POLITICS AND COMPETITION BETWEEN PROFESSIONS OF PHARMACY PRACTICE IN DEVELOPING COUNTRIES

At the World Health Assembly in 1994, WHO discussed elements related to the role of pharmacists in a revised drug strategy solution (World Health Organization, 1994). This resolution recognizes the pivotal role of the pharmacists in public healthcare team. It emphasizes the responsibility of pharmacists to provide professional and objective advice on medicines and to participate actively in the prevention of disease and health activities.

The healthcare team consists of patients and all the healthcare professionals responsible for the health of patients. The role of members of this team needs to be clearly defined. After physicians and nurses, pharmacists constitute the third largest group of health professionals. Moreover, professional pharmacy is responsible for educating, communicating, and exchanging information with patients and their family members, prescribers, and other healthcare professionals.

Pharmacists play an important role in the public healthcare team increasingly, especially in the developed countries. In 2007, there were approximately 253,000 pharmacist jobs in the United States, while the employment rate of pharmacists was expected to increase by 22% between 2006 and 2016, much faster than the average for all occupations (Bureau of Labor Statistics, 2008, 2016, pp. 29–1051). A Gallup's survey shows that the pharmacists are always the highest trust of the professionals in the United States (Jones, 2017). The availability and affordability of essential medicines continues to be a major problem in developing countries (Mendis et al., 2007). As a result, the role of pharmacists in counseling, prevention, and healthcare was still not the primary consideration for policy makers and other relevant stakeholders.

On the other hand, many developed countries, such as the United States, Japan, the United Kingdom, France, Germany, Sweden, Denmark, Switzerland, Italy, Spain, Canada, Australia, New Zealand, Singapore, Korea, and so on, have licensed pharmacists' laws, which regulate pharmacists' behavior and also ensure that the legal status of pharmacists (Fang et al., 2011). However, in many developing countries, the legislation of pharmacists is still very backward, which is in large part difficult to ensure the status of pharmacists in the professional competition. The rights, duties, and role of pharmacists are not clearly defined by the law. Some pharmaceutical practices cannot get the guarantee by law. For example, medication education and medication advice of pharmaceutical care have not been set out in the law. Pharmaceutical practice will bear the corresponding legal risks.

At present, therefore, clarifying the status of pharmacists and practice behavior by legislation is the top priority for many developing countries. The charges for pharmacists' service also need legal support.

In the healthcare field, it is expected and assumed that physicians, pharmacists, nurses, and others professionals make clinical decisions anchored in a strong ethical perspective. In addition, there is an increasing interest among healthcare professionals to optimize patient care by applying a teamwork approach.

The healthcare team consists of the patient and all the healthcare professionals who have responsibility for patient care. This team needs to be well defined, and collaboration needs to be actively sought. It is believed that pharmacists have an important role to play in this team. However, they will need to adapt their knowledge, skills, and attitudes to this new role, which integrates traditional pharmaceutical science knowledge with clinical aspects of patient care, namely, clinical, management, and communication skills, ability to actively collaborate with medical teams, and competence to prevent and resolve medicine-related problems.

It should be highlighted that the practice of pharmaceutical care does not exist and should not exist in isolation from other healthcare services. It must be provided in collaboration with patients, physicians, nurses, and other healthcare providers. The pharmaceutical care practitioner develops a partnership with the patient and other providers to ensure patients get the most benefit from all their medications. The roles of the physicians and pharmacists are complementary, and it has been established that the expertise of pharmacists when channeled through a cooperative relationship with physicians has a positive impact on patient outcomes (Nijjer, Gill, & Nijjer, 2008).

Insufficient communication between pharmacists and physicians occurs for several reasons. One barrier that has been cited is pharmacists expressed lack of confidence in their ability to persuade physicians to accept their recommendations. Another possible cause is ineffective or needless communication initiated by pharmacists, which makes physicians less willing to listen to pharmacists during future interactions. With communication so limited, physicians are unable to benefit from pharmacists' suggestion about drug therapy.

Pharmacists must demonstrate how important they are for patients in terms of improving their clinical outcomes and quality of life. We believe that this is the only way pharmacists will be able to gain the confidence of physicians, nurses, and the health system in general. It is the time for pharmacists to take the challenge that society has presented to them and organize their time to undertake clinical and cognitive functions, which means working directly with patients and other providers, delivering the best possible care, and documenting and evaluating the care provided. This is the only way to obtain social recognition and the identity of a healthcare provider (Niurka María Dupotey Varela et al., 2011).

SCOPE OF PHARMACY PRACTICE IN THE FUTURE

THE GAP BETWEEN EIGHT-STAR PHARMACISTS AND PHARMACISTS IN DEVELOPING COUNTRIES

The WHO has proposed the eight-star pharmacist model to describe various roles of pharmacists in providing better pharmaceutical care and decision-making. Considering this, if practiced under a well-trained pharmacy professional, there is a possibility of achieving a better impact in the healthcare system (Wiedenmayer et al., 2006). The eight-star pharmacists' elements are as follows.

Caregiver: Pharmacists provide patient care services. They must keep their pharmacy practice up-to-date with the highest quality healthcare professionals.

Decision-maker: Appropriate, efficient, safe, and cost-effective use of resources should be the basis for the work of pharmacists. Pharmacists play an important role in the formulation of drug policies at the local and national levels.

Communicator: Pharmacists are ideally placed to increase the links between physicians and patients and to communicate information about health and medicines to the public. They must also have the knowledge and confidence to interact with other health professionals and the public at the same time.

Manager: Pharmacists must be able to effectively manage resources and information and must also be managed by others, whether by the employer or by the manager/leader of the healthcare team.

Lifelong learner: It is not possible to obtain all the knowledge and experience required for a lifelong career as a pharmacist in the school of pharmacy. The concepts, principles, and commitments of lifelong learning must begin to emerge from the time they enter the school of pharmacy and must be supported throughout the pharmacists' career. Pharmacists should learn how to keep their knowledge and skills updated.

Teacher: Pharmacists are responsible for assisting the new generation of pharmacists and the public in their education and training. Participation as a teacher not only imparts knowledge to others but also provides opportunities for practitioners to acquire new knowledge and adapt existing skills.

Leader: In some areas where multidisciplinary care or other healthcare providers are in short supply, pharmacists should assume a leadership positions in the overall well-being of patients and communities. Leadership skills include compassion and empathy, effective decision-making, communicating, and managing effectively. The pharmacist with a recognized leadership role must have vision and leadership and other additional capabilities.
Researcher: Pharmacists should be able to use evidence effectively to advise on the rational use of drugs. Pharmacists can also contribute to the evidence base by sharing and documenting experiences to optimize patient care and outcomes. As a researcher, a pharmacist can provide to the public and other healthcare professionals with fair and unbiased health and drug-related information without personal preference.

There is still a big gap between the pharmacists in developing countries and the eight-star pharmacists. The field of pharmacy is a rapidly changing field, which will continue to introduce new information, new technologies, and new products. All health workers, including pharmacists, must constantly face new challenges that need to be filtered, absorbed, and used to improve their pharmaceutical practice. How to filter the information and get the accurate information is the barrier to become an eight-star pharmacist.

Keeping up-to-date scientific and professional knowledge may be the most important needs of a pharmacist throughout his or her career. As the pharmacists' role is more focused on pharmaceutical care, drug treatment outcomes and the management of individual patient medications also require greater involvement of pharmacists. Pharmacists are also faced with new opportunities in all areas of pharmacy practice and the volume of new drug information. If pharmacists want to keep up with the changing demands, continuing learning is essential for becoming an eight-star pharmacist. In developing countries, continuing learning is still strange for a pharmacist who wants to become an eight-star pharmacist. In addition, pharmacists are reluctant to move forward and grow. It is an effective means to help pharmacists continue to learn and become more professional in their workplace. Continuing learning, unlike continuing education, does not indicate the time to attend the lectures, courses, or Web education. The literature analysis shows that while education cannot change professional practice through individual lectures, intervention workshops can lead to improvements (Orien et al., 2001). Pharmacists are often unable to continue learning. After leaving the school, knowledge cannot be effectively updated, which has become a barrier for the pharmacists to become the eight-star pharmacists.

THE SCOPE OF PHARMACY PRACTICE IN THE FUTURE

Pharmacy practice will be carried out at different levels in the future. The ultimate goal of pharmaceutical activities is to maintain their health literacy through improving and benefit to patients. A well-placed pharmacist can meet the needs of professionals and ensure safe and effective drug usage. For this reason, the pharmacists must assume greater responsibility than the current management of the patients' medication, which will far exceed that of traditional medicines and this has long been a pillar of pharmacy practice. While the supervision of routine drug distribution in the future remains the responsibility of the pharmacists, their direct involvement in drug distribution will be reduced as these routine activities will be handled by qualified pharmaceutical assistants and automated dispensing equipment. Many hospitals have already equipped with fully automatic dispensing equipment. In China, hospitals must be equipped with automatic drug dispensing equipment because of the requirement for hospital accreditation (Rayes, Hassali, & Abduelkarem, 2015). The manual labor of the pharmacists will gradually be replaced by the machine. However, the number of monitoring activities will increase. Therefore, the responsibility of pharmacists will have to be expanded to include monitoring the progress of treatment, counseling prescribers, and working with other healthcare practitioners. In 2000, the UK Department of Health published a publication called "Pharmacy of the Future" (Silcock, Raynor, & Petty, 2004), which clarified the need for pharmacists to provide structured professional support to improve and expand the range of pharmacy services provided to patients, including meeting individual drug needs, developing partnerships in drug use, coordinating the repetition of prescribing and dispensing processes, and targeting therapeutic reviews. This approach may also provide a reference for the future development of pharmaceutical practice in developing countries.

The practice of pharmaceutical care may be a new concept for pharmacists in developing countries. Whether pharmacists are reviewing a prescription or documenting medications, talking to patients, or answering symptoms, they should automatically assess the need to prioritize and develop treatment plans to meet patients' needs. What they often fail to do is to accept responsibility for this care currently.

The practice of pharmaceutical care has made pharmacists more accountable for patients' medicine-related issues. In the future, the pharmacists should evaluate the patients' medication needs and then determine if there are one or more drug treatment problems and, if so, work with the patient and other health professionals to design, implement, and follow up a treatment plan. This plan can be designed with reference to the relevant guidelines but should be as simple as possible (Supplementary Prescribing by Nurses and Pharmacists within the NHS in England, 2003). The treatment plan for pharmacists will address the actual drug therapy problems and prevent potential drug treatment problems becoming reality. The pharmacists' primary role is clinical pharmacy practice, including working with the healthcare team, diagnosing patients, proposing specific drug recommendations, monitoring patient response to medication, and providing medication information. In the future, clinical pharmacies will be more and more important for the developing countries. The focus of pharmaceutical practice will change from dispensing drugs to pharmaceutical care and clinical pharmacy.

In the future, for the whole care system, pharmacist practice and involvement in patient-centered care will improve health outcomes, reduce medical-related adverse events, improve quality of life, and reduce morbidity and mortality (Berenguer, La, De la Matta, & Martin-Calero, 2004; Strand, Cipolle, Morley, & Frakes, 2004). These achievements will be gained through the gradual expansion of the role of traditional pharmacists. By influencing the health state of individual patients, pharmaceutical care enhances the quality and cost-effectiveness of the entire healthcare system.

In the future, pharmacy practice will include providing and managing all aspects of patients' drug therapy. At individual level, decisions will be made on issues of pharmaceutical classification. At the institutional level, such as hospitals, clinics, or managed healthcare institutions, pharmaceutical tools will be used for drug selection, including formulations, standard treatment guidelines, and drug use monitoring. These tools are generally developed by drug and therapeutics committees (Quick et al., 1997; World Health Organization, 2004a, 2004b) or national essential medicines committees. The development process will no longer be limited to the pharmacists, but to all levels of medical professionals, and gradually based on clinical evidence, rather than purely expert advice. These tools should be accepted by pharmacists and should be implemented in the future.

At the system level, for example, at national or district level, an enabling environment for the development of healthcare systems includes planning, management, legislation, regulations, and policies. And it also includes standards of practice and mandates for pharmacy which managed by system level depending on different countries. National medicines policies (World Health Organization, 2001) will become an important part of national health policies in many developing countries. At the international level, action will be taken to harmonize approaches around the world and this approach deserves more attention, given the global impact of the pharmaceutical industry and pharmacy practice.

At the level of community and population, pharmaceutical practice will include the activities that support the other levels (World Health Organization, 2004a, 2004b). Promoting health, preventing disease, and changing lifestyles are activities at the population level that will be the focus of public health. The focus of pharmacy practice will no longer be solely on drug-related issues. Pharmacists will provide public health services more easily than other healthcare members because they are easily supported and recognized as health professionals, and they will become experts who can provide trusted health and drug information and advice. However, they cannot work independently and must share responsibility with other health professionals to serve public health.

THE POLITICS AND COMPETITION BETWEEN PROFESSIONS OF PHARMACY PRACTICE IN THE FUTURE

As a medical expert, a pharmacist has long been considered a counselor who can provide credible advice and treatment advice. Today, they are making new contributions to healthcare to guide patients in rational use of medicines and support clinical decision-making in their areas of expertise. They also can provide special skill and service, such as pharmacokinetic dosing and monitoring. Clinical pharmacists are often active members of the medical team and are involved with the physician in the rounds to facilitate the discussion of clinical treatment decisions.

They should apply their knowledge and skills to this new role, combining traditional pharmacy sciences with clinical patient care, clinical skills, and management and communication skills, actively collaborating with medical teams and solving medical-related problems. To become a highly effective healthcare team member, pharmacists need to master high skills and attitudes to enable them to take on many different functions. While change may pose a potential threat, it can also bring great opportunities. Pharmaceutical professions have a responsibility to identify new opportunities for pharmacy practice in the context of changing health sectors and to assess and test these opportunities to demonstrate their ability.

At the same time, the pharmacist law in all countries (both developed and developing countries) will be able to develop and to ensure the basic rights of the pharmacists in the industry competition.

HOW TO EXPAND THE SCOPE OF PHARMACY PRACTICE IN DEVELOPING COUNTRIES

The essential element of all healthcare services and pharmacy practice is ensuring the quality of the patient care process. The quality of pharmacy practice cannot be guaranteed in many developing countries. The deficiency of pharmacist education is the most important problem.

Drug shortage was always very rampant for many developing countries. To ensure adequate supply of drugs, the main responsibility of pharmacists is recognized as production and supply of drugs by government. Courses for pharmacy education are mainly pharmaceutical chemistry, pharmaceutical analysis, pharmacology, and other courses-related drug production. At the school stage, the pharmacy students are rarely able to accept the clinical knowledge. Therefore, the quality of pharmaceutical care will be inadequate. This is the era of great changes in the field of healthcare and pharmacy. In the recent history, this profession at any time did not face with such challenges and opportunities. While pharmacists will make a major contribution to future social development, pharmacy education will need to develop the outcomes, capabilities, content, and processes of educational curricula that prepare students for the healthcare systems needed for drug care at the time of enrollment.

Improving the education of pharmacists in developing countries not only can improve the pharmacy practice but also can help pharmacists in competing with the other professions. The pharmacist stands between the patient and the medicine itself. WHO has called on pharmacists to become more involved in the regular health system and to make more extensive use of their professional backgrounds to serve patients. The International Pharmaceutical Federation (FIP) announced that the changes in the role of the pharmacist must be reflected in the basic pharmacists' foundation and continuing education (Austin et al., 2005), with a greater focus on student course. The future model of pharmacy requires more than pharmacists' expertise in pharmaceutical chemistry and production. They have to understand and apply the principles behind all the activities, which are necessary to manage drug therapy. More clinical knowledge, communication skills, and humanistic knowledge need to be mastered by pharmacists in developing countries.

In 1999, the European Association of Faculties of Pharmacy has proposed a shift from laboratory-based science to practice-based and clinical-based science in pharmacy research programs (Van Mil, Schulz, & Tromp, 2004). In some developed countries, such as the United Kingdom and the United States, the patient care approaches have evolved to varying degrees (Anton Calis et al., 2004; Bradley, 1992; Chiquette, Amato, & Bussey, 2000; Nemire & Meyer, 2006). The change of pharmacy curriculum structure is an important method to improve the quality of pharmacy practices.

The educational change will require not only the revision and reorganization of the curriculum but also a major commitment to faculty development to prepare teachers so that teachers can teach pharmacists in different methods. The type and depth of teaching experience and materials will be different. The School of Pharmacy should establish and evaluate models of pharmacy practice that can be used in continuous development (Tromp, 1999). The introduction of the course should take into account the needs of the target audience, learning outcomes, course content, teaching methods, learning resources, participant evaluation, curriculum assessment, and quality assurance (Wuliji & Airaksinen, 2005). Pharmacist qualification access is too easy in developing countries. Many people who have not got a higher education can qualify for a pharmacist. The quality of the pharmacist is not high enough to provide good pharmacy practice. Improving the access threshold of pharmacists is a way to improve the pharmacy practice quality. In the United States, many schools of pharmacy have introduced the corresponding courses and require all pharmacology students to study clinical pharmacy, which is a PhD in clinical pharmacy.

Pharmacists should get enough financial compensation to ensure that they can move toward good pharmacy practice, especially for pharmaceutical care. But pharmaceutical care in many developing countries is free of charge. However, ensuring that the pharmacists have adequately compensated will require an effective record of what the pharmacist actually did to improve the outcome of the treatment, as well as the recipients who believe that what they do has economic value.

ACHIEVEMENTS

Pharmacy practice in developing countries has played a significant role in the past and present in ensuring the quality of pharmaceuticals in the production, circulation, and supply chain. Pharmacy practice is working to shift from product-centered pharmacy practices to patient-centered pharmacy services, which will enable pharmacy practice makes a greater contribution in the future.

CHALLENGES

In developing countries, demand for pharmacy practice is not limited to the supply of drugs and has become increasingly biased patient-centered pharmaceutical care, for example, medication consultation and therapeutic drug monitoring. However, there is a big gap between the ability of the pharmacist and the requirements of the patient, which is mainly reflected in the gap between pharmacists in developing countries and eight-star pharmacists. How to narrow this gap and meet the needs of patients is a major challenge in the current practice of pharmacy in developing countries.

RECOMMENDATIONS: THE WAY FORWARD

The ways to narrow the gap between the pharmacists in developing countries and eight-star pharmacists and to meet the needs of patients may mainly include change the structure of pharmacy education, increase the knowledge related to clinical pharmacy, raise the access threshold of pharmacists, protect the rights of pharmacists, and clarify the obligations of pharmacists by legislation.

CONCLUSIONS

In developing countries, although pharmaceutical practice is moving from a drug-centered profession to a patient-centered pharmaceutical care model, the pharmacists still have a very big development space, according to the "eight-star pharmacist" standards. There are many reasons for this discrepancy. Pharmacy education that mainly confined to the knowledge about pharmaceutical production of the chemical synthesis and no financial incentives toward pharmaceutical practice may be the important reasons. The most important way to reverse this situation is to change the way and content of pharmacy education, such as increase the training opportunities in clinical pharmacy–related knowledge, raise the access threshold of pharmacists to enhance the overall quality of pharmacists, improve the relevant laws of the pharmaceutical practice to protect the rights of pharmacists, and clarify the obligations of pharmacists.

LESSONS LEARNED

- In developing countries, the content of pharmacy education should be more involved in clinical pharmacy–related knowledge, rather than confined to pharmaceutical production-related chemical knowledge.
- The threshold of access to pharmacists cannot be reduced, which ensures that only those who have received higher education can take part in pharmacy title examination and eventually become a pharmacist.
- The evolution of pharmacy practice offers pharmacists many new opportunities for performing functions and providing services that are not considered traditional roles.
- The pharmacy profession is striving to achieve universal patterns and standards of care to meet the needs of patients and populations.
- The imperfection of the legal system of pharmaceuticals is a common problem in many developing countries. Therefore, the state should protect the rights of pharmacists and clarify the obligations of pharmacists through legislation.

REFERENCES

Albanese, N. P., Rouse, M. J., Schlaifer, M., et al. (2010). Scope of contemporary pharmacy practice: Roles, responsibilities, and functions of pharmacists and pharmacy technicians. *Journal of the American Pharmacists Association*, *50*(2), 35–69.

Anderson, S. (2005). *Making medicine: A brief history of pharmacyand pharmaceuticals*. London, UK: Pharmaceutical Press London.

Anton Calis, K., Elliott, M. E., Poirier, T., et al. (2004). Healthy people 2010: Challenges, opportunities, and a call to action for America's pharmacists. *Pharmacotherapy*, *24*(9), 1241–1294.

Austin, Z., Marini, A., Glover, N. M., et al. (2005). Continuous professional development: A qualitative study of pharmacists' attitudes, behaviors, and preferences in Ontario, Canada. *American Journal of Pharmaceutical Education*, *69*(1–5), 25.

Berenguer, B., La, C. C., De la Matta, M. J., & Martin-Calero, M. J. (2004). Pharmaceutical care: Past, present and future. *Current Pharmaceutical Design*, *10*(31), 3931–3946.

Bradley, V. (1992). Healthy America: Practitioners for 2005. *Journal of Emergency Nursing Jen Official Publication of the Emergency Department Nurses Association*, *18*(5), 365–367.

Bureau of Labor Statistics. (2008). *U.S. Department of Labor: Occupational outlook handbook*. 2008–09 edition http://liberty.state.nj.us/health/surv/documents/cfoi98.pdf.

Bureau of Labor Statistics. (2016). *Occupational employment statistics*. Pharmacists. https://www.bls.gov/oes/tables.htm.

Chiquette, E., Amato, M. G., & Bussey, H. I. (2000). ACCP white paper a vision of Pharmacy's future roles, responsibilities, and manpower needs in the United States. *Pharmacotherapy*, *20*(8), 991–1020.

Fang, Y., Yang, S. M., Feng, B. L., et al. (2011). Pharmacists' perception of pharmaceutical care in community pharmacy: A questionnaire survey in Northwest China. *Health and Social Care in the Community*, *19*(2), 189–197.

Hasan, S., Sulieman, H., Chapman, C., et al. (2011). Community pharmacy in the United Arab Emirates: Characteristics and workforce issues. *International Journal of Pharmacy Practice*, *19*(6), 392–399.

Hasan, S., Sulieman, H., Chapman, C. B., et al. (2012). Community pharmacy services in the United Arab Emirates. *International Journal of Pharmacy Practice*, *20*(4), 218–225.

Hepler, C. D. (2004). Clinical pharmacy, pharmaceutical care, and the quality of drug therapy. *Pharmacotherapy, 24*(11), 1491–1498.

Hepler, C. D., & Strand, L. M. (1990). Opportunities and responsibilities in pharmaceutical care. *American Journal of Pharmaceutical Education, 47*(3), 533–543.

Jones, J. M. (2017). *Lobbyists Debut at Bottom of Honesty and Ethics list; Gallup.* http://www.highbeam.com/doc/1G1-185510755.html.

Mendis, S., Fukino, K., Cameron, A., et al. (2007). The availability and affordability of selected essential medicines for chronic diseases in six low- and middle-income countries. *Bulletin of the World Health Organization, 85*(4), 279–288.

Nemire, R. E., & Meyer, S. M. (2006). Educating students for practice: Educational outcomes and community experience. *American Journal of Pharmaceutical Education, 70*(1), S1.

Nijjer, S., Gill, J., & Nijjer, S. (2008). Effective collaboration between doctors and pharmacists. *Hospital Pharmacist, 15*, 179–182.

Niquille, A., Lattmann, C., & Bugnon, O. (2010). Medication reviews led by community pharmacists in Switzerland: A qualitative survey to evaluate barriers and facilitators. *Pharmacy Practice, 8*(1), 35–42.

Niurka María Dupotey Varela, Djenane Ramalho de Oliveira, Caridad Sedeño Argilagos., et al. (2011). What is the role of the pharmacist? Physicians' and nurses' perspectives in community and hospital settings of Santiago de Cuba. *Brazilian Journal of Pharmaceutical Sciences, 47*(4), 709–718.

Orien, T., Freemantle, N., Oxman, A. D., et al. (2001). .Continuing education meetings and workshops: Effects on professional practice and health care outcomes (Cochrane review). *Cochrane DatabaseSystematic Reviews, 2*, CD003030.

Peterson, A. M., & Kelly, W. N. (Eds.). (2004). *Managing pharmacy practice: Principles, strategies, and systems.* CRC Press.

Quick, J. D., Rankin, J. R., Laing, R. O., et al. (1997). *Managing drug supply* (2nd ed.). Hartford, CT, USA: Kumarian Press.

Rayes, I. K., Hassali, M. A., & Abduelkarem, A. R. (2015). The role of pharmacists in developing countries: The current scenario in the United Arab Emirates. *Saudi Pharmaceutical Journal, 23*(5), 470–474.

Silcock, J., Raynor, D. K. T., & Petty, D. (2004). The organisation and development of primary care pharmacy in the United Kingdom. *Health Policy, 67*(2), 207–214.

Strand, L. M., Cipolle, R. J., Morley, P. C., & Frakes, M. J. (2004). The impact of pharmaceutical care practice on the practitioner and the patient in the ambulatory practice setting: Twenty-five years of experience. *Current Pharmaceutical Design, 10*(31), 3987–4001.

Supplementary Prescribing by Nurses, Pharmacists within the NHS in England. (2003). *A guide for implementation.* London: Department of Health. Available at http://www.doh.gov.uk/supplementaryprescribing/implementation.

Tromp, T. F. J. (1999). *Report of the Task Force for implementing pharmaceutical care into the curriculum.* European Association of Faculties of Pharmacy.

Van Mil, J. W., Schulz, M., & Tromp, T. F. (2004). Pharmaceutical care, European developments in concepts, implementation, teaching, and research: A review. *Pharmacy World &Science, 26*(6), 303–311.

WHO Policy Perspectives on Medicines. (2004). *Pharmacovigilance: Ensuring the safe use of medicines.* Available at http://www.who.int/medicines/.

WHO. (1988). *The role of the pharmacist in the health care system.Geneva.* World Health Organization.

WHO. (1996). *Good pharmacy practice: Guidelines in community andhospital pharmacy settings.* Geneva: World Health Organization.

Wiedenmayer, K., Summers, R. S., Mackie, C. A., Gous, A. G. S., Everard, M., Tromp, D., World Health Organization, & International Pharmaceutical Federation (2006). *Developing pharmacy practice: A focus on patient care: Handbook.*

World Health Organization. (1994). Role of the pharmacist in support of the WHO revised drug strategy. *In Executive Board Session, 93*(14).

World Health Organization. (2004a). *A practical guide. Drug and therapeutics committees.* Available at http://www.who.int/medicines/.

World Health Organization. (2004b). *How to investigate the use of medicines by consumers.* Available at http://www.who.int/medicines/.

World HealthOrganization. (2001). *How to develop and implement a national drug policy.* Available at http://www.who.int/medicines/.

Wuliji, T., & Airaksinen, M. (2005). *Counselling, concordance and communication innovative education for pharmacists.* International Pharmaceutical Students' Federation and International Pharmaceutical Federation.

SECTION

8

MEDICINE QUALITY: SUBSTANDARD AND COUNTERFEIT MEDICINE IN LOW- AND MIDDLE-INCOME COUNTRIES

CHAPTER

21 PERSPECTIVE, KNOWLEDGE, ATTITUDE, AND BELIEF OF VARIOUS STAKEHOLDERS ON MEDICINES QUALITY: COUNTERFEIT AND SUBSTANDARD MEDICINES

Abubakr A. Alfadl

Qassim University, Unaizah, Kingdom of Saudi Arabia

CHAPTER OUTLINE

INTRODUCTION

Provision of affordable, effective, and high-quality drugs is particularly a difficult task (Milovanovic, Pavlovic, Folic, & Jankovic, 2004). This task is more difficult in developing countries where the pharmaceutical market has experienced significant vulnerability to substandard and counterfeit drugs. However, in tackling this problem of high prevalence of substandard and counterfeit drugs in developing countries' markets, the supply side of the problem has received high attention, while very little is

Social and Administrative Aspects of Pharmacy in Low- and Middle-Income Countries. http://dx.doi.org/10.1016/B978-0-12-811228-1.00021-2

known about the demand side, although it is reported in the literature that problem of counterfeiting is "fuelled by consumer demand" (International Anticounterfeiting Coalition, 2012). This is also supported by another study, which concluded that governments and businesses must put more effort to eliminate the demand side of the problem of substandard and counterfeit. Even, the study went further to emphasize that money spent to stop or reduce demand for counterfeit will most likely be wasted without more research be conducted to specify the best way to approach consumers and best appeal that could be used to convince them not to purchase counterfeits (Bloch, Bush, & Campbell, 1993). May be that is why, although the WHO and governments in developing countries are making a lot of efforts to combat substandard and counterfeit drugs at both the manufacturing and distribution levels, substandard and counterfeit drugs continue to have a high presence in the market of these countries. May be this is because the root of all this is on the demand side. Therefore, to slow the wide distribution of substandard and counterfeit drugs in the market of developing countries with a huge number of vulnerable consumers, it is critical to develop new measures that can target the demand side. With this in mind, this chapter is written to gain better understanding of the demand side of the problem and, consequently, specify the most effective measures to slow the rapid progression of substandard and counterfeit drugs sale.

The demand side of the problem of substandard and counterfeit drugs is clearly an issue of consumer behavior. Consumers play a decisive role in the trade of substandard and counterfeit drugs, and their willingness to purchase counterfeit products was reported worldwide (Cordell, Wongtada, & Kieschnick, 1996). Although substandard and counterfeit drugs are compromising the quality, consumer may show willingness to overlook this due to attitudinal and/or motivational factors. A study conducted in some countries revealed an alarming finding that consumers perceive purchasing, as well as disseminating to peers, substandard, and/or counterfeit medicines as acceptable practice (Wertheimer & Wang, 2012). This mounting literature ensures that if consumers' perceptions and attitude toward substandard and counterfeit drugs problem are not factored into the analysis of the problem, then strategies to combat this problem will remain ineffective. This is supported by the director of the Nigerian regulatory authority, NAFDAC: "Having analyzed the past interventions to enforce the regulation in Nigeria, we arrived at the conclusion that they were rather ad-hoc measures, and as such, their impact, if any, was not sustainable. Consequently, we deemed it more effective to embark on the massive enlightenment campaign, dialogue, education and persuasion in our regulatory activities, because this strategy addresses the fundamental issue at stake, which is behavioural change" (Akunyili, 2005, pp. 10).

In fact, despite the fact that counterfeiting has existed a long time ago, knowledge about consumer behavior toward counterfeit products and the influencing factors that motivate willingness to purchase counterfeits are still very limited (Eisend & Schuchert-Güler, 2006). This is in spite the fact that consumers remain both the root problem and the ultimate destination of counterfeit products.

This lack of information about the demand side is even more serious in developing countries for two reasons. First, in developing countries, there is a strong link between high drug prices and counterfeiting of medicines (European Generic Medicines Association, 2007). Nonavailability or unaffordability of essential medicines causes a desperate need-driven demand for life-saving drugs that are unavailable or unaffordable through the legitimate distribution channels. This need allows the counterfeiters to exploit this gap. Therefore, for a successful anticounterfeiting policy, there is a need for better understanding of the demand side of the problem. Second, in developing countries, drug regulatory authorities work in a limited resource setting. This lack of resources necessitates the selection of suitable strategies to protect public health. Without the essential knowledge of the characteristics of counterfeit drug buyers, it will be difficult for these drug regulatory authorities to prioritize their options.

The purpose of this chapter is to establish this necessary knowledge about the perceptions of various stakeholders in general, and consumers in specific. This is expected to help drug regulatory authorities as well as pharmaceutical industry understand the main factors influencing consumer behavior toward counterfeit drugs and hence, create effective anticounterfeiting strategies.

BACKGROUND

Unfortunately, research studies in a developing countries' context, studying perceptions of various stakeholders about substandard and counterfeit drugs are scarce. May be that is the reason behind the tendency in most research studies addressing consumers' perceptions toward the purchase of substandard and counterfeit drugs to maximize the same attributes, in fighting against these drugs, throughout the world. However, due to contextual variations, this may fail to address the fundamental differences in the nature of pharmaceutical counterfeiting among countries at different stages of economic development. Currently, most of the research studies exploring substandard and counterfeit drugs from the consumer perspective use data collected in the advanced world (Bloch et al., 1993; Tom, Garibaldi, Zeng, & Pilcher, 1998). However, substandard and counterfeit drug problem has developed differently in different regions (Bate, 2008), and there is no indication whether or not consumers living in areas and/or coming from different backgrounds perceive it similarly (Veloutsou & Bian, 2008). To develop appropriate countermeasures, it is necessary to understand the reasons why people in a specific region buy these products.

There has been various published works (theoretical and empirical) on exploring, measuring, or combating substandard and counterfeit drugs. However, these research studies are seldom based on theoretical reasoning and are strongly data driven. As reminded by Hoe, Hogg, and Hart (2003), those studies focus on facts without investigating why substandard and counterfeit drugs are purchased. Marketing scholars have expressed concern over the lack of research available for studying the patterns of counterfeit-buying consumers. Problem is even deeper when it comes to developing countries as the existing literature on measuring the prevalence of substandard and counterfeit drugs in developing countries has primarily focused on withdrawing samples from the market and running laboratory tests. Although those efforts may, to some extent, succeed in measuring or describing the prevalence of substandard and counterfeit drugs, these studies fail to consider the factors contributing to the prevalence of these drugs and, consequently, the steps which should be taken to arrive at a policy to root them out. As a result, most remedies to curb the problem of substandard and counterfeit drugs in developing countries are a simple extension of remedies followed in developed countries and are mostly geared toward limiting the supply.

Significantly, there is evidence that remarkable distinctions necessitate a more fine-tuned approach in combating substandard and counterfeit drugs in different regions. However, these differences between developed and developing countries are generally not seriously considered in the available literature. This is an important shortcoming, as an understanding of the factors that influence the distribution and sale of substandard and counterfeit drugs in a particular economic region is tremendously valuable. Solutions that specifically act in response to such factors can make strategies that are far more efficient. To combat substandard and counterfeit drugs in developing countries, it is important to understand the underlying reasons for the differences between developed and developing countries before trying to extend strategies developed in the advanced world to the developing world. If such distinctions or differences are ignored, there is a risk that the problem will not be sufficiently addressed in the developing countries. By addressing these differences, this chapter will offer the necessary information needed to better target the problem of substandard and counterfeit drugs. In other words, by addressing perspective, knowledge, and attitude of various stakeholders toward substandard and counterfeit drugs in developing countries, specific theoretical knowledge can be generated that helps tailoring more fine-tuned strategies to combat substandard and counterfeit drugs.

PERCEPTIONS

Studying perceptions of stakeholders about substandard and counterfeit drugs may be a valuable step toward effective combating efforts. It is reported in the literature that counterfeit drugs influence economy of developing countries due to many factors, one among them is perception (Muthiani & Wanjau, 2012). Therefore, the development of effective organizational and technical countermeasures requires thorough understanding of the perspective, knowledge, and attitude of various stakeholders. Unfortunately, currently, particularly in developing countries, most of the efforts are directed toward countermeasures based on lawful and administrative techniques (reducing the supply) (Bloch et al., 1993), while perspective, knowledge, and attitude toward substandard and counterfeits (the demand)-oriented approach is still scarce (Ang, Cheng, Lim, & Tambyah, 2001; Bloch et al., 1993; Dubinsky, Nataraajan, & Huang, 2005; Stöttinger & Penz, 2003). In an effort to fill this gap, we will try in this chapter to shed lights on those understudied areas.

PERCEPTION WITH REGARD TO UNDERSTANDING OF THE TERMS "SUBSTANDARD AND COUNTERFEIT DRUG"

In developing countries, there are great differences and mix-up in the understanding of both the terms "substandard drug" and "counterfeit drug" not only among public, but even among policy makers and healthcare practitioners. Many do not differentiate between counterfeit and substandard drugs. A survey conducted in Sudan showed that knowledge about counterfeit drugs among laymen, and even health personnel is weak, if not totally absent (Alfadl, Ibrahim, & Hassali, 2012). But this is not surprising as literature reveals that even in the developed world, one of the most challenging obstacles in understanding the terms substandard and counterfeit drugs is the confusion and disagreement on the meaning of both terms (Bosworth, 2006; Jacobs, Samli, & Jedlik, 2001; Nogues, 1990). The language used to distinguish between these products is inherently confusing. In the literature there is much confusion between the words counterfeit, fake, illicit, and substandard. In fact, this confusion comes largely from the presence of different elements in defining these products depending on whether a definition stems from a public health discussion or to answer an inquiry raised in a case of infringement on an intellectual property right (IPR). In other words, confusion in definition comes from whether the definition is a public health–oriented approach or an IPR-oriented approach to the problem of distribution and sale of substandard and counterfeit drugs. However, whatsoever the cause, this inconsistency in the definition is a real problem urging the need for a wider consensus.

PERCEPTION WITH REGARD TO VULNERABILITY TO SUBSTANDARD AND COUNTERFEIT DRUGS

The general perception among consumers, healthcare professionals, policy makers, and other stakeholders in developing countries is that the major reason for the increasing vulnerability to substandard and counterfeit drugs is the unaffordable prices of medicines. Perceiving price as the most obvious determinant for purchasing substandard and counterfeit drugs may be in line with what was concluded by other researchers that price appears to be the sole determinant of purchasing decisions and that little more need be discussed (Eisend & Schuchert-Güler, 2006). Link between prices and consumers willingness to purchase a substandard or counterfeit has strong support in the literature (Bloch et al., 1993; Cespedes, Corey, & Rangan, 1988; Cordell et al., 1996; Schlegelmilch, Stottinger, & Nill, 2015; Stöttinger & Penz, 2003).

Nonetheless, when it comes to medicines, major difference between consumers in developed and developing countries is clearly noticed. Literature reported that, regardless their prices, substandard or counterfeit drugs were the least among other products to be knowingly purchased by consumers in developed countries (Anti-Counterfeiting Group, 2003). May be the reason behind this is that while consumers in developed countries make their purchase decision of counterfeit for saving purposes, although they can afford buying the genuine (Gentry, Putrevu, & Shultz, 2006; Prendergast, Hing Chuen, & Phau, 2002), in developing countries the main motivation for purchasing fake drugs is to find a cheaper alternative for the unaffordable, impossible-to-purchase, legitimate medicine. In other words, poor consumers in developing countries have no choice other than the substandard or counterfeit because the genuine life-saving medicine is not affordable. In developing countries, for many consumers the price of the legitimate, badly needed, drug is out of reach. Therefore, for those consumers suffering, for example, from malaria, even if the risk of harm from counterfeit consumption is significant, it may be less than the risk of harm arising from forgoing medication altogether for the sake of not taking a substandard or counterfeit drug. This problem is further complicated by the fact that even modestly priced drugs affordable by western standards may be out of reach for most of the developing countries' consumers who live in poverty.

PERCEPTION WITH REGARD TO PRESENCE AND SOURCE OF SUBSTANDARD AND COUNTERFEIT DRUGS IN DEVELOPING COUNTRIES' MARKET

Despite the scarcity of the official data, documenting the presence of substandard and counterfeit drugs in developing countries' market, but the general belief is that they are widely distributed in the market because factors encouraging and facilitating their presence are well documented. A study conducted in Tanzania reported that consumers perceived the presence of counterfeit drugs in the community to be a big problem (Mhando, Jande, Liwa, Mwita, & Marwa, 2016).

PERCEPTION WITH REGARD TO PRICE–QUALITY INFERENCE

Literature documents that consumers in developing countries strongly link price and quality, with high price means high quality and vice versa. No different from that belief between educated and noneducated, and maybe the educated consumers link more strongly between quality and price (Alfadl, Hassali, & Ibrahim, 2013). Although this contradicts their behavior as they willingly purchase substandard and counterfeit drugs, but anyhow, this is a common belief among consumers worldwide (Chapman & Wahlers, 1999; Tellis & Gaeth, 1990).

PERCEPTION WITH REGARD TO SUBJECTIVE NORMS

Perceptions of policy makers and healthcare providers about peer pressure support the belief that it has huge effect leading community pharmacists in developing countries to source their medicines from suspected sources (Alfadl et al., 2013). Engagement in illicit behavior due to peer pressure is widely reported in the literature. It is documented that not only a person may exhibit a deviant behavior because he has friends exhibiting the same, but moreover, he could tolerate and accept that behavior if he found peer support (Albers-Miller, 1999; Ang et al., 2001; Kallis, Krentler, & Vanier, 1986; Powers & Anglin, 1996). Regarding social stigma, it is also documented that community pharmacists working in pharmacies do not feel any wrongdoing in selling counterfeit drugs if quality is assured (Alfadl et al., 2013). Interestingly, this is also the case in developed countries as a study conducted there reported that both buyers and nonbuyers of counterfeit music did not believe the counterfeit buyers had low morals (Ang et al., 2001). This strengthening the belief that counterfeits selling and purchasing in general lack a significant social stigma.

On the other hand, in developing countries, consumers' decision to purchase substandard or counterfeit drugs is significantly influenced by pressure exerted through family and friends, interesting enough, in favor not to purchase (Alfadl et al., 2012). This is consistent with the literature on the influence of family and friends on a consumer's decision to engage or not in a deviant behavior (Albers-Miller, 1999; Ang et al., 2001; Kallis et al., 1986; Powers & Anglin, 1996).

PERCEPTION WITH REGARD TO AWARENESS ABOUT THE SOCIETAL CONSEQUENCES

The general perception is that raising awareness of the societal consequences does not look like a promising avenue to combat the problem. A study conducted in Sudan reported that from all anticounterfeiting campaigns used in the developed countries (Chakraborty, Allred, & Bristol, 1996), both policy makers and community pharmacists believe that the only possible cause which may discourage consumers in Sudan from buying counterfeit drugs is to convince them that those drugs threaten their health and safety (Alfadl et al., 2013). Messages highlighting societal consequences such as its chilling effect on the economy; its tendency to discourage companies from investments in research and developments; the hazardous labor conditions found in countries engaged in drug counterfeiting; undermining the official health system; loss of jobs; illegal nature of the behavior (buying counterfeit) implying social stigma; and the potential link to organized crime that would profit from counterfeit purchases (Ang et al., 2001; Wee, Ta, & Cheok, 1995) might be effective in western countries where counterfeiters targeting the so-called life-style drugs (e.g., Viagra) (Bate, 2008). However, in developing countries, for impoverished consumer infected with HIV AIDS, for whom purchasing the counterfeit may be the only viable alternative, social stigma and other similar messages might be the last thing that could discourage him from buying the counterfeits.

Also, it is reported in the literature that the increased use of counterfeit drugs in poor countries had created them a serious macroeconomic problem (Wertheimer & Norris, 2009), but still community pharmacists continue to find excuses for both their peers and consumers not to believe in what they call the "assumed" societal consequences. They stated that both pharmacists and doctors strongly believe as long as they do not put their customers at risk, no harm in selling them what assumed a counterfeit (Alfadl et al., 2013), an excuse used in Western countries as well (Anti-Counterfeiting Group, 2003). Also, this perception has been documented even in the literature generated among consumers from developed countries. It was found in a study conducted in the United States, which investigated the effect of awareness of societal consequences on the purchase intent of a counterfeited Tylenol (a pain reliever) that the awareness has no significant effect on purchase intent of the counterfeit drug (Leisen & Nill, 2001, p. 271). However, tendency to rationalize misbehavior whenever a person is actively or passively benefiting from that behavior or believing in what is known as "no harm/no foul" is well documented in the literature (Muncy & Vitell, 1992; Strutton, Pelton, & Ferrell, 1997; Strutton, Vitell, & Pelton, 1994).

KNOWLEDGE

EDUCATION PERTAINING TO SUBSTANDARD AND COUNTERFEIT DRUGS

In developing countries, education pertaining to substandard and counterfeit drugs is not a priority, or more accurately, is a neglected issue. Consequently, knowledge about substandard and counterfeit drugs is very weak between both consumers and healthcare providers, which resulted in what stated by some researchers that consumers in developing countries purchase substandard and counterfeit drugs due to ignorance about the health implications (Asuamah, Prempeh, & Boateng, 2013). This is a very serious problem, especially in the light that it seems there is no clear strategy on how to mitigate this problem. The main problem pertaining to this weak knowledge about substandard and counterfeit drugs is that it could negatively affect all combating efforts. A study highlighted this problem and mentioned the need for campaigns to increase awareness among all concerned parties (Abu Taleb & Almadadha, 2013). This was supported by another study that reported that consumers view campaign announcements as an effective strategy in increasing their awareness about substandard and counterfeit drugs (Abdoulaye, Chastanier, Azondekon, Dansou, & Bruneton, 2006). However, for any campaign to discourage consumers from buying substandard and counterfeit drugs to be effective there should be in the first place reasonable knowledge and awareness about the drawbacks of substandard and counterfeit drugs. Another factor complicating the problem of weak knowledge about substandard and counterfeit drugs is the disagreement about their definition. In fact, the educational efforts to raise the awareness about substandard and counterfeit drugs problem are jeopardized by differing national definitions of these products adopted by different countries. However, this problem of weak knowledge about substandard and counterfeit drugs seems to be not restricted to developing countries, but common and hindering the efforts to combat the problem even in developed countries. For example, a survey conducted in Europe revealed that only 18% of the respondents were aware of the presence of counterfeit pharmaceuticals in the market (Anti-Counterfeiting Group, 2003).

However, educational strategies are still mentioned as a tool to combat substandard and counterfeit drugs. For example, one of the educational strategies reported in the literature for shifting consumer from buying substandard and counterfeit drugs is highlighting the risks that accompany fake drugs (Tom et al., 1998). This could be accomplished through publicizing tragedies encountered from consuming substandard and counterfeit drugs such as injuries or death. Nonetheless, although this strategy could be effective in the West, but the same strategy in the developing countries may not be without negative impact. Some policy makers in developing countries expressed concern over using this last education strategy (highlighting risk) as it may discourage, especially in remote rural areas, modern medication and encourage alternative medicine, hence exacerbate an already existing problem. Some of those policy makers explicitly mentioned the presence of markets where conventional and alternative medicines are often sold alongside in the same outlet with conventional medicines sold in simple, or even no packaging at all (Alfadl et al., 2013). While selling medicines with no package cause suspicion to a Western consumer, consumers in developing countries, especially in rural areas, are accustomed to it because alternative medicine is popular with them. Unfortunately, as packaging is an important feature to differentiate between genuine and fake products, stripping-off medicines from their original packaging, enables counterfeit drugs to be easily leaked and sold in those markets without any cues for a consumer to evaluate whether the product is genuine or counterfeit. These problems of alternative medicine and buying drugs from nonlegitimate outlets in developing countries are clearly problems of the poor education that need to be addressed and, cautiously, tackled. Interestingly, concerns of those policy makers are supported by a study that noticed the sale of medicines might fall because of campaigns raising awareness of consumers on the dangers of substandard and counterfeit drugs, which consequently aggravate the problem of lack of access to good quality medicines (Lybecker, 2007).

Other educational option to move consumers not to buy substandard and counterfeits may be accomplished through educational programs highlighting the illegal nature of the activity, implying the presence of social stigma, and explaining the negative impact of buying counterfeit on the national economy. However, such educational programs may not be useful in developing countries as it was reported in a study conducted in Sudan that some community pharmacists stated clearly that as long as consumers assured about the quality of the drugs they would not care for other considerations. Moreover, even if they were noticed about the negative impact of purchasing counterfeit drugs in the official health system and national economy, they may buy them as retaliation on what they believed an inequity in health services and national wealth distribution (Alfadl et al., 2013). Interestingly, this has supported even in developed countries as it was reported in the literature that some consumers in developed countries purchase counterfeit products as an expression of their anti–big business feelings (Tom et al., 1998).

Nevertheless, still weak knowledge and the absence of education pertaining to substandard and counterfeit drugs are a serious problem that needs to be addressed and seriously tackled worldwide. No excuse to continue neglecting this problem, especially in the light of the findings of some studies revealed that counterfeiting could be curtailed through changing consumers' behavior through finely tailored campaigns to shape attitudes and beliefs (Wee et al., 1995).

ATTITUDE

Against the expectation, and reported literature in developed countries, attitude has no significant effect on the consumers' purchase intention of counterfeit drugs in developing countries. Previous studies reported that the negative perception toward counterfeiting consistently influenced the intention to purchase across all products studied by researchers (Wee et al., 1995). This contradiction in consumers' attitude toward substandard and counterfeit drugs between consumers in developed and developing countries may be explained by the fact that knowledge about substandard and counterfeit drugs among consumers in developing countries, as mentioned earlier, is very weak. Attitude is dependent on the previous knowledge and beliefs about the specific thing or product, therefore, might be, most probably, this weak knowledge about the counterfeit drugs in developing countries had weakened the effect of consumers' attitude on their purchase intention of substandard and counterfeit drugs.

This reveals that substandard and counterfeit drugs can be combated through what public health officers do best through educating consumers about the dangers of substandard and counterfeit drugs. Such efforts can at least have effects on consumers' attitudes and therefore, their purchase intention toward these drugs. However, in a study conducted in Sudan, some policy makers and healthcare givers raise concern about the tools used for educating people. They anticipate that using the media to publicize the fact that drugs could be subject to counterfeiting can generate distrust in the minds of consumers and lead them away from conventional drugs toward alternative medicine, as highlighted earlier. However, apart from the most suitable tool that could be used, it is evident that the issue of educating people on substandard and counterfeit drugs aspects can no longer be taken lightly. From another perspective, achieving better response from consumers could be introduced through anticounterfeit drugs advertisements showing imminent health hazards and long-term negative impact on the health system and national economy (Ang et al., 2001; Tom et al., 1998; Wang, Zhang, Zang, & Ouyang, 2005; Wee et al., 1995).

However, for efficient, more finely tuned strategies targeting changing attitude of the highly vulnerable groups, close understanding of the characteristics of those groups seems indispensable.

SOCIODEMOGRAPHIC CHARACTERS

In developing countries, there is a general belief that with the exception of economic status, all other demographic factors such as education, age, and gender have no effect on substandard and counterfeit drugs purchase decision. This complies with a study in a developing country mentioning poverty as a main cause for the decision to purchase substandard or counterfeit drug (Asuamah et al., 2013). This perception is logical taking into account the potential high prices of many drugs. In addition, most probably, economic status is perceived as the determinant factor of purchase intention because drugs counterfeited are mainly lifesaving, unlike those counterfeited in the developed countries, which are mainly life-style drugs (Bate, 2008). Therefore, if the counterfeited drug treats a life-critical illness, the economically weak consumer will buy the drug no matter what is the risk. He will see this purchase decision rational as even a tiny chance of improved health may be better than no chance at all. This is aggravated by the fact that most of the consumers in developing countries are without health insurance or the ability to pay out-of-pocket for drugs, therefore they are left out of the market.

Perceiving economic status as the determinant sociodemographic factor should be reflected in designing combating efforts. Policy makers should be aware that even raising awareness of risk associated with consumption of substandard or counterfeit drugs may not be sufficient to shift those economically constrained consumers to the more expensive legitimate drugs. Therefore, to move those consumers not to buy substandard or counterfeit drugs, may be the only viable solution in the provision of legitimate versions of the life-saving drugs at affordable prices. This is consistent with a previous study, which investigated Chinese consumers and concluded that if prices could be lowered and made more affordable, there might be less tendency for consumers to purchase counterfeit products and instead purchase the original (Phau & Teah, 2009).

Interestingly, perceiving economic status as the determinant sociodemographic factor is consistent even with literature generated in developed countries. For instance, some studies conducted in the West have found that consumers who purchase counterfeit products are of lower social status (Tom et al., 1998; Wee et al., 1995).

EFFECT OF DIVERSE PERCEPTIONS ON COMBATING STRATEGIES

There have been many attempts and methods to combat substandard and counterfeit drugs through a number of different strategies and techniques, but due to contextual differences that create differences in how substandard and counterfeit drugs viewed or perceived; efficiency of these methods in developing countries is questioned. On one hand, different views and perspectives affect countermeasures at legal provision and the law enforcement level. For example, World Health Organization (WHO) promotes a lot of strategies and proposals that pursue legal provisions and law enforcement (World Health Organization (WHO), 2011), but such proposals are undermined by how substandard and counterfeit drugs are perceived, which inhibits their realization in developing countries. This is because law enforcement is dependent on the resources available, and in countries facing urgent economic problems and severely limited resources, perception of the importance of law enforcement will likely come very low on the list of priorities.

At the other hand, as mentioned earlier under subheading "understanding the terms substandard and counterfeit drugs," it is apparent that one of the most challenging obstacles in combating substandard and counterfeit drugs is the confusion and disagreement on the meaning of the terms "substandard/counterfeit drug" even among policy makers. Although the WHO definition (WHO, 2007) is widely disseminated, but, unfortunately, there is no consensus about it. Countries issuing their own regulations against counterfeiting have their own definitions, making information exchange among them difficult and hindering the development of global anticounterfeiting strategies. The WHO admits that the definition of counterfeit drug used in practice based on the laws of different countries differs enough to create problems in the collection of data and the implementation of global measures to combat counterfeit drugs (Nogues, 1990). This may be the main reason undermining the effectiveness of the prominent initiative toward measuring and combating of counterfeit drugs in Southeast Asia called Rapid Alert System (RAS). It was developed by the WHO and aims mainly to "establish an IT communication network for rapid dissemination of reported counterfeit drugs; and propose strategy for advocacy and identify appropriate advocacy materials" to combat counterfeit drugs (Ibrahim, 2004, p. 2). This is because the efforts to collect and disseminate information and reports about counterfeit drugs are jeopardized by differing national definitions of counterfeit drugs among different countries, something makes law enforcement and cooperation across national borders very difficult particularly when the counterfeit drug that meet one country's definition do not meet that of another.

This lack in the uniformity in the definition as well as the confusion in determining a specific meaning for the term "counterfeit drug" creates real obstacles hindering the possibility of developing global strategies for combating drug counterfeiting. This problem remained unsolved and was highlighted by

Attaran and colleagues stating that "The most fundamental reason for current and past inaction is a failure to recognise shared goals" (Attaran et al., 2012, p. 1). Because of these differences, a debate flared in 2008 about IMPACT's definition of counterfeit medicine, which was opposed by some countries (mainly developing) and organizations arguing that it confused a public health issue with an IPR issue. This has ended with the whole issue of counterfeits being dropped from the 2009 World Health Assembly.

Hence, it is clear that developing new policies and strategies considering the distinction between developed and developing countries market and consumer perspectives with regard to counterfeit and substandard medicines may offer a possibility of a more efficient combating of substandard and counterfeit drugs, especially in developing countries.

INTEGRATING KNOWLEDGE AND PERCEPTIONS ABOUT SUBSTANDARD AND COUNTERFEIT DRUGS INTO PRACTICE

Some researchers proposed and validated a conceptual model that empirically investigates Sudanese consumers' perspectives of their purchase intention of counterfeit drugs. Creation of this conceptual model may aid a deeper understanding of the connections linking consumers' perspectives about counterfeit drugs and their purchase intention by examining the association between attitude, subjective norm, motivation, and purchase intention in one single model. Despite the fact that there could be variables other than those highlighted in the model, the proposed conceptual model incorporated variables that have proved to offer successful relationships (Alfadl et al., 2012) (Fig. 21.1).

Achievements:

- Considerable awareness about substandard and counterfeit drugs was achieved through media, campaigns in schools, and others, but still a lot is needed.

Challenges:

- Confusion regarding the definition of substandard and counterfeit drugs directly contributes to the serious barriers hindering the fight against the problem.
- Conflict of interest between different stakeholders (e.g., industry and public health activists) negatively affects the efficacy of policies and strategies adopted in the fight against substandard and counterfeit drugs.
- Current strategies or campaigns that are geared toward raising awareness of consumers about dangers of substandard and counterfeit drugs may result in leading consumers away from conventional medicines toward alternative and fake drugs, which consequently lead to lack of access to good quality medicines.

Recommendations:

- Lack in the uniformity in the definition as well as the confusion in determining a specific meaning for the terms "substandard" and "counterfeit drug" creates real obstacles hindering the possibility of developing global strategies for combating drug counterfeiting. Therefore, clarifying and unifying the definition of substandard and counterfeit drugs should be a top priority for efficient, global combating of the problem.

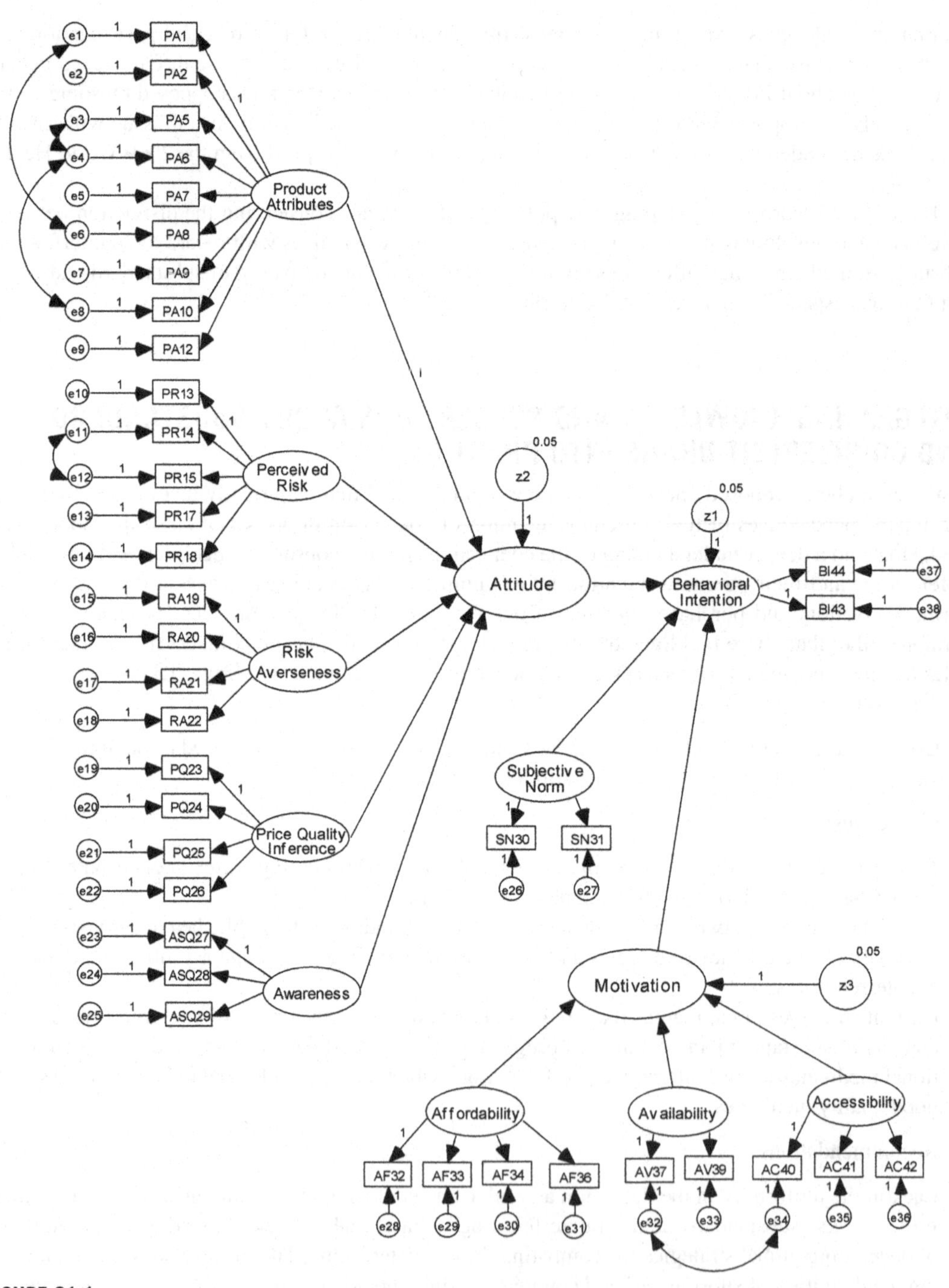

FIGURE 21.1

Relationships among beliefs, attitudes, subjective norms, motivations, and intention with respect to purchase of counterfeit drugs.

- To move economically constrained consumer not to buy counterfeit drugs may be the only viable solution in the provision of legitimate versions at affordable prices. Therefore, weak accessibility of drugs in developing countries should be highlighted as a main cause for distribution of substandard and counterfeit drugs in the pharmaceutical market.
- As societal pressure from family or friends was found to have great impact on substandard and counterfeit drugs purchase intent, in favor of not to purchase, this could be exploited in designing combat strategies. The power of those who are against the purchase of substandard and counterfeit drugs has on their families and friends should be utilized in discouraging this behavior.
- Education programs targeting consumers, industry, health personnel, as well as medical students should be developed. Public health policy makers should educate health professionals about the dangers of nonlegitimate drugs. A policy should be implemented to (1) publicize criminal prosecutions of illegal health professionals' behavior to spread the notion among peer groups that sourcing medicines through illegal drug supply channels is no longer acceptable; (2) promote social disapproval of dispensing of nonlegitimate drugs from pharmacies and clinics.
- Policy makers should reexamine the loose rules, or the relaxed rules governing the alternative or traditional medicines, as the culture of alternative medicines seems to encourage purchase of substandard and counterfeit drugs as well.

CONCLUSIONS

In summary, it may be better to include measures specifically tailored to suit consumers in developing countries context for more effective strategies to combat substandard and counterfeit drugs. In addition, enhancing accessibility to low price, legitimate drugs seem indispensable for combating substandard and counterfeit drug problem in developing countries.

Lessons learned:

- It seems that disagreement on single definition for both terms, i.e., "substandard" and "counterfeit drug," inversely affects combating strategies of the problem. Therefore, agreement on a definition to be universally accepted and adopted is a prerequisite for effectively combating the problem.
- Although it is not clear to what extent current programs designed for raising awareness about substandard and counterfeit drugs are effective in combating the problem, it seems that developing educational programs finely tailored to suit developing countries' context is extremely needed.
- It seems that most strategies to combat drug counterfeiting in developing countries failed because stakeholders', and in specific consumers' perceptions, knowledge, and attitudes toward substandard and counterfeit drugs are factored inadequately, if at all, into the analysis of the problem. However, remedies require long-term policy making, planning, and efficient strategies that directly address the need of vulnerable consumers who have a real demand for affordable and cheap drugs in developing countries.

REFERENCES

Abdoulaye, I., Chastanier, H., Azondekon, A., Dansou, A., & Bruneton, C. (2006). Evaluation of public awareness campaigns on counterfeit medicines in Cotonou, Benin. *Medecine tropicale: revue du Corps de sante colonial, 66*(6), 615–618.

Abu Taleb, Y., & Almadadha, R. (2013). Pharmacists' awareness about counterfeit medications in Jordan. *Journal of the Royal Medical Services, 20*(2), 57–70.

Akunyili, D. (March 2005). Counterfeit and substandard drugs, Nigeria's experience: Implications, challenges, actions and recommendations. In *Talk for NAFDAC at a meeting for Key interest groups on health.*

Albers-Miller, N. D. (1999). Consumer misbehavior: Why people buy illicit goods. *Journal of Consumer Marketing, 16*(3), 273–287.

Alfadl, A. A., Hassali, M. A., & Ibrahim, M. I. M. (2013). Counterfeit drug demand: Perceptions of policy makers and community pharmacists in Sudan. *Research in Social and Administrative Pharmacy, 9*(3), 302–310.

Alfadl, A. A., Ibrahim, M. I. M., & Hassali, M. A. (2012). Consumer behaviour towards counterfeit drugs in a developing country. *Journal of Pharmaceutical Health Services Research, 3*(3), 165–172.

Ang, S. H., Cheng, P. S., Lim, E. A. C., & Tambyah, S. K. (2001). Spot the difference: Consumer responses towards counterfeits. *Journal of Consumer Marketing, 18*(3), 219–235.

Anti-Counterfeiting Group. (2003). *Why you should care about counterfeiting.*

Asuamah, S. Y., Prempeh, V. O., & Boateng, C. A. (2013). A study of the purchase and consumption of counterfeit drugs in Ghana: The case of marketing students in Sunyani Polytechnic? *International Journal of Innovative Research and Development, 2*(5).

Attaran, A., Barry, D., Basheer, S., Bate, R., Benton, D., Chauvin, J., Midha, K. (2012). How to achieve international action on falsified and substandard medicines. *Bmj: British Medical Journal, 345*, 1–6.

Bate, R. (2008). *Making a killing: The deadly implications of the counterfeit drug trade.* Washington, D.C.: AEI Press.

Bloch, P. H., Bush, R. F., & Campbell, L. (1993). Consumer "accomplices" in product counterfeiting: A demand side investigation. *Journal of Consumer Marketing, 10*(4), 27–36.

Bosworth, D. (May 2006). Counterfeiting and piracy: The state of the art *Intellectual property in the new Millennium Seminar, Oxford intellectual property research Centre, St. Peter's College* (Vol. 9).

Cespedes, F. V., Corey, E. R., & Rangan, V. K. (1988). Gray markets-causes and cures. *Harvard Business Review, 66*(4), 75–82.

Chakraborty, G., Allred, A. T., & Bristol, T. (1996). Exploring consumers' evaluations of counterfeits: The roles of country of origin and ethnocentrism. *Na-advances in Consumer Research Volume, 23.*

Chapman, J., & Wahlers, R. (1999). A revision and empirical test of the extended price-perceived quality model. *Journal of Marketing Theory and Practice, 7*(3), 53–64.

Cordell, V. V., Wongtada, N., & Kieschnick, R. L. (1996). Counterfeit purchase intentions: Role of lawfulness attitudes and product traits as determinants. *Journal of Business Research, 35*(1), 41–53.

Dubinsky, A. J., Nataraajan, R., & Huang, W. Y. (2005). Consumers' moral philosophies: Identifying the idealist and the relativist. *Journal of Business Research, 58*(12), 1690–1701.

Eisend, M., & Schuchert-Güler, P. (2006). Explaining counterfeit purchases: A review and preview. *Academy of Marketing Science Review, 2006*, 1.

European Generic Medicines Association. (2007). *Position paper on anti-counterfeiting.* Retrieved from http://www.egagenerics.com.

Gentry, J. W., Putrevu, S., & Shultz, C. J. (2006). The effects of counterfeiting on consumer search. *Journal of Consumer Behaviour, 5*(3), 245–256.

Hoe, L., Hogg, G., & Hart, S. (2003). Fakin'it: Counterfeiting and consumer contradictions. *E-European Advances in Consumer Research Volume, 6.*

Ibrahim, M. I. (2004). *Regional rapid alert system (RAS). WHO/WPRO/2004.*

International Anticounterfeiting Coalition. (2012). *About counterfeiting*. Retrieved from https://iacc.org/about-counterfeiting/.

Jacobs, L., Samli, A. C., & Jedlik, T. (2001). The nightmare of international product piracy: Exploring defensive strategies. *Industrial Marketing Management*, *30*(6), 499–509.

Kallis, M. J., Krentler, K. A., & Vanier, D. J. (1986). The value of user image in quelling aberrant consumer behavior. *Journal of the Academy of Marketing Science*, *14*(1), 29–35.

Leisen, B., & Nill, A. (January 2001). Combating product counterfeiting: An investigation into the likely effectiveness of a demand-oriented approach. *American marketing association. Conference Proceedings* (Vol. 12). American Marketing Association, 271.

Lybecker, K. M. (2007). Rx Roulette: Combating counterfeit pharmaceuticals in developing nations. *Managerial and Decision Economics*, *28*(45), 509–520.

Mhando, L., Jande, M. B., Liwa, A., Mwita, S., & Marwa, K. J. (2016). Public awareness and identification of counterfeit drugs in Tanzania: A view on antimalarial drugs. *Advances in Public Health, 2016*.

Milovanovic, D. R., Pavlovic, R., Folic, M., & Jankovic, S. M. (2004). Public drug procurement: The lessons from a drug tender in a teaching hospital of a transition country. *European Journal of Clinical Pharmacology*, *60*(3), 149–153.

Muncy, J. A., & Vitell, S. J. (1992). Consumer ethics: An investigation of the ethical beliefs of the final consumer. *Journal of Business Research*, *24*(4), 297–311.

Muthiani, M., & Wanjau, K. (2012). Factors influencing the influx of counterfeit medicines in Kenya: A survey of pharmaceutical importing small and medium enterprises within Nairobi. *International Journal of Business and Social Science*, *3*(11).

Nogues, J. (1990). *Notes on patents, distortions, and development (No. 315)*. The World Bank.

Phau, I., & Teah, M. (2009). Devil wears (counterfeit) Prada: A study of antecedents and outcomes of attitudes towards counterfeits of luxury brands. *Journal of Consumer Marketing*, *26*(1), 15–27.

Powers, K. I., & Anglin, M. D. (1996). Couples' reciprocal patterns in narcotics addiction: A recommendation on treatment strategy. *Psychology & Marketing*, *13*(8), 769–783.

Prendergast, G., Hing Chuen, L., & Phau, I. (2002). Understanding consumer demand for non-deceptive pirated brands. *Marketing Intelligence & Planning*, *20*(7), 405–416.

Schlegelmilch, B. B., Stottinger, B., & Nill, A. (2015). Why are Counterfeits so Attractive to Consumers? An Empirical Analysis. In *Proceedings of the 1998 Academy of Marketing Science (AMS) Annual Conference* (pp. 395–396). Springer International Publishing.

Stöttinger, B., & Penz, E. (2003). *The demand for counterfeits: are consumers across borders triggered by the same motives?*.

Strutton, D., Pelton, L. E., & Ferrell, O. C. (1997). Ethical behavior in retail settings: Is there a generation gap? *Journal of Business Ethics*, *16*(1), 87–105.

Strutton, D., Vitell, S. J., & Pelton, L. E. (1994). How consumers may justify inappropriate behavior in market settings: An application on the techniques of neutralization. *Journal of Business Research*, *30*(3), 253–260.

Tellis, G. J., & Gaeth, G. J. (1990). Best value, price-seeking, and price aversion: The impact of information and learning on consumer choices. *The Journal of Marketing*, 34–45.

Tom, G., Garibaldi, B., Zeng, Y., & Pilcher, J. (1998). Consumer demand for counterfeit goods. *Psychology & Marketing*, *15*(5), 405–421.

Veloutsou, C., & Bian, X. (2008). A cross-national examination of consumer perceived risk in the context of non-deceptive counterfeit brands. *Journal of Consumer Behaviour*, *7*(1), 3–20.

Wang, F., Zhang, H., Zang, H., & Ouyang, M. (2005). Purchasing pirated software: An initial examination of Chinese consumers. *Journal of Consumer Marketing*, *22*(6), 340–351.

Wee, C. H., Ta, S. J., & Cheok, K. H. (1995). Non-price determinants of intention to purchase counterfeit goods: An exploratory study. *International Marketing Review*, *12*(6), 19–46.

Wertheimer, A. I., & Norris, J. (2009). Safeguarding against substandard/counterfeit drugs: Mitigating a macroeconomic pandemic. *Research in Social and Administrative Pharmacy*, *5*(1), 4–16.

Wertheimer, A. I., & Wang, P. G. (2012). *Counterfeit Medicines: Policy, economics, and countermeasures* (Vol. 1). ILM Publications.

World Health Organization. (2007). Quality assurance of pharmaceuticals: A compendium of guidelines and related materials. *Good manufacturing practices and inspection* (Vol. 2). World Health Organization.

World Health Organization. (2011). *WHO's role in the prevention and control of medical products of compromised quality, safety and efficacy such as substandard/spurious/falsely-labelled/falsified/counterfeit medical products*. Geneva: World Health Organization.

SECTION 9

MEDICINE INFORMATION AND HEALTH LITERACY IN LOW- AND MIDDLE-INCOME COUNTRIES

CHAPTER

22

ISSUES ON SOURCE, ACCESS, EXTENT, AND QUALITY OF INFORMATION AVAILABLE AMONG PHARMACISTS AND PHARMACY PERSONNEL TO PRACTICE EFFECTIVELY

Ahmed I. Fathelrahman

Qassim University, Buraidah, Kingdom of Saudi Arabia

CHAPTER OUTLINE

Social and Administrative Aspects of Pharmacy in Low- and Middle-Income Countries. http://dx.doi.org/10.1016/B978-0-12-811228-1.00022-4

INTRODUCTION

Providing information about medicines to the prescribers and to other healthcare providers was the earliest task undertaken by pharmacists while making the dramatic transformation in the pharmacy profession by shifting the orientation of practice from focusing mainly on the medicine itself to focusing on the patient who uses medicine and later on focusing also on the community. Such huge change ended by establishing clinical pharmacy practice during the period of 1960s and 1970s and led later on to founding pharmaceutical care (Elenbaas & Worthen, 2009). The new trend of practice, which was started early in the United States and transferred to other countries, represents a way of practice dominating worldwide. Since then, pharmacists became the main source of information on medicines and gained the appreciation and respect of the healthcare team members everywhere in the world. Information on medicines is provided by individual pharmacists during medical rounds and scientific meetings such as conferences, workshops, and seminars or within official bodies such as medicines information centers and hospital committees. Trust and appreciation extended to the general public because of pharmacists' contribution to the awareness campaigns, patients counseling, pharmacists-run clinics, and participation in wellness programs.

Our world today witnesses huge advancements in the information-related technologies and in the amount of medicines information available and accessible by all healthcare providers as well as the public. This represents great challenge for pharmacists and puts more responsibility on them as medicines information specialists. To remain in the front line as information providers and as information experts, pharmacists need to provide specific, objective, up-to-date, and unbiased information and be very efficient, competent, and skillful while searching for and providing the information.

This chapter describes various medicines information sources and their availability, accessibility, and quality based on research conducted worldwide with a more focus on the studies performed in developing countries. When describing the characteristics of a particular medicines information source and the potentialities for improvement in a certain area, we may rely on some researches conducted in developed countries due to scarcity of evidence from developing countries and because evidences can be generalized to other countries given that the basic requirements for establishing a particular initiative exist. Information on novel initiatives from developed countries can be used as valued lessons and learning experiences that can be replicated elsewhere.

It is important to make a note here that using the descriptions "medicines information centers" and "medicines information services" is chosen throughout the chapter consistently with the terminology used in the whole book. However, some resources cited here were using the descriptions "drug information centers" and "drug information services." We tried to be consistent in using the description "medicines information" whenever possible unless the term was linked in the original resource to a name of a particular service or center; in such cases we used the word "drug" to illustrate such descriptions.

SOURCES OF MEDICINES INFORMATION AVAILABLE TO PHARMACISTS IN DEVELOPING COUNTRIES

Pharmacists should identify and be able to use credible, up-to-date, and high-quality information resources while practicing. The information will be used to build pharmacists' own competencies to practice efficiently and ethically and to provide high-quality services. The information will be needed to effectively manage drug supply, monitor and assess medication use, evaluate medications, counsel patients, promote rational use of medicines, and perform administrative works besides other activities. However, acting as a primary source of medicines information for healthcare providers and the public is the job most done by all pharmacists working in different settings of practice in a formal or in an informal manner. This is why this chapter is focusing mainly on the issues related to the source, access, extent, and quality of medicines information available among pharmacists and pharmacy personnel. Nevertheless, any other type of information ahead from medicines information is also applicable to what is described in the chapter.

SCIENTIFIC JOURNALS

Scientific biomedical journals represent the core source of our knowledge about medicines. Published research papers are called primary literature because they are the primary source of newly discovered and recently revealed information that is established from research and investigations before such information becomes well known and later on all other sources of information are built based on them. Previously, all journals are published as printed material. Nowadays, journals are published as print and as online digital copies, and some journals are online-only. This has increased accessibility of the journal materials to the readers. In terms of accessibility, journals are either subscription based (i.e., users' payments) or freely accessed (i.e., publication fees are paid by the individual researchers or their institutions). When we describe the availability of biomedical journals in a particular institution, we mean their availability within the library databases of that institution, which requires the subscription of such institution with the database that includes the required journals. If a journal is available free to the readers, then there is no problem with accessibility to its content and the content can be downloaded and easily used by anyone. However, with subscription-only journals' content, there may be a problem in the accessibility to such information among pharmacists in the poorest developing countries (i.e., low- to middle-income countries).

TEXTBOOKS, BOOKS, AND HANDBOOKS

For a user who needs to establish basic information about certain topic, textbooks and books represent the cornerstone, particularly when the topic is very broad and the information user has little or no background about the topic. However, a major limitation of textbooks and books is that some included details must be updated from other resources depending on the nature of the information and on how progressive the research in the particular scientific field is. This is like statistics on the epidemiology of a fast-spreading disease. On average, for a book to be written and published, it requires a period ranges from 3 to 5 years. If some references included in a book at the book preparation time were 5 years back, then such information will be about 10 years backdated when the book becomes firstly available in the market. In our rapidly changing world today, 10 years-back information might be totally obsolete. A study conducted by Novo Nordisk Inc. to assess the accuracy of information about Novo Nordisk products in 37 common drug and medical references identified some errors in such references including outdated product information (Lum & Ahn, 2012).

However, textbooks, books, and handbooks still remain important sources of medicines information. A survey conducted in Nigeria among practicing pharmacists revealed that text books such as *Index of Essential Medicines* (*Emdex*, first published in 1991 as Nigeria's Essential Drugs (NED)

Guide), *British National Formulary*, and others are among most used sources of medicine information (Udezi, Oparah, & Enyi, 2007). In Jordan, a study conducted by Wazaify, Maani, and Ball (2009) reported that all private community pharmacies had at least one reference book, but most were outdated. In Singapore, reference texts are still trusted by pharmacists (Wong, Ko, & Sklar, 2009). Even in the United States, a survey performed among Alabama pharmacy facilities indicated a high use of textbooks as medicine information resources such as *Drug Facts and Comparisons* and *Physician's Desk Reference* (Schrimsher, Freeman, & Kendrach, 2006). Clauson, Fass, and Seamon (2008a) explored the legal requirements for maintaining medicines information resources in pharmacies across the 50 states in the United States and found that two states, Minnesota and South Dakota (3.8% of states), required print references. The availability of digital copies of textbooks, books, and monographs has increased the availability and the wide usage of such resources since they are portable and they are convenient while used (Hughes, Kendrach, Schrimsher, Wensel, & Freeman, 2011).

THE INTERNET (THE WORLD WIDE WEB)

The emergence of the Internet, which had begun on small scale in the mid-1960s as part of the US Department of Defense's projects and propagated outside the United States as a worldwide service in the early 1990s by establishing the World Wide Web, had changed life of the people and the communities all around the globe and played huge roles in science advancement and sharing (Abate, 2001, pp. 1–27). Today, the Internet is the most commonly used source of information for a variety of uses and topics. This is because it is fast in information retrieval and is convenient and enjoyable in its use. Moreover, it is a good medium for information storage and exchange and almost all known types of medicines information resources have been transformed into Web-based products. However, a major limitation of some Internet-based resources is the uncertainty of quality, accuracy, and credibility of the information.

Digital versions of textbooks and books are easily uploaded to and downloaded from websites. Interactive versions of such resources provide more opportunity for information search, processing, and recovery. Surveys from both developed and developing countries indicated that online medicines information resources are widely utilized by pharmacists. In Malaysia for example, the majority of pharmacists preferred online medicines information resources (Khan, Emeka, & Khan, 2013).

DATABASES (WEB BASED AND CD BASED)

Databases are large collections of data that are organized in a way that facilitates processing, searching, and retrieval of the required information. The use of databases, which are either CD based or Web based (the later format becomes more prominent), requires the availability of computers facilities, which are considered a basic requirement of any medicines information center (MIC). An online collection of thousands of journals' contents represents a database, such as MEDLINE, ScienceDirect, Scopus, Springer Link, and ProQuest. Cochrane Database for Systematic Reviews represents an example of evidence-based resources that is very useful for practitioners, academician, and researchers.

MEDICINES INFORMATION CENTERS

The year 1962 witnessed the establishment of the first medicines information center in the world at the new University of Kentucky Medical Centre by Paul Parker (Elenbaas & Worthen, 2009). An MIC is a unit or a department having specific physical setting, supported with certain facilities (such as computers and Internet, print and digital library, a telephone line and a fax) and dedicated staff specialized in the area of medicines information services provision. MICs are commonly localized or affiliated to hospitals, academic institutions, Ministries of Health, medicines manufacturers, health professional associations, and community pharmacies. In hospitals, which are the primary setting of MIC, if no center exists, there should be at least a medicines information service provided by pharmacy department, individual clinical pharmacists, or ordinary pharmacists. Sometimes, an MIC serves the poison information needs of its users and it may be referred to as a medicines and poisons information center. In some situations, there is a need for a regional MIC that covers with its services a large region or a state from a country. This is particularly needed in the poorest countries and it should be encouraged to overcome problems of shortage in infrastructures, facilities, funding, qualified personnel, and other resources.

The prescribers should be the primary target of the services provided by the MICs, and the utilization of such services by the prescribers is a good indicator of the success of a particular center.

The literature available in our hand indicates the presence of MICs in a variety of countries from the developing world. Such literature represented reporting of the activities undertaken by the centers, rates of medicines information inquiries, classification of requests made, classification of the information users, the satisfaction of the information users, and the impact of the information provided. It is important to notice that some reports presented here are 20 years back since very recent studies are scarce. Also, what is presented here only indicates the availability of the services and describes the pattern of the available reports and does not represent a conclusive listing of the actually available services as some services might be available but not reported.

1. A study was conducted in Saudi Arabia to evaluate electronic information resources for questions received by King Saud University College of Pharmacy Medicines Information Centre (Alnaim & Abuelsoud, 2007). The evaluation included time spent to get an answer, ease of use, comprehensiveness, and availability of information in *Drugdex, Lexi-Drugs*, and the Internet search engine *AltaVista*. Investigators concluded that *Drugdex* and *Lexi-Drugs* are faster, more efficient medicines information databases and all of the three databases were comparable regarding comprehensiveness and availability of information. Using the Internet through the search engine *AltaVista*, in addition to print drug information resources, appears to be a suitable substitute to *Drugdex* and *Lexi-Drugs* when they are not available.
2. A study assessed the utilization of MICs located in four public hospitals of Addis Ababa, Ethiopia, found that most of the queries made came from the public hospitals (69%) and likely from healthcare professionals (94.9%) (Samuel, Dawit, & Ashenef, 2014). Physicians were ranked first in making queries (49.7%) followed by pharmacists (32.8%). The highest number of questions was categorized under therapeutic use followed by general product information and product availability.
3. A telephone interviews were conducted using a semistructured questionnaire to assess the user satisfaction with the services provided by an MIC affiliated with Ministry of Health Khartoum State, Sudan (Fathelrahman, Awang, Bashir, Taha, & Ibrahim, 2008). Most of calls came from within Khartoum State (89.6%). Pharmacists were ranked first in making calls (36.1%), followed by physicians (29.5%) and the public (22.3%). Almost one-fifth, one-half, and one-third of users had made inquiries more than five times, two to five times, and once, respectively. Overall, users reported very high satisfaction with the services received and with the way how the medicines information pharmacists treated them.

4. Another study from Zimbabwe assessed the utilization of the national drugs and poisons information center in Harare, the capital city (Ball, Tagwireyi, & Maponga, 2007). Most of the requests came from within Harare (67%). Pharmacists were ranked first in making medicines information calls (40%), whereas physicians were ranked first in making toxicology-related calls (49%). Among medicines information inquiries, systemic antiinfective (24%) and nervous system agents (20.4%) predominated. Among toxicological inquiries, pesticides (28%) and pharmaceuticals (21%) predominated.
5. A review on records of medicines information inquiries received by the Hospital Universiti Sains Malaysia Drug Information Unit was performed (Ab Rahman and Abu Samah, 1998). Among main findings were the quantity and type of questions received and the categories of users remained relatively constant during a period of 6 years. Most of the requests were directly related to patient care and they came within the university hospital. The use of textbooks as sources for answering questions was the most common practice during the first years of the unit start and it became less common during the subsequent years. This was associated with a gradually increased use of *MICROMEDEX* drug database, which became the most consulted source of information at the end of the studied period.
6. A study was performed to identify the characteristics of the medicines information provided by an MIC of a university hospital in Brazil (Silva et al., 2011 available only as an abstract). There was a variation in the rate and nature of the received inquiries and in the categories of requesters during a period of only 2 years.
7. An assessment of medicines information services provided by pharmacy practice department in Kasturba Hospital, Manipal, a South Indian teaching hospital, was made (George & Rao, 2005). Evaluation included the nature of queries and the quality of the provided services. The majority of the service users were physicians (82%) and medical postgraduate students (16%). Feedback from users indicated their regular use and their high satisfaction with the services provided.
8. After promoting the services of the MIC of Karnataka State Pharmacy Council, India, to healthcare professionals and patients, a dramatic increase in the number of queries received by the center was eminent (Lakshmi, Rao, Gore, & Bhaskaran, 2003). Pediatricians, general physicians, dermatologists, and gynecologists constituted the bulk of the doctors using the center services. Queries received from doctors represented 41.3% after the promotion of the service, while they represented only 13.2% at the beginning. Other requests were from patients, pharmacists, and drug regulatory authorities (Table 22.1).

MANUFACTURERS-BASED INFORMATION SOURCES

Manufacturers of medicines usually represent an important source of information on medicines specifically about the labeled and off-label indications, potential toxicities, and adverse reactions of the medications newly introduced to the market and on other pharmacoepidemiologic information. However, the major limitation of the manufacturers-based information is the potentiality of bias involved in such information. Bias here simply means declaring the information that is considered positive from the provider point of view and hiding the information that is seemed to be negative.

The *MIMS* (i.e., Monthly Index of Medical Specialties) is an inevitable source of information needed by prescribers and pharmacists about products marketed in a particular country or region (Management Sciences for Health, 2012). It is a pocket-size book reference that represents a compilation of technical information prepared originally by the medicines manufacturers at the registration

Table 22.1 Examples of a Variety of Medicines Information Centers-Related Studies and Reports Published From Developing Countries During a Period of 20 Years

Region	The Study	Country	Reported Information
Africa	Samuel et al. (2014)	Ethiopia	Assessment of the utilization of medicines information centers located in four public hospitals of Addis Ababa.
	Ball et al. (2007)	Zimbabwe	Assessment of the utilization of the national drug and poisons information center in Harare, the capital city.
	Fathelrahman et al. (2008)	Sudan	Evaluating user satisfaction with services provided by medicines information center affiliated with Ministry of Health.
Middle East	Alnaim and Abuelsoud (2007)	Saudi Arabia	Evaluation of electronic information resources for question received by a college of pharmacy medicines information center.
Southeastern Asia	Ab Rahman and Abu Samah (1998)	Malaysia	Reviewing records of medicines information inquiries received by the Hospital Universiti Sains Malaysia Drug Information Unit located in Kota Bharu, Kelantan, Malaysia.
Southern Asia	George and Rao (2005)	India	An assessment of medicines information services provided by pharmacy practice department in Kasturba Hospital, Manipal. Evaluation included the nature of queries and the quality of the provided services.
	Lakshmi et al., 2003	India	The utilization of the medicines information center of Karnataka State Pharmacy Council, India.
	Shankar et al. (2007)[a]	Nepal	Describing the scope of the activities and the achievements of drug information center at Manipal Teaching Hospital, Pokhara, Nepal.[a]
Latin America	Silva et al. (2011)	Brazil	Identifying the characteristics of the medicines information provided by a medicines information center of a university hospital in Brazil.
	Hall et al. (2006)[a]	Costa Rica	Describing the operations, activities, and resources of seven medicines information centers and services affiliated with public institutions in Costa Rica[a]

[a]*Such studies are described under the "Achievements" section.*

stage of every medication and has been approved by the regulatory authority in the particular country. It provides basic information on medicines indications, contraindications, dosing, side effects, toxicity, price, etc. *MIMS* can be a country-specific or a regional edition such as *MIMS* Middle East, *MIMS* Asia–Pacific, *MIMS* Africa, and *MIMS* Caribbean and can be a specialty-specific edition such as *MIMS* cardiology, *MIMS* pediatric, and *MIMS* obstetrics and gynecology. A study conducted in community pharmacies in Amman, Jordan, revealed that *MIMS* was the most commonly found medicines information resource (64.7%), whereas 19.2% of respondents declared getting medicines information directly from the pharmaceutical companies representatives (Wazaify et al. 2009).

MEDICINES INFORMATION SOURCES USED BY PRESCRIBERS AND OTHER HEALTHCARE PROVIDERS IN DEVELOPING COUNTRIES

Surveys conducted among prescribers to reveal their information seeking habits and usage patterns of information resources is useful for pharmacists while providing the medicines information services to them. Being aware of the information needs of the healthcare professionals is also helpful in tailoring the necessary assistance.

In Ethiopia, prescribers from different categories of hospitals (i.e., specialized referral, zonal, and district hospitals) are four to six times more likely to consult medicines information resources than the prescribers from healthcare centers (Hussien, Musa, Stergachis, Wabe, & Suleman, 2013). The prescribers complained from difficulty in accessing the required medicines information resources.

In Uganda, the sources of medicines information reported by physicians from district hospitals to be most available were colleagues, and those reported by the physicians from the regional and university hospitals were pharmaceutical companies literature and hard copies of research publications. However, the most commonly used sources in district and regional hospital at one hand and in university hospitals at the other hand, respectively, were National Standard Treatment Guideline and colleagues. Physicians reported difficulty in accessing medicines information from printed and digital research publication in medical journals, MIMS, and pharmacists (Tumwikirize et al., 2009).

In Estonia, main information sources used by healthcare professionals were the datasheet compendium *Pharmaca Estica*, specialty handbooks, medical journals, and medicines manufacturers' representatives (Raal, Fischer, & Irs, 2006). Healthcare professionals surveyed considered manufacturers-based medicines information sufficient according to their needs. However, substantial proportion of them declared that medicines information centers are necessary.

It is clear from the previous reports that the pharmaceutical manufacturers represent an influential source of medicines information among prescribers in various countries, especially when other resources are scarce or absent. Such influence is made via medical representatives' regular visits and communications with prescribers, promotional activities during conferences and medical gatherings. The Internet represents today an additional medium for communicating the manufacturers information. Some multinational companies established professional product information websites that are designed to provide clinicians with the same information that would otherwise be provided in response to a telephone call or a written inquiry (Kennedy, Baker, Riccio, & Song, 2001).

On the other hand, a survey was conducted among emergency medicine clinicians in an academic teaching center located in Brooklyn, New York City, the United States, to identify the medicines information references used for prescribing in pregnant patients (Jellinek, Cohen, Stansfield, Likourezos, & Sable, 2010). The study revealed the reliance of emergency medicine clinicians on general references rather than pregnancy-specific references to prescribe for pregnant patients. An important note to be made here is that such general references include Micromedex, Tarascon Pocket Pharmacopeia, and Epocrates. We know that Micromedex is a very useful and highly updated medicines information resource; however, it is still considered a general reference in a case of pregnancy and more specialized references should be used.

MEDICINES INFORMATION SOURCES USED BY THE PUBLIC IN DEVELOPING COUNTRIES

Understanding the public needs and use of the medicines information and their views and perceptions about various information sources is essential for understanding consumers' behaviors regarding the use, misuse, and abuse of the medications. Due to scarcity in research studies from developing countries, we present here some studies conducted in a number of developed countries. Despite the possible variability between consumers from various countries due to cultural reasons, some attitudes and behaviors are expected to be common and similar.

Mass media, especially the newspapers, used to play great roles in the wide spread of the information and sometimes the perceptions about medicines, medicines use, and their effects among the public. This was true worldwide and it remains true in most of the developing countries in the world today. The Internet and its various applications have reduced such role in some countries. Nevertheless, electronic newspapers are making use of the Internet huge capacity to extend the roles played by traditional newspapers. This makes research studies conducted earlier in the area of journalism and newspapers still useful in understanding the influences and effects of such media on the general public knowledge and their information about medicines.

Moynihan et al. (2000) reviewed a sample of 180 newspaper articles and 27 television reports that appeared between 1994 and 1998 in the United States, covering information about three medications that are used for preventing major diseases, namely, pravastatin, alendronate, and aspirin. The researchers reported that news media stories about medications may include inadequate or incomplete information about the benefits, risks, and costs of the drugs. The researchers reported presence of financial ties between the study groups or experts cited in news media stories and pharmaceutical manufacturers. Another study from the Netherlands revealed that pharmaceutical industry represented the third most frequently cited source of information in the newspaper articles (van Trigt, Haaijer-Ruskamp, Willems, & Tromp, 1994).

Evidences revealed high popularity of online applications of drug information resources among the public. A survey from the United States for example showed Wikipedia and the National Library of Medicine rank highly in online drug searches (Law, Mintzes, & Morgan, 2011).

A study was conducted among consumers visiting community pharmacies in Brisbane, Australia, to assess their perspectives of medication information sources (Tio, LaCaze, & Cottrell, 2007). Written information was ranked first by the majority of them (90%) as a source of information followed by their doctors (83%) and the pharmacists (78%). The consumer perceived that doctors and pharmacists, as information sources, have good knowledge, are trained, and are trusted.

A study from South Africa evaluated the effect of patient information leaflets on acquisition and recall of information about medicines. Researchers compared a simple, shorter patient information leaflet that included descriptive pictograms with two types of text-only patient information leaflets varying in length and complexity. Findings revealed that patient information leaflet incorporating pictograms resulted in better knowledge gain and understanding of medicines information (Mansoor & Dowse, 2007). Another study from the United Kingdom assessed the effectiveness of the information leaflets as a source of information about medicines and addressed the need for additional verbal information. The investigators reported that a large minority of patients have poor reading skills but when the medicine information leaflet is designed to be easy to read, patients gain significant amounts of knowledge. Providing additional verbal clarifications tends to increase patients' knowledge about the medicines (Hill & Bird, 2003).

A survey conducted among adolescents in Uganda found that four-fifth of the adolescents reported that parents, teachers, and other adults represent important sources of their information about health. About half and more than one-third of the adolescents, respectively, reported that they tend to read a book/went to the library and use the computer and Internet to get needed information (Ybarra, Emenyonu, Nansera, Kiwanuka, & Bangsberg, 2008).

ACCESS TO VARIOUS MEDICINES INFORMATION SOURCES IN THE DEVELOPING COUNTRIES

The availability of a medicines information resource does not indicate the usage or the usefulness of such resource. The accessibility and the quality of information are having great effects on the use and the full utilization of such resource. An information user may not be aware of the availability of a particular resource close to him or her. This is why medicines information pharmacists have the responsibility of raising awareness among information users about available resources. This is especially important in the case of a newly established medicine information center or a service. Outreach activities and proactive approach are necessary for marketing a medicines information service. Outreach activities include organizing awareness programs, participating in media campaigns, and publishing locally prepared printed materials such as brochures, medicines information bulletins, and newsletters. This is called proactive approach contrasting the reactive approach, which means merely responding to the inquiries received from information requesters.

The accessibility of an information resource is affected by various factors such as whether such resource is a subscription based or freely available and whether the usage of the resource requires the availability of other facilities such as computers and Internet. In a developing country with limited funds available for healthcare systems, the access to medicine information databases is very difficult. This is further worsened if there is limited or no Internet and/or electricity. Table 22.2 shows examples of some useful online resources for information on medicines and toxicology.

HINARI

Hinari was developed in the framework of the Health InterNetwork, introduced by the UN Secretary General Kofi Annan at the UN Millennium Summit in the year 2000. Hinari was launched in January 2002, with some 1500 journals from six major publishers: Blackwell, Elsevier Science, the Harcourt Worldwide STM Group, Wolters Kluwer International Health & Science, Springer Verlag, and John Wiley, following the principles in a Statement of Intent signed in July 2001. Since that time, the numbers of participating publishers and of journals and other full-text resources have grown continuously. To date, 180 publisher partners and up to 400 publishers' content are offering more than 60,000 information resources in Hinari and many others are joining the program (information copied from Hinari website http://www.who.int/hinari/en/). Any institution from countries eligible for receiving its service (only low- to middle-income countries) can get access to Hinari after registering using an online registration form.

Table 22.3 shows useful sources for providing access to free full-text articles besides Hinari.

Table 22.2 Selected Useful Online Resources for a Variety of Health and Medical Information[a]

Source and Website Address	Primary Users	Sponsored	Nature of Information
PubMed www.pubmed.gov	Medical practitioners and researchers	The US National Library of Medicine	Bibliographic and abstracting information of biomedical literature. It is a secondary resource that contains abstracts of the research and review articles included in MEDLINE database in addition to numerous other resources.
Medline Plus www.medlineplus.gov	Consumers		General medical information for healthcare professionals and consumers and information about prescription and over-the-counter (OTC) medications, dietary supplements, and herbal medicines in language suitable for lay persons.
Clinical Trials.gov http://clinicaltrials.gov	Medical practitioners and researchers	The US National Library of Medicine in collaboration with FDA	An electronic registry of clinical trials conducted in the United States and other countries. The website provides abstracts of study protocols including information such as the study aims, participants' inclusion criteria, location of trial, investigator contact information, study design, and the condition and therapy being studied.
TOXNET: Toxicology Data Network http://toxnet.nlm.nih.gov	Practitioners and poison information specialists and toxicologists	The US National Library of Medicine	Toxic effect of drugs and chemicals including household products and information on general environmental health.
US Food and Drug Administration www.fda.gov	Practitioners and regulators	US Food and Drug Administration	Information on approved drugs, recalls, safety warnings.
Cochrane Database of Systematic Reviews www.thecochranelibrary.com	Medical practitioners and researchers	The Cochrane Library, a production of Cochrane Collaboration	Contains over 5000 systematic reviews and metaanalyses answering clinical questions (only abstracts are freely available, but full-text access requires a subscription). Contents can be accessible in selected situations in low- to middle-income countries.
Google Scholar http://scholar.google.com	Medical practitioners and researchers		Secondary resource/scholarly literature on the Internet.
Medscape www.medscape.com	Healthcare professionals	WebMD	Large database organized by medical specialty. General medical information accessed by registered users only (i.e., contents are freely accessible but require registration).

Continued

Table 22.2 Selected Useful Online Resources for a Variety of Health and Medical Information[a]—cont'd

Source and Website Address	Primary Users	Sponsored	Nature of Information
Mayo Clinic. Drugs and Supplements http://www.mayoclinic.com/health/drug-information/DrugHerbIndex	Consumers and healthcare professionals	Mayo Clinic Foundation	Provides information on OTC and prescription drugs, herbs, supplements, and vitamins. Information on medicines is provided by Micromedex database for drug information.
The International Pharmaceutical Abstracts (IPA) database	Practicing pharmacists and researchers	Established by the American Society of Health-System Pharmacists (ASHP) in 1964, and later on its ownership was transferred to Thomson Scientific, a business of the Thomson Corporation	A comprehensive database provides indexing and abstracts for pharmaceutical and medical journals published worldwide.

[a]For more information, refer to Grossman and Zerilli, (2013) and Lapidus and Dryankova-Bond (2014).

QUALITY OF MEDICINES INFORMATION SOURCES IN THE DEVELOPING COUNTRIES

ASSESSING THE QUALITY AND THE IMPACT OF A MEDICINES INFORMATION SERVICE

Providing high-quality medicines information services and having an access to high-quality medicines information sources should be ultimate goals of every pharmacist, especially those officially involved in the provision of medicines information. The quality of information provided can be measured in terms of satisfying certain standard criteria or in terms of satisfying the needs of the information user. The later varies widely according to the characteristics of the information user whether he or she is a consumer, a patient, or a healthcare provider. The standard criteria of good medicines information include being evidence-based, accurate, up-to-date, objective, unbiased, user-specific, and clinically relevant. Satisfying the needs of a medicines information user means providing the information in a timely manner and providing concise and complete information that is tailored to their actual needs.

Studies evaluating the quality of the information services or resources are focusing mainly on one out of three aspects: (1) the characteristics of the information provided including the accuracy, the appropriateness, and the validity of the information; (2) the users' satisfaction, or (3) the impact of the medicines information on patient care and on population health (Bertsche, Hämmerlein, & Schulz, 2007; Hands, Stephens, & Brown, 2002; Spinewine & Dean, 2002). The impact of a medicines information service is clinical, economic, or humanistic (i.e., patients' quality of life and satisfaction).

Table 22.3 Useful Sources for Providing Access to Free Full-Text Articles (Primary Biomedical Literature)

Source and Website Address	Sponsored	Nature of Information
WHO's Hinari http://www.who.int/hinari/en/	Hinari Programme set up by WHO together with major publishers	Hinari enables low- and middle-income countries to gain access to one of the world's largest collections of biomedical and health literature. Up to 15,000 journals (in 30 different languages), up to 47,000 e-books, up to 100 other information resources are now available to health institutions in more than 100 countries, areas, and territories benefiting many thousands of health workers and researchers, and in turn, contributing to improve world health.
Free Medical Journals http://www.freemedicaljournals.com		Up-to-date it covers 4832 journals. It provides free access to the full texts of contents that are made free by the original publisher immediately, after 1–6 months, after 7–12 months, or later. Some well-known subscription-only journals such as New England Journal of Medicine and British Medical Journal make certain contents available free after certain period.
Directory of Open Access Journals (DOAJ) https://doaj.org/		DOAJ is a community-curated online directory that indexes and provides access to high-quality, open-access, peer-reviewed journals. Up-to-date it includes 9400 journals and about 2.4 million articles from 128 countries.
BioMed Central journals (BMC journals) https://www.biomedcentral.com/journals	BioMed Central is owned by Springer Nature	A publisher with a large portfolio of peer-reviewed open-access journals that cover all areas of biology, medicine, and health. The BMC series of journals is a collection of 65 online research journals published by BMC.
PubMed Central (PMC) https://www.ncbi.nlm.nih.gov/pmc/	The US National Institutes of Health's National Library of Medicine (NIH/NLM)	PMC is a free full-text archive of biomedical and life sciences journal literature. Full text available can be freely accessed via links from PubMed. Up-to-date it includes 4.1 million articles.

ASSESSING THE QUALITY OF PRIMARY LITERATURE

A basic skill for every medicines information provider should be an ability to assess the quality of the primary literature, which is the original research published in the peer-reviewed journal. Despite the filtering process of the peer review system undertaken by biomedical journals, still there are various limitations in the published literature. Accumulating evidence indicates that a significant proportion of the studies published in a variety of biomedical journals cannot be trusted regarding validity and accuracy, and there is a need for establishing some critical appraisal skills to differentiate between high-quality and low-quality studies. Developing critical appraisal skills depends mainly on familiarity with research methodology, study designs, and statistics (the scope of the chapter does not allow for further elaboration on such point and an interested reader should consult a specialized reference).

ASSESSING THE QUALITY OF THE INTERNET-BASED INFORMATION

The major limitations of the medicines information resources available in the Internet are the wide variability in the quality of the information and the uncertainty about its validity and accuracy. This requires that an Internet user be aware of such limitations and be skilled and knowledgeable about approaches that may be used to discern trustable high-quality information from untrusted low-quality information.

The first concern should be identifying the nature and the ownership of the website from which the information is derived, is it a government website (website address ends with .gov), an educational institution (website address ends with .edu), an organization (website address ends with .org), or a commercial website (website address ends with .com)? Grossman and Zerilli (2013) raised the attention of the Internet users to discern the purpose of the site and whether it provides objective information. Grossman and Zerilli ranked websites developed and/or sponsored by an educational institution (.edu), a nonprofit medical organization (.org), or a governmental agency (.gov) first in the likelihood of providing high-quality information compared with commercial websites (.com).

A second concern should be rating the quality of the contents of the website based on availability of the names of the authors/editors of the material, the good referencing, and citation, being regularly updated with dates of publication clearly indicated, having a controllable access policy that requires subscription or prior registration, and displaying the names of the sponsoring and funding bodies (Grossman & Zerilli, 2013). Clauson, Polen, Boulos, and Dzenowagis (2008b) evaluated the scope, completeness, and accuracy of drug information in Wikipedia compared with that of Medscape Drug Reference (MDR). Investigators concluded that Wikipedia has a more narrow scope, is less complete, and has more errors of omission than the comparator database. However, they also concluded it may be a useful point of engagement for consumers.

The American Medical Association (AMA) established guidelines that help in developing and posting contents of websites targeting professionals and consumers with certain standards that satisfy quality, ethical principle, and professionalism (Winker et al., 2000). The guidelines covered aspects such as site ownership; website policy toward site viewing, viewer access, payment, and privacy if applicable; funding and sponsorship of specific contents; quality of editorial content, linking to intrasite contents; intersite navigation; instructions regarding downloadable contents, and navigation of contents.

A medical or a health-related website certified by what is called Health on the Net Foundation (HON) will be trusted since it has been reviewed, approved, and regularly monitored by this noncommercial organization, which is based in Geneva, Switzerland. The HON has established Health on the Net Foundation Code of Conduct (HONcode) to assist with standardizing the reliability and credibility of medical and health information available on the World Wide Web (more information may be sought from the website https://www.hon.ch/). HONcode certification is voluntary, so some health-related websites with an excellent reputation might not be certified as they might not apply for certification (Grossman & Zerilli, 2013). Moreover, a certification does not indicate that all contents of a particular website are reliable, rather it indicate that such website, in general, fulfilled the minimum requirement of quality and ethical standards (Grossman & Zerilli, 2013).

MEDICINES INFORMATION EDUCATION IN DEVELOPING COUNTRIES

Education on medicines information should be well established in the curricula of pharmacy colleges to prepare future pharmacists with the required knowledge and skills needed for good practicing. Basic level courses should be developed both at PharmD and bachelor programs, and advanced level courses can be made available for postgraduate students. Topics to be covered can include types and sources of medicines and medical literature, skills needed for effective searching and retrieval of information, critical appraisal of the literature for evaluating the quality of information, how to receive medicines information calls, how to deliver the information to the user, and how to prepare medicines information publications such as medicines information bulletins and newsletters.

For a college of pharmacy with a PharmD program, medicines information training should be a core component of an advanced pharmacy practice experience (APPE) training in addition to the education provided to the students as a didactic course during years of study. Residencies (postdoctoral programs) in medicines information can be made available as another opportunity for advanced training and specialization. Both opportunities for training (i.e., during APPE and as a residency) had become widely established in the western countries, in particular the United States. In the following we will try to highlight some of the research findings in this regard to assist in establishing similar trends in the developing countries and strengthening such sort of training if already available.

Sixty colleges of pharmacy in the United States were surveyed using an online survey to determine the contents of drug information education (Wang, Troutman, Seo, Peak, & Rosenberg, 2006). Study indicated that 70% of these colleges are having a didactic course on drug information and 85% of the colleges offer an APPE training in drug information.

Graduates of Samford University Mc Whorter School of Pharmacy residing in southeastern states were surveyed to determine whether types of questions received by the respondents during their drug information APPE training at Samford University Global Drug Information Centre are similar to those received while practicing in community settings. The study identified various differences in types of questions received, expected speed of response, and reference utilization. Accordingly, some changes were incorporated into the drug information APPE to solve discrepancies identified by the study (Lauderdale, Kendrach, & Kelly Freeman, 2007).

The University of Tennessee Health Science Centre, College of Pharmacy, in Memphis, Tennessee, developed an industry-based drug information rotation at a medical information company in affiliation with the college of pharmacy. The purposes were to offer pharmacy students during APPE an opportunity of exposure in medicines information training within a pharmaceutical industry setting and to secure additional practice sites for training to face problems associated with the growing number of pharmacy schools (Hurley & Miller, 2009).

In addition, the University of Tennessee Health Science Centre, College of Pharmacy, in Memphis, Tennessee, established a postdoctoral residency with collaborative training from the college of pharmacy, a pharmaceutical industry–based medical information firm and a children's research hospital. This is to offer the trainee an opportunity of exposure to the medicines information service provision in different settings of practice (Tadrous, Gharbawy, Hurley, Miller, & Suda, 2011).

A 2-year, post-PharmD drug information center–based fellowship in natural product research was developed and implemented in the University of Missouri–Kansas City School of Pharmacy Drug Information Centre to address an increased need for evidence-based information about consumer use of natural products (Bryant & McQueen, 2001).

The above reports do not represent a conclusive listing of the only APPE training programs or residencies available in the United States and they are not necessarily be the first colleges to introduce such programs, but rather they represent examples of the variety of options available in the United States.

ACHIEVEMENTS

Reporting about the important achievements of developing countries in the area of medicines information is not easy since it stems from evaluating overall performances across different countries and judging what is coming first and what is the next in terms of importance and impact. In the following we are providing snapshots of nice experiences from a variety of countries from the developing world. The purpose of this description is to offer others an opportunity to learn such experiences and replicating them in their own way.

1. On April 6, 1998, in recognition for its contribution and services in the field of drug and poison information, the National Poison Centre of Malaysia, which is based in Universiti Sains Malaysia, was designated as a WHO Collaborating Centre for Drug Information. The founding of the WHO Collaborating Centre for Drug Information was meant: (a) To establish, develop and facilitate a system of electronic information exchange among member states of Western Pacific Region (WPR) in particular, and WHO in general. (b) To develop, update and implement training modules on Drug Information in developing countries with emphasis on the needs of the Western Pacific Region. (c) To arrange and conduct fellowship training in drugs as well as poison information in support of the concept of rational drug use. (d) To collaborate with the Western Pacific Regional Office in developing computer applications relating to drug information and pharmacoinformatics. (e) To collaborate with the Western Pacific Regional Office in initiating a systematic data and information collection on activities related to the drug utilization, management and policies for identification of priorities and forecasting of needs. (f) To support countries and areas in the region to conceptualize, plan and set up Drug Information Services tailored to individual needs. (g) To undertake relevant drug utilization studies in support of promoting rational use of medicines, develop focused drug information intervention for providers and consumers to improve prescribing and drug use practices, and to undertake proper evaluation of the impact of drug information on rational use of medicines (Information copied from the website of the National Poison Centre of Malaysia http://www.prn.usm.my/who_collaborating_centre.php accessed December 28, 2016).
2. Going beyond medicines information: The drug information center at Manipal Teaching Hospital, Pokhara, Nepal, founded in November 2003 succeeded in providing activities besides the provision of medicines information services such as running a pharmacovigilance center and a medication counseling center (Shankar, Mishra, Subish, & Upadhyay, 2007). The center resources are used for teaching of the undergraduates and for continuing pharmacy education program of pharmacists. The center publishes a quarterly bulletin and support research activities.
3. Between 1983 and 2000, seven public medicines information units have been established in Costa Rica (Hall, Gomez, & Fernandez-Llimos, 2006). Of those, four are MICs and three are medicines information services. The seven MICs and services followed the guidelines established by Pan-American Health Organization (PAHO), and the seven units provide almost comparable wide scope types of activities including as examples answering inquiries from

user from inside as well as outside hospitals; preparation of technical reports for hospital committees; conducting research about drug use and adverse drug reactions; delivering lectures and seminars; participation in continuing education activities; conducting educational programs for patients and high-risk groups; publication of drug bulletins, papers, and booklets; supporting rotation programs for trained students; and preparation of guides on drug use for healthcare team.

4. Information sharing systems: A possible compensation for the lack and the scarcity of information is to establish an information sharing system by constructing a national or a regional medicines information database. The database may contain information needed by all stakeholders in the country or the region similar to the national information sharing system suggested by Muangchoo and Kritchanchai (2015) to serve the healthcare supply chain in Thailand.

CHALLENGES

1. Securing enough funding for establishing and running an MIC in the poorest countries represents a great challenge: A developing country with very limited financial resources will not be able to establish and then run an MIC easily. Even if establishment is achieved via donations or other sources, running the center will not be easily achieved without proper solutions. One of the strategies that should be followed is to build up one regional center instead of establishing a couple of centers that grow weak and become unable to survive. Then the limited scarce resources can be saved to strengthen the center and ensure sustainability of its services. One of the possible solutions is to implement a fee-for-service policy. Several Western countries are having an experience in this regard. A survey sent to medicines information centers in Canada, the United Kingdom, and the United States revealed that 18% of the centers use a fee-for-service system (Ansong, Moody, & Stachnik, 2003). For a developing country, the payers can be the private sector and the industry, which will be willing to pay if their information needs are secured by the medicines information service provider
2. The full access to biomedical literature in the poorest countries: The full access to biomedical literature in the poorest countries where basic resources and infrastructures are lacking represents a challenge to the practicing pharmacists in general and to the medicines information specialists in particular. Pharmacists in such countries are advised to seek access to the required medicines information via registering with WHO's Hinari program.
3. Provision of medicines information about off-label use of medicines: "Off-label medicines use" refers to using a medication for an indication or in a dosage form or for a group of patients, which is not indicated when approved by the regulatory authority. It is very common practice worldwide and it may be unavoidable with a rate reaching 15% to 20% in western settings. It is most common among the groups of patients who are not normally included in the clinical trials that are conducted to evaluate the efficacy and safety of the medications. Those groups included pediatric patients, particularly neonates, adolescents, pregnant women, and psychiatric patients. There is a lack of evidence-based information on the efficacy and safety of a particular medication among the stated groups, and possible information available represents an extrapolation of the evidence generated from research conducted among other groups of patients. Manufacturers' sources of information can be useful in these situations, although such information should be used cautiously.

4. Provision of medicines and toxicological information during bioterrorism and biologic weapons attacks and other emergencies: An attack with a biologic weapon during a terrorism event or a biologic war is a special medical emergency that requires special readiness with poisoning and toxicology information. In such situation a medicines information pharmacist or an MIC is expected to provide the suitable support to the healthcare team and the attacked victims in a timely and an efficient manner.
5. Provision of medicines information during a pandemic: A pandemic is an epidemic of infectious diseases, such as H5N1 avian flu, Zika virus, Ebola virus disease, Rift Valley fever, and severe acute respiratory syndrome, which have spread through human populations across a large geographical areas including multiple continents or even worldwide. During such situations, a medicines information pharmacist or an MIC experiences a rush of high-frequency calls from healthcare providers asking for treatment information, especially at the beginning of an outbreak when healthcare providers are still not fully aware and may be lacking basic information about the disease.

RECOMMENDATIONS: THE WAY FORWARD

1. Poorest countries with limited resources should work on establishing national medicines information centers to cover the needs of the whole country.
2. Different institutions within the same country can work on establishing an information sharing system to facilitate information exchange and building up huge medicines information databases.
3. Collaboration among countries from the same region provides great opportunities to save resources and strengthening the capacities for attaining sustainable high-quality services. This can be achieved via sharing available experiences and resources and can be maximized by building collaborative regional MICs.
4. Institutions from developing countries with no or limited access to high-quality medicines information resources should seek assistance from supportive organizations such as the WHO, which can offer free access to the Hinari database. Other freely available resources should be also sought.
5. Medicines information education should be promoted among colleges of pharmacy at various levels including didactic courses during undergraduate studies, during APPE training of PharmD students and as postgraduate studies and training (i.e., residencies, fellowships, and masters programs).
6. Training for developing and strengthening the medicines information skills should be provided regularly to all practicing pharmacists as part of the continuing professional development (CPD) programs
7. Advanced training can be scheduled for pharmacists working on the provision of medicines information services as part of CPD activities to build their capacities and to raise their competencies.
8. Countries with limited experiences in the area of medicines information should work on to learn from countries having well-established systems of medicines information and try to copy successful innovations.
9. There is a need to monitor and evaluate various resources of medicines information available in the developing countries as well as evaluating the services provided by the medicines information centers. This is very useful for improvement and for the expansion and the sustainability of the services. Evaluations are done by conducting scientific research studies. Such researches should be published to allow others make use of the established evidence.

CONCLUSIONS

Pharmacists should identify and be able to use credible, up-to-date, and high-quality information resources while practicing. The information will be used to build pharmacists own competencies to practice efficiently and ethically and to provide high-quality services. The quality of information can be measured in terms of satisfying certain standard criteria and in terms of satisfying the needs of the information user. Being aware of the information needs of the healthcare professionals is helpful in offering the required assistance that is tailored to the users' needs. The availability of a medicine information resource does not indicate the usage or the usefulness of such resource. The accessibility and the quality of information are having great effects on the use and the full utilization of such resource. Securing enough funding for establishing and running an MIC in the poorest countries represents a great challenge. Education on medicines information should be well established in the curricula of pharmacy colleges to prepare future pharmacists with the required knowledge and skills needed for good practicing.

LESSONS LEARNED

- Collaboration between academia, hospitals, and industry provides great opportunity to achieve distinguished successes in research and for securing resources in the area of medicines information.
- Implementation of a fee-for-service system where the payer can be the private sector and the industry, which will be willing to pay if their information needs are secured by the medicines information service provider.
- Publications documenting the source, access, extent, and quality of information available among pharmacists and pharmacy personnel in developing countries are scarce, and this needs the attention of medicines information specialists, educators, researchers, and policy makers

REFERENCES

Ab Rahman, A., & Samah, N. A. A. (1998). The drug information service at a university hospital in Malaysia: Characteristics of drug inquiries. *Drug Information Journal*, *32*(1), 293–298.

Abate, M. A. (2001). Drug information resources and literature retrieval. In *American college of clinical pharmacy, PSAP pharmacotherapy self-assessment program* (4th ed.). Kansas City, MO: ACCP.

Alnaim, L. S., & Abuelsoud, N. N. (2007). Evaluation of electronic information resources for questions received by a college of pharmacy drug information center. *Drug Information Journal*, *41*(4), 441–448.

Anonymous. (2012). Chapter 34: Medicine and therapeutics information. In *Management sciences for health, MDS-3: managing access to medicines and health technologies*. Arlington, VA: management Sciences for Health pp. 34.1–34.16.

Ansong, M. A., Moody, M. L., & Stachnik, J. (2003). Fee-for-service drug information centers. *Drug Information Journal*, *37*(2), 233–239.

Ball, D. E., Tagwireyi, D., & Maponga, C. C. (2007). Drug information in Zimbabwe: 1990–1999. *Pharmacy World & Science*, *29*(3), 131–136. http://dx.doi.org/10.1007/s11096-007-9110-6.

Bertsche, T., Hämmerlein, A., & Schulz, M. (2007). German national drug information service: User satisfaction and potential positive patient outcomes. *Pharmacy World & Science*, *29*(3), 167–172. http://dx.doi.org/10.1007/s11096-006-9041-7.

Bryant, P. J., & McQueen, C. E. (2001). Conception and implementation of a drug information center based fellowship in natural product research. *Journal of Herbal Pharmacotherapy*, *1*(3), 17–24.

Clauson, K. A., Fass, J. A., & Seamon, M. J. (2008a). Legal requirements for drug information resources maintained by pharmacies. *Drug Information Journal*, *42*(6), 569–582.

Clauson, K. A., Polen, H. H., Boulos, M. N. K., & Dzenowagis, J. H. (2008b). Scope, completeness, and accuracy of drug information in Wikipedia. *Annals of Pharmacotherapy*, *42*(12), 1814–1821.

Elenbaas, R. M., & Worthen, D. B. (2009). Transformation of a profession: An overview of the 20th century. *Pharmacy in History*, *51*(4), 151–182.

Fathelrahman, A. I., Awang, R., Bashir, A. A., Taha, I. A. M., & Ibrahim, H. M. (2008). User satisfaction with services provided by a drug information center in Sudan. *Pharmacy World & Science*, *30*(6), 759–763. http://dx.doi.org/10.1007/s11096-008-9245-0.

George, B., & Rao, P. G. (2005). Assessment and evaluation of drug information services provided in a South Indian teaching hospital. *Indian Journal of Pharmacology*, *37*(5), 315.

Grossman, S., & Zerilli, T. (2013). Health and medication information resources on the world wide web. *Journal of Pharmacy Practice* 0897190012474231.

Hall, V., Gomez, C., & Fernandez-Llimos, F. (2006). Situation of drug information centers and services in Costa Rica. *Pharmacy Practice*, *4*(2), 83–87.

Hands, D., Stephens, M., & Brown, D. (2002). A systematic review of the clinical and economic impact of drug information services on patient outcome. *Pharmacy World and Science*, *24*(4), 132–138. http://dx.doi.org/10.1023/A:1019573118419.

Hill, J., & Bird, H. (2003). The development and evaluation of a drug information leaflet for patients with rheumatoid arthritis. *Rheumatology*, *42*(1), 66–70.

Hughes, P. J., Kendrach, M., Schrimsher, R. H., Wensel, T. M., & Freeman, M. K. (2011). Assessment of electronic drug information resource availability in Alabama pharmacies. *Drug Information Journal*, *45*(6), 797–803.

Hurley, A. M., & Miller, E. S. (2009). Establishing an industry-based drug information pharmacy student rotation. *Drug Information Journal*, *43*(2), 151–158.

Hussien, N., Musa, S., Stergachis, A., Wabe, N. T., & Suleman, S. (2013). Drug information prescribers' need for and access to drug information resources in Ethiopia. *Therapeutic Innovation & Regulatory Science*, *47*(2), 219–225.

Jellinek, S. P., Cohen, V., Stansfield, L., Likourezos, A., & Sable, K. N. (2010). A survey of drug information references emergency medicine clinicians utilize for prescribing in pregnant patients. *Annals of Pharmacotherapy*, *44*(3), 456–461.

Kennedy, A. M., Baker, R. P., Riccio, K. J., & Song, K. H. (2001). Development and implementation of a drug information Web site for health care professionals. *Drug Information Journal*, *35*(2), 561–568.

Khan, T. M., Emeka, P., & Khan, A. H. (2013). Drug information activity and nonprescription requests over the Malaysian counter. *Therapeutic Innovation & Regulatory Science* 2168479012462214.

Lakshmi, P. K., Rao, D. G., Gore, S. B., & Bhaskaran, S. (2003). Drug information services to doctors of Karnataka, India. *Indian Journal of Pharmacology*, *35*(4), 245–247.

Lapidus, M., & Dryankova-Bond, I. (2014). Free drug information resources on the internet. *Journal of Consumer Health on the Internet*, *18*(4), 367–376.

Lauderdale, S. A., Kendrach, M. G., & Kelly Freeman, M. (2007). Preparing students for community pharmacy practice during a drug information advanced practice experience. *American Journal of Pharmaceutical Education*, *71*(2), 25.

Law, M. R., Mintzes, B., & Morgan, S. G. (2011). The sources and popularity of online drug information: An analysis of top search engine results and web page views. *Annals of Pharmacotherapy*, *45*(3), 350–356.

Lum, C., & Ahn, S. M. (2012). The correction of product information in drug references and medical textbooks. *Drug Information Journal*, *46*(1), 94–98.

Mansoor, L., & Dowse, R. (2007). Written medicines information for South African HIV/AIDS patients: Does it enhance understanding of co-trimoxazole therapy? *Health Education Research*, *22*(1), 37–48.

Moynihan, R., Bero, L., Ross-Degnan, D., Henry, D., Lee, K., Watkins, J., … Soumerai, S. B. (2000). Coverage by the news media of the benefits and risks of medications. *New England Journal of Medicine*, *342*(22), 1645–1650.

Muangchoo, S., & Kritchanchai, D. (2015). National drug information sharing in the Thailand health care supply chain. *Therapeutic Innovation & Regulatory Science*, *49*(6), 920–928.

Raal, A., Fischer, K., & Irs, A. (2006). Determination of drug information needs of health care professionals in Estonia. *Medicina*, *42*(12), 1030–1034.

Samuel, F., Dawit, H., & Ashenef, A. (2014). Utilization of recently established drug information centers located in the public hospitals of Addis Ababa, Ethiopia an assessment. *Therapeutic Innovation & Regulatory Science*, *48*(3), 378–385.

Schrimsher, R. H., Freeman, M. K., & Kendrach, M. (2006). A survey of drug information resources in Alabama pharmacy facilities. *Drug Information Journal*, *40*(1), 51–60.

Shankar, P. R., Mishra, P., Subish, P., & Upadhyay, D. K. (2007). The drug information center at the Manipal teaching hospital—going beyond drug information. *Drug Information Journal*, *41*(6), 761–768.

Silva, V. N., Diniz, R. S., Egito, E. S., Azevedo, P. R., Vidotti, C. C., & Araujo, I. B. (2011). A way to evaluate the peculiarities of drug information centers in university hospitals. *Latin American Journal of Pharmacy*, *30*(5), 902–907.

Spinewine, A., & Dean, B. (2002). Measuring the impact of medicines information services on patient care: Methodological considerations. *Pharmacy World and Science*, *24*(5), 177–181. http://dx.doi.org/10.1023/A:1020575031753.

Tadrous, M., Gharbawy, D. E., Hurley, A. M., Miller, E. S., & Suda, K. J. (2011). Establishing a complete drug information Triad: Academic, Industry, and Hospital Training. *Drug Information Journal*, *45*(5), 641–644.

Tio, J., LaCaze, A., & Cottrell, W. N. (2007). Ascertaining consumer perspectives of medication information sources using a modified repertory grid technique. *Pharmacy World & Science*, *29*(2), 73–80. http://dx.doi.org/10.1007/s11096-006-9076-9.

Tumwikirize, W. A., Ogwal-Okeng, J. W., Vernby, A., Anokbonggo, W. W., Gustafsson, L. L., & Lundborg, C. L. (2009). Access and use of medicines information sources by physicians in public hospitals in Uganda: A cross-sectional survey. *African Health Sciences*, *8*(4), 220–226.

Udezi, W. A., Oparah, A. C., & Enyi, K. U. (2007). An investigation of drug information needs of Nigerian pharmacists. *Drug Information Journal*, *41*(4), 471–479.

van Trigt, A. M., Haaijer-Ruskamp, F. M., Willems, J., & Tromp, T. F. (1994). Journalists and their sources of ideas and information on medicines. *Social Science & Medicine*, *38*(4), 637–643.

Wang, F., Troutman, W. G., Seo, T., Peak, A., & Rosenberg, J. M. (2006). Drug information education in doctor of pharmacy programs. *American Journal of Pharmaceutical Education*, *70*(3).

Wazaify, M., Maani, M., & Ball, D. (2009). Drug information resources at community pharmacies in Amman, Jordan. *International Journal of Pharmacy Practice*, *17*(3), 151–155.

Winker, M. A., Flanagin, A., Chi-Lum, B., White, J., Andrews, K., Kennett, R. L., … Musacchio, R. A. (2000). Guidelines for medical and health information sites on the internet: Principles governing AMA web sites. *JAMA*, *283*(12), 1600–1606.

Wong, P. S. J., Ko, Y., & Sklar, G. E. (2009). Identification and evaluation of pharmacists' commonly used drug information sources. *Annals of Pharmacotherapy*, *43*(2), 347–352.

Ybarra, M. L., Emenyonu, N., Nansera, D., Kiwanuka, J., & Bangsberg, D. R. (2008). Health information seeking among Mbararan adolescents: Results from the Uganda media and you survey. *Health Education Research*, *23*(2), 249–258.

SECTION 10

GOOD GOVERNANCE AND PHARMACEUTICAL POLICY IN LOW- AND MIDDLE-INCOME COUNTRIES

CHAPTER

23

PROBLEMS AND OBSTACLES OF POOREST COUNTRIES IN HAVING GOOD GOVERNANCE AND QUALITY AND EFFECTIVE PHARMACEUTICAL POLICY

Sonak Pastakia[1,2], Benson Njuguna[2], Dan N. Tran[1,2]

[1]Purdue University College of Pharmacy, Eldoret, Kenya; [2]Moi Teaching and Referral Hospital, Eldoret, Kenya

CHAPTER OUTLINE

Social and Administrative Aspects of Pharmacy in Low- and Middle-Income Countries. http://dx.doi.org/10.1016/B978-0-12-811228-1.00023-6

INTRODUCTION

Pharmaceutical policy is the framework which guides the practice of global and regional health organizations, country governments, and hospitals in their quest to promote access to and rational use of quality-assured medicines to the populations they serve (WHO, 2001). Effective pharmaceutical policies should enable the provision of a reliable, adequate, and consistent access of quality-assured medicines that patients can afford and use as required (WHO, 2001). As with any other policy document, it is possible to formulate a framework for action that works extremely well in theory but may never materialize into practice. Indeed, for many pharmaceutical policies, despite extremely well-researched and thought-out pharmaceutical policy statements, the objectives set out by such policies remain suboptimally implemented for a majority of low- and middle-income countries (LMICs) (Hoebert, van Dijk, Mantel-Teeuwisse, Leufkens, & Laing, 2013; Tran & Bero, 2015).

To judge the effectiveness of a pharmaceutical policy, one must first identify what the intended goals of the policy are and then use these as a yard stick to compare how the current state of affairs reflects the intentions of these policies. The goals of pharmaceutical policies vary based on available resources, prevailing population healthcare needs, and the socioeconomic status of the intended population (Hoebert et al., 2013). The focus of this chapter (and book) is on the poorest world settings. In this respect, we consider these settings to be countries that, at this point in time, are classified by the World Bank as being low-income countries (LICs) or lower-middle-income countries (LMICs). For these settings, the overarching goal of pharmaceutical policy is to ensure (1) equitable availability and affordability of medicines, (2) safe and efficacious medicines, and (3) therapeutically sound and cost-effective use of medicines and healthcare providers and patients in the entire population (WHO, 2001, 2016b). The desired outcomes of these goals are to promote better individual and public health by preventing, treating, and limiting the complications of the major diseases that afflict LICs and LMICs. Table 23.1 summarizes a few highlighted pharmaceutical policies that were developed by international agencies with these goals and anticipated impacts in mind.

However, an appropriate starting point for this discussion is to assess how effective have pharmaceutical policies been thus far in LMICs. Given implementation barriers described in the above table with highlighted policy examples, it is inevitable that translating pharmaceutical policy from a document into practice requires good governance (Fig. 23.1). According to the World Health Organization (WHO), good governance refers to a fundamental need to have in place laws, regulations, policies, and procedures based on ethical principles to improve the management of pharmaceutical systems and create a corrupt-free environment to promote realization of the goals of pharmaceutical policy (WHO, 2014). However, significant obstacles to good governance, and consequently, obstacles to effective pharmaceutical policy, exist in LMICs with the consequence of poor health outcomes for these populations (Fig. 23.1).

Table 23.1 Highlighted Pharmaceutical Policies, Their Anticipated Impacts, and Challenges to On-The-Ground Implementation

Policy Statement	Anticipated Impact	Implementation Challenges
WHO Essential Medicines List (WHO, 1977)	A list of minimum medicine needs for a basic healthcare system, listing the most efficacious, safe, and cost-effective medicines for priority conditions.	Most countries follow this list; however, they have not been able to ensure reliable access for patients in the public sector. Barriers at all health system levels must be addressed to improve access and quality use of medicines.
WHO Operational Principles for Good Pharmaceutical Procurement (WHO, 1999)	A list of 4 strategic objectives and 12 operational principles to improve good pharmaceutical procurement practices.	Inefficient consumption forecasting techniques, stock deficiencies of certain pharmaceuticals in some facilities and excesses in others in "push system," absence of real-time documentation and integration of information up and down the supply chain leading to low availability of medicines in "pull system."
Doha Declaration ("WHO: The Doha Declaration on the Trips Agreement and Public Health," 2001)	Declaration ensures that governments may issue compulsory licenses on patients for medicines or take other steps to protect public health.	Legal right to obtain a product does not mean that it can afford the product, especially if start-up costs must be covered. Manufacture of drugs under compulsory license for countries that may lack the capability to manufacture the drugs.
WHO Guidelines for Medicines Donation (WHO, 2011a)	Improve the quality of medicine donations in international development assistance and emergency aid. Promote good medicine donation practice in both donors and recipients.	Inefficiency in coordinating donations, inadequate staffing by pharmacists and logistics experts, poor communication with donating agencies. Emergency drug donations are not guided by essential medicines lists or adherent to the guidelines.
WHO Good Governance for Medicines (GGM) (WHO, 2014)	A framework that focuses on fundamental laws and regulations, policies, and procedures to improve the management of pharmaceutical systems and create a corrupt-free environment to promote access to quality-assured medicines.	Corruption, GGM framework not fully developed, endorsed, or adopted implementation gaps.
WHO Guidelines for Country Pharmaceutical Pricing Policies (WHO, 2015b)	A set of policy interventions regarding pharmaceutical pricing, tax exemptions or reductions for pharmaceutical products, cost-plus pricing formula, external reference pricing, promotion of generic drug use, and health technology assessment to guide national policy makers to managing pharmaceutical pricing.	Low drug availability (low supply) coupled with high rates of out-of-pocket purchases (high demand) drives up pricing of drugs above the international reference prices.
WHO Regional Strategy for Human Resources for Health (WHO, 2015a)	Policy options and practical guidance to develop and sustain health workforces that enhance health systems performance and service quality and improve health outcomes.	Inadequate human resources for health and inefficient utilization of trained health workers.

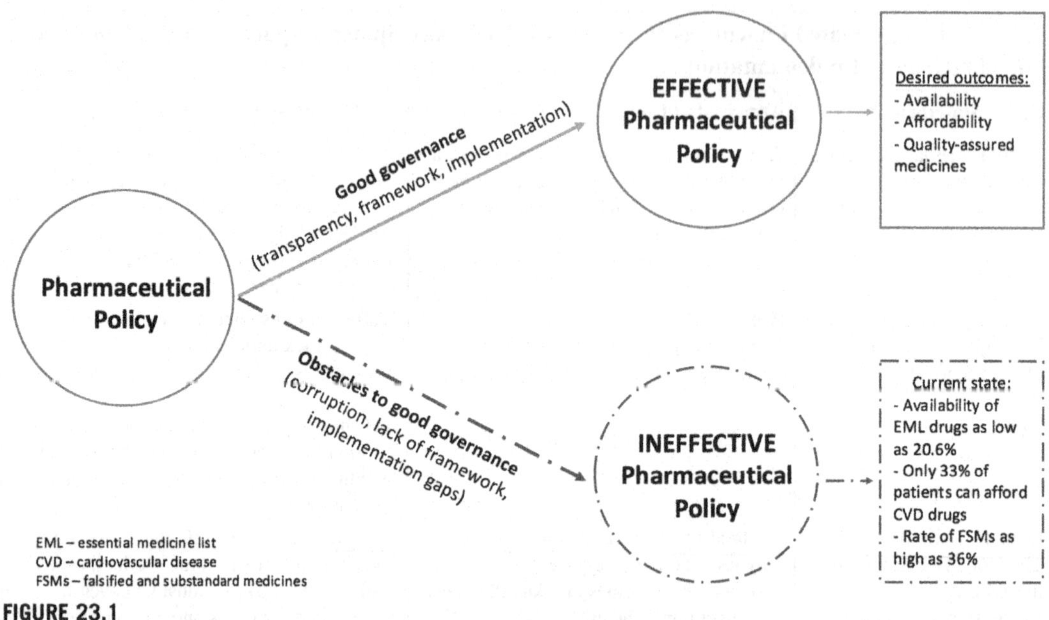

FIGURE 23.1

Pathway to effective and ineffective pharmaceutical policy and governance.

In part 1 of this chapter, we will discuss the challenges and obstacles of good governance and effective pharmaceutical policy that LMICs face. We will limit our discussion to "on-the ground" obstacles faced by everyday healthcare personnel and patients and those that cut across most such settings. Our focus is informed by the need to stimulate discussion on finding simple solutions that can be applied to similar settings and that can readily be implemented to achieve high impact at low cost. In part 2, we will present a case vignette to exemplify initial achievements from how the world responded to the need for effective pharmaceutical policy to ensure the health of millions of HIV patients in LMICs through demonstrating good governance and filling implementation gaps.

PART 1: CHALLENGES—OBSTACLES TO GOOD GOVERNANCE AND QUALITY AND EFFECTIVE PHARMACEUTICAL POLICY

HEALTHCARE FINANCING

Financing in pharmaceutical care and healthcare is an important component of policy governance and implementation to ensure access to affordable essential medicines and health services. Under the Abuja Declaration in 2001, the African Union pledged to spend at least 15% of annual expenditure on health (WHO, 2011b). Over the years, we have seen an improvement in budget allocations to health, evidenced by an average annual public expenditure on health of 10% (ranging from 4% to 17%) in the African region (WHO, 2016a). However, this increase in domestic resources, coupled with a rise in external aid, still has not adequately helped the African region to meet its target goal. Even though LMICs may have limited resources with many other competing priorities besides healthcare financing, it is argued that the inefficient management system of public finance is one of the major rate limiting steps to better health budget planning and utilization decisions (WHO, 2016a).

Suboptimal Health Budget Allocation

As revenues and resources become more available to LICs, one might suspect that these countries may choose to focus prioritizing health spending. On the contrary, it has been shown that some LIC governments have in fact deprioritized health expenditure because of country instability, poor governance, and corruption (Liang & Mirelman, 2014; WHO, 2016a). As a result, financial support for the healthcare sector has suffered from funding instability, making it difficult for effective planning and implementation in many aspects of pharmaceutical supplies and health service delivery.

Ineffective Management of Health Budgets

In addition to suboptimal financial support, budgets that are not well managed due to public financial management deficiencies can lead to health budget underspending. Underspending can be due to unpredictable allocations (unpredictable revenue sources lead to health budget cuts), mismatch between policy and budget allocations (budget allocations do not meet national priorities), inappropriate budget structures (rigidities in line-item budgeting), and underperforming execution system in health (the use of discretionary or nonwage expenditures) (WHO, 2016a).

Inefficient Use of Resources for Health

As primary care has not been prioritized in many LICs, public health budgets tend not to be as accessible for vulnerable populations such as rural patient populations who are financially unstable. In Africa, it has been estimated that patients who are financially advantaged are able to access healthcare services two to seven times more often than patients who are from financially unstable areas (WHO, 2016a). Within the supply chain management of pharmaceuticals, corruption and diversion of funds represent some of the most significant barriers to increasing transparency and ultimately access to medicines for vulnerable patient populations.

Current pharmaceutical governance efforts exist to enhance transparency and minimize corruption. For example, the WHO's Good Governance for Medicines (GGM) program has recommended the development of a stepwise framework to assess transparency, develop a national GGM framework, and implementation of the GGM program (WHO, 2014). Although successes have been recognized in many countries, common challenges that prevent GGM from working effectively in other countries include low priority of good governance by ministries of health, poor understanding of the culture of transparency, resistance to change, lack of adequate monitoring, and evaluation tools for follow-up (WHO, 2014).

SUPPLY CHAIN MANAGEMENT

Existence of Parallel Systems

Parallel systems in pharmaceutical supply chains refer to having nonintegrated systems for the delivery of one or more commodities. An example of a parallel system includes drug donations to LMICs. Drug donations are medicines that are given at no cost by nongovernment organizations, other resource-rich countries, or other donors (Bero, Carson, Moller, & Hill, 2010). Drug donations can be useful in many situations by providing assistance in emergencies, supplying long-term use for chronic disease medicines, or recycling medicines that have short expiry dates (Bero et al., 2010). Despite the WHO Guidelines for Drug Donations and the establishment of the Partnership for Quality Medical Donations, it has been reported that several donations do not comply with these guidelines (Bero et al., 2010; Fire, 2016). It is important to note that even though no changes needed to be made with policy documents, difficulties in enforcing the guidelines are due to lack of infrastructure for monitoring donated medicines (WHO, 2011a). Even though this nonintegrated approach may improve the supply chain for a specific disease of interest or a specific occasion, it does not provide a comprehensive and cost-effective solution for the lack of access to medicines in LMICs.

Poor Stock Management Practices

In 1999, WHO, United Nations Children's Fund, United Nations Population Fund, and the World Bank issued a statement with recommendations for 12 operational principles for good pharmaceutical procurement. These principles include strategies for efficient and transparent management, drug selection and quantification, financing and competition, and supplier selection and quality assurance (WHO, 1999). Despite these efforts, many challenges still exist with pharmaceutical procurement and stock management. Firstly, inefficient consumption forecasting techniques hamper the ability to anticipate and stock adequate quantities of pharmaceuticals that are required to serve the population (Yadav, 2015). This dynamic leads to consistently reported low availability of pharmaceutical stocks (Yadav, 2015). Secondly, push systems of stock management utilized in some LMIC supply chain systems lead to excesses and deficiencies in stock. In a push system, the central health store (CHS), usually a government entity, distributes drugs to the facilities it serves based on availability of commodities in the CHS without regard for the stock status of "pushed items" in the receiving facilities (Yadav, 2015). This setup often leads to stock deficiencies of certain pharmaceuticals in some facilities and excesses in others. For example, a recent WHO study found that in the public sector, the availability of noncommunicable disease medicines is much less than that for communicable diseases (36% vs. 53%) (Hanna & Kangolle, 2010). Thirdly, in settings that operate using the "pull" system (whereby facilities request for drug stock based on their consumption and current levels), absence of real-time documentation and integration of information up and down the supply chain in stock management delays decision-making in supplying pharmaceuticals, leading to low availability of pharmaceuticals in some facilities because of time lags between demand/order placement and supply (Yadav, 2015). Part of this problem is that most facilities are required at the end of a given time period (monthly or quarterly) to conduct a physical stocktake, generate reports on stock status, estimate consumption, and place new drug orders for the next period of time. Not only does this system create a redundancy that results in business and personnel outage for the period of the stocktake, but also orders are often placed at prespecified intervals rather than based on medication availability (Yadav, 2015). This dynamic often leads to a lag time between when the order is made and when delivery occurs, leading to stock outages.

SELECTION OF ESSENTIAL MEDICINES AND MEDICINE AFFORDABILITY

The WHO Essential Medicines List (EML) was developed in 1977 with the goal of guiding the development of national and institutional EMLs to improve access to medicines, availability, safety, and cost-effectiveness. Even though the EML has been adapted in several countries, studies have reported dismal drug availability and unaffordability for essential drugs in LMICs. It was estimated that drug availability of essential drugs in LMIC health facilities was as low as 20.6% in

2014 (Bazargani, Ewen, de Boer, Leufkens, & Mantel-Teeuwisse, 2014). Finally, an analysis of affordability of four CVD medicines in 18 different communities in LMICs revealed that only 33% of households in low-income countries and 60% of LMICs were able to afford these medicines (Yusuf et al., 2011). The WHO Guideline on Country Pharmaceutical Pricing Policies recommended sound and rational policy interventions on regulation of markups in the pharmaceutical supply and distribution chain, tax exemptions/reductions for pharmaceutical products, use of external reference pricing, promotion of use of generic medicines (WHO, 2015b). However, as exemplified by the above studies, which are by no means exhaustive, essential medicines are still largely unaffordable and account for substantial family expenditure. Countries such as India have a long history of introducing regulations which cap the price of certain essential medications; however, adaptation of these policies across other LMICs has not been adequate (Swain, 2014). Ensuring access, quality, and affordability to all essential medicines requires that barriers and implementation gaps at all health system levels be adequately addressed.

HUMAN RESOURCE

Health workforce has been described as one of the six crucial system building blocks within the WHO health systems framework (WHO, 2015a). There is still a global shortage of health workers estimated at more than 4 million doctors, pharmacists, nurses, midwives, and others (Gall, Bates, & Bruno, 2012; Hawthorne & Anderson, 2009; WHO, 2015a). Low numbers of health workers are invariably found where health needs are greatest, hence the need to frame policies and actions for human resources for health (HRH) within the context of "equity and health." The Regional Strategy on Human Resources for Health, published by the WHO Western Pacific Region, recommended three key focus areas within their framework of action: (1) health workforce response to population health needs; (2) health workforce development, deployment, and retention; and (3) health workforce governance and management (WHO, 2015a) Despite these calls for action, the health workforce crisis still exists, partly due to the reasons discussed below.

Inadequate Human Resources for Health

Delivery of optimal healthcare services in a majority of developing countries has been hampered by many factors with the lack of HRH being one of the main challenges. Inadequate or lack of sufficient human resources results in a decline in quality and quantity of the services provided. In most LMICs, the lack of human resources hinders the implementation of numerous healthcare interventions (Chen et al., 2004). In achieving the goals of effective pharmaceutical policy, limited HRH hampers the ability to deliver pharmaceutical care due to a lack of trained providers such as pharmacists and pharmaceutical technologists, as well as undermining effective commodity management due to lack of trained pharmacists and supply chain officers (Ssengooba et al., 2007).

A picture commonly observed in a majority of developing countries is the presence of a high concentration of highly trained professionals in urban centers and private institutions and a low concentration of the same in the rural areas where a majority of the population who needs health services is concentrated (Hongoro & McPake, 2004). The lower World Bank Income Status Classification of a country, the fewer pharmacists, and pharmacies are present to serve the population (Gall et al., 2012). This lower density of care providers and pharmacy access points in LMICs is unable to reliably provide access to medicines to the population.

Inefficient Utilization of Human Resources for Health

Variance in skill levels of different healthcare professionals is a key component of the deficiencies in the HRH. Qualifications well above the minimum are routinely being utilized at skill levels that are well below what the healthcare personnel are trained. In some cases, there are an excess of particular specialties. This in turn leads to duplication of roles and insufficient utilization of the available human resources (Ssengooba et al., 2007). In some settings, for instance, a pharmacy degree is acquired over 4 years of specialty training, whereas a diploma in pharmacy is acquired over 3 years of less specialized training. At the end of the training, however, these two different cadres, which demand different rates of recompense, end up often doing similar jobs. Some countries have noticed this gap and have attempted to shift the role of pharmacists into management of supplies, which, although reasonable, then creates redundancies with supply chain officers.

QUALITY ASSURANCE

Regulatory Agencies Weak or Nonexistent

Although resource-rich settings have developed robust structures to counter the falsified and substandard medicine (FSM) threat and assure the quality of medicines provided to their populations, these structures are largely absent in lower resource settings. In a report analyzing poor-quality antimalarial medicines in Southeast Asia and sub-Saharan Africa, up to 36% of medicines were classified as falsified (Nayyar, Breman, Newton, & Herrington, 2012). Recently, 16.3% of medications for cardiovascular diseases were deemed to be of poor quality in a study assessing quality of CVD medicines in sub-Saharan Africa (Antignac et al, 2016). The limited ability of LMICs to battle the FSM burden is due to underdeveloped medication regulatory infrastructure that is characterized by lack of, and/or weakly implemented, regulatory policies and a limited number of WHO prequalified laboratories (Ranieri et al., 2014).

High Costs of Operation (Testing and Personnel)

Where testing infrastructure is available, chemical analysis of medications is quite expensive and requires advanced technical training, which is challenging (Eliasson & Matousek, 2007; Ranieri et al., 2014). Inadequate financing toward healthcare comprises one major factor limiting the ability of country health organizations to build their capacity to more effectively identify and halt FSMs in their market, particularly in the context of competing health priorities for limited resources.

Corruption

Although the above two factors lead to the introduction of FSMs into the market, this propagation of weak regulation and cost-inefficient operation is further enhanced by corrupt dealings in the registration of drugs, drug manufacturers, distributors, and sellers with the consequence of creating and sustaining a supply chain for FSMs that goes unchecked (Ranieri et al., 2014).

IRRATIONAL DRUG USE

Irrational drug use broadly refers to the inappropriate prescription, dispensing, sale, and use of drugs (van Mourik, Cameron, Ewen, & Laing, 2010). Although effective pharmaceutical policy in LMICs should ensure universal access to essential drugs, irrational drug use undercuts this objective in various ways. Brand prescribing of expensive brand name drugs and overprescribing of drugs are potential factors for patients' noncompliance to prescribed medicines. Consequently, this may lead to poor treatment outcomes and complications requiring higher cost interventions.

Brand Prescribing

Brand prescribing refers to a practice whereby patients are instructed to seek a particular brand of medicine. Brand name drugs are typically more expensive to acquire for patients in LMICs (Flegel, 2012). In addition to prescribing specific brand name drugs, some clinicians may even warn against lower cost substitutes. Although brand prescribing may be required with some medications where there may be concern over generic bioequivalence, such as with antiepileptics, generic prescribing is appropriate in most instances as quality-assured generics work just as well as branded medications (Rascati, Richards, Johnsrud, & Mann, 2009). Although prescribers may prescribe branded products based on their own experience or perceptions of efficacy and safety in healthcare systems, which lack proactive quality assurance, for some, it may be as a result of influence from pharmaceutical representatives who may offer incentives for them to prescribe their products such as emoluments to attend conferences (Flegel, 2012). Clinicians, particularly in the public sector who are responsible for raising prescriptions for their patients, should focus on generic prescribing, using drugs on the EML to ensure that drug policies in place are adequately addressing the population drug needs. This promotion of lower-cost generic substitutes could be greatly enhanced if proactive monitoring of medication quality implemented to assure both the patients and providers of the integrity of the supply chain.

Overprescribing

This refers to the prescription of drugs in cases where they are not clinically indicated, such as prescription for antibacterials for viral illnesses. Overprescribing may reflect inadequate diagnostic practices, a lack of knowledge on appropriate use of medicines by the clinician, or a perceived pressure to prescribe medicines to a patient seeking healthcare (Seiter, 2010). In some instances, however, conflicts of interest may be the driving factor, such as when prescribers are also dispensers and therefore seek increased revenue by prescribing unnecessary drugs (Parker, Wardle, Weir, & Stewart, 2011). All of these factors combine to lead to increases in irrational use of medications, which carries considerable expense for patients and the health system at large, which is seeing a rise in antimicrobial resistance due in large part to irrational use.

Patient Nonadherence

Patient nonadherence is another example of irrational drug use that in the long run has an impact on the effectiveness of pharmaceutical policy. When patients fail to take their medications as required, the detrimental health outcomes that occur may lead to higher costs of care associated with complications. For example, a patient with uncontrolled hypertension due to medication nonadherence could subsequently develop chronic kidney disease requiring more costly interventions such as kidney transplant and future use of pricey immunosuppressant drugs. Without the consideration of the importance of adherence within pharmaceutical policy and governance, we will limit the gains we can achieve in patient outcomes. By targeting the barriers that continue to impede adherence, we can make our supply chains more responsive to patient needs and reduce the overall costs to the healthcare system.

MONITORING AND EVALUATION

Most developing countries have adopted some form of monitoring and evaluation to assess the progress of the different interventions being carried out. Most of these monitoring and evaluation systems fail to provide the right data at the right time to the policy makers. Paper-based reporting tools are still being utilized in some developing countries resulting in delayed transmission of information to policy makers who in turn utilize this outdated information in making decisions. Consequently, there is a disintegration of the reports from the whole process of monitoring and evaluation. This creates a scenario whereby additional steps need to be performed for decisions to be made.

Lack of inclusion of all stakeholders in the decision-making process hinders the implementation of laid out policies. In most developing countries, there is limited participation of civil societies as well as governments in formulation, implementation, and monitoring of health policies. In those cases, with participation from both sectors, there is inadequate coordination of the whole monitoring and evaluation process, which in turn defeats the purpose of such a measure. In the absence of effective monitoring, there is corruption and mismanagement of healthcare resources. Similarly, failure to routinely assess, report, communicate, document, and report cases of mismanagement and corruption from all levels of management results in untimely recognition and lack of prevention of such practices (WHO, 2014). LMICs tend not to have a robust legal and regulatory framework in place to act as a foundation for the evaluation of the progress of execution of the policies put forth to safeguard good health practices.

PART 2: ACHIEVEMENTS

HIV IN SUB-SAHARAN AFRICA—THE INTERSECTION OF POLICY, GOVERNANCE, AND IMPLEMENTATION

The unique ongoing story of HIV provides an informative case to analyze because we consider the policy, governance, and implementation gaps continue to plague LMICs. The HIV burden has a long history of preferentially afflicting LMICs, especially Sub-Saharan Africa (SSA), because it was the number 1 killer in SSA in 1998 and SSA continues to bear 71% of the world's burden of people living with HIV (Pastakia, Njuguna, Le, Singh, & Brock, 2015; UNAIDS, 2014).

However, what started as a ravaging pandemic, unlike anything the world had ever seen, has been transformed into another chronic disease in most parts of the world where policy, governance, and local implementers work in unison to create responsive healthcare systems. With the continued reliance on uninterrupted treatment with antiretroviral medications to stave off the preventable progression of HIV to AIDS, a strong supply chain has become the cornerstone of health systems tackling HIV.

It is through the policy and governance activities related to HIV, and its treatment specifically, which local implementers have been able to expand treatment broadly and foresee an end to the HIV pandemic (Jamieson & Kellerman, 2016).

When the HIV pandemic was decimating populations in SSA in the late 1990s and early 2000s, the cost of HIV medications was out of reach for almost the entire population in need because stringent patent protections meant a year's worth of anti-retroviral therapy (ART) cost over $10,000 per year (Holmes et al., 2010; MSF, 2002).

With the exorbitant costs of patent-protected HIV medications, many LMICs all over the world saw an overwhelming burden of HIV that not only stretched already fragile healthcare systems but also destabilized the economies of entire countries because HIV predominantly affected young adults soon to enter or already in the workforce (UNAIDS, 2016).

However, one of the major policy events to help demonstrate the potential of universal HIV treatment to stem the tide of HIV can be seen through legal proceedings, which occurred in Brazil in the late 1990s and early 2000s. Through the country-specific patent laws of Brazil, Brazil allowed local generic production of any medication patented before 1997. This local manufacturing of HIV medications dramatically reduced the price of HIV medications to less than $3000 a year and was utilized to support the provision of HIV medications to any Brazilian citizen needing treatment. This strategy of universal treatment is largely credited for the >50% reduction in HIV-associated mortality seen in Brazil between 1996 and 1999 and saved Brazil over $472 million (USD) in AIDS-related infections and hospital costs. Despite the remarkable gains seen with this strategy, Brazil's unique patent laws were later challenged in 2001 by the United States because they believed that they contravened the key protections guaranteed within the World Trade Organization–supported TRIPS agreement. Through political advocacy and a public outcry, the United States later dropped their lawsuit and Brazil was able to continue to build on the gains of their highly successful HIV program (Barton, 2004).

As the world continued to watch the growing toll of HIV in SSA, the US government decided to make a resolute commitment to address the HIV pandemic by launching the President's Emergency Plan for AIDS Relief (PEPFAR), which committed an unparalleled $15,000,000,000 over 5 years to 15 focus countries in Africa to fight HIV (Venkatesh, Mayer, & Carpenter, 2012). However, with the United States being one of the primary signatories to the TRIPS agreement and Doha Declaration, PEPFAR-supported programs were required to obtain the costly original HIV medications only from manufacturers who had received FDA approval. At the time, there were no generic HIV medications which had received FDA approval because these antiretroviral compounds were still protected during the period of patent exclusivity granted to pharmaceutical manufacturers under US law. This provision prevented the sale of generic HIV medications in the United States until the period of patent exclusivity for the original manufacturers had lapsed. As PEPFAR continued to advance prevention of HIV in SSA and subsequently identified ever-growing numbers of patients, the need to access higher quantities of ART at a more reasonable price became a major priority. This realization led to increased pressure from advocacy and development organizations such as the Clinton Foundation and Medicines Sans Frontieres (MSF) to provide creative solutions for the policy challenges, which limited access to HIV medications. As a result of this growing need, recognized through implementation, the FDA developed an expedited review process that could be extended to manufacturers all over the world with the primary concentration being in India. Although several manufacturers have been periodically banned from supplying medications to PEPFAR because of poor performance, this program was able to dramatically reduce the cost of HIV treatment and rapidly meet the demand for low-cost HIV medications in this market (Fleck, 2004; Johnston & Holt, 2014). By 2008, up to 90% of antiretroviral medications procured by PEPFAR-supported programs in SSA were supplied by generic manufacturers and there was a mean price difference of 50% between the generic and proprietary medication (Bartlett & Muro, 2007; Holmes et al., 2010; Kumarasamy, 2004; Venkatesh et al., 2012).

The description of the intersection between policy, governance, and implementation with this HIV example illustrates what is possible through the multiple layers of feedback among the different stakeholders involved with the crucial policy, governance, and implementation aspects of medication access. Through this concerted effort on improving medication access, there has been a 39% reduction in

AIDS-related deaths in SSA between 2005 and 2013. The shifting and adaptive policy and governance landscape in this short period has also led to dramatic increases in access because only 1 in 10 people in need had access to treatment in 2010 compared with 4 in 10 in 2013 (UNAIDS, 2014).

Although we have not yet achieved the medication access goals set forth in the 90-90-90 vision to end the HIV pandemic by 2030 (90% diagnosed, 90% on ART, and 90% achieving sustained virologic suppression by 2020), we have made great strides in overcoming barriers, which were once thought insurmountable. Continued emphasis on enhancing the efficacy of the supply chain to meet patient needs is essential to permanently end the HIV pandemic while also addressing emerging health needs beyond HIV (Jamieson & Kellerman, 2016, p. 90).

RECOMMENDATIONS: THE WAY FORWARD

Although there are still many challenges to overcome, the recent infrastructural advancements made to address the HIV epidemic as described above present a compelling example of how policy, governance, and implementation can be aligned to achieve dramatic life-changing outcomes for patients in LMICs in desperate need of lifesaving medications. As shown in Fig. 23.1, we propose that the path from making pharmaceutical policy to having *effective* pharmaceutical policy requires a good governing body that must take into consideration on-the-ground, practical, and real-world challenges. With good governance that addresses transparency, ensures framework for action, and foresees implementation challenges, we will be one step closer to achieving pharmaceutical policies with desired outcomes of increased availability, affordability, and quality-assured medicines for those who need them most.

CONCLUSIONS

Throughout this chapter, we have discussed many challenges faced when trying to turn well-intentioned pharmaceutical policies into impactful, well-governed programs, which are responsive to populations residing in LMICs. These practical challenges exist in every step of the way to create effective national pharmaceutical policies such as healthcare financing, supply chain management, selection of essential medicines, affordability, human resource, rational drug use, and monitoring and evaluation. To address these challenges, good governance must be in place to address the lack of transparency, the lack of framework for action, as well as gaps in implementation.

LESSONS LEARNED

- Effective pharmaceutical policy must exist to achieve these desired outcomes: adequate availability, equitable affordability, and quality-assured medicines.
- In LMICs, obstacles to effective pharmaceutical policy may be a result of barriers to good governance such as corruption, lack of framework, and implementation gaps.
- To overcome these obstacles, there is a need to address these challenges from a practical and contextualized standpoint to create sustainable, high-impact, and low-cost solutions.

ACKNOWLEDGMENTS

Beatrice Jakait PharmD, Imran Manji BPharm, Benson Njuguna BPharm, Paul Wasike BPharm, Dan Tran PharmD.

REFERENCES

Antignac, M., Diop, B. I., Macquart De Terline, D., Do, B., Ikama, M. S., N'guetta, R., … Jouven, X. (2016). *Quality assessment of 7 cardiovascular drugs in SubSaharan African countries: results of the seven study by drug and version of drug*. Mexico City, Mexico: Presented at the World Congress of Cardiology and Cardiovascular Health.

Bartlett, J. A., & Muro, E. P. (2007). Generic and branded drugs for the treatment of people living with HIV/AIDS. *Journal of the International Association of Physicians in AIDS Care (Chicago, IL : 2002)*, *6*(1), 15–23. https://doi.org/10.1177/1545109707299856.

Barton, J. H. (2004). TRIPS and the global pharmaceutical market. *Health Affairs*, *23*(3), 146–154. https://doi.org/10.1377/hlthaff.23.3.146.

Bazargani, Y. T., Ewen, M., de Boer, A., Leufkens, H. G. M., & Mantel-Teeuwisse, A. K. (2014). Essential medicines are more available than other medicines around the globe. *PLoS One*, *9*(2), e87576. https://doi.org/10.1371/journal.pone.0087576.

Bero, L., Carson, B., Moller, H., & Hill, S. (2010). To give is better than to receive: compliance with WHO guidelines for drug donations during 2000–2008. *Bulletin of the World Health Organization*, *88*(12), 922–929. https://doi.org/10.2471/BLT.10.079764.

Chen, L., Evans, T., Anand, S., Boufford, J. I., Brown, H., Chowdhury, M., … Wibulpolprasert, S. (2004). Human resources for health: overcoming the crisis. *The Lancet*, *364*(9449), 1984–1990.

Eliasson, C., & Matousek, P. (2007). Noninvasive authentication of pharmaceutical products through packaging using spatially offset Raman spectroscopy. *Analytical Chemistry*, *79*(4), 1696–1701. https://doi.org/10.1021/ac062223z.

Fire, C. (2016). Partnership for quality medical donations. Retrieved from: http://www.pqmd.org/.

Fleck, F. (2004). Ranbaxy withdraws all its AIDS drugs from WHO list. *BMJ : British Medical Journal*, *329*(7476), 1205.

Flegel, K. (2012). The adverse effects of brand-name drug prescribing. *CMAJ : Canadian Medical Association Journal*, *184*(5), 616. https://doi.org/10.1503/cmaj.112160.

Gall, D., Bates, I., & Bruno, A. (2012). *FIP global pharmacy workforce report 2012*. Retrieved from: http://discovery.ucl.ac.uk/1369202/.

Hanna, T. P., & Kangolle, A. C. T. (2010). Cancer control in developing countries: using health data and health services research to measure and improve access, quality and efficiency. *BMC International Health and Human Rights*, *10*, 24. https://doi.org/10.1186/1472-698X-10-24.

Hawthorne, N., & Anderson, C. (2009). The global pharmacy workforce: a systematic review of the literature. *Human Resources for Health*, *7*(1). https://doi.org/10.1186/1478-4491-7-48.

Hoebert, J. M., van Dijk, L., Mantel-Teeuwisse, A. K., Leufkens, H. G., & Laing, R. O. (2013). National medicines policies–a review of the evolution and development processes. *Journal of Pharmaceutical Policy and Practice*, *6*(1), 1.

Holmes, C. B., Coggin, W., Jamieson, D., Mihm, H., Granich, R., Savio, P., … Dybul, M. (2010). Use of generic antiretroviral agents and cost savings in PEPFAR treatment programs. *JAMA*, *304*(3), 313–320. https://doi.org/10.1001/jama.2010.993.

Hongoro, C., & McPake, B. (2004). How to bridge the gap in human resources for health. *Lancet (London, England)*, *364*(9443), 1451–1456. https://doi.org/10.1016/S0140-6736(04)17229-2.

Jamieson, D., & Kellerman, S. E. (2016). The 90 90 90 strategy to end the HIV Pandemic by 2030: Can the supply chain handle it? *Journal of the International AIDS Society*, *19*(1), 20917.

Johnston, A., & Holt, D. W. (2014). Substandard drugs: a potential crisis for public health. *British Journal of Clinical Pharmacology*, *78*(2), 218–243. https://doi.org/10.1111/bcp.12298.

Kumarasamy, N. (2004). Generic antiretroviral drugs–will they be the answer to HIV in the developing world? *Lancet (London, England)*, *364*(9428), 3–4. https://doi.org/10.1016/S0140-6736(04)16605-1.

Liang, L.-L., & Mirelman, A. J. (2014). Why do some countries spend more for health? An assessment of socio-political determinants and international aid for government health expenditures. *Social Science & Medicine (1982)*, *114*, 161–168. https://doi.org/10.1016/j.socscimed.2014.05.044.

MSF. (2002). *The impact of patents on access to medicines*. Retrieved from: http://www.msfaccess.org/content/impact-patents-access-medicines.

Nayyar, G. M. L., Breman, J. G., Newton, P. N., & Herrington, J. (2012). Poor-quality antimalarial drugs in south-east Asia and sub-Saharan Africa. *The Lancet Infectious Diseases*, *12*(6), 488–496. https://doi.org/10.1016/S1473-3099(12)70064-6.

Parker, M. H., Wardle, J. L., Weir, M., & Stewart, C. L. (2011). Medical merchants: conflict of interest, office product sales and notifiable conduct. *The Medical Journal of Australia*, *194*(1), 34–37.

Pastakia, S., Njuguna, B., Le, P. V., Singh, M. K., & Brock, T. P. (2015). To address emerging infections, we must invest in enduring systems: the kinetics and dynamics of health systems strengthening. *Clinical Pharmacology and Therapeutics*, *98*(4), 362–364. https://doi.org/10.1002/cpt.182.

Ranieri, N., Tabernero, P., Green, M. D., Verbois, L., Herrington, J., Sampson, E., … Witkowski, M. R. (2014). Evaluation of a new handheld instrument for the detection of counterfeit artesunate by visual fluorescence comparison. *The American Journal of Tropical Medicine and Hygiene*, *91*(5), 920–924. https://doi.org/10.4269/ajtmh.13-0644.

Rascati, K. L., Richards, K. M., Johnsrud, M. T., & Mann, T. A. (2009). Effects of antiepileptic drug substitutions on epileptic events requiring acute care. *Pharmacotherapy*, *29*(7), 769–774. https://doi.org/10.1592/phco.29.7.769.

Seiter, A. (2010). *A practical approach to pharmaceutical policy*. The World Bank. Retrieved from: http://elibrary.worldbank.org/doi/book/10.1596/978-0-8213-8386-5.

Ssengooba, F., Rahman, S. A., Hongoro, C., Rutebemberwa, E., Mustafa, A., Kielmann, T., & McPake, B. (2007). Health sector reforms and human resources for health in Uganda and Bangladesh: mechanisms of effect. *Human Resources for Health*, *5*(1). https://doi.org/10.1186/1478-4491-5-3.

Swain, S. (2014). Pharma regulations for generic drug products in India and US: case studies and future prospectives. *Pharmaceutical Regulatory Affairs: Open Access*, *3*(2). https://doi.org/10.4172/2167-7689.1000119.

Tran, D. N., & Bero, L. A. (2015). Barriers and facilitators to the quality use of essential medicines for maternal health in low–resource countries: an Ishikawa framework. *Journal of Global Health*, *5*(1). https://doi.org/10.7189/jogh.05.010406.

UNAIDS. (2014). *UNAIDS Gap report 2014*.

UNAIDS. (2016). *Global AIDS update*.

van Mourik, M. S. M., Cameron, A., Ewen, M., & Laing, R. O. (2010). Availability, price and affordability of cardiovascular medicines: a comparison across 36 countries using WHO/HAI data. *BMC Cardiovascular Disorders*, *10*, 25. https://doi.org/10.1186/1471-2261-10-25.

Venkatesh, K. K., Mayer, K. H., & Carpenter, C. C. J. (2012). Low-cost generic drugs under the President's Emergency Plan for AIDS Relief drove down treatment cost; more are needed. *Health Affairs (Project Hope)*, *31*(7), 1429–1438. https://doi.org/10.1377/hlthaff.2012.0210.

WHO. (1977). The selection of essential drugs: Report of a WHO expert committee. (Tech Rep Ser WHO no. 615). Geneva: World Health Organization.

WHO. (1999). *Operational principles for good pharmaceutical procurement*. Retrieved from: http://wwwlive.who.int/entity/hiv/pub/amds/who_edm_par_may99.pdf.

WHO. (2001). *How to develop and implement a national drug policy* (2nd ed.). Retrieved from:http://apps.who.int/medicinedocs/en/d/Js2283e/.

WHO. (2011a). *Guidelines for medicine donations: Revised 2010*. Geneva: World health organization.

WHO. (2011b). *The Abuja declaration: Ten years on*.

WHO. (2014). *Good governance for medicines: Model framework, updated version 2014*. Retrieved from: http://apps.who.int/iris/handle/10665/129495.

WHO. (2015a). *Regional strategy on human resources for health 2006-2015*. Retrieved from: http://iris.wpro.who.int/handle/10665.1/5566.

WHO. (2015b). *WHO guideline on country pharmaceutical pricing policies*. Retrieved from: http://apps.who.int/iris/bitstream/10665/153920/1/9789241549035_eng.pdf?ua=1.

WHO. (2016a). *Public financing for health in Africa: From Abuja to the SDGs*. Retrieved from: http://apps.who.int/iris/handle/10665/249527.

WHO. (2016b). *WHO | essential medicines*. Retrieved from: http://www.who.int/topics/essential_medicines/en/.

Yadav, P. (2015). Health product supply chains in developing countries: diagnosis of the root causes of underperformance and an agenda for reform. *Health Systems & Reform*, *1*(2), 142–154. https://doi.org/10.4161/23288604.2014.968005.

Yusuf, S., Islam, S., Chow, C. K., Rangarajan, S., Dagenais, G., Diaz, R., … Prospective Urban Rural Epidemiology (PURE) Study Investigators (2011). Use of secondary prevention drugs for cardiovascular disease in the community in high-income, middle-income, and low-income countries (the PURE Study): a prospective epidemiological survey. *Lancet*, *378*(9798), 1231–1243.

FURTHER READING

Wang, Z., Norris, S. L., & Bero, L. (2015). Implementation plans included in World Health Organisation guidelines. *Implementation Science*, *11*(1). https://doi.org/10.1186/s13012-016-0440-4.

CHAPTER

PHARMACOGOVERNANCE: ADVANCING PHARMACOVIGILANCE AND PATIENT SAFETY

24

Kathy Moscou[1,2,3], Jillian C. Kohler[1,4]

[1]University of Toronto, Toronto, ON, Canada; [2]York University, Toronto, ON, Canada; [3]Brandon University, Brandon, MB, Canada; [4]Munk School of Global Affairs, Toronto, ON, Canada

CHAPTER OUTLINE

Social and Administrative Aspects of Pharmacy in Low- and Middle-Income Countries. http://dx.doi.org/10.1016/B978-0-12-811228-1.00024-8

INTRODUCTION

Governance is defined by the UN Economic and Social Council (2006, p. 3) as the "exercise of economic, political and administrative authority to manage a country's affairs at all levels. It comprises the mechanisms, processes and institutions through which citizens and groups articulate their interests, exercise their legal rights, meet their obligations and mediate their differences". Governance influences national and subnational policy choices (or lack thereof) and allocation of resources necessary to achieve its policy agenda. In this chapter, we focus on how governance has had an impact on the pharmaceutical sector. Specifically, the relationship between the postmarket drug safety issues facing developing countries and pharmacogovernance is described. Pharmacogovernance is defined as the manner in which governing structures, policy instruments, and institutional authority (e.g., ability to act, implement, and enforce norms, policies, and processes) are managed to promote societal interests for patient safety and protection from adverse drug events (Moscou, 2016; Moscou, Kohler, & MaGahan, 2016). The case studies presented in the chapter illuminate the implications of pharmacogovernance on postmarket drug safety.

A framework for assessing pharmacogovernance is also presented. A pharmacogovernance framework would inform decision-making regarding policy choices to best protect patient safety nationwide. The absence of a pharmacogovernance framework disproportionately affects developing countries, as will be illustrated in the examples provided in this chapter. The chapter concludes with recommendations for a way forward to improve pharmacogovernance and pharmacovigilance.

GOVERNANCE AND POSTMARKET DRUG SAFETY IN DEVELOPING COUNTRIES

Governance is essential to ensure that government institutions have the institutional authority, will, and capacity to effectively implement policies and enforce law to be held accountable to their constituents. Weak governance negatively affects policy, laws, and regulations that would strengthen drug safety. In many low- and middle-income countries (LMICs), weak governance is endemic, particularly in the face of uncertain economies, unstable political regimes, and low per capita incomes (Mulili & Wong, 2011). A survey of sub-Saharan countries found that fewer than one-third had sufficient laws and regulations to mandate pharmacovigilance activities, although 78% had a national medicines policy (Strengthening Pharmaceutical Systems (SPS) Program, 2011). In many LMICs, there were no legal requirements for adverse drug reaction (ADR) reporting and pharmaceutical manufacturers were not required to undertake postmarket surveillance (Strengthening Pharmaceutical Systems (SPS) Program, 2011). Weak governance has fostered conditions, which permit drugs such as sibutramine (a weight loss medicine) to remain on the market in Brazil and India, despite being withdrawn in Europe and the United States where clinical trial data show that the use of such drugs increases the risk of heart attack and stroke (Moscou, Kohler, & Lexchin, 2013; Moscou et al., 2016).

Weak governance can also create an environment where corruption can thrive. Corruption is defined as the "misuse of entrusted power for private gain" (Transparency International http://www.transparency.org/what-is-corruption/). Corruption is costly. It is estimated to cost billions of dollars each year globally (Mackey & Liang, 2012). It wastes limited healthcare resources that might otherwise be used to provide quality and affordable care by increasing the cost of medicines, some of which may be unsafe or ineffective (Kohler, Martinez, Petkov, & Sale, 2016). Corrupt practices (e.g., extortion and bribes) can emerge in the absence of transparency, accountable regulatory control, and adequate law enforcement, thereby reducing access to safe and effective essential drugs (Kohler et al., 2016; Mackey & Liang, 2012), as an example, falsified antiretrovirals that entered the medicines supply chain in Kenya and the drugs that were visually indistinguishable from the actual generic product but differed in product deterioration. What was egregious about the Kenya example is that the drugs were inadvertently distributed to patients by Médicins Sans Frontières, a credible and well-respected nongovernment organization (Attaran et al., 2012). When substandard, spurious, falsely labeled, falsified, and counterfeit (SSFFC) medicines enter the drug supply chain, the risk for ADRs, morbidity, and death rises.

PHARMACOGOVERNANCE AND POSTMARKET DRUG SAFETY

Key features of pharmacogovernance are effective institutional authority, legislation, and policy instruments to strengthen drug safety. Weak pharmacogovernance can result in limited oversight and accountability that undermines stewardship for postmarket drug safety; creates opportunities for corruption to emerge (Baghdadi-Sabeti, Cohen-Kohler, & Wondemagegnehu, 2009; Garuba, Kohler, & Huisman, 2009; Mackey & Liang, 2012); creates institutional conflicts of interest (Gava, Bermudez, Pepe, & Reis, 2010; Miranda, 2010; Silva, 2011); and deincentivizes the adoption of legislation and norms for pharmacovigilance.

REGULATORY AUTHORITIES' INSTITUTIONAL POWERS

In many countries, pharmacovigilance policy is delegated to a national regulatory authority. The following examples show how regulatory powers influence strategies for postmarket surveillance and funding for pharmacovigilance. First, the Food and Drug Administration (FDA) (United States) and the European Medicines Agency (EMA) (Europe) have the authority to require drug companies to submit a risk minimization plan as part of the market authorization process. The EMA approves Risk Management Plans (RMPs) for drugs approved in European Union Member States. The FDA approves the Risk Evaluation and Mitigation Strategy (REMS) for drugs marketed in the United States. REMS and RMPs are policy instruments that outline the strategies to employ to further characterize drug safety risks or mitigate adverse events that may occur by taking a marketed medicine. REMS and RMPs may include postmarket requirements for safety studies and/or product labeling. This authority has been described as advancing pharmacovigilance by regulators. However, Wiktorowicz, Lexchin, and Moscou (2012) and Davis and Abraham (2011) have suggested that RMPs and REMS have hindered pharmacovigilance because the relaxation of FDA and EMA requirements for market approval and renewal of medicines have occurred in tandem with their adoption.

Regulatory authorities' institutional powers extend to the adoption of policy norms that affect resources to fund pharmacovigilance. In the United States, policies have been adopted that tie funding of pharmacovigilance to industry drug approval times (Frau, Pous, Luppino, & Conforti, 2010; Vernon, Golec, Lutter, & Nardinelli, 2009; Wieseler, McGauran, Kerekes, & Kaiser, 2012; Wiktorowicz et al., 2012). Critics of the *Prescription Drug User Fee Act* (PDUFA), which allows the US FDA to collect fees in exchange for expedited premarket review, have argued that drug approval times have shortened since the passage of PDUFA (Frank et al., 2014). At present, there is a greater reliance on gathering data about adverse drug events and other drug safety issues in the postmarket period.

Regulators' decisions are influenced by the regulator–industry relationship. The firm's brand recognition, perceptions of safety, and information asymmetry between the drug company and regulator, influence regulatory decisions to renew product registration or require postmarket safety studies (Carpenter, 2004). Postmarket safety studies are typically conducted by the drug company. Studies have shown industry bias in reporting study results (Lexchin, 2012; Lundh, Sismondo, Lexchin, Busuioc, & Bero, 2012). Lundh et al. (2012) and found that industry-sponsored studies produced more favorable results than non–industry-funded studies. These studies suggest that guidelines and regulatory norms regarding the use of industry-conducted safety studies as a basis for decisions pertaining to postmarket requirements are needed (Batt, 2016; Lundh et al., 2012; Wiktorowicz et al., 2012). Thus, the choice to base regulatory decision-making on industry-sponsored studies is influenced by pharmacogovernance.

POLICY INSTRUMENTS

Policy instruments that have the potential to strengthen postmarket drug safety processes may apply specifically to pharmacovigilance or more broadly to regulatory governance. RMPs and REMS, described earlier in this chapter, are policy instruments aimed at improving pharmacovigilance. The debate about the effectiveness of these pharmacovigilance policy instruments in improving postmarket drug safety versus legitimizing the collection of safety information in the postmarket period continues (Davis & Abraham, 2011; Frau et al., 2010).

Examples of policy instruments that aim to strengthen regulatory accountability are found in Brazil. The regulatory agenda and regulatory impact analysis (RIA) are policy instruments adopted by the Agência Nacional de Vigilância Sanitária (ANVISA). The regulatory agenda is adopted annually, and citizens may contribute to the process of setting priorities. Assessment of regulator progress in meeting the regulatory agenda and the effectiveness of policies are evaluated as part of the RIA (Moscou et al., 2016).

ASSESSING NATIONAL PHARMACOGOVERNANCE

All of the above suggest the importance of a pharmacogovernance framework. A pharmacogovernance framework serves as a guide for making choices that advance pharmacovigilance. The domains of the pharmacogovernance framework are informed by the United Nations Economic and Social Commission for Asia and the Pacific (UNESCAP) characteristics of good governance. Good governance, according to UNESCAP, is participatory, consensus oriented, accountable, transparent, responsive, effective and efficient, equitable, and inclusive and follows the rule of law (United Nations Economic and Social Commission for Asia and the Pacific, n.d.). The pharmacogovernance framework domains are policy, law, and regulation; transparency and accountability; participation and representation; equity and inclusiveness; effectiveness and efficiency; intelligence and information; ethics; responsiveness; and stakeholder coordination (Moscou, 2016; Moscou et al., 2016) (see Fig. 24.1).

POLICY, LAW, AND REGULATION

Good governance follows the rule of law whereby "fair legal frameworks are enforced impartially" requiring "an independent judiciary and an impartial and incorruptible police force" (United Nations Economic and Social Commission for Asia and the Pacific, n.d.). The pharmacogovernance domain "policy, law, and

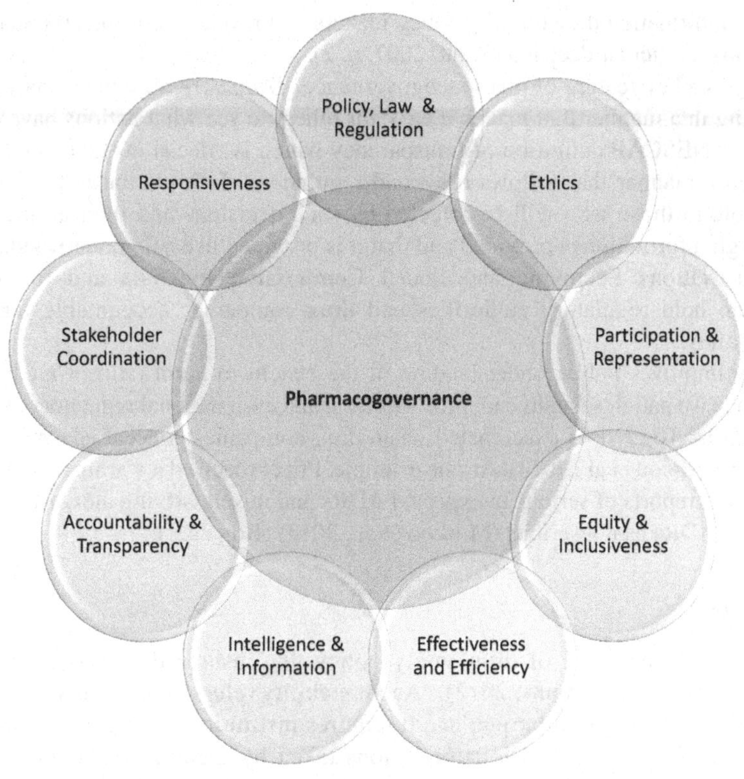

FIGURE 24.1

Pharmacogovernance framework.

Adapted from: Moscou K, Kohler J, MaGahan A. Governance and pharmacovigilance in Brazil: a scoping review. Journal of Pharmaceutical Policy and Practice. 2016; 9(3).

> **BOX 24.1 POLICY, LAW, AND REGULATION**
>
> Legislation requiring pharmacovigilance is an important measure of pharmacogovernance. In Brazil, laws have been passed requiring each pharmaceutical company to establish a pharmacovigilance program and report adverse drug reactions (ADRs). In Kenya, where fewer laws have been adopted, some drug companies have a single person responsible for managing pharmacovigilance for up to 46 countries. ADR reporting is also not legally mandated.

regulation" is defined as laws, bills, and resolutions that are intended to support the regulatory authority mandate to assure access to safe medicines, health products, and services (Box 24.1).

TRANSPARENCY

Transparency requires that citizens are fully informed as to how and why public policy decisions are taken. Understanding how decisions are made requires information about the procedures followed and the criteria used by policy makers to reach decisions. Understanding why decisions are made requires disclosure of the information drawn on by policy makers and revelation of the arguments adduced in favor of and against particular decision (Scott, 2007, p. 2).

Transparency is a key feature of pharmacogovernance. *Transparency* entails sharing of information and operating in a manner that makes it easy for others to see what actions have occurred. It is aligned with the UNESCAP definition of transparency which is "decisions taken and their enforcement are done in a manner that follows rules and regulations. Information is freely available and directly accessible to those who will be affected by such decisions and their enforcement. It also means that enough information is provided and that it is provided in easily understandable forms and media" (United Nations Economic and Social Commission for Asia and the Pacific, n.d.). Transparency can hold regulatory authorities and drug companies accountable for their actions related to drug safety.

Transparency improves public understanding of the benefit to harm ratio of medicines. Lack of transparency can leave patients, healthcare professionals, and even national regulatory authorities uninformed about ADRs. The risk is exacerbated when drug companies conceal adverse effects of their drugs (Batt, 2016; Moscou et al., 2013). As one example, Pfizer received a warning letter from the FDA for failing to submit reports of serious unexpected ADRs and misclassifying atorvastatin (Lipitor) and sildenafil (Viagra) ADRs as nonserious (Moscou et al., 2013) (Box 24.2).

ACCOUNTABILITY

Accountability is a cornerstone of drug safety policy. It "ensures the exercise of discretion is checked" (Brandsma & Schillemans, 2012). "Accountability refers to mechanisms that make institutions responsive to their particular publics. It requires institutions or organizations to answer to those who will be affected by decisions or actions taken by them. Accountability can improve health system performance by reducing abuses (including corruption), assuring compliance with standards and procedures, and improving performance and organizational learning" (Brinkerhoff, 2004; Vian & Kohler, 2016, p. 9). The enforcement of accountability relies heavily on transparency and the rule of law (United Nations Economic and Social Commission for Asia and the Pacific, n.d.). In the absence of mechanisms for accountability, corruption may flourish. As one example, bribes paid by vendors to government officials in order to win a bid to supply medicines, represents corruption in the drug procurement process (Kohler et al., 2016). The awarding of government tenders by officials as a political favor is another example of a corrupt drug procurement process (Otieno, Odundo, & Rambo, 2014; Rich & Gomez, 2012). Weak pharmacogovernance, in particular, poor transparency regarding contract tenders, weak monitoring and enforcement of regulations, and failure to adopt penalties large enough to incentivize ethical behavior (accountability), increases the risk of corruption (Box 24.3).

BOX 24.2 TRANSPARENCY

In an effort to increase transparency, public access to FDA warning letters to pharmaceutical companies is readily available on the FDA website. The public may view letters describing violations and noncompliance with FDA requirements. See http://www.fda.gov/Drugs/GuidanceComplianceRegulatoryInformation/EnforcementActivitiesbyFDA/WarningLettersandNoticeofViolationLetterstoPharmaceuticalCompanies/default.htm

BOX 24.3 ACCOUNTABILITY

The April 2016 decision by the Brazilian congress to resume the production and distribution of phosphoethanolamine (a drug used to treat cancer), even though the drug was not approved by Agência Nacional de Vigilância Sanitária (ANVISA) and human safety and efficacy studies had not been conducted, represents a failure of government accountability to assure that marketed drugs are safe and effective. The drug is produced in Brazil, prompting questions about to whom does Congress perceive it is accountable. By requiring patients to sign informed consent prior to receiving the drug, government accountability is shifted to medicines users. Kuchenbecker and Mota (2016) argue that in Brazil, drug regulation and health and technology assessment are threatened by weak governance, economic crisis, and political interference (Marowits, 2016).

BOX 24.4 PARTICIPATION AND REPRESENTATION

In Brazil, ANVISA's (Agência Nacional de Vigilância Sanitária) regulatory governance includes spaces for social participation (e.g., public hearings and consultations) to debate its regulatory agenda as a mechanism for transparency and accountability (ANVISA, n.d.; Lagerquist, 2016; Miranda, 2010). Social participation is also codified in Brazil's Federal Constitution of 1988, laws and ordinances. This gives legitimacy to public stakeholder engagement in decision-making spaces.

PARTICIPATION AND REPRESENTATION

UNESCAP suggests that participation is a characteristic of good governance. "Participation could be either direct or through legitimate intermediate institutions or representatives. It is important to point out that representative democracy does not necessarily mean that the concerns of the most vulnerable in society would be taken into consideration in decision making" (United Nations Economic and Social Commission for Asia and the Pacific, n.d.). Pertaining to pharmacogovernance, inclusive representation aims to actively seek input about drug safety policy from traditionally unrepresented voices. Public input in setting the regulatory agenda establishes greater assurance of regional equity in drug safety.

In practice, actors with perceived expertise (e.g., pharmaceutical industry representatives and global donors) have greater access to regulators than citizens, particularly in developing countries. Therefore regulatory policy may be skewed toward industry interests (Davis & Abraham, 2011; Frank et al., 2014; Hochstetler, 2013). When citizens participate in decision-making forums (e.g., participatory health councils in Brazil), the effect of their participation may be marginalized by their lack of education, training, and technical knowledge or coopted by political patronage, especially during elections (Kohler & Martinez, 2015; Lima, 2013; Otieno et al., 2014) (Box 24.4).

EQUITY AND INCLUSIVENESS

UNESCAP defines equity and inclusiveness as "all members feel that they have a stake in it and do not feel excluded from the mainstream of society. This requires [that] all groups, but particularly the most vulnerable, have opportunities to improve or maintain their wellbeing" (United Nations Economic and Social Commission for Asia and the Pacific, n.d.). Pharmacogovernance expands this definition beyond representation in decision-making to include equitable allocation and distribution of resources to ensure that all regions within the country have access to safe medicines and resources to detect and act on drug safety signals (Box 24.5).

BOX 24.5 EQUITY AND INCLUSIVENESS

In Brazil and Kenya, the distribution of sentinel surveillance sites and resources to monitor and assess drug safety is inequitable. The concentration of sentinel hospitals is greatest in large urban centers that are highly resourced (e.g., São Paulo, Rio de Janeiro, and Minas Gerais) (IBGE, n.d.) and Kenyan counties (e.g., Nairobi and Uasin Gishu). The pharmacovigilance units with the greatest resources and autonomy to set state pharmacovigilance priorities were located in states with a large pharmaceutical industry (e.g., Sao Paulo) (IBGE, n.d.).

BOX 24.6 RESPONSIVENESS

In the United States, the Food and Drug Administration Amendments Act (2007) gives the FDA the authority to require drug manufacturers to conduct postmarket safety studies and clinical trials to assess possible serious risks associated with the drugs. A 2013 audit of FDA postmarket requirements (PMRs) and postmarket commitments found that only 10% of requirements were fulfilled. 24% of studies were ongoing and 16% of the open studies were delayed in starting, completing or submitting required reports. In 2014, 13% of PMRs were delayed. The lack of responsiveness in meeting postmarket requirements leads to a lack of data that would inform market authorization decisions. See http://www.fda.gov/downloads/Drugs/GuidanceComplianceRegulatoryInformation/Post-marketingPhaseIVCommitments/UCM527213.pdf.

BOX 24.7 EFFECTIVENESS AND EFFICIENCY

In Brazil, the Regulatory Process Improvement Programme (PRO-REG) and regulatory impact analysis have been introduced as policy instruments for accountability. Although they aim to measure ANVISA's (Agência Nacional de Vigilância Sanitária) responsiveness in meeting the regulatory agenda (Silva, 2011), neither they have yet been applied to pharmacovigilance nor they have been used to evaluate the effectiveness of ANVISA's postmarket drug safety policies.

RESPONSIVENESS

Responsiveness is defined as policies and regulations that address drug safety issues within a reasonable timeframe. This definition is consistent with "responsiveness" as defined by UNESCAP, which states that good governance requires that institutions and processes try to serve all stakeholders within a reasonable timeframe (Box 24.6).

EFFECTIVENESS AND EFFICIENCY

Effectiveness and efficiency is defined as "processes and institutions that produce results that meet the needs of society while making the best use of resources at their disposal" by the UNESCAP. As related to pharmacogovernance, effectiveness and efficiency is defined as the capacity to evaluate the utility of pharmacovigilance policies and monitor pharmaceutical industry compliance with policy, law, and regulation pertaining to postmarket drug safety. Regulatory authority effectiveness may be challenged by fragmented establishment of norms, a cultural disregard for rules of the State, unnecessary or overlapping regulations, ineffective monitoring and enforcement, and poor design and/or implementation of norms leading to high costs for compliance (Ramalho, 2009) (Box 24.7).

BOX 24.8 ETHICS

High-profile examples of price gouging have recently been publicized, which affect the treatment of diseases endemic in developing countries and impoverished inner cities in developed countries. Turing Pharmaceutical raised the price of pyrimethamine (Daraprim), a drug approved by the FDA in 1953, which is used to treat malaria and toxoplasmosis, from $13.50 per tablet to $750 per tablet. Mylan Pharmaceutical raised the price of Epipen (used to treat life-threatening allergic reactions) from $94 per 2-dose package to $608. Valeant Pharmaceuticals raised the price of calcium EDTA (a drug used to treat lead poisoning) from $950 to $26,927 per treatment. A lawsuit was filed against Valeant alleging the company violated the Racketeer Influenced and Corrupt Organizations Act and the New York Deceptive Practices Act (Jalonick, 2016; Lagerquist, 2016; Marowits, 2016; Pollack, 2015).

BOX 24.9 CORRUPTION

In 2014, a procurement corruption scandal was discovered in Uasin Gishu County, Kenya. Drugs valued at 40 million Kenyan schillings (Ksh) were not delivered to Uasin Gishu hospitals or purchased at an exaggerated price. Drugs to treat malaria accounted for nearly 8 million shillings of the drugs involved in this scandal (Ndanyi, 2014).

The US Department of Justice and SEC investigated Pfizer for improper transactions with foreign governments. In China, subsidiaries paid bribes to doctors and government officials to influence regulatory decisions, drug formulary approvals, purchase decisions, and prescription choices. The SEC investigated Eli Lilly China for bribing physicians and government officials to expand access to Lilly products in China by listing Lilly products on government reimbursement lists. Eli Lilly & Co. agreed to pay $29 million to settle the case. China's Ministry of Public Security accused GSK China of bribing government officials and doctors over drug prices and product sales using a corrupt cooperative agreement between GSK China and Chinese travel agency to hide transactions (Rose-Ackerman & Tan, 2014).

ETHICS

Embedded in the definition of the pharmacogovernance domain "policy, law, and regulation" and UNESCAP definition of "follows the rule of law" is the fair and impartial enforcement of national pharmaceutical policy and national pharmacovigilance policy. This suggests that a separate domain of "ethics" may be warranted. "Ethics" is defined as respect for justice, autonomy, nonmaleficence, and beneficence to safeguard patient interests, right to safe medicines, and health.

Pharmacogovernance influences decisions to adopt policy and law that requires a code of conduct to address conflicts of interest to ensure ethical practice (Kohler et al., 2016; Moscou et al., 2013, 2016). Ethical issues arise when pharmaceutical firms that are the sole supplier of a medication charge exorbitant prices for their product. As an example, Valeant Pharmaceuticals increased the price of one drug more than 2700% (Lagerquist, 2016). The higher prices increase healthcare system costs and limit access to medicines (Box 24.8).

A government may face conflicts insofar as it seeks to promote its domestic drug industry, which may also undercut public health goals (Miranda, 2010; Silva, 2011). There may also be reluctance to implement policies perceived to deter multinational drug companies' investments. Cross-purpose interests regarding economic and public health policy may impede drug safety by hindering adoption of drug policy and legislation, monitoring pharmaceutical industry compliance, and enforcement of laws pertaining to pharmacovigilance. The risk of corruption may increase if necessary checks and balances are not in place and the number of suppliers is small (Kohler et al., 2016). Procurement corruption can result in inflated drug prices, stock shortages, and the introduction of SSFFCs into the supply chain (Box 24.9).

BOX 24.10 INTELLIGENCE AND INFORMATION

In Kenya, the Pharmacy and Poisons Board launched an online reporting system and mobile phone application in 2014. The e-reporting systems are designed to capture reports of adverse drug reactions and poor quality medicine. The introduction of e-reporting has made Kenya a regional leader in pharmacosurveillance technology. The data collected can increase the pool of information about adverse drug reactions that can be mined for signals of drug safety issues, thereby aiding regulators' drug approval decisions.

INTELLIGENCE AND INFORMATION

The safe use of medicines is supported by sound intelligence and information that strengthens communication among national regulatory authorities, state pharmacovigilance centers, patients, healthcare professionals, policy makers, and the general public. Pharmacogovernance influences the laws, regulations, and policies governing the collection of data needed to support regulatory decisions. It also influences the resources required to design and implement information technology to collect and analyze reports of ADRs. Ministry of Health and drug benefit managers' decision-making related to drugs being considered for addition to essential medication lists or drug benefit plan formularies is also affected by intelligence and information (Lexchin, Wiktorowicz, Moscou, & Silversides, 2013; Wiktorowicz, Lexchin, Moscou, Silversides, & Eggertson, 2010). In many LMICs, the national medicines regulator lacks sufficient data to inform its decision-making about marketed drugs, and the information gap is exacerbated by the absence of legislation requiring the pharmaceutical industry to report ADRs (Ministry of Health, 2015). Kenya has addressed intelligence and information challenges by establishing an online system where health professionals and consumers can report ADRs (Box 24.10).

STAKEHOLDER COORDINATION

The pharmacogovernance domain "stakeholder coordination" is defined as domestic and global actors that coordinate activities for the purpose of strengthening the national regulatory authority and human resources to benefit pharmacovigilance. Global pharmacogovernance favors state and exogenous actors' engagement to reduce drug safety risks by strengthening pharmacovigilance because the risks for ADRs and other drug safety issues extend beyond national boundaries. The UN sustainable development goals (SDGs) call for strengthening multistakeholder partnerships (SDG 17) to support sustainable development (Mackey et al., 2016). Global partnerships can contribute to pharmacogovernance and sustainable institutional capacity to prevent, detect, and respond to drug safety issues through resource development (e.g., Regional Centre of Regulatory Excellence (RCORE)) and advocacy for adoption of a national pharmacovigilance system, pharmacovigilance laws, regulations, and policy norms (World Health Assembly, May 26, 2012) (Box 24.11).

ACHIEVEMENTS

Globally, countries are increasingly recognizing the importance of pharmacovigilance (Olsson, Pal, & Dodoo, 2015; Olsson, Pal, Stergachis, & Couper, 2010; Strengthening Pharmaceutical Systems (SPS) Program, 2011). Pharmacogovernance embraces a culture that supports pharmacovigilance, contributing to drug safety and the right to the highest attainable standard of health as expressed in

BOX 24.11 STAKEHOLDER COORDINATION

Pharmaceutical sector support that has specifically targeted pharmacogovernance includes Global Fund grants for assessment of countrywide systems for pharmacovigilance, instruments to assess the countrywide pharmacovigilance systems (e.g., WHO comprehensive tool for assessing pharmacovigilance systems and the USAID/MSH Indicator-based Pharmacovigilance Assessment Tool (IPAT)) and resources to strengthen regulatory institutions and governance (Management Sciences for Health, 2009; World Health Organization, 2015). In the report, Experience with supporting pharmaceutical policies and systems in Kenya: Progress, lessons and the role of WHO (2009), the WHO found that their support (e.g., funding and technical guidance), "coupled with support from other partners, is contributing to ongoing policy interventions that could positively impact on access to essential medicines" by targeting critical pharmaceutical sector gaps and providing guidance for adapting norms and standards. This model of global actor engagement has been employed throughout Latin America and Africa to strengthen pharmacogovernance and pharmacovigilance (Mbindyo et al., 2010; Organización Panamericana de la Salud, 2011).

BOX 24.12 WORLD HEALTH ASSEMBLY DECLARATION (2012)

"Acknowledging the need for improving access to affordable, quality, safe and efficacious medicines as an important element in the effort to prevent and control medicines with compromised quality, safety and efficacy and in the decrease of "substandard/spurious/falsely-labelled/falsified/counterfeit medical products" (the 65th World Health Assembly):

2. REITERATES that WHO should continue to focus on and intensify its measures to make medical products more affordable, strengthening national regulatory authorities and health systems that include national medicine policies, health risk management systems, sustainable financing, human resource development and reliable procurement and supply systems; and to enhance and support work on prequalification and promotion of generics, and efforts in rational selection and use of medical products. In each of these areas, WHO's function should be: information sharing and awareness creation; norms and standards and technical assistance to countries on country situation assessment; national policy development; and capacity building, supporting product development and domestic production" (World Health Assembly, 26 May 2012, pp. 1–2).

the World Health Organization's (WHO's) Constitution (Moscou et al., 2013, 2016). In 2012, the 65th World Health Assembly reaffirmed the role of the WHO in supporting regulatory authorities to ensure quality, safe, and efficacious products, responding to the report of the Working Group of Member States on SSFFC medical products (Box 24.12). LMICs are addressing gaps in pharmacogovernance by strengthening regulatory governance at the national and subnational level (Kohler et al., 2016; Olsson et al., 2015), collaborating with global actors to build capacity for pharmacovigilance (Moscou et al., 2016; Olsson et al., 2015), developing technology to expand ADR data collection and reduce corruption via e-procurement (Prasad & Shivarajan, 2015), and creating advocacy networks to adopt stronger pharmacovigilance regulations and laws (Olsson et al., 2015). As an example, in 2014, the Kenyan Pharmacy and Poison Board received funding from the New Partnership for Africa's Development (NEPAD) African Medicines Regulatory Harmonization (AMRH) Programme to create a RCORE for pharmacovigilance. The aim of the RCORE is to boost regulatory governance in Africa. The AMRH supports harmonization of regulation pertaining to the approval of medicines and reporting formats for ADR case reports (Olsson et al., 2015). Collaborative engagement with global civil society may further strengthen pharmacogovernance and fight corruption by delegitimizing the societal and political patronage incentives that hinder pharmacovigilance (Mackey et al., 2016).

CHALLENGES

Despite addressing some of the gaps in pharmacogovernance, there are many challenges remaining that impede national capacity to meet societal interests for patient safety and protection from adverse drug events. Countrywide gaps in the pharmacogovernance exist in policy; law and regulation; equity and inclusion; and ethics that challenge postmarket drug safety. Conflicting policies, laws, and regulations hinder enforcement of drug safety laws negatively affecting access to safe medicines (Mbindyo, Okello, & Kimani, 2010; Sessional Paper No. 1 on the National Pharmaceutical Policy, 2010). Regional inequities in the distribution of sentinel pharmacosurveillance sites remain a challenge for developing countries. Regional disparities in pharmacovigilance are exacerbated by inadequate, human resources, sustainable funding, and resource allocation decisions (Olsson et al., 2010; Pal, Dodoo, Mantel, & Olsson, 2011). Gaps in ethics, conflicts of interest, cross-purpose interests, and/or corruption can also reduce access to safe and effective essential drugs, as shown by the examples in this chapter. Most noteworthy, is the negative impact of corrupt practices on public resources in further impoverishing fragile health systems (Mackey & Liang, 2012). The population in LMICs is disproportionately affected by the challenges posed by the gaps in ethics; however, developed economies should not falsely believe that they are spared because the drug supply chain is global and interdependent.

RECOMMENDATIONS: THE WAY FORWARD

To be sure, adoption of laws and regulations is key to strengthening pharmacogovernance. They codify institutional authority to act, implement, and enforce norms, policies, and processes in line with societal interests for patient safety and protection from adverse drug events. However, gaps in other pharmacogovernance areas may still hinder postmarket drug safety, as shown by the examples presented in this chapter. Civil society can improve drug safety by combating deficiencies in pharmacogovernance when present. Civil society can act as a watchdog and help promote transparency and accountability in drug safety policy making. Citizen participation in establishing the regulatory priorities for postmarket drug safety is a characteristic of pharmacogovernance that assures the voice of medicine's users is considered in policy enactment. Training in participatory governance is necessary, particularly in developing countries with limited experience with social participation, to overcome barriers to citizen participation (Kohler & Martinez, 2015). The gap in funding also threatens pharmacovigilance in developing countries. Pharmacogovernance would address this gap by ensuring sustainable, public funding models to support ongoing, rather than ad hoc, pharmacovigilance. Additionally, pharmacogovernance would assure equitable resource allocation to combat regional disparities in pharmacosurveillance and risk communication (Moscou et al., 2016).

CONCLUSIONS

Pharmacogovernance can improve postmarket drug safety in developing countries and address current challenges by strengthening pharmacogovernance institutions; governing structures; policy instruments; and institutional authority to act, implement, and enforce norms, policies, and processes. Specifically, pharmacogovernance can improve postmarket drug safety by establishing (1) an internal

BOX 24.13 KEY POINTS

- Pharmacogovernance and strong institutions are ensuring access to safe and effective medicines
- Postmarket drug safety is advanced by strong pharmacogovernance at the national, subnational, and supranational level.
- Pharmacogovernance advances the adoption of regulatory policy instruments (e.g., regulatory impact analysis) that improve transparency, accountability, and effectiveness of pharmacovigilance policies and practice.
- Adoption of laws and regulations are key to strengthening pharmacogovernance; however, gaps in other pharmacogovernance areas may still hinder postmarket drug safety.
- Sustainable public funding of regulatory authorities can reduce vulnerability to conflicts of interests affecting patient safety.
- Collaborative partnerships among national and global actors in line with sustainable development goals to improve governance will strengthen pharmacogovernance.

policy framework for drug safety, (2) the active cultivation of organizational capabilities, (3) sustainable funding, and (4) external partnerships for drug safety. The use of a pharmacogovernance framework can contribute to a holistic assessment national/subnational structures and institutions that impact pharmacovigilance.

LESSONS LEARNED

The lessons we have learned about the influence of governance on national and subnational policy choices for governing structures, policy instruments, institutional authority, and resource allocation to promote societal interests for patient safety and protections from adverse drug events are shown in Box 24.13.

ACKNOWLEDGMENTS

This chapter is based on the doctoral thesis of Dr. Kathy Moscou, Pharmacogovernance in low- and middle-income countries: a case study of Brazil and Kenya. University of Toronto, 2016.

REFERENCES

ANVISA. (n.d.). ANVISA Stratégias prioritárias da gestão institucional. Agência Nacional de Vigilância Sanitária. Retrieved from http://www.anvisa.gov.br/divulga/noticias/2009/pdf/cartilha_pmg.pdf.

Attaran, A., Barry, D., Basheer, S., Bate, R., Benton, D., Chauvin, J., … Mckee, M. (2012). How to achieve international action on falsified and substandard medicines. *BMJ: British Medical Journal, 345*(e7381), 1–6.

Baghdadi-Sabeti, G., Cohen-Kohler, J., & Wondemagegnehu, E. (2009). *Measuring Transparency in the Public Pharmaceutical Sector- Assessment Instrument*. Geneva: World Health Orgranization, Departments of Essential Medicines and Pharmaceutical Policies & Ethics, Equity, Trade and Human Rights.

Batt, S. (2016). Pharmaceutical company corruption and the moral crisis in medicine. *Hastings center report 46* (vol. 4. Hastings Center Report 46, 10–13.

Brandsma, G. J., & Schillemans, T. (2012). The accountability cube: Measuring accountability. *Journal of Public Administration, Research and Theory, 23*, 953–975.

Brinkerhoff, D. (2004). Accountability and health systems: Toward conceptual clarity and policy relevance. *Health Policy and Planning. Oxford University Press, 19*(6), 371–379. http://dx.doi.org/10.1093/heapol/czh052.

Carpenter, D. (2004). Protection without Capture: Product approval by a politically responsive, learning regulator. *American Political Science Review, 98*(4).

Davis, C., & Abraham, J. (2011). A comparative analysis of risk management strategies in European Union and United States pharmaceutical regulation. *Health, Risk & Society, 13*(5), 413–431. http://dx.doi.org/10.1080/13698575.2011.596191.

Frank, C., Himmelstein, D. U., Woolhandler, S., Bor, D. H., Wolfe, S. M., Heymann, O., … Lasser, K. E. (2014). Era of faster fda drug approval has also seen increased black-box warnings and market withdrawals. *Health Affairs, 33*(8), 1453–1459. http://dx.doi.org/10.1377/hlthaff.2014.0122.

Frau, S., Pous, M. F., Luppino, M. R., & Conforti, A. (2010). Risk management plans: Are they a tool for improving drug safety? *European Journal of Clinical Pharmacology, 66*, 785–790.

Garuba, H., Kohler, J., & Huisman, A. (2009). Transparency in Nigeria's public pharmaceutical sector: Perceptions from policy makers. *Globalization and Health, 5*(14). http://dx.doi.org/10.1186/1744-8603-5-14.

Gava, C. M., Bermudez, J. A. Z., Pepe, V. L. E., & Reis, A. L. A.D. (2010). Novos medicamentos registrados no Brasil: Podem ser considerados como avanço terapêutico?/new medicines registered in Brazil: Can they be considered as a therapeutic advance? *Ciência & Saúde Coletiva, 15*(supp.3), 3403–3412.

Hochstetler, K. (2013). Civil society and the regulatory state of the South. In N. Dubash, & B. Morgan (Eds.), *The rise of the regulatory state of the South: Infrastructure and development in emerging economies*. Oxford Scholarship Online. http://dx.doi.org/10.1093/acprof:oso/9780199677160.001.0001.

IBGE. (n.d.). States@. Retrieved from http://www.ibge.gov.br/estadosat/index.php.

Jalonick, M. C. (August 23, 2016). *U.S. lawmakers demand information on massive EpiPen price increase*. The Associated Press. Retrieved from CTVNews.ca website http://www.ctvnews.ca/health/u-s-lawmakers-demand-information-on-massive-epipen-price-increase-1.3040752.

Kohler, J. C., & Martinez, M. G. (2015). Participatory health councils and good governance: Healthy democracy in Brazil? *International Journal for Equity in Health, 14*, 21. http://dx.doi.org/10.1186/s12939-015-0151-5.

Kohler, J., Martinez, M., Petkov, M., & Sale, J. (2016). *Corruption in the pharmaceutical Sector: Diagnosing the challenges*. Transparency International UK. http://www.transparency.org.uk/publications/corruption-in-the-pharmaceutical-sector/.

Kuchenbecker, R. S., & Mota, D. M. (2016). Miracle drug: Brazil approves never-tested cancer medicine. *Journal of Oncology Pharmacy Practice*, 1–2. https://doi.org/10.1177/1078155216665246.

Lagerquist, J. (October 11, 2016). *Valeant hiked lead poisoning drug price by 2,700 per cent*. CTVNews. Retrieved from CTVNews.ca website http://www.ctvnews.ca/business/valeant-hiked-lead-poisoning-drug-price-by-2-700-per-cent-report-1.3111322.

Lexchin, J. (2012). Sponsorship bias in clinical research. *International Journal of Risk and Safety in Medicines, 24*(4), 233–242. http://dx.doi.org/10.3233/JRS-2012-0574.

Lexchin, J., Wiktorowicz, M., Moscou, K., & Silversides, A. (2013). Provincial drug plan officials' views of the Canadian drug safety system. *Journal of Health, Politics, Policy and Law, 38*(3), 545–571.

Lima, M. I. (2013). *Alternatives to Decentralization of pharmaceutical policies in Brazil: Case studies of HIV/AIDS and Tuberculosis*. University of Toronto. Masters of Law.

Lundh, A., Sismondo, S., Lexchin, J., Busuioc, O. A., & Bero, L. (2012). Industry sponsorship and research outcome (Review). *The Cochrane Library*.

Mackey, T. K., Kohler, J. C., Savedoff, W. D., Vogl, F., Lewis, M., Sale, J., … Vian, T. (2016). The disease of corruption: Views on how to fight corruption to advance 21st century global health goals. *BMC Medicine, 14*, 149.

Mackey, T., & Liang, B. (2012). Combating healthcare corruption and fraud with improved global health governance. *BMC International Health and Human Rights, 12*(23), 1–7. http://dx.doi.org/10.1186/1472-698X-12-23.

Marowits, R. (August 29, 2016). *Valeant accused of racketeering in class-action lawsuit from N.Y. health funds.* The Canadian Press. Retrieved from http://www.ctvnews.ca/business/valeant-accused-of-racketeering-in-class-action-lawsuit-from-n-y-health-funds-1.3049284.

Mbindyo, R., Okello, D., & Kimani, F. (2010). *Experience with supporting pharmaceutical policies and systems in Kenya- Progress, lessons and the role of WHO. WHO/EMP/MPC/2010.2.* WHO.

Ministry of Health. (2015). *Pharmacy and poisons board strategic plan 2014-2019.* Nairobi: Republic of Kenya Ministry of Health.

Miranda, A. (2010). *Transparência na gestão da Anvisa: uma análise dos espaços de participação social [transparency in the management of Anvisa: An analysis of opportunities for social participation]* (Masters of Science Dissertation), Fundação Oswaldo Cruz. LILACS database.

Moscou, K. (2016). *Pharmacogovernance in low- and middle-income countries: A case study of Brazil and Kenya.* Toronto: University of Toronto. Ph.D. Doctoral.

Moscou, K., Kohler, J., & Lexchin, J. (2013). Drug safety and corporate governance. *Global Health Governance, 7*, 56–79.

Moscou, K., Kohler, J., & MaGahan, A. (2016). Governance and pharmacovigilance in Brazil: A scoping review. *Journal of Pharmaceutical Policy and Practice, 9*(3). http://dx.doi.org/10.1186/s40545-016-0053-y.

Mulili, B. M., & Wong, P. (2011). Corporate governance practices in developing countries: The case for Kenya. *International Journal of Business Administration, 2*(1).

Ndanyi, M. (April 8, 2014). Uasin Gishu Sh40 million drug scandal. *The Star.* Retrieved from http://www.the-star.co.ke/news/2014/04/08/uasin-gishu-probes-sh40-million-drugs-scandal_c921992.

Olsson, S., Pal, S., & Dodoo, A. (2015). Pharmacovigilance in resource-limited countries. *Expert Review of Clinical Pharmacology, 8*(4), 449–460.

Olsson, S., Pal, S. N., Stergachis, A., & Couper, M. (2010). Pharmacovigilance activities in 55 low- and middle-income countries a questionnaire-based analysis. *Drug Safety, 33*(8), 689–703.

Organización Panamericana de la Salud. (2011). *Buenas Prácticas de Farmacovigilancia [Good pharmacovigilance practices for the Americas] (pp. 78).* Washington, DC.

Otieno, J. O., Odundo, P. A., & Rambo, C. M. (2014). Influence of local authority transfer fund on service delivery by local government authorities in Kenya. *International Journal of Management and Marketing Research, 7*(1).

Pal, S., Dodoo, A., Mantel, A., & Olsson, S. (2011). *The World medicines situation 2011: Pharmacovigilance and afety of medicines* (3rd ed.). Geneva: World Health Organization.

Pollack, A. (September 20, 2015). Drug goes from $13.50 a tablet to $750, overnight. *The New York Times.* Retrieved from http://www.nytimes.com/2015/09/21/business/a-huge-overnight-increase-in-a-drugs-price-raises-protests.html?_r=0.

Prasad, A., & Shivarajan, S. (2015). Understanding the role of technology in reducing corruption: A transaction cost approach. *Journal of Public Affairs, 15*(1), 19.

Ramalho, P. I. S. (2009). *Chapter 5: Regulação e agências reguladoras: Reforma regulatória da década de 1990 e desenho institucional das agências no Brasil Regulação e Agências Reguladoras: Governança e análise de impacto regulatório [regulation and agency Regulators: Analysis of the impact of regulatory governance].* Brasilia: Agência Nacional de Vigilância Sanitária/Pedro Ivo Sebba Ramalho Org).

Rich, J. A., & Gomez, E. J. (2012). Centralizing decentralized governance in Brazil. *The Journal of Federalism, 42*(4), 636–661. http://dx.doi.org/10.1093/publius/pjs002.

Rose-Ackerman, S., & Tan, Y. (June 2, 2014). Corruption in the procurement of pharmaceuticals and medical equipment in China: The incentives facing multinationals, domestic firms and hospital officials. *Social Science Research Network (Yale Law & Economics Research Paper No. 498).*

Scott, C. (2007). *Figuring out accountability: Selected uses of official statistics by civil society to improve public sector performanceQ Squared working Paper No. 37.* Toronto: Centre for International Studies, University of Toronto. Retrieved from https://www.trentu.ca/ids/documents/Q2_WP37_Scott.pdf.

Sessional Paper No. 1 on the national pharmaceutical policy. (2010). Office of the Prime Minister Ministry of State for Planning.

Silva, G. H. (2011). *Agenda Regulatória e Análise de Impacto Regulatório: A Experiência da Agência Nacional de Vigilância Sanitária na Aplicação Práctica de Instumentos Inovadores de Previsibilidade, Transparência e Accountability. Paper presented at the IV Congresso CONSAD de Gestao Publica*. Brasilia: Centro de Convencoes Ulysses,Guimaraess.

Strengthening Pharmaceutical Systems (SPS) Program. (2011). *Safety of medicines in sub-Saharan Africa: Assessment of pharmacovigilance systems and their performance*. Arlington: US Agency for International Development by the Strengthening Pharmaceutical Systems (SPS) Program.

UN Economic, Social Council. (2006). *Compendium of basic terminology in governance and public administration, Fifth session. (E/C.16/2006/4)*. New York City: United Nations.

United Nations Economic and Social Commission for Asia and the Pacific. (n.d.). What Is Good Governance? Retrieved from http://www.unescap.org/sites/default/files/good-governance.pdf.

Vernon, J. A., Golec, J. H., Lutter, R., & Nardinelli, C. (2009). An exploratory study of FDA new drug review times, prescription drug user fee acts, and R&D spending. *The Quarterly Review of Economics and Finance*, *49*, 1260–1274.

Vian, T., & Kohler, J. (May 2016). *Medicines transparency alliance (MeTA): Pathways to transparency, accountability and access: Cross-case analysis and review of phase II*. Geneva: WHO Publications.

Wieseler, B., McGauran, N., Kerekes, M. F., & Kaiser, T. (2012). Access to regulatory data from the European medicines agency: The times they are a-changing. *Systematic Reviews*, *50*(1). http://dx.doi.org/10.1186/2046-4053-1-50. http://www.systematicreviewsjournal.com/content/1/1/50.

Wiktorowicz, M., Lexchin, J., & Moscou, K. (2012). Pharmacovigilance in Europe and North America: Divergent approaches. *Social Science & Medicine*, *75*, 165–170.

Wiktorowicz, M., Lexchin, J., Moscou, K., Silversides, A., & Eggertson, L. (2010). *Keeping an eye on prescription drugs, keeping Canadians safe. Active monitoring systems for drug safety and effectiveness in Canada and Internationally*. Toronto: Health Council of Canada.

World Health Assembly. (May 26, 2012). Substandard/spurious/falsely-labelled/falsified/counterfeit medical products. In *WHA65.19 Sixty-fifth World Health Assembly. Tenth Plenary Meeting A65/VR/10 (Vol. Agenda item 13.13)*.

CHAPTER

PHARMACEUTICAL POLICY: SYNTHESIS, THEMES, AND FUTURE DIRECTIONS

25

Zaheer-Ud-Din Babar[1,2], **Shane L. Scahill**[3]

[1]*University of Huddersfield, Huddersfield, United Kingdom;* [2]*University of Auckland, Auckland, New Zealand;* [3]*Massey University, Auckland, New Zealand*

CHAPTER OUTLINE

Social and Administrative Aspects of Pharmacy in Low- and Middle-Income Countries. http://dx.doi.org/10.1016/B978-0-12-811228-1.00025-X

This book presents key issues related to pharmaceutical policy and practice in countries with developing healthcare systems. Themes that warrant consideration are dealt with across a range of countries. This chapter synthesizes the information provided in this book and presents the key emergent themes that have developed within the body of work outlined in this book. Topics that represent the work in this chapter are the "use of medicines," "economic evaluation," "generic medicines," "pharmacovigilance," "quality of pharmacy services," "quality of medicines," "future scope of pharmacy practice" and "information resources available on the Internet that are relevant to Pharmacy." Each of these themes will be critiqued in turn, with a view to providing the reader with a synthesis of the entire book.

USE OF MEDICINES

The use of medicines theme draws from Chapters 3, 4, 17, 18, and 19. The corresponding topic areas are (1) patients', consumers', and healthcare professionals' (HCPs') perceptions, beliefs, knowledge, and attitudes toward the use of medicines, (2) the use of measurements and health behavioral models to improve medication adherence, (3) misconceptions and misuse of drugs by prescribers, dispensers, and consumers, (4) strengths and weaknesses of pharmaceutical policy in relation to rational and responsible medicines use, and (5) rational and responsible use of medicines.

PATIENTS', CONSUMERS', AND HEALTHCARE PROFESSIONALS' PERCEPTIONS, BELIEFS, KNOWLEDGE, AND ATTITUDES TOWARD THE USE OF MEDICINES

The process of ensuring the delivery and appropriate use of medicines by patients is complex and involves multiple stages and health professionals from different disciplines. The appropriateness, effectiveness, and safety of the medication use process are largely determined by several factors. These are attributable to HCPs, patients, and organizational or institutional frameworks within which the process of medication use exists (Institute of Medicine, 1999). Nadzam (1991), while developing medication use indicators, suggested medication use processes as consisting of five sequential succeeding steps including prescribing, dispensing, administering, monitoring, and systems and management control (Nadzam, 1991).

Ross and Loke (2009) and Dornan et al. (2009) reported that physician attitudes and behaviors toward prescribing are determined by a number of factors. These include things such as the quality, content, and depth of medical education and postgraduate training. These have been identified as critical determinants of physicians' medication use behaviors (Dornan et al., 2009, Ross & Loke, 2009). The dispensing process is a critical determinant of the effectiveness, safety, and convenience of medication use, and pharmacists play critical "care-defining roles" in ensuring that medication choice is effective and safe and that it meets patient-specific therapeutic needs and achieves set therapeutic goals. This chapter also illustrates that patient medication use behaviors are influenced by several factors including ethnic culture and religious beliefs, levels of patient health literacy, and self-efficacy and effectiveness of self-management practices. Furthermore, patients' understanding of the educational information provided by HCPs during the counseling process and the cognitive association of the therapeutic benefits inherent in using prescribed medicines for achieving specific therapeutic goals are important determinants of patient medication use behavior.

THE USE OF MEASUREMENTS AND HEALTH BEHAVIORAL MODELS TO IMPROVE MEDICATION ADHERENCE

Patients are commonly nonadherent and take fewer medications than they have been prescribed, or they prematurely discontinue therapy. To enhance medication adherence, the multifactorial causes of nonadherence must be understood, e.g., patient characteristics, patient beliefs, patient–healthcare provider relationships, stigma, therapy schedules, drug regimens, information, side effects, access to medicines, and so forth.

A report by the WHO (2003) classifies factors causing nonadherence into three categories: patient-related, physician-related, and health system/team building–related factors. Sociobehavioral models identify the factors that influence the expected behaviors to enable outcomes to be achieved and sustained. Such models allow us to make sense of the complex causes of outcomes, the associated behaviors, and other influential factors. According to Newman, Steed, and Mulligan (2008), the health belief model, the theory of reasoned action, the theory of planned behavior, the transtheoretical model, and the information–motivation–behavioral skills model all deal with the concept of change and have been widely used to develop behavioral interventions (Newman et al., 2008). Hence, multifaceted and tailored adherence interventions should be implemented in developing health systems to enhance medication adherence. Although studies centering on medication adherence have increased, there is no single international guideline available for enhancing medication adherence.

MISCONCEPTIONS AND MISUSE OF DRUGS BY PRESCRIBERS, DISPENSERS, AND CONSUMERS

Problems have been noted with the use of medicines at touch points including prescribers, dispensers, consumers, and other individuals, all over the world. Homedes, Ugalde, and Chaumont (2001) report that most developing countries waste a lot of scarce healthcare resources on medicines that are of doubtful therapeutic value. A number of medicines-related problems (MRPs) have been noted among consumers in developing nations. Specifically, problems with the use of antibiotics, analgesics, and potential interactions from concomitant use of allopathic and complementary and alternative remedies (CAMs) have been observed. Self-medication when carried out responsibly for certain self-limiting illnesses is the recommended way to save resources and improve patient self-care. But self-medication carries a number of risks when undertaken in an inappropriate manner. These risks include adverse effects, drug interactions, and the development of antimicrobial resistance. Using studies from the literature, misconceptions about medicines among prescribers, dispensers, and consumers were examined in this chapter, with a special emphasis on generic medicines, CAM, self-medication, and adverse drug reactions. Antimicrobial resistance is an important consequence of improper use of these medicines through prescribing by doctors and inappropriate over-the-counter use by consumers in emerging countries where there are lower levels of pharmaceutical regulation.

STRENGTHS AND WEAKNESSES OF PHARMACEUTICAL POLICY IN RELATION TO RATIONAL AND RESPONSIBLE USE OF MEDICINES

Medicines are the most commonly used intervention in healthcare being a key technology that plays an important role in improving public health outcomes around the globe. However, the use of medicines is not without risks. Problems with medicines, also known as "medication incidents," are the most common safety issues in healthcare. Where assessable, problems with medicine use are still common, with one estimate suggesting that more than 50% of all medicines are prescribed, dispensed, or sold inappropriately by healthcare providers (WHO, 2002).

Ratanawijitrasin, Soumerai, and Weerasuriya (2001) concluded that to improve medicine use, governments in many countries have policies and strategies in place to ensure the availability, accessibility, and quality use of affordable medicines that have reasonable quality, efficacy, and safety. The WHO Guidelines for developing national drug policies (1988) highlight that quality use of medicines is dependent on the availability of affordable essential medicines, at the very least. Policies to improve the use of medicines need to be considered within the broader context of other activities to strengthen the pharmaceutical sector. Optimally, this should occur under the umbrella of a national medicines policy (WHO, 1988). Monitoring the implementation and policy evaluation through strategic research and routine data collection should be the building blocks for this work within the framework of a national medicines policy and broader national health policies.

RATIONAL AND RESPONSIBLE USE OF MEDICINES

The appropriate supply and use of medicines in the last decade has had some positive influence on health resulting in decreased disease burden and reduced mortality and has also improved the overall quality of life (World Health Organization, 2012). Interestingly, Morris and Yoritomo (2015) found that global health spending is growing, having increased from 2% in 2012 to 2.8% in 2013. However, the significant progress in health outcomes over recent decades has been inequitable. According to Smith (2015, p. 103), health provision varies throughout the world and is challenging, particularly in developing countries because of the associated costs and the influence of cultural, political, and socioeconomic conditions.

Medicine use is influenced by many interrelated factors that make up the therapeutic process that involves prescribers, patients, dispensers, health systems, and the community at large. Diminished quality of care results directly in increased morbidity and mortality, increased costs, and wastage of resources, which limits the availability of essential medicines and increases the risk of adverse events. Many intervention studies conducted to promote the rational use of medicines have lacked reproducibility and sustainability (Thawani, 2010). Successful interventions require "political willingness" with the consequent enactment of laws and regulations and these processes are often lacking in developing countries. In addition, developing countries fall short in providing adequate education and training to healthcare workers on the rational use of medicines, as well as regular updates to standard treatment guidelines and the development of adequate systems to monitor and regulate how medicines are used.

ECONOMIC EVALUATION OF MEDICINES AND DISEASES IN DEVELOPING COUNTRIES

The second theme, which has emerged out of this book, centers on economic evaluation. This is a significant requirement in developed countries, but there has been some debate as to the extent that economic evaluation is relevant within countries that have developing healthcare systems.

This section provides a summary of economic evaluation by drawing together the material found in Chapters 8 and 10. The section covers the economic evaluation of medicines, in general, in developing countries and specifically in diabetes management. The reader can see by the fact that there are only two chapters making up this theme that there is a relative dearth of information in this area. There is a rich opportunity for ongoing development of a research agenda.

ECONOMIC EVALUATION AND MEDICINES EXPENDITURE IN DEVELOPING COUNTRIES

Chootipongchaivat, Tritasavit, Luz, Teerawattanon, and Tantivess (2015) studied different factors related to the development of health technology assessment (HTA) in particular Asian countries, and they report that South Korea, Malaysia, Taiwan, and Thailand have already accomplished almost full health coverage and this has been going on for more than 15 years. Other countries such as China, Indonesia, and Vietnam aim to reach this goal by the beginning of the next decade, i.e., beyond 2020 (Chootipongchaivat et al., 2015).

An interesting study by Augustovski, Melendez, Lemgruber, and Drummond (2011) reports that in Latin America, the healthcare systems are fragmented and public social security is the most significant healthcare provider complemented by private systems. The health services in these countries consist mainly of compulsory benefits packages and formularies of essential medicines for public subsidy (Augustovski et al., 2011). Continuing in Latin America, Vanegas (2016) presented facts about the healthcare system in Columbia and states that The Institute of Health Technology Assessment (IETS) has carried out 148 evaluations, mainly related to medicines. They found that through the use of an HTA-based systems, patient out-of-pocket expenses dropped from 50% in 1995 to 16% in 2015 (Vanegas, 2016). Hence, in many emerging countries where health priorities have already been identified and systems put in place to manage the institutionalization of HTA as an evaluative framework, the pricing and reimbursement policies have been an effective step to streamline the allocation of resources. This is no difference with the developed world with regard to this and in those emerging countries that have stable pharmaceutical systems and access to essential medicines, it is likely that we will see the increasing use of HTA as more high-cost medicines (HCMs) become available in these emerging economies.

ECONOMIC EVALUATION OF DIABETES AS A DISEASE

The global disease burden is significant and has changed dramatically in terms of chronic disease over the past two decades. Lozano et al. (2012) estimated that mortality from communicable diseases has decreased by at least 17%, whereas the mortality from noncommunicable chronic diseases has increased by 30%. The developing nations are not free from this shift and collectively they face significant challenges in sustaining operable healthcare systems in the face of the changing epidemiology of chronic disease. This is underpinned by an overwhelming and difficult economic climate in many of these nations. In a number of developing countries, economic evaluation is increasingly being advocated as a tool to ensure the efficient use of resources particularly when addressing chronic disease (Babar, 2016).

Diabetes is a major contributor to the global health burden from chronic disease. The prevalence of diabetes was studied by Wild, Roglic, Green, Sicree, and King (2004) across all age groups and it was predicted to be 4.4% in 2030, which will translate to 366 million people worldwide. Insulin is the mainstay treatment for type 1 and advanced stage type 2 diabetes mellitus. At present, there is no evidence on the cost-effectiveness of short-acting insulin analogues for type 2 diabetes mellitus in developing countries. There is moderate evidence of the cost-effectiveness of long-acting insulin analogues; however, given the small incremental benefit gained with the insulin analogue, it is critical for future studies to investigate the impact of varying the effectiveness on their results (Home, Baik, Galvez, Malek, & Nikolajsen, 2015). Hence, it is important to allocate sufficient resources to fund local economic evaluation studies and proactively detect the availability of new technologies through horizon scanning activities.

PHARMACOVIGILANCE

Pharmacovigilance is certainly on the increase and there is considerable direction being provided by organizations such as the World Health Organization (WHO). This section includes a summation of Chapters 12, 13, 30, and 31; making it a significant theme. In this section, coverage includes the behavioral aspects and practices, alongside the governance of pharmacovigilance.

BEHAVIORAL ASPECTS OF PHARMACOVIGILANCE

Pirmohamed, Atuah, Dodoo, and Winstanley (2007) presented data suggesting that low-income countries share 90% of the global disease burden and are also major consumers of prescription medicines. Therefore, establishing safety profiles of medicines specific to diseases that are endemic to the developing world is very important. Equally, historically it has been challenging due to a lack of effective and efficient pharmacovigilance systems or there being systems in place that were not being used due to low levels of engagement. The emerging concept of pharmacovigilance in developing countries captures wider aspects of safety related to the prescribing, dispensing, storage, administration, and consumption of medicines.

A report by the WHO (2009) actively promotes the establishment of national and local pharmacovigilance programs, thereby enabling the identification of pharmacovigilance issues specific to the local and national populations of emerging nations (World Health Organization (WHO), 2009). International consortiums are being established to enable greater use of technology for reporting and management of data related to pharmacovigilance in both specific and broad therapeutic categories (Pal, Olsson, & Brown, 2015). Moreover, a research agenda around the behavioral aspects of pharmacovigilance in the developing context could range from review of current research evidence; exploring the current state of practice; exploring policy priorities in local and national contexts; development, implementation, and evaluation of novel pharmacovigilance systems; and researching patient, HCP, and stakeholder perspectives of their participation in pharmacovigilance. CAMs and traditional medicines would also be the significant topics for research in the pharmacovigilance space. These topics in turn may inform the development, implementation, and evaluation of interventions that would be expected to positively impact on pharmacovigilance practices in developing countries.

KNOWLEDGE, ATTITUDES, AND PRACTICES OF PHARMACOVIGILANCE

In many developed countries, pharmacovigilance is a normal practice; in fact more often than not it is a regulated practice for which there is associated legislation. Social and administrative pharmacists work in close contact with consumers, HCPs, healthcare agencies, regulators, and other administrators in this pharmacovigilance space. It is important to consider the knowledge, attitudes, and practices (KAP) of those involved in pharmacovigilance, particularly from a societal perspective. Knowledge and attitudes underpin behavior and therefore influence practice. They are hierarchical in a sense that knowledge influences the development of attitude, and attitude influences behavior and therefore practice. Knowledge and attitudes can be reinforced with ongoing practice. It is also possible that new knowledge and attitudes can develop through practical experiences. In this way the relationship between knowledge, attitudes and behavioral practice is recursive; one affects the other in a cyclical manner. The KAP aspects of pharmacovigilance within the context of developing country require significant attention to improve. Despite positive attitudes, health professionals in developing countries have poor knowledge and therefore suboptimal practices. The relevant professionals have poor to moderate knowledge, a positive attitude, and poor practice.

There has been an increase in the number of developing countries that have become members of the WHO Program for International Drug Monitoring (PIDM). As of October 2016, the number of associate members was 28, and the majority of these are low- and middle-income countries (LMICs) (UMC, 2016b). In fact, most developing countries are members or associate members of the WHO PIDM. The key features of pharmacovigilance operations in developing countries include, at a macrolevel, coordination by drug regulatory agencies, support from funding agencies, and support from developed countries. This is especially the case for Africa. There are better-established pharmacovigilance in some national public health programs in these nations but insufficient regional or peripheral centers to support these national centers. Olsson, Pal, Stergachis, and Couper (2010a, 2010b) report that most of the centers in their study involving 55 LMICs were also involved in other activities such as drug information, rational drug use, poison information, and so forth. A study by Moscou, Kohler, and Lexchin (2013) found that even though pharmaceutical companies produce and market medicines, their contributions to pharmacovigilance in developing countries are insufficient. Strong policy reforms are required to force pharmaceutical companies to improve their pharmacovigilance support for products that they distribute (Moscou et al., 2013).

PHARMACOGOVERNANCE: ADVANCING PHARMACOVIGILANCE AND PATIENT SAFETY

The UN Economic and Social Council (2006) defines governance as the "exercise of economic, political and administrative authority to manage a country's affairs at all levels. It comprises the mechanisms, processes, and institutions through which citizens and groups articulate their interests, exercise their legal rights, meet their obligations and mediate their differences". Governance influences national and subnational policy choices (or lack thereof) and allocation of resources necessary to achieve defined policy agendas.

Key features of pharmacogovernance include effective institutional authority, legislation, and policy instruments to strengthen drug safety processes. Weak pharmacogovernance can result in limited oversight and accountability that undermines stewardship for postmarket drug safety. This also creates opportunities for corruption to emerge, creates institutional conflicts of interest, and deincentivizes the adoption of legislation and norms for pharmacovigilance at the macrolevel. This strong governance also needs to filter down to the mesolevel policy and microlevel practices. Specifically, pharmacogovernance improves postmarket drug safety by establishing (1) an internal policy framework for drug safety, (2) the active cultivation of organizational capabilities at the mesolevel, (3) sustainable funding for pharmacovigilance activities, and (4) external partnerships. Moscou, Kohler, and MaGahan (2016) concluded that pharmacogovernance would assure equitable resource allocation to combat regional disparities in pharmacosurveillance and risk communication.

Governance is essential to ensuring that government institutions have the institutional authority, will, and capacity to effectively implement policies and enforce the law to be held accountable to their constituents. Weak governance negatively affects policies, laws, and regulations. Weak governance also impacts on mesolevel organizational policy, which is likely to also influence microlevel individual pharmacovigilance behaviors. In their study, Mulili and Wong (2011) found that in many LMICs, weak governance is endemic. This was the case particularly in the face of uncertain economies, unstable political regimes, and countries with low per capita incomes (Mulili & Wong, 2011).

The key features of pharmacogovernance at a macrolevel include an effective institutional authority, legislation, and policy instruments to strengthen drug safety processes. A pharmacogovernance framework serves as a guide for making choices that advance the practice of pharmacovigilance. Countrywide gaps that challenge postmarket drug safety include whether pharmacogovernance exists in policy, law and regulation, equity and inclusion, and ethics. Various studies have concluded that regional disparities in pharmacovigilance are exacerbated by inadequate human resources, lack of sustainable funding, and poor resource allocation decisions (Olsson et al., 2010a, 2010b; Pal, Dodoo, Mantel, & Olsson, 2011). Pharmacogovernance would address this gap by ensuring sustainable, public funding models to support ongoing, rather than ad hoc pharmacovigilance systems. Moscou et al. (2016) concluded in their scoping review of Brazilian literature that pharmacogovernance would assure equitable resource allocation to combat regional disparities in pharmacosurveillance and risk communication.

IMPROVING ACCESS THROUGH GENERIC MEDICINES USE

The use of generic medicines over originator brands has always been a strategy for improving access to medicines. There has been plenty written about this topic, and the research agenda is ongoing. This section draws on subthemes related to generic medicines including an overview of challenges and consideration of policies.

OVERCOMING CHALLENGES OF GENERIC MEDICINES UTILIZATION IN LOW- AND MIDDLE-INCOME COUNTRIES

Around the globe, escalating healthcare costs are the major challenge faced by governments and specifically healthcare providers and policy makers (Borger et al., 2006; Steinwachs, 2002). Marchildon and DiMatteo (2011) report that the budget for pharmaceuticals constitutes the second largest cost in healthcare provision after staffing costs. Thorpe (2005, 2006) reminds us that the rise in disease prevalence changes the clinical threshold for treatment, and the emergence of new medical treatments has contributed to an escalation of pharmaceutical expenditures. Together with the current financial situation, policy makers face challenges in ensuring access to affordable medicines within limited healthcare budgets in a sector where there are competing demands for very scarce resources.

There are challenges faced during the provision of pharmaceutical products to consumers. These supply-side challenges in LMICs include such issues as unsecured intellectual property and the access to medicines narratives. This involves complex issues surrounding the link between multinational pharmaceutical company patents and delays in generic medicine approvals, weak patent examination, and granting procedures that allow the patenting of noninventive aspects alongside a lack of clarity in legal regulation. On the other hand, demand-side challenges in LMICs include a lack of clarity in the legal regulations, rules permitting physicians to dispense medicines that can result in a lower utilization rate of generic medicines, low markups during the dispensing of generic medicines, and concerns about the quality, safety, and efficacy of generic medicines among healthcare stakeholders. Hence, to boost the generic utilization in health systems of LMICs, there is a need to implement coherent generic medicine policies that address both supply- and demand-side pressures.

ASSESSMENT OF POLICIES, DETERMINANTS, AND CHARACTERISTICS OF GENERIC MEDICINES ENTRY INTO PHARMACEUTICAL MARKETS

The availability of generic medicines provides opportunities for the containment of pharmaceutical costs through savings in the differential cost between generic and originator brands. Outcomes for generic medicines are expected to be the same, as the originator brand and the cost of competing products can be compared using HTA and cost-effectiveness ratio. However, there has been some debate as to whether pharmacoeconomics is a priority in healthcare systems in developing nations, which are still struggling to achieve basic access to essential medicines (Babar & Scahill, 2010) when the strength of pharmacoeconomics is in assessing HCMs. This is especially important in developing countries where the greatest proportion of payment for medicines is largely "out of pocket" for most consumers. However, Sheppard (2010) recommends that to derive the maximum benefit from generic medicines, prompt market entry following patent expiration of the originator brand is crucial. According to findings by González, Fitzgerald, and Rovira (2008), policies relating to generic medicines in Latin America are highly diverse in nature with policy measures implemented to meet the overall objectives of drug affordability and accessibility, including promoting the domestic pharmaceutical industry. Kaplan, Ritz, Vitello, and Wirtz (2012) comments that although many of these policy measures are in place in developing countries, they are much less robust compared with those in developed countries. The degree to which policies encourage generic entry and uptake in developing countries is less than satisfactory (Kaplan et al., 2012).

Many factors influence whether generic medicines entry is promoted or not. These are both direct and indirect including market size of originator medicines, regulatory exception provision, fast-track generic approval, differential registration fees, and whether existing technical capabilities represent the most relevant in the context of developing countries. The strength of barriers to entry is one of the most important determinants for a firm to enter a given market. The features characterizing generic entry in the pharmaceutical market, with potential impact on price-lowering competition, include the time of entry and number of generic entrants, following patent expiration of originator products, and the effect of generic entry and resultant competition around drug prices.

QUALITY OF PHARMACY SERVICES

There is a single chapter that contributes to themes relating to pharmacy service quality. Hepler and Strand (1990) defined the role of the pharmacist as "the responsible provision of drug therapy for the purpose of achieving definite outcomes that improve a patient's quality of life." The past two decades have seen rapid changes in how services are delivered. Currently the pharmacy profession is experiencing significant development and growth in terms of providing a higher quality of pharmaceutical care services. This is in line with the reprofessionalization agenda that started in the United States in the early 1990s and the increasing drive from policy makers, who are pushing for the better use of pharmacists to optimize medicines use and improve health outcomes.

Pharmacists are increasingly adopting patient-centric approaches due to the poor adherence of prescribed medicine and increase in health demands, along with an ever-increasing and complex range of medicines (WHO, 2006).

WHO has played a significant role in promoting and defending the role of pharmacists around the world and has taken into account that almost all healthcare providers and the public are rationally involved in the use of medicines (World Health Organization, 2006). Therefore, when considering the need for quality in pharmacy health services and the safe and effective administration of drugs, the WHO has rightly acknowledged a special role for pharmacists (Dunlop & Shaw, 2002). In LMICs the profession is still under significant evolution, and health demands are requiring a change in the pharmacists' role toward patient-centered approaches. The quality of pharmacy services is significantly variable, and pharmacists in developing countries are still struggling with their identity and the gaining of recognition. Healthcare systems without pharmacists are not capable of managing health-related issues. High-quality pharmacy services can only be achieved through the proper implementation of pharmaceutical care services. To push the present role of pharmacists forward, there is a need for pharmacists in LMICs to take up the challenge, gain confidence, and proactively assert the role and be focused toward a patient-centered approach.

PHARMACEUTICAL CARE INTERVENTIONS

Public health interventions, pharmaceutical care interventions, and effective medicines supply management are key components to the rational use of drugs and promoting health. Aslani et al (2012) identified that attempts to convey the correct information to patients are equally important as providing the medicine(s) themselves to patients.

The concept of pharmaceutical care intervention (PCI) was introduced and became established and practiced in the developed world in daily hospital and community pharmacy practice. Pharmaceutical care has failed miserably in the United States and in Western Europe. Hepler, himself, stated this: These chapters are really about clinical pharmacy practice, which is what is growing around the world—successfully! The implementation of either a variant of PCI or clinical pharmacy practice is still in the dormant stage in developing countries. Barriers to the implementation of PCI in developing countries include the attitude of pharmacists, lack of pharmacists' advanced practice skills, lack of time, and resource- and system-related constraints. Educational obstacles also come into play. Berenguer et al. (2004) highlighted in a commentary that the traditional culture or mind-set of pharmacists has to be renewed and changed. Efforts are needed within the profession to understand the lack of advancement in pharmacy practice within LMICs. The profession may need to seek technical assistance from global bodies such as WHO and International Pharmaceutical Federation (FIP), who have been working on relevant models and have developed a number of strategies to deal with these barriers and provide services to the appropriate patient populations.

FUTURE SCOPE OF PHARMACY PRACTICE

POLITICS AND COMPETITION BETWEEN PROFESSIONS: FUTURE SCOPE OF PHARMACY PRACTICE

In developing countries, pharmacists are still unable to shift from drug-centered pharmacy practice to patient-centered care. The WHO has proposed an eight-star pharmacist model to describe the various roles of a pharmacist as caregiver, decision-maker, communicator, manager, learner, teacher, leader, and researcher in providing better pharmaceutical care and decision-making. Taking this into account, if practiced under a well-trained pharmacy professional, there is the possibility of achieving greater impact within healthcare systems (World Health Organization, 2006). In 2000, the UK Department of Health published "Pharmacy of the Future" (Pharmacy in the Future – Implementing the NHS Plan, 2000), which clarified the need for pharmacists to provide structured professional support to improve and expand the range of pharmacy services provided to patients, including meeting individual drug needs, development of partnerships in the drug use process, coordinating of prescribing and dispensing processes, and conducting therapeutic reviews (Pharmacy in the Future – Implementing the NHS Plan, 2000). Strand, Cipolle, Morley, and Frakes (2004) and Berenguer et al. (2004) predicted that in the future, for the whole care system, pharmacist practice and involvement in patient-centered care will improve health outcomes, reduce medical-related adverse events, improve the quality of life, and reduce morbidity and mortality.

QUALITY OF MEDICINES

PERSPECTIVES, KNOWLEDGE, ATTITUDES, AND BELIEFS REGARDING MEDICINES QUALITY

Milovanovic, Pavlovic, Folic, and Jankovic (2004) highlight that the provision of affordable, effective, and high-quality medicines is important but challenging. Provision of high-quality medicines is more difficult in developing countries where the pharmaceutical market has experienced significant vulnerability to substandard and counterfeit drugs. It is reported in the literature that the problem of counterfeiting is "fueled by consumer demand" (Anti-Counterfeiting Group, 2003). Unfortunately, research in the context of developing country, which explores perceptions of various stakeholders regarding substandard and counterfeit medicines, is scarce. This is an important research gap, which when addressed will be a valuable step toward combating these practices.

Muthiani and Wanjau (2012) reported that counterfeit drugs impact on the economies through many factors including perception. Consequently, knowledge about substandard and counterfeit drugs is very weak with both consumers and healthcare providers, which results in consumers in developing countries purchasing substandard and counterfeit drugs due to ignorance about the health implications of doing so (Asuamah, Prempeh, & Boateng, 2013). Contrary to what would be expected and what is reported in the literature on developed countries, attitude has no significant effect on consumers' purchase intentions when it comes to counterfeit drugs in developing countries. An interesting study by Wee, Ta, and Cheok (1995) suggested that the negative perception toward counterfeiting consistently influenced the intention to purchase products. However, remedying this situation requires long-term policy making, planning, and efficient strategies to directly address the need of vulnerable consumers who have a real demand for affordable and cheap drugs in developing countries.

ISSUES ON SOURCE, ACCESS, EXTENT, AND QUALITY OF INFORMATION AVAILABLE TO PHARMACISTS AND PHARMACY PERSONNEL TO PRACTICE EFFECTIVELY

Our world today is witnessing huge advancements in information-related technologies and in the volume of medicines information available and accessible by healthcare providers and the public. There is the very real scenario of "information overload" through information made available on the Internet from both reliable and unreliable sources. This represents a great challenge for pharmacists and puts more responsibility on them as medicines information specialists. To remain in the front line as information providers and as information experts around medicines, pharmacists need to provide specific, objective, up-to-date, and unbiased information. They need to be very efficient, competent, and skillful in searching for and providing information in a manner that is easily digestible by patients. Elenbaas and Worthen (2009) studied the establishment of clinical pharmacy practice during the period of 1960s and 1970s as a platform for the founding of pharmaceutical care soon after.

As pharmacists, medical and pharmacy journals represent the core source of clinical knowledge about medicines. This is because they are the primary source of newly discovered and recently revealed information based on findings from primary research. Guidelines, text books, Internet sites, databases, and medicines information centers are generated from these primary sources. The accessibility and quality of information available has significant effects on the extent to which patients approach their health professionals with queries. Of course, with the increased availability of information, there is a need to teach biostatistics to pharmacy students in developing nations, so they can read and interpret findings from international journals and incorporate those findings in their own practices.

Having access to high-quality medicines information sources and providing high-quality medicines information services should be an ultimate goal of every pharmacist, especially those officially involved in the provision of medicines information. Hands, Stephens, and Brown (2002), Bertsche, Hämmerlein, and Schulz (2007), and Spinewine and Dean (2002) have evaluated the quality of information resources, focusing on different aspects including the characteristics of accurate and valid information, user satisfaction, and the impact of the medicine information on patient care and on population health.

OTHER THEMES THAT WARRANT CONSIDERATION

While we have cogently identified eight main themes mentioned in the chapters making up the main body of this book, there are some additional themes that cannot be ignored even though the chapter authors have not mentioned them. These considerations include the following:

- The application of tools from social and organizational sciences that can be applied to pharmacy practice research
- The substantive issue of counterfeit and substandard drug quality
- Efforts to locate new pharmacy roles and transition pharmacy education away from chemistry and the physical sciences to a more clinical focus
- Efficiency, automation, and cost savings

In part, these themes suggest an ongoing research agenda relating to pharmaceutical policy in LMICs, which also impact in a significant way on knowledge generation in the developed world.

TOOLS FROM THE SOCIAL, BEHAVIORAL, AND ORGANIZATIONAL SCIENCES LITERATURES

Tools and theories from the social and behavioral sciences and policy theory literatures can help with understanding patient–pharmacist communication, compliance enhancement efforts, the function of pharmacy at the organizational level, and the development, implementation, and evaluation of macrolevel policy. One of the earlier themes touches on this but it could do with expansion at this point. There has been some application from the social and behavioral sciences in the area of pharmacy practice and patient interaction (Guirguis & Chewning, 2005), chronic disease management (Bane, Hughe, & McElnay, 2006; Feletto, Lui, Armour, & Saini, 2013; Smith et al., 2007), addiction and mental health (Hattingh, Scahill, Fowler, & Wheeler, 2016; Scahill, Fowler, Hattingh, Kelly, & Wheeler, 2015), and HIV/AIDS (Rovers, 2011), to name but a few disease areas. In addition to applying theory to change management in patient behavior, there is a literature on change in pharmacist intentions and behavior (Herbert, Urmie, Newland, & Farris, 2006; Roberts et al., 2003; Walker, Watson, Grimshaw, & Bond, 2004). Of course, both these streams of work have been applied in the context of high-income countries. This approach needs to be applied to low-income countries where the cultures (both national and organizational) are likely to be different and so applying the social sciences should be central to this (Scahill, 2013). Pharmacy practice researchers have been relatively naïve to the application of organizational theories and constructs to their pharmacy practice research, and there is a call to do more of this in research pertaining to the high- and low-income contexts. Again, most of the work has been undertaken in the context of the development world using theories founded on cognitive behavior, social network theory, and organizational culture (Scahill, 2015).

Another area of significance is the information technology area and particularly the use of big data analytics. Many emerging countries have started the development of their IT infrastructure from scratch (from the ground up) and as a result the latest technology is often available. As soon as systems and policies are put in place to better capture data in the developing world, there will be tremendous volumes of real-time data available. Increasingly in high-income countries, these data are informing practices and decision-making in healthcare (Beal, 2015) and there is no reason why the same would not be true for the pharmacy sector in developed and developing nations (Stokes, Rogers, Hertig, & Weber, 2016).

THE ISSUE OF COUNTERFEIT AND SUBSTANDARD DRUGS

There are huge worldwide problems with counterfeit and substandard drugs, and strategies to counter this criminal epidemic need to be further explored. In a book titled *Fake Meds Online*, Hall and Antonopoulos (2016) highlight the burgeoning trade of counterfeit and substandard medications being made available online. Estimates from this book suggest that with the explosion of the Internet, "the trade" has increased by as much as 90% since 2005 with an approximate turnover of 200 billion, suggesting it is big business. This book is a grounded social science analysis of the online trade in illicit medicinal products. It uses the United Kingdom as a case study. The book explores supply and demand dimensions of trade in this high-income country. The book lies at the intersection of research on illicit markets, cybercrime, intellectual property crime, medical sociology, and digital culture. These exact same issues need to be looked into in the context of LMICs.

In a systematic review on substandard and counterfeit medicines, Almuzaini, Choonara, and Sammons (2013) found that fairly much of all the published research has been conducted in LMICs. The focus of studies has been largely around prevalence of this issue, with around one-third (Chootipongchaivat et al., 2015) of the 44 papers they identified being of good quality. The majority of studies (93%) contained samples with inadequate amounts of active ingredients. The prevalence of substandard/counterfeit antimicrobials was significantly higher when purchased from unlicensed outlets ($P < .000$; 95% CI 0.21 to 0.32). The limitations of this body of work include the poor methodological quality of most of the studies. The majority did not differentiate between substandard and counterfeit medicines. Most studies assessed only a single therapeutic class of antimicrobials only. Studies on more toxic agents, those with low therapeutic index or that treat critical organs such as heart, could possibly have a more significant impact on patient outcomes. Having said that, antibiotics are freely available and extensively used within LMICs.

There are two important considerations that seem to be missing from this literature stream and these warrant more thought. Firstly, there is a scarce literature regarding the prevalence of counterfeit or substandard medicines in upper middle- and high-income countries. In these high-income countries, considerable volumes of medicines are imported from LMICs. There are often strict regulations in these nations relating to the registration and import. However, in New Zealand as an example, both patients and health professionals are in the position where they can import medicines for their own use or the use of individual named patients (Section 29 of the Medicines Act 1981). One published report from a collaborative project between the Pharmacy School at the University of Auckland and Medicines Control at the New Zealand Ministry of Health identified that counterfeit medications were being inadvertently imported by unsuspecting consumers. More studies of this nature need to be undertaken to understand the prevalence in high-income countries.

There has been some work undertaken, which investigates the inspection processes in middle-income countries but these are of established pharmaceutical companies (Garg, Hasan, Scahill, & Babar, 2013). Studies need to be thought about and set up, which research strategies that reduce this criminal intent and assist in the reduction of these criminally based clandestine activities outlined by Hall and Antonopoulos (2016) previously.

EFFICIENCY, AUTOMATION, AND COST SAVINGS

Being commercial enterprises, most change in community pharmacy is due to policy drivers calling for increased clinical work and a drive for the efficient use of money and resource within the business. This is why automation and technicians are widely used to save money. However, automation is barely mentioned in this book. Unit dose, unit-of-use, and the like are all implemented to save money. Medication therapy management is undertaken to save money and that is why most other changes are accepted—if they are cost-effective and policy makers are prepared to reimburse pharmacy owners for this work. The focus on savings and resource use tends to be through economic analysis, but perhaps more research needs to be undertaken in the economics of technological innovation, workforce delegation, and process design and automation.

REFERENCES

Almuzaini, T., Choonara, I., & Sammons, H. (August 1, 2013). Substandard and counterfeit medicines: A systematic review of the literature. *BMJ Open*, *3*(8), e002923.

Anti-Counterfeiting Group. (2003). *Why you should care about counterfeiting*. https://www.a-cg.org/guests/news-desk/acg-press-releases#.WSL1AOvyuHs.

Aslani, P., Leucero, E., et al. (2012). *Counselling, concordance and communication: Innovative education for pharmacists* (2nd ed.). International Pharmaceutical Students' Federation (IPSF) and International Pharmaceutical Federation (FIP).

Asuamah, S. Y., Prempeh, V. O., & Boateng, C. A. (2013). A study of the purchase and consumption of counterfeit drugs in Ghana: the case of marketing students in Sunyani polytechnic? *International Journal of Innovative Research and Development*, *2*(5).

Augustovski, F., Melendez, G., Lemgruber, A., & Drummond, M. (2011). Implementing pharmacoeconomic guidelines in Latin America: Lessons learned. *Value in Health: the Journal of the International Society for Pharmacoeconomics and Outcomes Research*, *14*(Suppl. 5), S3–S7.

Babar, Z. U., & Scahill, S. (2010). Is there a role for pharmacoeconomics in developing countries? *Pharmacoeconomics*, *28*(12), 1069–1074.

Babar, Z. U. D. (2016). *Economic evaluation of pharmacy services*. Elsevier Monographs.

Bane, C., Hughe, C. M., & McElnay, J. C. (September 1, 2006). Determinants of medication adherence in hypertensive patients: An application of self-efficacy and the theory of planned behaviour. *International Journal of Pharmacy Practice*, *14*(3), 197–204.

Beal, S. (2015). *Business Time. Big data has potential to improve health care*. Pharmacy Today accessed from https://www.pharmacytoday.co.nz/business-time/2015/september-2015/30/big-data-has-potential-to-improve-healthcare.aspx.

Berenguer, B., La Casa, C., De la Matta, M. J., & Martin-Calero, M. J. (2004). Pharmaceutical care: Past, present and future. *Current Pharmaceutical Design*, *10*(31), 3931–3946.

Berenguer, B., La Casa, C., et al. (2004). Pharmaceutical care: Past, present and future. *Current Pharmaceutical Design*, *10*(31), 3931–3946.

Bertsche, T., Hämmerlein, A., & Schulz, M. (2007). German national drug information service: User satisfaction and potential positive patient outcomes. *Pharmacy World & Science*, *29*(3), 167–172. http://dx.doi.org/10.1007/s11096-006-9041-7.

Borger, C., Smith, S., Truffer, C., Keehan, S., Sisko, A., Poisal, J., & Clemens, M. K. (2006). Health spending projections through 2015: Changes on the horizon. *Health Affairs*, *25*(2), w61–w73.

Chootipongchaivat, S., Tritasavit, N., Luz, A., Teerawattanon, Y., & Tantivess, S. (2015). Factors conducive to the development of health technology assessment in Asia. *Policy Brief*, *4*(2), 1–57.

Dornan, T., Ashcroft, D. M., Heathfield, H., Lewis, P. J., Miles, J., Taylor, D., Wass, V. (2009). FINAL report. In *An in-depth investigation into causes of prescribing errors by foundation trainees in relation to their medical education – EQUIP study*. General Medical Council, United Kingdom.

Dunlop, J. A., & Shaw, J. P. (2002). Community pharmacists' perspectives on pharmaceutical care implementation in New Zealand. *Pharmacy World & Science*, *24*(6), 224–230.

Elenbaas, R. M., & Worthen, D. B. (2009). Transformation of a profession: An overview of the 20th century. *Pharmacy in History*, *51*(4), 151–182.

Feletto, E., Lui, G. W., Armour, C., & Saini, B. (February 1, 2013). Practice change in community pharmacy: Using change-management principles when implementing a pharmacy asthma management service in NSW, Australia. *International Journal of Pharmacy Practice*, *21*(1), 28–37.

Garg, S., Hasan, R., Scahill, S., & Babar, Z. U. D. (2013). Investigating inspection practices of pharmaceutical manufacturing facilities in selected Arab countries: Views of inspectors and pharmaceutical industry employees/Enquete sur les pratiques d'inspection des etablissements de production pharmaceutique dans des pays arabes selectionnes: Opinions des inspecteurs et des employes de l'industrie pharmaceutique. *Eastern Mediterranean Health Journal*, *19*(11), 919.

González, C. P., Fitzgerald, J. F., & Rovira, J. (2008). Generics in Latin America: Trends and regulation. *Journal of Generic Medicines*, *6*, 43–56.

Guirguis, L. M., & Chewning, B. A. (December 31, 2005). Role theory: Literature review and implications for patient-pharmacist interactions. *Research in Social and Administrative Pharmacy*, *1*(4), 483–507.

Hall, A., & Antonopoulos, G. A. (2016). *Introduction. Fake Meds online pp. 1–17*. London: Palgrave Macmillan.

Hands, D., Stephens, M., & Brown, D. (2002). A systematic review of the clinical and economic impact of drug information services on patient outcome. *Pharmacy World and Science*, *24*(4), 132–138. http://dx.doi.org/10.1023/A:1019573118419.

Hattingh, H. L., Scahill, S., Fowler, J. L., & Wheeler, A. J. (November 1, 2016). Exploring an increased role for Australian community pharmacy in mental health professional service delivery: Evaluation of the literature. *Journal of Mental Health*, *25*(6), 550–559.

Hepler, C. D., & Strand, L. M. (1990). Opportunities and responsibilities in pharmaceutical care. *American Journal of Hospital Pharmacy*, *47*, 533–543.

Herbert, K. E., Urmie, J. M., Newland, B. A., & Farris, K. B. (September 30, 2006). Prediction of pharmacist intention to provide Medicare medication therapy management services using the theory of planned behavior. *Research in Social and Administrative Pharmacy*, *2*(3), 299–314.

Home, P., Baik, S. H., Galvez, G. G., Malek, R., & Nikolajsen, A. (2015). An analysis of the cost-effectiveness of starting insulin detemir in insulin-naive people with type 2 diabetes. *Journal of Medical Economics*, *18*(3), 230–240. http://dx.doi.org/10.3111/13696998.2014.985788.

Homedes, N., Ugalde, A., & Chaumont, C. (2001). Scientific evaluations of interventions to improve the adequate use of pharmaceuticals in third world countries. *Public Health Reviews*, *29*, 207–230.

Institute of Medicine. (1999). To Err is Human: Building a safer health system. In L. T. Kohn, J. M. Corrigan, & M. S. Donaldson (Eds.), *Report of the committee on quality of health care in America.* Washington, DC: National Academy Press.

Kaplan, W. A., Ritz, L. S., Vitello, M., & Wirtz, V. J. (2012). Policies to promote use of generic medicines in low and middle income countries: A review of published literature, 2000–2010. *Health Policy*, *106*, 211–224.

Lozano, R., Naghavi, M., Foreman, K., Lim, S., Shibuya, K., Aboyans, V., … Murray, C. J. L. (2012). Global and regional mortality from 235 causes of death for 20 age groups in 1990 and 2010: A systematic analysis for the global burden of disease study 2010. *Lancet*, *380*(9859), 2095–2128.

Marchildon, G., & DiMatteo, L. (2011). *Health care cost drivers: The facts.* Retrieved from https://secure.cihi.ca/free_products/health_care_cost_drivers_the_facts_en.pdf.

Milovanovic, D. R., Pavlovic, R., Folic, M., & Jankovic, S. M. (2004). Public drug procurement: The lessons from a drug tender in a teaching hospital of a transition country. *European Journal of Clinical Pharmacology*, *60*(3), 149–153.

Morris, M., & Yoritomo, W. (2015). *Global health care outlook: Common goals, competing priorities.* Retrieved from deloitte. com http://www2.deloitte.com/au/en/pages/life-sciences-and-healthcare/articles/global-health-care-sector-outlook.html.

Moscou, K., Kohler, J. C., & Lexchin, J. (2013). Drug safety and corporate governance. *Global Health Governance*, *VII*(1), 56–79 Retrieved from http://pharmacy.utoronto.ca/sites/default/files/upload/faculty-staff/faculty/kohler/GHGFall2013Issue.pdf.

Moscou, K., Kohler, J., & MaGahan, A. (2016). Governance and pharmacovigilance in Brazil: A scoping review. *Journal of Pharmaceutical Policy and Practice*, *9*(3). http://dx.doi.org/10.1186/s40545-016-0053-y.

Mulili, B. M., & Wong, P. (2011). Corporate Governance Practices in Developing Countries: The Case for Kenya. *International Journal of Business Administration*, *2*(1).

Muthiani, M., & Wanjau, K. (2012). Factors influencing the influx of counterfeit medicines in Kenya: A survey of pharmaceutical importing small and medium enterprises within Nairobi. *International Journal of Business and Social Science*, *3*(11).

Nadzam, D. M. (1991). Development of medication-use indicators by the Joint Commission on Accreditation of health organization. *American Journal of Health- System Pharmacy*, *48*, 1925–1930.

Newman, S., Steed, E., & Mulligan, K. (2008). *Chronic physical illness: Self-management and behavioral interventions.* Maidenhead, UK: Open University Press.

Olsson, S., Pal, S. N., Stergachis, A., & Couper, M. (2010a). Pharmacovigilance activities in 55 low- and middle-income countries. *Drug Safety*, *33*(8), 689–703. http://doi.org/10.2165/11536390-000000000-00000.

Olsson, S., Pal, S. N., Stergachis, A., & Couper, M. (2010b). Pharmacovigilance activities in 55 low- and middle-income countries a questionnaire-based analysis. *Drug Safety*, *33*(8), 689–703.

Pal, S., Dodoo, A., Mantel, A., & Olsson, S. (2011). *The world medicines situation 2011: Pharmacovigilance and safety of medicines* (3rd ed.). Geneva: World Health Organization.

Pal, S. N., Olsson, S., & Brown, E. G. (2015). The monitoring medicines project: A multinational pharmacovigilance and public health project. *Drug Safety*, *38*, 319. http://dx.doi.org/10.1007/s40264.

Pharmacy in the Future – Implementing the NHS Plan. (2000). *A programme for pharmacy in the national health service.* London: Department of Health.

Pirmohamed, M., Atuah, K. N., Dodoo, A. N. O., & Winstanley, P. (2007). Pharmacovigilance in developing countries. *BMJ: British Medical Journal*, *335*(7618), 462.

Ratanawijitrasin, S., Soumerai, S. B., & Weerasuriya, K. (2001). Do national medicinal drug policies and essential drug programs improve drug use?: a review of experiences in developing countries. *Social Science & Medicine*, *53*(7), 831–844.

Roberts, A. S., Hopp, T., Sørensen, E. W., Benrimoj, S. I., Williams, K., Chen, T. F., Herborg, H. (October 1, 2003). Understanding practice change in community pharmacy: A qualitative research instrument based on organisational theory. *Pharmacy World & Science*, *25*(5), 227–234.

Ross, S., & Loke, Y. K. (2009). Do educational interventions improve prescribing by medical students and junior doctors? A systematic review. *British Journal of Clinical Pharmacology*, *67*, 662–670.

Rovers, J. (2011). Advancing pharmacy practice through social theory. *Innovations in Pharmacy*, *2*(3). Article 53. http://pubs.lib.umn.edu/innovations/vol2/iss3/7.

Scahill, S. L. (2015). Applying organisational theory in pharmacy practice research. In Z. U. D. Babar (Ed.), *Pharmacy practice research methods*. http://dx.doi.org/10.1007/978-3-319-14672-0.

Scahill, S. L. (January 1, 2013). Placing "culture" at the center of social pharmacy practice and research. *Research in Social and Administrative Pharmacy*, *9*(1), 1–3.

Scahill, S., Fowler, J. L., Hattingh, H. L., Kelly, F., & Wheeler, A. J. (September 12, 2015). Mapping the terrain: A conceptual schema for a mental health medication support service in community pharmacy. *SAGE Open Medicine*, *3* 2050312115603002.

Sheppard, A. (2010). *Generic medicines: Essential contributors to the long-term health of society*. London: IMS Health. Retrieved from http://www.medicinesforeurope.com/wp-content/uploads/2016/03/IMS_Generic_Medicines_Essential_contributors.pdf.

Smith, F. (2015). *Chapter 7 pharmacy in developing countries*. Pharmacy Practice.

Smith, L., Bosnic-Anticevich, S. Z., Mitchell, B., Saini, B., Krass, I., & Armour, C. (April 30, 2007). Treating asthma with a self-management model of illness behaviour in an Australian community pharmacy setting. *Social Science & Medicine*, *64*(7), 1501–1511.

Spinewine, A., & Dean, B. (2002). Measuring the impact of medicines information services on patient care: Methodological considerations. *Pharmacy World & Science*, *24*(5), 177–181. http://dx.doi.org/10.1023/A:1020575031753.

Steinwachs, D. M. (2002). Pharmacy benefit plans and prescription drug spending. *Journal of the American Medical Association*, *288*(14), 1773–1774.

Stokes, L. B., Rogers, J. W., Hertig, J. B., & Weber, R. J. (July 2016). Big data: Implications for Health system pharmacy. *Hospital Pharmacy*, *51*(7), 599–603.

Strand, L. M., Cipolle, R. J., Morley, P. C., & Frakes, M. J. (2004). The impact of pharmaceutical care practice on the practitioner and the patient in the ambulatory practice setting: Twenty-five years of experience. *Current Pharmaceutical Design*, *10*(31), 3987–4001.

Thawani, V. (2010). Rational use of medicines: Achievements and challenges. *Indian Journal of Pharmacology*, *42*(2), 63.

Thorpe, K. E. (2005). The rise in health care spending and what to do about it. *Health Affairs*, *24*(6), 1436–1445.

Thorpe, K. E. (2006). *Factors accounting for the rise in health-care spending in the United States: The role of rising*.

UMC. (2016b). *WHO programme members*. Uppsala Monitoring Center. Retrieved from http://www.who.umc.org/DynPage.aspx?id=100653&mn1=7347&mn2=7252&mn3=7322&mn4=7442.

UN Economic, Social Council. (2006). *Compendium of basic terminology in governance and public administration, Fifth session. (E/C.16/2006/4)*. New York City: United Nations.

Vanegas, G. (2016). *The institutionalization of health technology assessment in Colombia: Advancements and future challenges. News across Latin America: ISPOR Latin America consortium*. Available from http://press.ispor.org/LatinAmerica/2016/05/the-institutionalization-of-health-technology-assessment-in-colombia-advancements-and-future-challenges-2/.

Walker, A., Watson, M., Grimshaw, J., & Bond, C. (December 1, 2004). Applying the theory of planned behaviour to pharmacists' beliefs and intentions about the treatment of vaginal candidiasis with non-prescription medicines. *Family Practice*, *21*(6), 670–676.

Wee, C. H., Ta, S. J., & Cheok, K. H. (1995). Non-price determinants of intention to purchase counterfeit goods: An exploratory study. *International Marketing Review*, *12*(6), 19–46.

WHO. (1988). *Guidelines for developing national drug policies*. Geneva: World Health Organization.

WHO. (2002). *Promoting rational use of medicines: Core components, in WHO policy perspectives on medicines*. Geneva: World Health Organization.

WHO. (2003). *Adherence to long-term therapies. Evidence for action*. Geneva.

WHO. (2006). *New tool to enhance role of pharmacists in health care*. http://www.who.int/mediacentre/news/new/2006/nw05/en/index.html.

Wild, S., Roglic, G., Green, A., Sicree, R., & King, H. (2004). Global prevalence of diabetes: Estimates for the year 2000 and projections for 2030. *Diabetes Care*, *27*, 1047–1053.

World Health Organization. (2006). *Developing pharmacy practice a focus on patient care*.

World Health Organization. (2012). *The pursuit of responsible use of medicines: Sharing and learning from country experiences*. Available at http://www.who.int/medicines/areas/rational_use/en/.

World Health Organization (WHO). (2009). *Supporting pharmacovigilance in developing countries the systems perspective [internet]*. Retrieved from http://apps.who.int/medicinedocs/documents/s18813en/s18813en.pdf.

Index

'*Note*: Page numbers followed by "f" indicate figures, "t" indicate tables and "b" indicate boxes.'

A

B

C

E

N

S

V

W

Y

Z

Printed in the United States
By Bookmasters